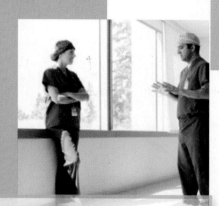

Nursing Documentation Using Electronic Health Records

Byron R. Hamilton, BA, MA

President, Virtual Classroom Academy
CEO, Med-Soft National Training Institute

Mary Harper, PhD, RN-BC

Clinical Faculty Coordinator
Western Governors University Pre-licensure BSN Program

Paul Moore, RN, BSN

Assistant Nursing Director—Orthopedics
St. John's Health System

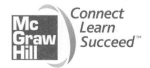

Connect
Learn
Succeed™

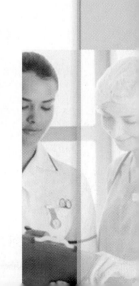

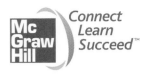

The McGraw-Hill Companies

Connect
Learn
Succeed™

NURSING DOCUMENTATION USING ELECTRONIC HEALTH RECORDS

Published by McGraw-Hill, a business unit of The McGraw-Hill Companies, Inc., 1221 Avenue of the Americas, New York, NY, 10020. Copyright © 2012 by The McGraw-Hill Companies, Inc. All rights reserved. No part of this publication may be reproduced or distributed in any form or by any means, or stored in a database or retrieval system, without the prior written consent of The McGraw-Hill Companies, Inc., including, but not limited to, in any network or other electronic storage or transmission, or broadcast for distance learning.

Some ancillaries, including electronic and print components, may not be available to customers outside the United States.

This book is printed on acid-free paper.

1 2 3 4 5 6 7 8 9 0 RMN/RMN 1 0 9 8 7 6 5 4 3 2 1

ISBN   978-0-07-337481-9
MHID   0-07-337481-4

Vice president/Editor in chief: *Elizabeth Haefele*
Vice president/Director of marketing: *Alice Harra*
Publisher: *Kenneth S. Kasee Jr.*
Managing developmental editor: *Kimberly D. Hooker*
Marketing manager: *Mary B. Haran*
Lead digital product manager: *Damian Moshak*
Director, Editing/Design/Production: *Jess Ann Kosic*
Project manager: *Kathryn D. Wright*
Buyer II: *Laura M. Fuller*
Senior designer: *Srdjan Savanovic*
Lead photo research coordinator: *Carrie K. Burger*
Photo researcher: *Danny Meldung/PhotoAffairs, Inc.*
Media project manager: *Brent dela Cruz*
Outside development house: *Andrea Edwards, Triple SSS Press*
Cover design: *Alexa Viscius*
Interior design: *PV Studios*
Typeface: *10/12 Times New Roman*
Compositor: *Laserwords Private Limited*
Printer: *R. R. Donnelley*
Cover credit: monitor: © Mike Kemp, Gettyimages; hand + files: © Stefan Klein, iStockphoto
Credits: The credits section for this book begins on page 305 and is considered an extension of the copyright page.

Library of Congress Cataloging-in-Publication Data

Hamilton, Byron R., author.
   Nursing documentation using EHR/Byron R. Hamilton, President, Virtual Classroom
   Academy CEO, Med-Soft National Training Institute, BA, MA, Mary Harper, Western
   Governors University, Paul Moore, St. John's Hospital.
        p.; cm.
   Includes index.
   ISBN-13: 978-0-07-337481-9 (alk. paper)
   ISBN-10: 0-07-337481-4 (alk. paper)
   1. Nursing records—Data processing. I. Harper, Mary, author. II. Moore, Paul, 1969- author. III. Title.
   [DNLM: 1. Electronic Health Records. 2. Nursing Records. WY 100.5]
RT50.H36 2012
610.285—dc22

                                                                                           2010050244

www.mhhe.com

Dedication

Nursing Documentation Using Electronic Health Records is dedicated to my wife Leesa and my children Jeremie, Joshua, and Kelsey. They are the inspiration and joy of my life. I can finally be a dad again!

My appreciation is extended to Jack B. Smyth, president and CEO of Spring Medical Systems Inc., and Ken Santoro, Director of Support and Operations at Spring Medical Systems Inc., for the contribution of the SpringCharts EHR program for every student. The incorporation of this full-featured, popular electronic health record software has taken the nursing student from a sterile, abstract setting to a dynamic, realistic learning environment. This hands-on experience will successfully equip each student with the knowledge and confidence necessary to contribute to the electronic health records in the medical field.

—Byron R. Hamilton

I'd like to dedicate this work to my staff at Florida Hospital Memorial System. Linda, Wendy, Debbie, Jen, and especially Sarah and Barb—you all struggled through the growing pains of implementing the EHR and figuring out how to ensure that the needs of our nursing students were met. Working with experts like you has been the highlight of my career!

I'd also like to dedicate this to my husband, Oscar, who has endured hours with me at the computer. You have been the highlight of my life!

—Mary Harper

Nursing Documentation Using Electronic Health Records is dedicated to my wife and children, Lisa, Jared, and Courtney. Lisa has been ultimately patient during the writing of the textbook, and is always my inspiration to achieve more than is at first glance possible.

—Paul Moore

Byron R. Hamilton

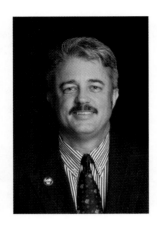

Byron R. Hamilton received a BA in Education from the College of Advanced Education in Australia and taught for several years in both private and public institutions. He earned an MA in Biblical Literature in Springfield, Missouri.

In 1997, Byron and his wife, Leesa, established *MedTech Medical Management Systems*, a medical billing and consulting company for both practice management software and electronic medical records. For the following decade they were involved with medical billing, supervision of healthcare information management, medical consultation, and training. Byron has been involved with electronic health record systems from the inception of the industry.

In 2004, he launched Med-Soft National Training Institute (MNTI), a software training group conducting onsite and online training on medical software, including Medisoft™ PMS and SpringCharts™ EHR, both nationally and internationally. He has written the product training manuals for several PMS and EHR programs and has authored numerous articles for professional magazines. MNTI also provides strategies for healthcare organizations in the selection, implementation, and project management of electronic health records.

In 2007, Hamilton authored *Electronic Health Records*, a textbook used in over 600 Allied Health programs across the country. Byron is a national speaker at career college workshops, business college associations, and medical professional groups.

Mary Harper

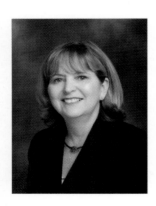

Dr. Harper obtained her MSN in Nursing Administration from the University of Florida and her PhD in Nursing from the University of Central Florida. Certified in Nursing Professional Development, Dr. Harper has participated in the development and implementation of electronic health records (EHR) for nursing in acute care settings. As the Director of Education for a three-hospital system, Dr. Harper collaborated with local colleges and schools of nursing to ensure that nursing students were educated on the use of the EHR in order to learn essential skills during their clinical rotations. In 2008, she presented a National League for Nursing workshop entitled "Student Use of the Electronic Health Record" during the national annual education summit.

In addition to her experience in the acute care setting, Dr. Harper has served as an instructor in prelicensure Bachelor of Science in Nursing programs. She currently works for Western Governors University's online prelicensure program where she educates nursing staff to serve as clinical coaches for students. In her academic positions, Dr. Harper has encountered various hospital regulations concerning student use of the EHR and understands the need for nursing students to understand the basic concepts of using an EHR.

Dr. Harper has published several articles in nursing journals and speaks nationally and internationally. She was on the work group that revised the Nursing Professional Development Scope and Standards, published in 2010. Her current research includes student encounters with substandard nursing care in the clinical setting and emotional intelligence of nursing students and successful nurses.

Paul Moore

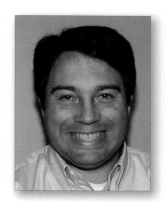

Paul B. Moore received a nursing diploma from St. John's School of Nursing and a BSN from Southwest Baptist University.

Paul obtained both Pediatric and Medical Surgical Certifications while working as an inpatient nurse for St. John's Hospital in Springfield, Missouri. Moving out of the hospital, he worked as a case manager for both CCO, Inc. and CorVel Corporation and earned CCM Certification. Paul was the president of the Case Management Society of America Springfield and Greater Ozarks chapter for 2001–2002 and served as board member for the following year. Paul was promoted to the branch manager position of the CorVel Springfield, Missouri, office.

Paul was an education consultant and Certified Web Instructor for McKesson Corporation, teaching Advanced Clinicals and Scheduling for the Horizon Homecare software utilized by home health care and hospice agencies. In 2005 and 2006, Paul received the Group President award from McKesson. At the annual users' conference he was selected as a speaker four consecutive years from 2005 to 2008. Paul was also team leader of the education department.

Paul became certified in Inpatient Orders for the *EPIC EHR* program while employed by Sisters of Mercy in 2008. He was a credentialed trainer for the program in 2009.

Brief Contents

Level I

Level II

Level III

Level IV

Contents

Level I — Introducing Electronic Health Records

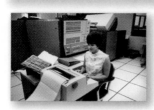

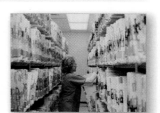

Level III

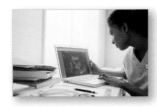
Level IV

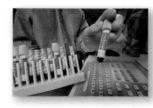

Chapter 14 Learning Assessment 238

Learning Outcomes 239

What You Need to Know 239

Exercises 240

Exercises

Introduction

Health information technology continues to expand rapidly across the entire spectrum of the healthcare community. Although electronic health records have been a part of the healthcare community since the 1960s, a major adoption of informatics in the general population has only recently been witnessed. Affordability in computer technology and healthcare software is now exerting a major influence on providers in private practice groups of eight or less to adopt electronic health records. This enclave of healthcare providers makes up nearly 78% of all practices in the United States. The availability and reliability of wireless computer networks, the public concern for patient safety, and the affordability of health information technology are being met with the federal government's involvement in coordinating and setting technical standards for electronic health records. These converging forces are bringing about a virtual explosion in the electronic healthcare industry, leading business experts to concur that in less than five years 90% of small- to medium-sized practices will be using electronic health record systems. The remarkable surge of interest in electronic health records (EHRs) is leading to further development in comprehensive clinical decision support that continues to enhance computerized knowledge management systems and create even more robust EHRs.

Never in the history of nursing has there been a greater need for the exposure to and hands-on experience with electronic documentation. Specialization of informatics that now manages and processes health data has created the urgent need to provide nursing students and educators with the ability to document patient care in an electronic health record system.

Nursing Documentation Using Electronic Health Records arose from the need to educate nurses for the anticipated phenomenal growth of electronic health records in the healthcare field. This text provides nursing students with an exceptional tool that integrates health informatics into the nursing curriculum. Twenty percent of the text is devoted to the theory, history, evolution, and legal/ethical considerations of electronic documentation and the remainder of the text provides nursing students with a technology-rich, hands-on, informatics environment. Students learn to document electronically using the SOAPIER format, NANDA-I nursing diagnoses, NOC, and NIC with the click of a mouse, and to document procedures, patient education, and care plans from pick lists. A wealth of resource material is provided to develop individualized electronic documentation.

Nursing Documentation Using Electronic Health Records provides a detailed history of the EHR from the inception of electronic records in the 1960s and traces the influence of several federal agencies and private-sector organizations from the Health Insurance Portability and Accountability Act of 1996, through the Certification Commission of Health Information Technology formed in 2004 to the HITECH ACT of 2009. This text devotes 11 chapters to practical, hands-on experience with *SpringCharts EHR™*, a popular electronic health records program used by a wide range of healthcare professionals in a variety of specialties both nationally and internationally. At the completion of this course, students are awarded a Completion Certificate acknowledging their successful training as *SpringCharts EHR* users.

Key Features:

- **The ONC Certified SpringCharts premium EHR program is available with each text at no additional cost to the student or school.** Students learn EHR documentation through this industry-standard software. It combines the right mix of rich functionality and intuitive ease of use to enable rapid and complete clinical and clerical documentation.

- An abundance of screen captures and menu icons from SpringCharts™ EHR software provide step-by-step instructions for easy reference and application.

"That is well thought through, provides the latest regulations with charting and is a comprehensive, integrated charting system."

—Donna Gloe, EdD, MSN, RN-BC, Missouri State University

"As an effective method of teaching EHR and documentation; provides the learner with a comprehensive course that facilitates practical application of EHR documentation in nursing practice."

—Donna Beuk, MSN, BSN, RN, Auburn University

"An activity-based learning tool that teaches electronic charting in a realistic setting. It gives the student the opportunity to learn and perform charting in a simulated, therefore less stressful environment than the hospital."

—Anita Fitzgerald, RN, MSN, California State University —Long Beach

- *Nursing Documentation Using Electronic Health Records* incorporates **four levels of nursing instruction** and arranges the material from the simple to the more complex, enabling the text to be used over a four-semester program.
- **Concept Checkups** follow each topic and break down learning outcomes into manageable components.
- **Focal Points, Documentation Tips, Legal/Ethical Considerations,** and **Evidence-Based Practices** appear in the margins throughout the text to spotlight critical data necessary to master end-of-chapter review quizzes. **Key Term Definitions** appear in the glossary.
- A **Certificate of Training** is available on McGraw-Hill's Online Learning Center (OLC) for each student completing the course.

Text Overview

Nursing Documentation Using Electronic Health Records is organized into four different levels of charting, moving from simple to complex.

Level 1—Level 1 includes Chapters 1, 2, 3, and 4. These chapters focus on the history and development of the electronic health record (EHR) and trace the impact of standards development, certification, and the government's involvement. The theory, purpose, and types of nursing documentation are discussed with a focus on the medication administration record (MAR) and the relevance of standardized nursing language. Students are introduced to SpringCharts™ and learn essential documentation on an industry standard EHR program. They are also introduced to the *Nurse Note* and are given hands-on practice in documenting chief complaints, vital signs, and physical assessments on 10 different patient case studies.

Chapter 1—An Introduction to Electronic Health Records

Chapter 1 provides a concise history of the EHR and unravels the multiple nomenclatures surrounding its evolution. It explores standards development and nursing's role in that development. Students learn about the benefits of EHRs in both inpatient and ambulatory settings. The chapter concludes with a discussion of EHR certification, the federal government's role in the promotion of the EHR, and the current financial remuneration available through the HITECH portion of the American Recovery and Reinvestment Act of 2009.

"I am impressed with the emphasis on nursing as it relates to electronic documentation. I am most impressed with the clarity that prevails throughout all chapters."

—Kate Lein, MS, FNP-BC, Michigan State University

Chapter 2—Nursing Documentation Overview

Chapter 2 examines the purpose and methods of nursing documentation. The MAR is examined and the importance of standardized nursing language for nursing diagnoses, nursing outcomes, and nursing interventions is highlighted.

Chapter 3—Essential EHR Documentation

This chapter initiates hands-on training in nursing documentation on Spring-Charts EHR program. Students learn to set up personal user preferences and create ten patients with different disease processes to be used throughout the remainder of the course. Students are also introduced to the electronic chart, specifically learning about the *Face Sheet* and *Care Tree*.

Note: The individual SpringCharts program must be downloaded from the text website www.mhhe.com/nursingehr or the networked program needs to be installed by the nursing school's IT department before students start this chapter.

Chapter 4—Nurse Note Documentation—Level 1

In Chapter 4, students begin to practice *Nurse Note* documentation. Students work with their patients with diabetes, congestive heart failure, and pneumonia and electronically document chief complaints, vital signs, and physical exams.

Level 2—Level 2 includes Chapters 5, 6, 7, and 8. These chapters take students deeper into the EHR features of documentation and enable them to enhance their *Nurse Note* documentation using these more advanced features. Students are introduced to the ambulatory healthcare setting and its documentation requirements. Exercises are provided for the student to create an *Office Visit Note* while assuming the roles of nurse and nurse practitioner.

Chapter 5—Fundamental EHR Documentation

Chapter 5 explains EHR features of documenting telephone calls, letters, diagnostic test reports, and excuse notes. Students are exposed to the Plan of Care Manager where they import practice guidelines. This chapter includes EHR utilities such as linking to favorite websites and using SpringCharts calculators.

Chapter 6—Nurse Note Documentation—Level 2

Here, students begin to use NANDA-I nursing diagnoses, identify patient goals using nursing outcomes classifications (NOC), and employ nursing interventions using nursing intervention classifications (NIC) verbiage from within the EHR program as they continue to build *Nurse Notes* on designated patients with different disease processes. Level two of the *Nurse Note* also deals with documentation on the electronic MAR and intake and output (I&O) forms.

Chapter 7—Ambulatory Healthcare

Chapter 7 introduces students to the ambulatory healthcare setting and its documentation requirements. Students learn the role of an ambulatory nurse, document in an *Office Visit Note,* and modify and make addendums to the note.

Chapter 8—Ambulatory Healthcare Exercises

This chapter provides students with eight ambulatory healthcare documentation exercises. Students practice documenting in the EHR program using features learned in Chapter 7. They create, modify, and make addendums to *Office Visit Notes.* Students also generate reports and excuse notes.

Level 3—Level 3 includes Chapters 9, 10, and 11. These chapters promote a deeper understanding of EHR features and enable students to add to their *Nurse Notes* using these advanced features. Students learn EHR administrative features such as working through a 'to do' list, and sending and receiving internal messages. Chapter 10 is devoted to patient education where students learn patients' rights and nurses' responsibilities. The *Nurse Note* documentation becomes increasingly complex and students complete notes created in Levels 1 and 2.

Chapter 9—Routine EHR Documentation

Chapter 9 exposes students to various administrative EHR functions. They learn how to use the *ToDo* feature, send and receive internal messages, complete immunization records, and create patient instruction sheets. Students also learn how to use the draw program to enhance nursing documentation within the EHR.

Chapter 10—Patient Education

This chapter focuses on patients' rights, nurses' responsibilities, and accreditation requirements related to patient education. Students learn how to apply appropriate NANDA-I nursing diagnoses, NOC, and NIC for patient education. They assess patients' learning needs then implement, evaluate, and document patient education.

Chapter 11—Nurse Note Documentation—Level 3

This chapter continues to take students deeper into the *Nurse Note,* moving from simple to complex. Students document patient education interventions, evaluate patient responses to nursing interventions, and make revisions to the plan of care as needed. The *Nurse Note* is built using stroke, cellulitis, and chest

"A great help in teaching the students to learn electronic charting and documentation. The exercises provided will be sure to provide adequate practice which will assist the student to function with EHR in the clinical setting."

—Carmen Vela, MSN, RN, Covenant School of Nursing

"Unifies electronic health record documentation applying nursing process and current regulatory requirements of nursing care including JCAHO requirements, NPSS, CDC requirements etc. The program is supported by threads of evidenced based practice, legal ethical, and documentation tips. The practical applications afford the student the opportunity to apply the concepts utilizing SpringCharts EHR. The program is well written, concise, and predictable in its applications as well as fun to use."

—Cynthia Neff, MSN, RN, Allegany College of Maryland

pain patient case studies. Students also create *ToDo* items and reminders from within the *Nurse Note*.

Level 4—Level 4 includes Chapters 12, 13, and 14. In this final level, students learn more complex EHR documentation functions. Level Four is the EHR capstone section. Chapters 13 and 14 present students with case studies that require them to navigate through all SpringCharts screens as they build *Nurse Notes* for multiple patients.

Chapter 12—Advanced EHR Documentation

Chapter 12 introduces students to more advanced EHR documentation features of SpringCharts. Students learn to order diagnostic tests, perform electronic chart evaluations, and export elements of the chart. They also create addendums to existing Nurse Notes.

Chapter 13—Nurse Note Documentation—Level 4

While no new information is introduced in the last two chapters, students are presented with exercises that take them through all the main screens of the EHR program. Students document Face Sheet information, build Nurse Notes, import documents, and print Nurse Notes. Screen shots are provided throughout the exercises, providing immediate feedback to students.

Chapter 14—Learning Assessment

This chapter consists of 15 documentation exercises. Students use copies of documents typically used in a paper environment to gather information and place it in an electronic format within the EHR program. These exercises take the students through multiple screens in SpringCharts as they build electronic records and Nurse Notes.

Instructor Support

Access instructor resources from the text website at www.mhhe.com/nursingehr.

- **PowerPoint® slide presentations,** available for every chapter, contain teaching notes keyed to learning outcomes, making the teaching and learning experience exciting for both the instructor and the student.
- The **Instructor's Manual** contains a course overview, chapter summaries, answer keys, and instructions for installing the SpringCharts EHR software.
- **Exercise Checkup References** are supplied via screen captures from SpringCharts EHR at critical points in each exercise to ensure that students are completing exercises accurately.
- McGraw-Hill's **EZ-Test Test Generator** is an electronic testing program that allows instructors to create tests from book-specific items. It accommodates a wide range of question types, and instructors may add their own questions. Multiple versions of the test can be created, and any test can be exported for use with course management systems such as WebCT, BlackBoard, or PageOut. EZ-Test Online is a new service that provides you with a place to easily administer the exams and quizzes you created with EZ-Test. The program is available for Windows and Macintosh environments.

Downloading SpringCharts Is Easy!
Overview

SpringCharts EHR is an electronic health records software suite based on the latest industry standard Java technology. It requires a very modest network system for installation. SpringCharts is available in two system configurations: single computer and network option.

Note: Before beginning to work on the exercises in *Nursing Documentation Using Electronic Health Records*, access and download both the SpringCharts EHR software and the *EHR Material* folder located on the OLC at www.mhhe.com/nursingehr. The *EHR Material* folder contains images, documents, and files to give students real scenarios for EHR documentation throughout the course.

Please follow the instructions below to download the Java Runtime Environment, the SpringCharts EHR program, and the *EHR Materials* folder onto your computer. For problems with the download, contact one of the support teams listed below.

Support

McGraw-Hill Higher Education technical support team: 1-800-331-5094

- 8 a.m.–11 p.m. CST, Monday–Thursday
- 8 a.m.–6 p.m. CST, Friday
- 6 p.m.–11 p.m. CST, Sunday
- www.mhhe.com/support
- Med-Soft National Training Institute textbook support: questions@spring medical.com

Single Computer Version

The single computer version of SpringCharts needs to be installed onto each student's computer in the classroom. We recommend that SpringCharts be installed to and run from a 2GB flash drive (see **Running SpringCharts from a Flash Drive** instructions below) to eliminate the need to back up and restore data on a daily basis. The use of a flash drive enables a portable application of SpringCharts on any computer that will accept the flash drive and enables students to work outside the classroom. The single computer version of SpringCharts is not networked; therefore, the instructor is unable to view the students' exercises online. Exercises must be printed and submitted, e-mailed in pdf format (see instructions below), or viewed by the instructor on the students' computers.

Network Version

The network version of SpringCharts EHR comes in two applications: SpringCharts server and SpringCharts client. The downloadable network version of SpringCharts EHR is provided via a personalized link. Upon receipt, open and save the zipped file, as shown in Figure 1.

Note: The network version SpringCharts file is large and may take 15 minutes or more to download.

SpringCharts server must be installed on the server in the network and SpringCharts client must be installed on all the computer workstations in the network. Since the instructor and students are on the same network, completed exercises can be

Figure 1 Saving SpringCharts file to the computer

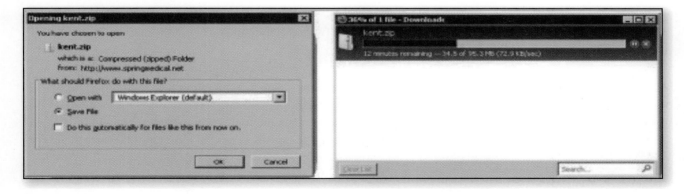

viewed across the network. The limitation of the local network version is that students cannot work on exercises outside of the classroom.

The optimum network configuration is to install SpringCharts server and SpringCharts client versions in the same local computer lab. Because the system requirements for SpringCharts EHR are very conservative, a local computer can be designated as the server and the other workstations pointed to this server within the SpringCharts client program.

System Requirements

The minimum requirements for **SpringCharts single** computer version are:

- An 800 MHz, or faster, processor.
- 400 MB of available disk space.
- 1 GB of memory (2 GB is preferable).
- A computer running one of the following operating systems: Windows 2000 or above, Mac OS 10.5 (Leopard) or above.

To complete all exercises in this text, access to a network printer and the Internet is required.

The minimum requirements for the **SpringCharts server** network option are:

- Pentium 4, or faster, processor (Xeon preferred).
- 150 GB of available disk space (after loading the JRE), primarily for the File Cabinet and local backups.
- 2 GB of memory (4 GB is preferable).
- Computer running the following operating systems: Windows 2000 or above, or MacOS Leopard (10.5) or above. (The network computers do not need to be running the same operating system.)
- **Note:** SpringCharts uses ports 4447 and 4448.

The minimum requirements for the **SpringCharts client** network option are:

- 800 MHZ, or faster, processor.
- 25 MB of available disk space.
- 1 GB of memory (2 GB is preferable).
- Workstation computers running the following operating systems: Windows 2000 or above, or MacOS Leopard (10.5) or above. (The network computers do not need to be running the same operating system.)

Operating Environment Notice

SpringCharts is an online system that requires uninterrupted access to a minimum level of system resources. As a result, it is recommended that SpringCharts server be located on a dedicated computer when possible.

It is also recommended that highly resource-intensive programs and/or programs that may intermittently use up the majority of system processing capacity or network bandwidth *not be run at the same time as SpringCharts.* Examples of these types of programs are:

- Virus scans of the entire hard drive (scans of individual files are acceptable).
- Music streaming programs.
- Certain backup programs (when activated).

Single Computer Installation

Installing Java Runtime Environment (JRE) 1.6

JRE 1.6.0_17 must be installed before running SpringCharts EHR.

- Access the following website on the Internet: www.java.com.
- Click the *Do I have Java?* link to test the computer system for the correct version of Java.
- If the computer has JRE 1.6_17, an upgrade is not needed.

- If the system does not meet the requirements of JRE 1.6, download JRE 1.6.0_17 from the online learning center. **Do not download the latest version of JRE from the Java website.**

Running SpringCharts from a Flash Drive

In a computer environment that uses a product like Deep Freeze™ to return the computer to its baseline configurations each day, all work in SpringCharts is eradicated when the computer is reset to its original state. To bypass the need to back up and restore SpringCharts data on a daily basis, the SpringCharts program can be run from a 2GB flash drive, as seen in Figure 2, that is placed into the computer's USB port daily. **If the school requires an administrative password to run programs from a flash drive, this method may not be feasible. Please consult with the school's IT department before proceeding.**

To use the alternate flash drive method, install JRE 1.6.0_17, SpringCharts EHR, and the *EHR Material* folder as outlined in the next sections; however, **install the Java Runtime (JRE) onto the computer**, and the SpringCharts program and *EHR Material* folder to the flash drive. When installing SpringCharts an option to change the default location of installation is presented (see Figure 3). To install SpringCharts to the flash drive, select this option, locate *My Computer*, and select the USB port where the flash drive is located. Once installed, a SpringCharts icon appears on the desktop. To access SpringCharts, place the flash drive into the computer's USB port and double-click on this icon. If the icon has been removed from the desktop, locate the flash drive and double-click the SpringCharts icon in the SpringCharts folder.

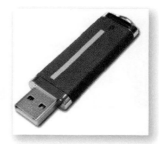

Figure 2 A flash drive is a portable device for memory storage. It can also be referred to as a jump drive or a thumb drive. Flash drives will fit into any USB (universal serial bus) port on a computer.

Figure 3 SpringCharts installation window

Note: Backing up and restoring SpringCharts data is not required when SpringCharts is operating from a flash drive.

When closing down the SpringCharts program the option to back up is given. If using a flash drive select **No**. The flash drive may be used in any computer's USB port to work on the exercises in this text.

Installing SpringCharts EHR on a Single Computer

The SpringCharts installation is accomplished in a few easy steps. Remember, the JRE must be installed before SpringCharts EHR will run.

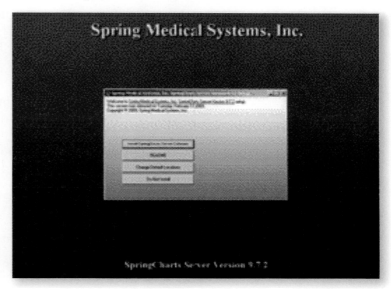

- Type the following address in the Internet browser: www.mhhe.com/nursingehr.
- Click the *SpringCharts* link in the menu on the left.
- Locate the *Downloading and Installing SpringCharts EHR* portion of the page.
- Click either the *SpringCharts PC Demo installer zip file* link or the *SpringCharts Mac Demo installer stuffed file* link as appropriate for the computer's operating system.
- Download the installer file to the computer desktop.
- Decompress the downloaded file (use a file program such as Winzip or StuffIt.)
- Double click either the **SpringChartsDEMOSetup.exe or SCDemoSetupMac** installation applications as appropriate for the computer's operating system.
- Follow the directions offered by the installer. A screen similar to the one displayed in Figure 3 appears.

Note: If you are using the Windows Vista Operating System, please see **Installing SpringCharts in Window Vista** section below.

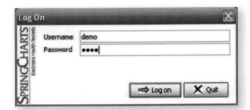

Figure 4 SpringCharts
Log on window

- SpringCharts program files are installed in the default location of C:\Program Files\SCDemo, the recommended installation location for a computer. To accept this default, click on the **Install Spring-Charts Demo Software** button. However, if installing SpringCharts to a flash drive, select the **Change Default Locations** button and select the appropriate drive.
- Accept the license agreement and the installation begins.
- After the files have been successfully installed, the final installation completion screen appears.
- Click on the **Thanks!** button and the installation is complete.
- Close open windows and a shortcut icon to SpringCharts appears on the desktop. Double-click on the SpringCharts icon to open the program. A *Log on* window appears as illustrated in Figure 4. The user name and password are hard coded; simply select the **Log on** button.

Downloading the EHR Material Folder

Note: Several files must be imported into the SpringCharts program to complete some of the exercises in the textbook. These files are contained in the folder titled *EHR Material* on the McGraw-Hill OLC.

- Access the following Website via the Internet browser: www.mhhe.com/ nursingehr.
- Click the *SpringCharts* link in the left-hand menu.
- Locate the *Downloading the EHR Material folder* portion of the page.
- Click the *EHR Material* link.
- Download the zip file to the computer desktop.
- Decompress the downloaded file (use a file decompression program such as Winzip or StuffIt.)
- Once the folder has been copied to the desktop or a flash drive, close the Web browser window.

Installing SpringCharts Network Option

Installing SpringCharts Server

The SpringCharts installation is accomplished in a few easy steps:

1. Verify hardware requirements (see above).
2. Ensure the correct version of JRE (see above).
3. Install SpringCharts server on the server.
4. Install SpringCharts client on all the client computers.
5. Set the IP address of SpringCharts server in SpringCharts client version.

When these steps are completed successfully, SpringCharts is ready to use!

Note: Download the SpringCharts program via the link provided by your McGraw-Hill sales representative. The zipped file contains the server folder, client folder, supplemental docs folder, and text file.

Double-click on the SCServer folder to see the following files: FileCabinet folder, MUData folder, PtData folder, and the compressed executable file **SpringChartsServer. exe, as seen in Figure 5.** Double-click on the executable program and extract the files to the *Program Files* folder on the C: drive (or other designated drive), illustrated in Figure 6. (See *Installing SpringCharts in Windows Vista* below for installation within the Vista operating system.)

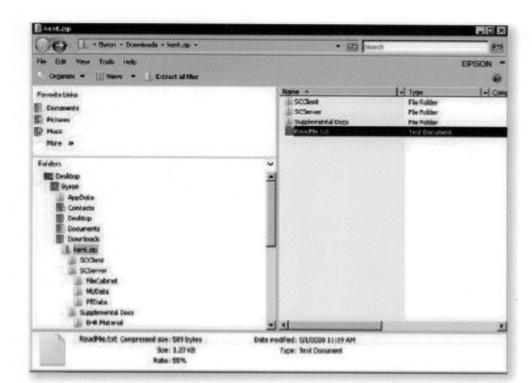

Figure 5 Downloaded file

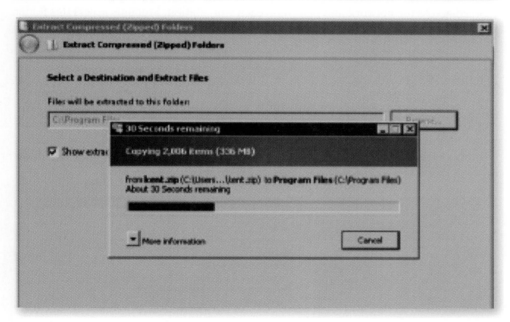

Figure 6 Extracting zipped SpringCharts program files

An SCServer folder and an SCClient folder are created in the *Program Files* folder containing the above-mentioned folders, and an SCServer folder is placed on the desktop. Double-click on **SpringCharts Server.exe** in this folder to launch the installation program, shown in Figure 7.

Note: The SpringCharts server program must be running at all times for the SpringCharts client program to access the database.

To locate the IP address of SpringCharts server, click on the *File* menu and select *SpringCharts Info*. The *Program Information* window contains the IP address needed when activating each SpringCharts client program for the first time, seen in Figure 8. Record this IP address for future reference.

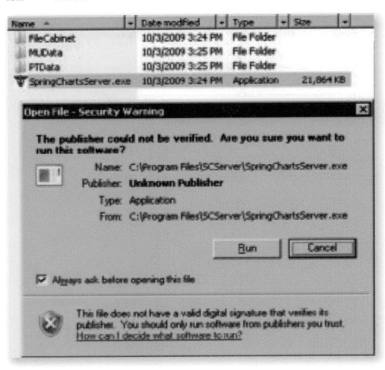

Figure 7 Installing SpringCharts server

Installing SpringCharts Client

The SCClient folder on the server can now be copied across the network and installed in the *Program Files* folder on the C: drive (or other designated drive) of each workstation, as seen in Figure 9. (See **Installing SpringCharts in Windows Vista** below for installation within the Vista operating system.)

Double-click on the **SpringCharts Client.exe** in this folder to launch the installation program. In the *Log on* window, seen in Figure 10, enter the following: **Username:** *demo* and **Password:** *demo*.

When asked for the IP address of SpringCharts server, enter the IP address recorded earlier in the *Program Information* window of SpringCharts server. You will be prompted to log on again.

Loading the EHR Materials Folder

The *EHR Materials* folder is in the *Supplemental Docs* folder that was downloaded earlier. The *EHR Materials* folder must be copied across the network and placed on each workstation. Students access this folder and retrieve files to complete various exercises.

Adding Additional Users

The network version of SpringCharts EHR that accompanies the *Nursing Documentation Using Electronic Health Records* textbook comes loaded with 50 user accounts and the accompanying pop-up text for each user. These 50 user licenses employ the same format for Username and Password, as follows: user1, password; user2, password; and so on. Each user account is already set up on the SpringCharts server under the **Users** button. Additional user accounts are required if more than 50 users are operating in SpringCharts

Figure 8 Locating SpringCharts server IP address

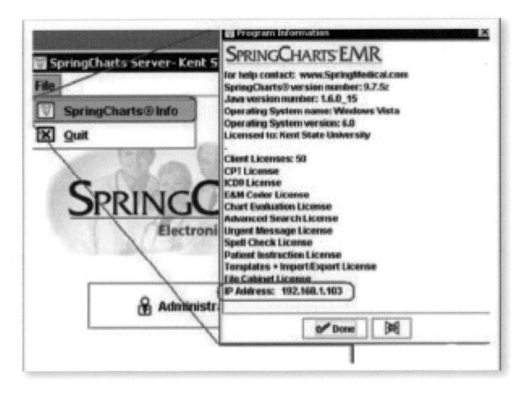

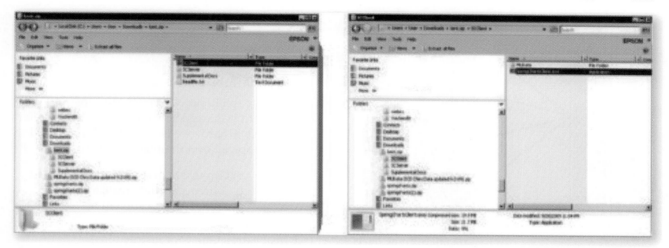

simultaneously. To add users, locate the **Adding Additional Users and PopUp Text.pdf** file in the *Supplemental Docs* folder of the downloaded file and follow the instructions.

Figure 9 Installing SpringCharts client program

Installing SpringCharts EHR on a Windows Terminal Server

SpringCharts can run on a Microsoft Windows Terminal server in one of two fashions, depending on the hardware resources available and the number of concurrent users expected to access SpringCharts during peak usage. In either case, the installation procedures are the same for installing the SpringCharts server or the SpringCharts client.

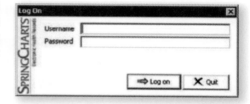

Single Server Method

If resources are not an issue, the Single Server Installation (Figure 11) is a good choice.

Figure 10 Logging on to SpringCharts client program

- Set up terminal services as instructed by Microsoft, and create a user account for each student accessing SpringCharts.
- Install SpringCharts server (see Installation Guide for instructions).
- Install SpringCharts client to the desired folder (see Installation Guide for instructions). Run the SpringCharts client once to configure the client with the server's IP address.

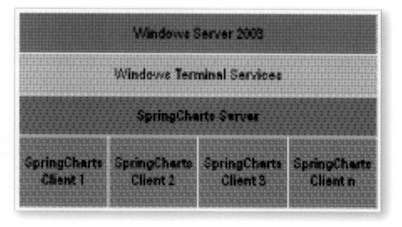

Note: The folder where the SpringCharts server was installed must have modified permissions for all users.

- Copy the SpringCharts client folder to each user's home directory, giving each user a copy of the SpringCharts client.
- Set the login script to run SpringCharts client whenever the user logs in (this is optional), or simply put a shortcut on each user's desktop.

Figure 11 Running SpringCharts on a single terminal server

System Requirements

The minimum requirements for running SpringCharts on a single terminal server are:

- (2) Dual Core 2.8 GHz Xeon Processors or comparable.
- 24+ GB RAM (1 GB per user plus 2 GB for the SpringCharts server).
- 10 GB of Free Disk Space.

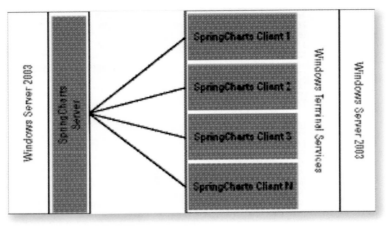

Figure 12 Running SpringCharts on multiple terminal server

This configuration should support 20 to 30 concurrent SpringCharts client users depending on the amount of physical memory.

Multiple Server Method

The multiple server method of installing SpringCharts, shown in Figure 12, is preferable if hardware is limited and users need to be spread over multiple resources.

- Set up terminal services as instructed by Microsoft, and create a user account for each student accessing SpringCharts.
- Install SpringCharts server (see Installation Guide for instructions).
- Install SpringCharts client to the desired folder (see Installation Guide for instructions). Run the SpringCharts client once to configure the client with the server's IP address.
- Copy the SpringCharts client folder to each user's home directory, giving each user a copy of the SpringCharts client.
- Set the login script to run SpringCharts client whenever the user logs in (this is optional) or simply put a shortcut on each user's desktop.

System Requirements

The minimum requirements for running SpringCharts on multiple servers are:

SERVER:

Dual Core Pentium 2 GHz or higher.
4 GB RAM (2 GB for SpringCharts Server and 2 for the OS).
10 GB of Free Disk Space.

CLIENTS:

(2) Dual Core 2.8 GHz Xeon Processors or comparable.
24+ GB RAM (1 GB per user plus 2 GB for the SpringCharts Server).

This configuration should support 20 to 30 concurrent SpringCharts client users depending on the amount of physical memory. As an option, server requirements for each client server may be decreased by splitting the clients over multiple terminal servers.

Backing Up Files

When working in a computer environment that uses a product like Deep Freeze™ to return the computer to its baseline configurations each day, all work in SpringCharts is eradicated when the computer is reset to its original state. It is important to back up SpringCharts at the close of each session. **A 2GB flash drive is needed.**

Note: If running SpringCharts from a flash drive, a backup of the program files is not necessary. See earlier section titled **Running SpringCharts from a Flash Drive** for details.

The SpringCharts application automatically activates the system backup each time the program is closed. The process may take several minutes. The MUData, PtData, and File Cabinet folders from the SpringCharts directory are included in the backup.

Use the following steps to back up and restore data:

1. Click on the main **File** menu option in the **Practice View** window.
2. Click on the **Quit** submenu option to exit the program. The following window opens.

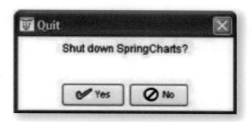

Figure 13 Shut down SpringCharts confirmation window

3. Click on the **Yes** button to close the program. The following window opens.

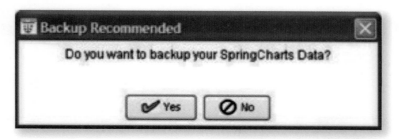

Figure 14 Backing up SpringCharts data option window

4. Click on the **Yes** button to start the backup process. The following window opens.

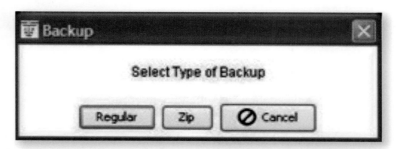

Figure 15 Regular or zip backup option window

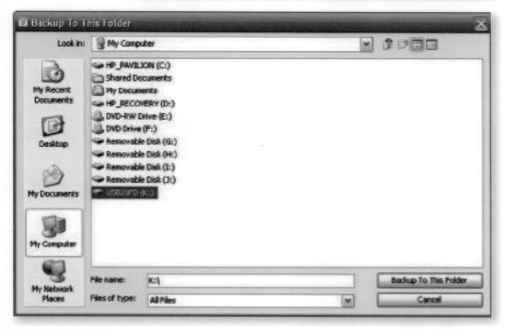

Figure 16 Backup destination window

5. Click on the **Zip** button.
6. Click on **My Computer** in the left column. Select the USB drive where the USB flash drive is placed. The drive name appears in the **File Name** field as seen in Figure 16.
7. Click on the **Backup To This Folder** button to start the backup process.

The program automatically shuts down when the backup is complete. Remove the flash drive.

Figure 17 Locating the restore data window

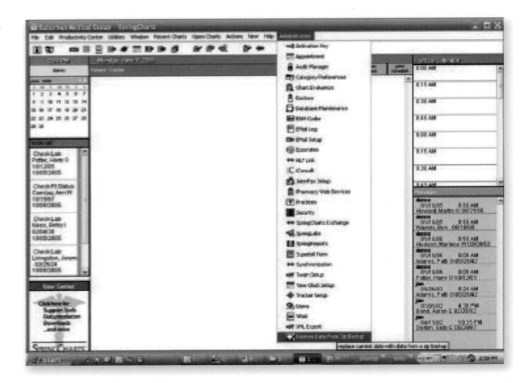

Restoring SpringCharts Files

SpringCharts data must be restored only if working in a computer environment that removes all added data to the program and restores the computer to its original configuration each day. To restore data follow these steps:

1. Open the SpringCharts program.
2. Click on the **Administration** menu. Select the **Restore Data From Zip Backup** option, seen in Figure 17.
3. In the subsequent **Restore from this zip file** window, click on **My Computer** in the left column. Double-click on the USB drive where the USB flash drive is placed. The next window displays the files on the flash drive. Select the backup zip file. The file name appears in the **File name** field, seen in Figure 18.

Figure 18 Locating the restore data file window

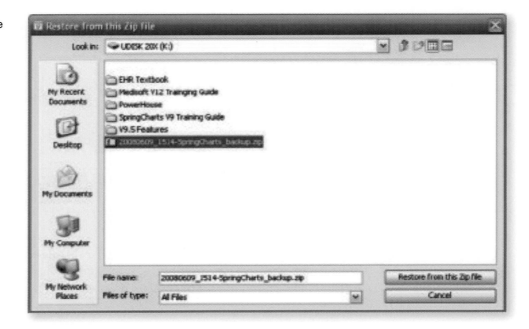

4. Click on the **Restore from this Zip file** button in the lower right corner as seen in Figure 18.

5. Confirm that data are to be restored from the backup zip file, seen in Figure 19. SpringCharts automatically shuts down to perform the restoration process.

6. Once the restoration of the backup data is completed, restart the SpringCharts program.

Figure 19 Restore backup confirmation window

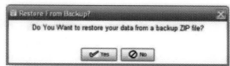

Installing SpringCharts in Windows Vista and Windows 7

SpringCharts is compatible with Microsoft Windows Vista and Windows 7; however, because of the added security features it is **not** recommended that SpringCharts be installed to the normal default location of **Program Files.** In order to configure SpringCharts client or SpringCharts single computer version to run on a Windows Vista or Windows 7 computer, follow the steps below:

Figure 20 Turning off user accounts

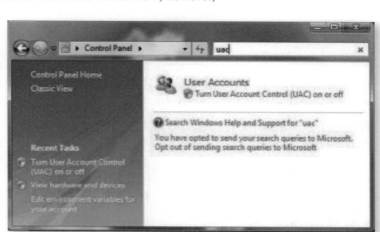

1. Turn off User Account Control (UAC). The easiest way to disable UAC is through the **User Account Control Panel** shown in Figure 20.

2. Make sure that the SpringCharts client folder (SCClient) or single computer version folder (SCDemo) is located in the Root folder (C:). If SpringCharts client or single computer version is already installed on the computer, simply cut and paste the corresponding folder to the C: drive. If this is a new installation, the location of the installation can be changed by clicking on **Change Default Location** on the first screen of the installation program.

Figure 21 Changing permission accounts window.

3. Finally, change the permissions on the folder to **Modify Access for Users and Everyone** by right-clicking on the folder and clicking on **Properties**. Then, click on the tab labeled **Security**. In this panel, make sure that Users and Everyone have modify access.

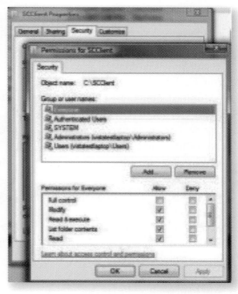

Submitting Assignments Electronically

Many of the exercises in this text instruct the students to print completed assignments and turn the document into the instructor. To submit coursework electronically, the student's computer must be able to create a .pdf file that can be e-mailed to the instructor. A free program that will re-create a word document in pdf format may be downloaded from http://www.primopdf.com/index.aspx. Once downloaded, *PrimoPDF* is installed as a printer option in the *Printer Select* window. To create a pdf document, the *PrimoPDF* printer is selected and the document appears on the screen viewed in *Acrobat Reader™*. Under the *File* menu the option to *attach to e-mail* allows the pdf document to be e-mailed to the instructor.

Acknowledgments

We would like to thank the following individuals who helped develop, critique, and shape our textbook and ancillary package:

The talented group of individuals at McGraw-Hill/Irwin who made all of this come together, especially Editor-in-Chief, Elizabeth Haefele; Publisher, Ken Kasee; Managing Developmental Editor, Kimberly Hooker; Marketing Manager, Mary Haran; Project Manager, Kathryn Wright; Publishing Systems Specialist, Christine Demma Foushi; Senior Designer, Srdjan Savanovic; Buyer, Laura Fuller; Media Project Manager, Brent Dela Cruz; Lead Photo Researcher, Carrie Burger; and Permission Researcher, Jolynn Kilburg of S4Carlisle Publishing Services. We would like to thank contributing author Rachael Christy, Missouri State University, for her valuable contribution to the Chapter 2 text and ancillaries and to her students—Shelley Bird, Sam Crowe, Kara Mattox, Casey Morrow, Savannah Radford, and Joanna Schroeder—who supported her throughout the project.

We also want to recognize the valuable input of all those who helped guide our developmental decisions.

Note to the Student

Technology is everywhere! From our cell phones to our laptops, we are all connected! Healthcare is no different. As the complexity of the healthcare environment increases, nurses must use technology to ensure safe, high-quality patient care.

Documentation is a key component of nursing care. As we move toward a nation with electronic health records (EHRs) for everyone, experience with the EHR is not optional for nurses. Fortunately, you are getting an introduction to this experience in nursing school. Here are a few tips to help you get the most from this book and this course to help ensure your success:

- Read the book. Seriously.
- ***Get the point.*** Even though you're going to read all the assigned chapters (right?), you'll want to know what's important and likely to be on your test. The learning outcomes tell you. Find them at the start of each chapter.
- Keep on track. The Concept Checkups gauge whether you've been thinking hard enough as you read. There's no point in blasting through the chapter just to finish. Check yourself after each section to make sure you understand the key points.
- Practice, practice, practice. Each chapter ends with review material you can use to test what you have learned. The review material in some chapters requires written answers; in other chapters it requires completing exercises in the Spring-Charts EHR program. Completing these exercises is key to ensuring you understand the material presented in each chapter.
- Get real-world experience. SpringCharts software, which is free with the purchase of this text, gives you access to over 100 hands-on exercises using authentic EHR software. Just follow the easy download instructions.
- Best of all, you can document your EHR knowledge by obtaining the Certificate of Completion at the end of your course!

All the Best!

Byron Hamilton
Mary Harper, PhD, RN-DC
Paul Moore

Walkthrough

Chapter Levels

The four levels in *Nursing Documentation* mirror the content typically used in the four semesters of nursing school, simplifying documentation instruction for the nursing instructor. Each level builds on the previous level until the student is documenting the entire nursing process in the electronic health record.

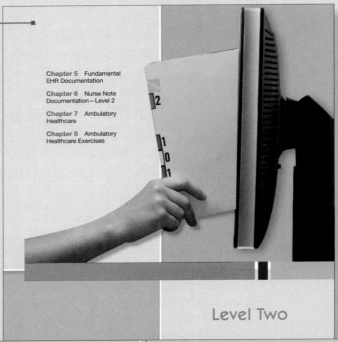

Chapter 5   Fundamental EHR Documentation

Chapter 6   Nurse Note Documentation—Level 2

Chapter 7   Ambulatory Healthcare

Chapter 8   Ambulatory Healthcare Exercises

Level Two

Chapter Openers

Every chapter of *Nursing Documentation* opens with a list of What You Need to Know, a list of Learning Outcomes, and Key Terms to help students identify what they need to understand from the chapter.

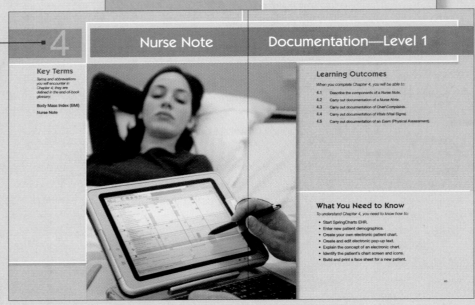

4 · Nurse Note · Documentation—Level 1

Key Terms

Terms and abbreviations you will encounter in Chapter 4; they are defined in the end-of-book glossary.

Body Mass Index (BMI)
Nurse Note

Learning Outcomes

When you complete Chapter 4, you will be able to:

4.1   Describe the components of a Nurse Note.
4.2   Carry out documentation of a Nurse Note.
4.3   Carry out documentation of Chief Complaints.
4.4   Carry out documentation of Vitals (Vital Signs).
4.5   Carry out documentation of an Exam (Physical Assessment).

What You Need to Know

To understand Chapter 4, you need to know how to:

- Start SpringCharts EHR.
- Enter new patient demographics.
- Create your own electronic patient chart.
- Create and edit electronic pop-up text.
- Explain the concept of an electronic chart.
- Identify the patient's chart screen and icons.
- Build and print a face sheet for a new patient.

Learning Outcomes

Each section heading, Concept Checkup, practice exercise, and review question is tied directly to the chapter's learning outcomes. This tagging allows instructors to move students from general theory to application in a step-by-step, logical manner.

Learning Outcomes

When you complete Chapter 5, you will be able to:

5.1	Use SpringCharts to record vitals.
5.2	Carry out documentation for telephone calls.
5.3	Use SpringCharts to create a letter to a patient and about a patient.
5.4	Use SpringCharts to create a letter unrelated to a patient.
5.5	Carry out sending a test report to a patient.
5.6	Use SpringCharts to create an excuse note and an order form for a patient.
5.7	Use the Plan of Care Manager.
5.8	Use *My Websites*.
5.9	Use the calculator utilities.

Concept Checkup 2.5

A. How are nursing diagnoses, NOC, and NIC relevant to nursing documentation?

B. In what settings can nursing diagnoses, NOC, and NIC be used by nurses?

C. List three benefits of documenting the nursing plan of care using standardized nursing diagnoses, NOC, and NIC.
1.
2.
3.

Concept Checkups

Research shows that students learn best when they are actively engaged in the learning process. This active learning feature engages the student, provides interactivity, and promotes effective learning. These checkups ask students to pause at strategic points throughout each chapter to ensure understanding of key points before moving ahead. Answers to all concept checkups are found in Appendix C.

Documentation Tip

Use quotation marks to document exactly what the patient says about the presenting problem.

Documentation Tip

Objective findings should be documented in clear, concise, and descriptive terms. Avoid using terms such as "apparently" or phrases like "appears to be."

Documentation Tips

These marginal tips provide quick bits of information intended to help students identify important aspects of nursing documentation.

FOCAL POINT

Pop-up text and customized lists allow rapid data entry when editing the face sheet.

FOCAL POINT

Healthcare lists and category preferences are set up on the server and are available on all client computers.

Focal Points

Focal Points appear in the margin throughout the text to spotlight crtical data necessary to master end-of-chapter review quizzes.

A. When is the *New Vitals Only* feature used in SpringCharts? _____

B. *True or False.* A user must manually calculate a patient's BMI once the height and weight are recorded. _____

Exercise 5.1

Recording and Viewing Vital Signs

1. Open your chart. Under the *New* menu select *New Vitals Only*.
2. Record a set of vital signs. Select verbiage from the pop-up text. Click the *Done* button and *Save* and *Skip Billing*.
3. Close and reopen your chart by selecting your name from the *Recent Charts* menu on the *Main* menu bar.
4. Open the *Actions* menu within the patient's chart. Select *Graph Vital Signs* and view the various graphed vital signs.
5. Open the *Body Mass Index* graph and print a copy. Write your name on the sheet and submit to your instructor. (See *Submitting Assignments Electronically* on page xxvii of the front material for electron submission instructions).

Legal/Ethical Considerations

This feature helps the student recognize the legal significance of nursing documentation and ensure that documentation is accurate yet nonjudgmental while protecting patients' right to privacy.

LO 5.2 Documenting Telephone Calls

Nurses often make telephone calls that require documentation. In the outpatient setting, the nurse may call to give a patient instructions, check on the patient's status after a procedure, or notify the patient of the date and time for a diagnostic test. In addition, the nurse may call in a prescription to the patient's pharmacy. In the inpatient setting, nurses call healthcare providers and patient families to inform them of

...ertification bodies continue to ...ld to a higher level of quality ...nd inpatient settings.

Concept Checkup 1.3

A. What is the mission of CCHIT?
_____
_____

B. List three requirements for CCHIT certification of EHR products.
1. _____
2. _____
3. _____

C. What is the purpose of the ONC-ATCB?
_____
_____

Evidence-Based Practices

Describe knowledge based on research that has been conducted in the area of nursing documentation and use of the Electronic Health Record.

Evidence-Based Practice 1.2

One VA medical center reported an increase in paper file generation nine years following initiation of a comprehensive, nationally used EHR (Saleem, Russ, Justice, et al., 2009). In another study, nurses reported documenting on paper then transferring documentation to the EHR due to crowded patient rooms that precluded use of the computer at the bedside (Moody, Slocumb, Berg, & Jackson, 2004). Other studies, however, have indicated reduced paperwork (Jamal, McKenzie, & Clark, 2009).

FOCAL POINT

LO 1.4 Benefits of The EHR

Although EHRs provide tremendous benefits to patients and healthcare providers, use of a paper chart remained common through the first decade of the use of the 21st century. Hindrances and concerns about the conversion from the traditional paper chart to electronic media are being overcome. Although the motivations vary from a private practice wanting to simply "become paperless" to a healthcare facility wanting to improve patient care, the benefits of EHRs are being quickly recognized.

Enhanced Accessibility to Clinical Information

EHRs provide enhanced accessibility of clinical information for the healthcare provider. Access to the patient's healthcare information is not limited to the location of the paper chart, but is available at the point of care. The healthcare provider can easily retrieve information such as past health history, family health history, and immunization records. Up-to-date data—including test results; current, routine medications; and allergy information—are crucial for informed decision making. For example, in the outpatient setting, if a patient calls with an issue concerning a current medication, the healthcare provider can instantly access the patient's medication information on the EHR (even if the provider is not in the office), make an informed decision, create a prescription, and document the consultation rapidly with a few mouse clicks or with the Tap&Go™ feature on a portable computer. In addition, information regarding drug interactions with current, routine medications; dosage information for the prescription being created; and instant alerts with allergy warnings are accessible within the EHR. In a paper chart, some information, such as drug interactions, is not present. In addition, the provider may not have access to the chart, making the process more complicated, time-consuming, and error-prone. In the inpatient setting, nurses and other staff have immediate access to information that has been collected in the past, such as allergies and past health history, and need only identify and document changes.

Key Terms

Key terms appear bold in text when a new term is introduced to give students a quick and easy reference. Definitions for the key terms appear in the Glossary at the back of the text.

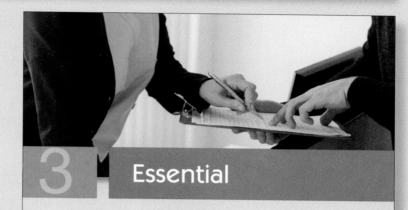

3 Essential

Key Terms

Terms and abbreviations you will encounter in Chapter 3; they are defined in the end-of-book glossary:

Care Tree
Category Preferences
Chart Alert
Electronic Chart
Encounters
Face Sheet

Family Medical History (FMHX)
Graphic User Interface
Imperial Units
Metric Units
Office Visit (OV)

Past Medical History (PMHX)
Practice Management Software (PMS)
User Preferences

Chapter 2 Review

Chapter Review

Many chapters conclude with practice reviews of the terminology and concepts using matching, fill-in-the-blank, and multiple choice questions to reinforce the learning outcomes presented in the chapter.

Using Terminology

Match the terms on the left with the definitions on the right.

_____ 1. NIC

_____ 2. eMAR

_____ 3. Computerized charting

_____ 4. Inpatient care

_____ 5. Quality improvement

_____ 6. Critical pathway

_____ 7. NOC

_____ 8. Ambulatory healthcare

_____ 9. Documentation

_____ 10. NANDA-I

A. Care provided to patients in a hospital involving overnight stays ordered by a primary care provider.

B. Use of electronic sources and databases to record data relating to patient care.

C. Provision of healthcare services to patients who are not admitted overnight to a hospital.

D. Act of recording patient information in written or electronic format; carries legal and ethical importance.

E. Electronic format for documentation of administering drugs.

F. Comprehensive preprinted interdisciplinary standardized plan of care for the average, stable patient experiencing a particular disease process or procedure with predictable outcomes.

G. Serves as an evaluative tool for the effectiveness of nursing interventions.

H. Responsible for developing diagnostic criteria for governing and guiding nursing care of the patient.

I. Provide nurses with standardized treatment options and activities for patients to assist the patients in attaining positive outcomes relating to their disease processes or medical interventions.

J. A formal process of collecting data about performance, comparing those data to accepted norms, and taking action to enhance performance.

Checking Your Understanding

Write "T" or "F" in the blank to indicate whether the statement is true or false.

_____ 11. Detailed and accurate nursing documentation within patient charts enables billing institutions to process claims in a timely manner.

_____ 12. Current Internet security systems are unable to handle the majority of issues surrounding confidentiality in electronic patient charting programs.

_____ 13. The nursing process fits with the SOAP(IER) charting method.

_____ 14. Documentation of general amounts of intake and output of fluid is sufficient to determine a patient's fluid balance.

_____ 15. Using eMARs allows the nurse to administer medications to a patient without the necessity of checking the five rights of medication administration.

_____ 16. Nursing documentation requirements for reimbursement do not change from payor to payor even though the paperwork may vary.

_____ 17. Precise and accurate documentation can be an effective mode of communi-

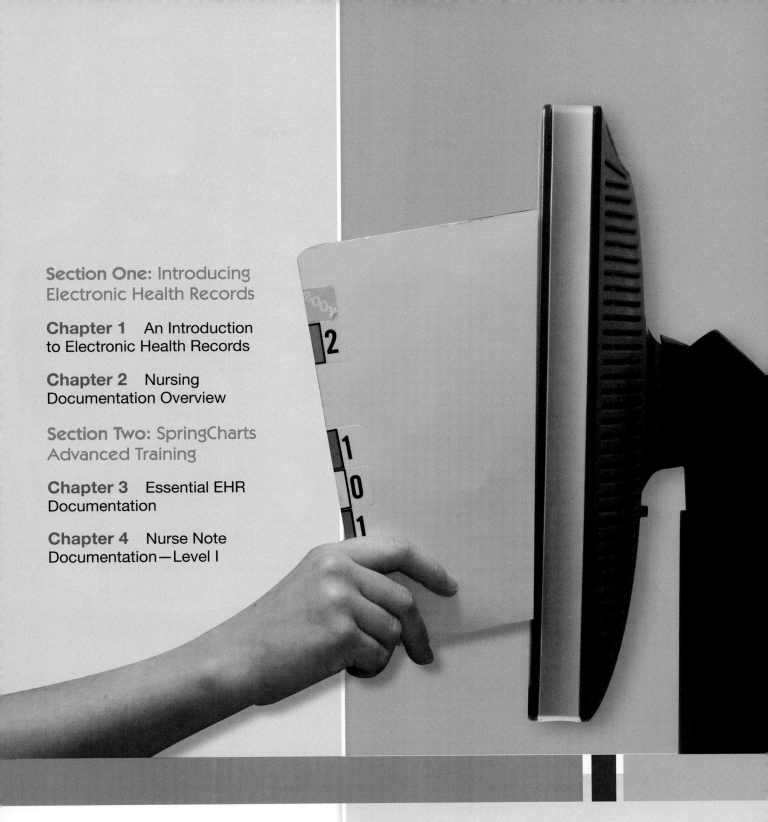

Level One

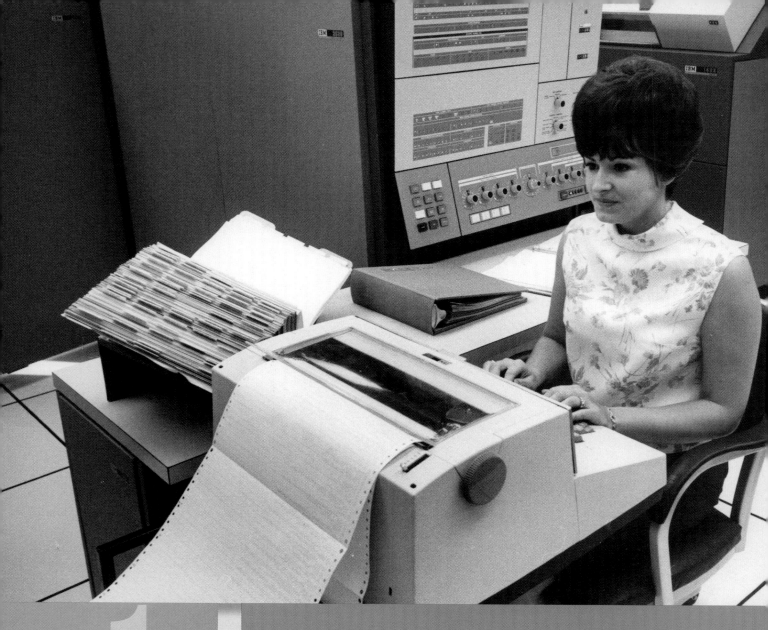

1

An Introduction to

Key Terms

Terms and abbreviations you will encounter in Chapter 1; they are defined in the end-of-book glossary:

Ambulatory	COW/WOW	Intranet Technologies	PHR
ARRA	DICOM	IOM	Point of Care
ASP	E&M Code	LAN	Server
CCD	EHR	Medicare Part A	Standards
CCHIT	Encrypted	Medicare Part B	Tablet PC
CHI	E-prescribing	MIPPA	Telehealth
CMS	HL7	Nursing Informatics	
Connectivity	Interoperability	ONC	

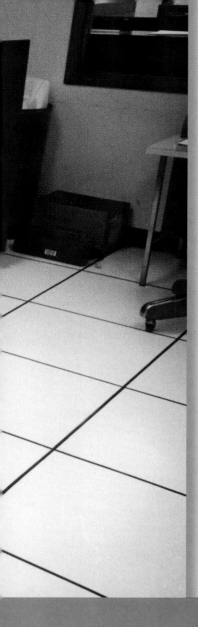

Learning Outcomes

When you complete Chapter 1, you will be able to:

1.1 Recall the history of electronic health records (EHRs).

1.2 Recall the history of standards development for the EHR and nursing's role in their development.

1.3 Identify certification bodies for the EHR.

1.4 Identify the benefits of the EHR.

1.5 Describe government involvement in the EHR.

1.6 Describe the role of nursing informatics in healthcare.

Electronic Health Records

What You Need to Know

To understand Chapter 1, you need to know:

• The role of a patient's chart in a healthcare encounter.

LO 1.1   The Electronic Health Record History

The concept of having a patient's health information stored electronically instead of on paper is not a new one. In the 1960s, as healthcare became more complex, healthcare providers realized that in certain situations the patient's complete health history may not be readily accessible to them. The potential for having comprehensive health information available when needed spurred the innovation of storing patient information electronically. Improvement of patient healthcare has been the catalyst for implementation of the electronic health record.

In the early 1960s the Mayo Clinic in Rochester, Minnesota, and the Medical Center Hospital of Vermont were among the first clinics to use an electronic medical record system, the predecessor of the electronic health record. Over the next two decades, as technology became available, more information and functionalities were added to the electronic medical record system in order to improve patient care. Information about drug dosages, side effects, allergies, and drug interactions became available electronically to healthcare providers, enabling its incorporation into electronic healthcare systems. Electronic diagnostic and treatment plans, which gave healthcare providers information for patient care, proliferated and were also integrated into electronic medical record systems. More academic and research institutes developed computerized health record systems as tools to track patient treatment. Each new enhancement promoted the quality of patient care.

A variety of acronyms are associated with the use of electronic health records. Some of these definitions reveal an evolution of terms and meanings of government agencies and independent associations that influence the field of electronic health records. The following terms are used often in the healthcare community.

CPR—Computer-Based Patient Record: This term was one of the first used to conceptualize the idea of an electronic health record. A computerized patient record is a lifetime patient record that includes all information from all specialties (including dental and psychiatry) and is available to all providers (potentially internationally). Because the CPR requires full **interoperability** between electronic health records, the CPR is not realistic in the foreseeable future. In the early 1990s the initiative to use the CPR caused the concept to evolve into the EMR.

EMR—Electronic Medical Record: This term was widely used as terminology migrated away from the computer-based patient record or CPR. However, as functions became more clearly delineated and complex, the electronic record industry began using the term EMR to refer to a program that *did not* offer certain high-end functionalities such as health maintenance and disease management, care alerts, the continuity of care record (CCR), personal health record functions, or interconnectivity with providers and diagnostic testing facilities outside the organization.

EHR—Electronic Health Record: Currently, this term is the most commonly accepted term for storing and accessing patient health information electronically. The **EHR** meets interoperability standards and therefore is able to be used across many healthcare organizations. The EHR encompasses a full range of functionalities and information, for both inpatient and outpatient settings. These functions include patient demographics, progress notes, problems, medications, vital signs, past health history, immunizations, laboratory data, radiology reports, scheduling, transcription, e-prescribing, evaluation and management coding, care alerts, chief complaints, evidence-based decision support, and health maintenance. In the near future, an EHR will include the continuity of care record and the personal health record; standards for these functionalities are still being developed.

CCD—Continuity of Care Document: The **CCD** is a health provider–oriented snapshot of a core set of data reflecting the most relevant and timely facts about a patient's healthcare. The CCD is a subset of the EHR. Typically, it includes patient information, diagnoses, recent procedures, allergies, medications, and

FOCAL POINT

Improvement of the quality of patients' healthcare has always been the catalyst for the development of the electronic health record.

future treatment plans. It should be accessible to all care providers whenever needed. The electronic CCD is designed to be vendor and technology neutral, that is, accessible and readable by other electronic systems. It provides a means for one healthcare practitioner, system, or setting to aggregate all pertinent data about a patient and forward it to another practitioner, system, or setting, whether inpatient, outpatient, or community-based to support the continuity of care. For patients, it provides continuity of care by allowing easier access to vital health information from other providers.

PHR—Personal Health Record: The **PHR** allows the patient to become an interactive source of health information and health management through an Internet-based patient portal to the healthcare facility. Through a secure connection, patients may schedule appointments, request medication refills, access lab or radiology results, and ask questions about their health. Some PHRs enable patients to complete or update family and social histories and even read their health records and notify providers of incorrect or missing information.

As computer technology continues to rapidly develop, the versatility of the EHR increases. Access to the patient's information, health alerts, warnings, drug information, and disease management becomes available at the **point of care** to the healthcare provider in a more user-friendly form. Modes of data entry into the EHR have also progressed. Traditionally, a keyboard was the only source for data entry. However, the need for convenience, efficiency, and speed has mandated other methods of input. Voice recognition systems adapt to a person's voice and speech patterns so that the computer inputs data as the operator speaks. Electronic handwriting recognition is now available. However, these two methods of data input are not commonly used because they require that the user repeat the same activity each time data are needed. Instead, large bodies of preset text known as "templates" can be used to easily input data into the patient's record. In lieu of typing, healthcare providers can enter data and access data via a few taps of a stylus pen on a touch screen or the click of a mouse. Touch screens are available on devices such as laptops, **Tablet PCs**, or iPads™, making the EHR portable. The ease of use and speed of the Tap&Go™ feature with portable computers has facilitated the use of EHRs, making them more desirable. Traditionally, a stationary computer workstation in each exam room has been cost-prohibitive for the independent healthcare provider. This lack of computer availability at the point of care resulted in delayed data entry. As a result, patient information was not readily available to other providers and healthcare staff. However, in recent years the increased use of laptops, computers on wheels **(COWs)**, workstations on wheels (WOWs), other portable computers, and wireless **connectivity** has resulted in greater mobility and lower costs.

Advances in security and reliability have promoted flexibility and mobility of the EHR. A local area network **(LAN)** enables computers to communicate and typically uses a main **server** for the database. The LAN system can be customized to the healthcare facility's needs. The LAN system may consist of wired connections and/or use a wireless network as illustrated in Figure 1.1. Wireless LAN networks enable healthcare providers to have full or open access to their EHR program from anywhere within the healthcare facility.

Internet and **intranet technologies** have increased the availability of healthcare databases that can be shared and accessed across large distances, giving healthcare providers accessibility to the EHR from remote locations such as nursing homes, a patient's home, a home office, or hospitals. Access to these networks is limited and data flowing on the network is **encrypted** for security. This configuration is ideal for home healthcare nurses

> ### Evidence-Based Practice 1.1
>
> In a pilot study exploring the use of a handheld computer, Baker and Copping (2009) found that participants perceived that the mobile point of care device improved efficiency, enhanced patient safety, and promoted quality care.

Figure 1.1

Hardwired and wireless LAN system.

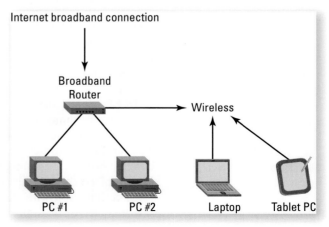

FOCAL POINT

The affordability of both hardware and software, and the reliability of Internet technology and wireless connectivity have enabled many independent practitioners to take advantage of the EHR in recent years.

who need to access patients' records that are stored on a remote server belonging to the healthcare provider. With the advent of portable wireless cards, data can be sent and received between the nurse's laptop and the network, giving access to the patient's record via the Internet in real time.

Another network option for a healthcare facility is the Web-based EHR or application server provider (**ASP**) where the EHR is accessed via the Internet using high-speed (broadband) connections. In this model, the software is not housed on a computer server at the healthcare facility. Maintenance, updates, and backups are conducted remotely by the EHR Web hosting company. Some concerns about Web-based EHRs expressed by healthcare professionals include the security of the EHR, the speed of downloading and uploading images or large files, and the availability of Internet connectivity (Melczer, Berkeyheiser, Miller, & Yeager, 2005).

Concept Checkup 1.1

A. What was the initial reason, and the ongoing reason, for the development of electronic health records?

_____

B. List four modes of data entry into EHR programs.
1. _____
2. _____
3. _____
4. _____

C. What two types of technologies have increased the availability of healthcare databases and access to the EHR?
1. _____
2. _____

D. What is the most commonly accepted term for electronically storing and accessing a patient's health information?

_____

LO 1.2   Development of EHR Standards

Understanding **standards** for EHRs seems to be a technical discussion with little relevance to nursing. However, since nursing is the largest group of healthcare professionals, knowledge of the need for standardization and current initiatives to achieve standardization is important as nurses advocate for quality care for the public. Since EHRs have the potential to improve the quality of healthcare, United States' government institutions, such as the Institute of Medicine (**IOM**), have been promoting their use for the last decade. Obstacles such as cost, organization, lack of unified standards, functionality, and interoperability have slowed the adoption of the EHR. Recommendations, reports, and standards from independent associations and federal government agencies have served as stepping stones to facilitate a wider usage of EHRs.

In May 2003, the U.S. Department of Health and Human Services requested the IOM, a governmental agency that provides information and advice about policies affecting public health, to provide guidance on the key capabilities for EHR systems. The IOM's Committee on Data Standards for Patient Safety identified key competencies that became the foundational benchmark for EHR development and programming (Board of Healthcare Services, 2003).

In conjunction with the IOM's EHR recommendations, the Consolidated Health Informatics (**CHI**) standards were initiated to enable federal agencies involved in

FOCAL POINT

The Institute of Medicine developed guidelines for key capabilities and functions that should exist in a quality electronic health record program.

healthcare and health-related missions to effectively share information. Some of these federal agencies included the Veterans Administration (VA), the Department of Health and Human Services, the Department of Defense, and the Social Security Administration. The CHI standards required common clinical vocabularies and standard methods for transmitting health information. By May of 2004, a set of 20 standards were announced and became the point of reference to standardize how information is coded or termed for use in exchanging data with an EHR (Presidential Initiatives, 2004).

CHI standards are not required by law. However, vendors doing business with the federal government voluntarily adopt these standards. The federal government, as the largest purchaser of healthcare services, uses these standards to promote interoperability between EHR systems. Some of these standards are as follows:

Health Level Seven (HL7) is a computer messaging and vocabulary standard for demographic information, units of measure, immunizations, clinical encounters, and clinical document architecture for text-based reports. Practically, it is the communication standard for the coordinated care of patients for scheduling, orders, tests, admissions, discharges, and transfers. HL7 enables clinical systems to communicate with each other, or interface, when they receive new information. HL7 is currently the standard for the interfacing of clinical data in most institutions.

National Council on Prescription Drug Programs (NCPDP) creates and promotes standards for the transfer of data to and from retail pharmacy services. NCPDP standards are focused on prescription drug messages and the activities involved in billing pharmacy claims and services, rebates, pharmacy ID cards, and standardized business transactions between pharmacies and the professionals who prescribe medications.

Institute of Electrical and Electronics Engineers (IEEE), pronounced as *eye-triple*-e, is an international organization for the advancement of technology related to electricity. The 11073 format is the *Point of Care Medical Device Communication Standards*, which addresses the interoperability of medical devices. (IEEE promulgates hundreds of standards; the standards/formats are numbered to keep them distinct.) IEEE sets electronic standards to allow connection of medical devices to information and computer systems, allowing healthcare providers to monitor information from intensive care units and from **telehealth** services, specifically on Native American tribal reservations.

Digital Imaging Communications in Medicine (DICOM) enables images and associated diagnostic information to be accessed and transferred from various manufacturers' devices as well as healthcare staff workstations.

The Laboratory Logical Observation Identifier Name Codes (LOINC) set standards for the electronic transfer of clinical laboratory results.

Systematized Nomenclature of Medicine Clinical Terms (SNOMED-CT) provides a common language that enables a consistent method of capturing, sharing, and aggregating health data across specialties and sites of care. It provides standard terminology for laboratory result contents, anatomy, diagnosis, healthcare problems, and nursing.

The Health Information Portability and Accountability Act's Transaction and Code Sets are the standards for electronic exchange of information for billing and administration.

The United States Food and Drug Administration (FDA) sets standards for medication names, codes for ingredients, manufactured dosage forms, drug products, and medication packages. The description of clinical drugs and drug classifications are set by the National Library of Medicine's RxNORM.

The Human Gene Nomenclature (HUGN) sets standards for the transfer of information about the role of genes in biomedical research.

The Environmental Protection Agency (EPA) sets standards for nonmedicinal chemicals that are important to healthcare through the Substance Registry System.

FOCAL POINT

Twenty Consolidated Health Informatics (CHI) standards were voluntarily adopted by vendors to promote interoperability between health information systems.

Nursing's Role in Setting Standards for EHRs

The nursing profession has recognized the importance of standardization in promoting the exchange of information since the days of Florence Nightingale (Ozbolt & Saba, 2008) and has taken steps to ensure nursing input into the standardization of the EHR. Standardization and interoperability promote safety, quality, cost savings, research, and identification of nursing's contribution to patient outcomes (Hallley, Brokel, & Sensemeier, 2009). Safety and quality are enhanced by the communication of information such as patient allergies, past health history, and current medications across organizations and from one level of care to another. Cost savings are achieved by reduction in duplicate tests and procedures. Finally, standardization promotes data collection for research purposes and allows nursing to identify the relationships among nursing interventions and patient outcomes.

Nurses have participated in and provided leadership for many of the national standards initiatives including SNOMED, **CCHIT**, HL7, and the Health Information Technology Standards Panel (HITSP). In 2006, the Technology Informatics Guiding Educational Reform (TIGER) Initiative summit brought together 100 nursing leaders to create "a vision for the future of nursing that bridges the quality chasm with information technology (IT), enabling nurses to use informatics in practice and education to provide safer, high-quality patient care" (TIGER, n.d., paragraph 2). One goal is to ensure nursing input into the standardization process for EHRs to reflect the work of nursing and its contribution to quality patient care. While nursing has developed standardized nursing terminologies, the American Nurses Association recognizes several different versions such as NANDA-International nursing diagnoses, nursing intervention classifications (NIC), nursing outcome classifications (NOC), and the International Classification of Nursing Practice (ICNP)® (Sensmeier, 2007). The TIGER Initiative calls for agreement on the standardized nursing terminology to promote interoperability. Clinical nurses, nurse leaders, and nurse educators must team with nursing informatics experts to ensure standardization and interoperability, guaranteeing that the needs of both patients and the nursing profession are met (Ozbolt & Saba, 2008; Fetter, 2009).

Concept Checkup 1.2

A. What was the purpose of the 20 criteria set up by the CHI by 2004?

_____

_____

B. List five of the standards and/or organizations that regulate the standards used to promote interoperability between EHR systems.

1. _____
2. _____
3. _____
4. _____
5. _____

C. Why are standardization and interoperability important?

_____

LO 1.3   EHR Certification Agencies

CCHIT®, The Certification Commission for Health Information Technology, was organized in July 2004 with support from the American Health Information Management Association (AHIMA), the Healthcare Information and Management Systems Society (HIMSS), and the National Alliance for Health Information Technology (NAHIT) (About the Certification Commission for Health Information Technology, 2009). These three organizations committed resources during the organizational phase to create the independent, nonprofit, private-sector organization called the *Certification Commission*. It is composed of 21 volunteer commissioners who guide the more than 100 work group members charged with the Commission's development work.

The Certification Commission states its mission is "to accelerate the adoption of health information technology by creating an efficient, credible and sustainable product certification program" (CCHIT, n.d.). In September 2005, the U.S. Department of Health & Human Services (HHS) awarded the Commission a contract to develop certification criteria, evaluate these standards, and create the inspection process for health information technology (HIT). The three specific HIT areas are (1) **ambulatory** care EHRs for the office-based healthcare provider, (2) inpatient EHRs for hospitals and health systems, and (3) network components through which EHRs interoperate and share information. Each year, the Commission develops and announces new criteria and features for EHRs. EHR companies must pay approximately $25,000 to go through the inspection process for their ambulatory EHR product for a three-year term of certification.

The Certification Commission provided an official recognition and approval that had been requested from both the private sector and government agencies. Such industry standards–based criteria for EHRs promoted confidence in their use. In the past, the lack of uniform requirements and standards was a considerable hurdle to the extensive adoption of EHRs. When HHS awarded the contract to the Certification Commission, this barrier was specifically addressed to promote the use of an EHR by primary care providers, hospitals, home-health, and other organizations.

Uniform EHR standards are primarily developed by the Health Information Technology Standards Panel (HITSP), a federally contracted standards development organization. The Certification Commission evaluated these standards as part of their development of conformance criteria and test scripts, and published the first set of 300 proposed ambulatory EHR criteria in May 2006. Each year since then, additional criteria and test steps have been added to the requirements for CCHIT certification.

CCHIT certification demonstrated that an EHR product met basic requirements for

- Functionality—ability to carry out specific tasks.
- Interoperability—compatibility and communication with other products.
- Security—ability to keep patients' information safe and private.

In 2004, the Office of the National Coordinator for Health Information Technology (**ONC**) was established within the Office of the Secretary for the U.S. Department of Health and Human Services. Its purpose was to serve as a resource to the entire health system, to support the adoption of health information technology, and to promote a nationwide health information exchange in order to improve healthcare in the United States (The Office of the National Coordinator for Health Information Technology, 2009).

The need to guarantee basic standards, implementation specifications, and functionality of EHR programs to the medical community spurred the ONC to launch a two-year temporary certification program in September 2010. Several IT organizations across the country were selected to fulfill the task of testing and certifying both ambulatory and inpatient EHR programs. Each entity is known as an ONC-Authorized Testing and Certification Body (ONC-ATCB). CCHIT became one of several ONC-ATCBs. After a two-year period, the ONC will move to a permanent certification program and select a few organizations that will be known as an ONC-Authorized Certification Body (ONC-ACB). EHR vendors are required to submit their EHR programs for testing and certification to one of these ONC-ATCBs. Products that were previously CCHIT certified must be resubmitted for ONC-ATCB certification.

With this certification process in place, providers and patients can be confident that electronic health information technology products and systems are secure, maintain data confidentially, perform a set of specified functions, and are interoperable with other systems to share medical information.

Regulations, government agencies, and recognized certification bodies continue to influence the EHR industry, bringing the healthcare field to a higher level of quality patient care and greater efficiency in both ambulatory and inpatient settings.

Concept Checkup 1.3

A. What is the mission of CCHIT?

_____

_____

_____

B. List three requirements for CCHIT certification of EHR products.

1. _____

2. _____

3. _____

C. What is the purpose of the ONC-ATCB?

_____

_____

Evidence-Based Practice 1.2

One VA medical center reported an increase in paper file generation nine years following initiation of a comprehensive, nationally used EHR (Saleem, Russ, Justice, et al., 2009). In another study, nurses reported documenting on paper then transferring documentation to the EHR due to crowded patient rooms that precluded use of the computer at the bedside (Moody, Slocumb, Berg, & Jackson, 2004). Other studies, however, have indicated reduced paperwork (Jamal, McKenzie, & Clark, 2009).

FOCAL POINT

Immediate access to all patient health information at the point of care promotes informed healthcare decision making.

LO 1.4 Benefits of the EHR

Although EHRs provide tremendous benefits to patients and healthcare providers, use of a paper chart remained common through the first decade of the 21st century. Hindrances and concerns about the conversion from the traditional paper chart to electronic media are being overcome. Although the motivations vary from a private practice wanting to simply "become paperless" to a healthcare facility wanting to improve patient care, the benefits of EHRs are being quickly recognized.

Enhanced Accessibility to Clinical Information

EHRs provide enhanced accessibility of clinical information for the healthcare provider. Access to the patient's healthcare information is not limited to the location of the paper chart, but is available at the point of care. The healthcare provider can easily retrieve information such as past health history, family health history, and immunization records. Up-to-date data—including test results; current, routine medications; and allergy information—are crucial for informed decision making. For example, in the outpatient setting, if a patient calls with an issue concerning a current medication, the healthcare provider can instantly access the patient's medication information on the EHR (even if the provider is not in the office), make an informed decision, create a prescription, and document the consultation rapidly with a few mouse clicks or with the Tap&Go™ feature on a portable computer. In addition, information regarding drug interactions with current, routine medications; dosage information for the prescription being created; and instant alerts with allergy warnings are accessible within the EHR. In a paper chart, some information, such as drug interactions, is not present. In addition, the provider may not have access to the chart, making the process more complicated, time-consuming, and error-prone. In the inpatient setting, nurses and other staff have immediate access to information that has been collected in the past, such as allergies and past health history, and need only identify and document changes.

Patient Safety

The EHR contributes to patient safety in several ways. For example, illegible handwriting is the source of many medical errors. The challenge of reading handwritten notes, orders, and prescriptions has been eliminated with the EHR. Patient information is clear and legible. Reports and letters to other specialists and patients are comprehensive, professional, and easy to create, promoting safe patient handoffs and continuity of care. As discussed earlier, information is readily accessible in the EHR. In paper charts, on the other hand, information may be easily misplaced.

EHRs also contribute to patient safety through various alert systems, particularly related to medications and allergies. Alerts appear when a medication order is not within normal prescribing parameters. Alerts can also signal drug interactions or food-drug interactions. Allergy alerts indicate when a contraindicated medication is ordered, preventing a possible allergic or anaphylactic reaction. National attention to patient safety is driving the healthcare industry toward drastically reducing errors through e-prescription and electronic provider orders.

Quality Patient Care

As healthcare becomes more complex, healthcare providers rely increasingly on evidence-based practice guidelines to support their practice. Through incorporation into the EHR as decision support systems, these guidelines are readily available to healthcare professionals and promote adherence, ensuring quality care for patients. Decision support systems allow healthcare professionals to easily access these guidelines and correlate them with past health history, family history, gender, age, and allergies, in order to make good clinical decisions. Nurses use clinical decision support systems for patient triage in the emergency department, for managing anticoagulants, and for pain management (Anderson & Wilson, 2008). Electronic reminders are available for routine screening and treatments, such as mammograms or immunizations, and may be individualized based on patient needs. For example, while a reminder for a colonoscopy may be set to appear for all patients older than 50 years, an EHR can also identify that a patient who is younger than 50, but has a family history of colon cancer, also needs to have a screening colonoscopy. These electronic reminders help prevent oversight by the practitioner and ensure optimal care for patients.

In addition to health promotion guidelines, over 2,000 best practice guidelines have been developed by reputable healthcare organizations to guide the diagnosis and treatment of many illnesses (AHRQ, 2010). Melczer, Berkeyheiser, Miller, and Yeager state:

> [P]ractice guidelines, based on "evidence-based medicine," often are very complex, with what is best for a patient with a particular condition depending on a variety of factors, including the patient's history, the patient's family history, other conditions of the patient and patient medications, and the availability of different modes of treatment in a community. No physician is able to keep up with all the latest practices and apply them to the particular conditions of each of his or her patients. (p. 4)

The EHR provides a mechanism to ensure that patients receive the most current standard of care consistently. EHRs incorporate evidence-based treatment protocols and also inform the healthcare provider of recommended diagnostic tests. Kaiser Permanente of Ohio saw the following practice guideline compliance improvements after implementing an automated health record system and adding reminders at the point of care:

- Aspirin use in patients with coronary artery disease increased from 56 percent to 82 percent in 27 months, whereas lipid-lowering agents increased from 10 percent to 20 percent in 7 months.
- ACE inhibitor use in patients with congestive heart failure increased from 54 percent to 66 percent.
- Stratification (staging) for patients with diabetes mellitus and asthma increased to 76 percent in 26 months and 65 percent in 29 months respectively. In addition, referrals to podiatry for medium- and high-risk diabetics increased from 14 percent to 66 percent in 12 months.
- Percentage of hypertensive patients taking nonrecommended medications decreased from 16 percent to 12 percent in 12 months.
- Percentage of patients older than 64 years of age who were offered an influenza vaccination during a primary care visit increased from 56 percent to 69 percent in 36 months (Scott, Rundall, Vogt, & Hsu, 2005).

EHRs also improve quality of care by providing information to patients concerning their diagnosis or the planned treatments. Instructions are easily accessed in the

---

FOCAL POINT

Automated alerts and the reduction in handwriting that may be illegible promote patient safety.

Evidence-Based Practice 1.3

In a review of studies of the effect of EHRs on quality of care, Jamal, McKenzie, and Clark (2009) found that adherence to guidelines improved in 14 of 17 studies. However, no consistent improvement in patient outcomes was evident in the studies reviewed.

FOCAL POINT

The availability of care plans and practice guidelines increase the accuracy of patient care. Rapid documentation and accurate coding have reduced costs and increased reimbursement as a result of the implementation of EHRs.

EHR by the provider and may be printed or e-mailed to the patient, giving the patient a resource to help manage an illness or prepare for a diagnostic procedure. The EHR records treatment plans and the instructions for procedural preparation or post-treatment care for the patient. As a result, patient care is enhanced and the healthcare provider may be safeguarded against liability.

Another mechanism to promote quality care is in the proficient handling of drug recalls. Reports generated through an EHR document signify which patients are currently taking specific medications. Form letters can be rapidly generated, alerting patients to the recall and requesting follow-up with their healthcare provider. The alternative process in a paper chart environment is time-consuming and prone to errors.

EHRs reduce the repetition of lab tests and other diagnostic studies through messages that inform the practitioner that a diagnostic procedure has already been ordered. Diagnostic test information is clearly displayed and readily accessed. Lost or delayed test and/or lab results are not as common with EHR programs, resulting in a quicker diagnosis and treatment plan for the patient, thus promoting patient satisfaction.

Efficiency and Savings

Major motivations for the increased use of an EHR are both efficiency and financial savings. As noted above, repetition of diagnostic testing is reduced. Another obvious financial saving is in the elimination of the paper-based chart's storage costs and retrieval costs. One study cites "that a chart pull costs $20 at Scott and White Memorial Hospital, Clinic, and Health Systems in Temple, Texas. Their electronic chart solution reduced electronic chart pulls to less than $1 apiece" (Stammer, 2001).

Simple uses of electronic messaging systems built into an EHR enable speedier communication between staff members. Communication to the healthcare provider concerning diagnoses, drug refills, pre-authorizations for treatments, and general patient concerns is expedited and simplified. Electronic communication among staff regarding referrals, phone call documentation, and letters to patients and other professionals is accelerated and the items are automatically saved into the patient's record.

Use of EHRs results in significant time saving for clinicians through streamlined job processes. Early studies by Dassenko and Slowinski (1995) reported a reduction in nurse intake time from 35 minutes to 20 minutes for initial office visits and from 35 minutes to 15 minutes for return visits at the University of Wisconsin Hospital and Clinics. The elimination of repeatedly collecting and entering information and the addition of the enhanced display of the patient's history, vital signs, weight, and health problems attributed to greater efficiency and time savings.

Reporting to public health organizations is expedited and facilitated with the reporting capabilities of EHRs. The simplification of this process for both ambulatory and inpatient settings is another example of time savings that translates into cost savings. Records are easily accessed and patient data sorted by diagnoses, treatments, or care plans and then sent to the appropriate agencies.

When healthcare providers complete documentation in an EHR, the need for a transcriptionist is often eliminated. This efficiency has generated an estimated savings of $300 to $1,000 or more per month per practitioner. In one six-provider practice, transcription took 150 hours per week. Initial studies looking at efficiency after implementing an EHR, that time was decreased by one-third. The turnaround time of the transcription went from seven days to one day. The time and money savings enabled the practice to add two additional providers (Mildon & Cohen, 2001).

In the private practice setting, EHRs' coding programs give healthcare providers confidence and support for coding Evaluation and Management (**E&M**) encounters with patients. Often, undercoding occurs by healthcare providers, resulting in reduced insurance reimbursement for services. However, with an EHR, more accurate level-of-care coding is based on documentation from the review of systems and examination within the office visit assessment, helping recover lost revenue for practices. In addition, some malpractice insurance carriers give discounts to their insureds when an EHR program is used because of more thorough documentation and improved patient care.

Melczer et al. reported the return on investment (ROI) of a Chicago-area hospital that implemented an EHR costing over $40 million:

The hospital estimates that it will save $10 million annually. The new system is substantially enhancing patient care. The turnaround time for obtaining test results has fallen significantly, with mammograms now taking a day compared to up to three weeks, and cardiographics reports dropping from as long as 10 days to one day. Entire categories of medication errors and potential errors have been eliminated, including transcription errors, errors due to misunderstood abbreviations and mix-ups due to look-alike drug names. In addition, delayed administration of patient medications has decreased 70 percent while omitted administration of medications has dropped 20 percent across the organization due to the electronic medication administration records and system tools that alert nurses of new patient orders and of overdue medications. (Melczer, Berkey-heiser, Miller, & Yeager, 2005)

Concept Checkup 1.4

List four benefits of implementing an EHR program.
A. _____
B. _____
C. _____
D. _____

LO 1.5 Government Involvement in the EHR

The promotion of the EHR concept by many organizations is related to the benefits EHRs bring to healthcare. The Institute of Medicine (IOM) recognized these benefits and in 1991 called for EHRs to be implemented with the elimination of paper-based patient records by 2001. President George W. Bush, in his 2004 State of the Union address stated, "By computerizing health records, we can avoid dangerous medical mistakes, reduce costs, and improve care" (Chin, 2004). President Bush subsequently created a sub-Cabinet-level position for a National Health Information Coordinator at the Department of Health and Human Services (HHS). Then in April of 2004, he outlined a plan "to ensure that most Americans have electronic health records within the next 10 years" (Associated Press, 2004). From that plan, government agencies have been able to promote the use of EHRs and overcome barriers to their use.

In 2008, concerns for reducing costs and improving patient care were echoed by the Obama presidential campaign. Mr. Obama promised to sponsor the adoption of EHRs through a sizable government financial commitment as part of a broader economic stimulus package. In the economic recovery plan of 2009, President Obama's administration outlined strategies to spend in excess of $19 billion to accelerate the use of computerized health records in physicians' offices and inpatient settings over a period of five years.

"Our recovery plan will invest in electronic health records and new technology that will reduce errors, bring down costs, ensure privacy, and save lives," President Obama stated in his speech to Congress in February 2009 (Obama, 2009).

Medicare Improvements for Patients and Providers Act of 2008

On July 15, 2008, the Medicare Improvements for Patients and Providers Act of 2008 (**MIPPA**) was enacted by Congress. Besides important changes that increase Medicare benefits to low-income beneficiaries, MIPPA provided positive incentives for practitioners who used **e-prescribing** beginning in 2009 through 2013. Electronic prescribing is intended to bring greater safety to patients by providing for automatic drug and allergy interaction checking and the elimination of medication errors due to poor handwriting. E-prescribing is also designed to bring greater efficiency to

FOCAL POINT

E-prescribing provides automatic drug and allergy interaction checking, reduces medical errors, and improves cost, quality, and patient safety.

the prescribing process for providers and pharmacists alike by dramatically decreasing communication from pharmacists requesting clarification of prescriptions. As a result, patients will receive their medications faster.

MIPPA defines e-prescribing as the ability to transmit prescriptions electronically and conduct all alerts. Alerts include automated prompts that offer information on the drug being prescribed and warn the prescriber of possible undesirable or unsafe situations, such as potentially inappropriate dosage or route of administration of the drug, drug-drug interactions, allergy concerns, or warnings/cautions (U.S. Department of Health and Human Services, 2010).

MIPPA impacted **Medicare Part A** by increasing payment to Community Health Centers and increasing healthcare accessibility to rural areas. Eligible providers who successfully reported e-prescribing in 2009 were eligible to receive an additional incentive payment equal to two percent of all of their **Medicare Part B** allowed charges for services furnished during the reporting year. These financial incentives continue through 2012. However, after 2014, the measure imposes penalties of two percent for practitioners who do not e-prescribe.

Surescripts™ is the national clearinghouse for e-prescribing. The company connects a network of thousands of prescribers, pharmacists, and payers nationwide enabling them to exchange health information and prescribe without paper. By adopting the NCPDP standard for data transfer, Surescripts collaborates with the national EHR vendors, pharmacies, and health plans to support practitioners using electronic health record software. With this network in place, healthcare providers are able to electronically access prescription information from pharmacies, health plans, and other providers to see the patient's total prescription history from all sources. Currently, prescribers are able to send e-prescriptions to any of the 51,000 retail pharmacies and six of the largest mail-order pharmacies. Through e-prescribing, EHRs are providing meaningful improvements in cost, quality, and patient safety. (For more details on the electronic prescribing network, please visit http://www.surescripts.com.)

American Recovery and Reinvestment Act

On February 17, 2009, President Obama signed the American Recovery and Reinvestment Act (**ARRA**) into law. The ARRA provided $787 billion to accelerate the nation's economic recovery through investments in infrastructure, unemployment benefits, transportation, education, and healthcare. The Health Information Technology for Economic and Clinical Health (HITECH) Act was passed as part of ARRA and included over $20 billion to aid in the development of a healthcare infrastructure and to assist individual providers and other entities such as hospitals in adopting and using health information technology, including EHRs. These incentives through the Medicare and Medicaid reimbursement systems have assisted providers in adopting EHRs.

In order to receive remuneration through the HITECH Act program, practitioners are required to demonstrate "meaningful use" of a "certified" EHR. Based on meeting certain requirements that began in 2011, providers receive a bonus or incentive payment from the Centers for Medicare and Medicaid Services (**CMS**).

An eligible provider who fully complies with the requirements in 2011 is qualified for payment the same year. Payments can be substantial, starting at $18,000 in 2011, with an accumulation of $44,000 over the life of the five-year program through Medicare or $63,750 available through Medicaid over a period of six years (CMS, 2010).

Because most EHRs follow the criteria, credentialing, and regulations reviewed in this chapter, the distinguishing factor between different software is not functionality. Certified EHRs have similar capabilities. However, each EHR is unique in data layout, ease of use, and accessibility for the user.

LO 1.6 | Nursing Informatics

While Florence Nightingale recognized the need for standardization of nursing language to facilitate communication and enhance quality care, Harriet Werley first provided nursing input for computer use in the healthcare arena in the 1950s (Ozbolt & Saba, 2008). In the 1970s, nursing applications for computers began to be developed, and in 1973, a group of nurses met and developed an initial set of nursing diagnoses.

This group became the North American Nursing Diagnosis Association (NANDA). In the 1980s, the development of personal computers promoted computer use in healthcare and nursing informatics courses were introduced in nursing programs and graduate schools. By 1994, **nursing informatics** was formally recognized as a nursing specialty when the scope and standards of nursing informatics practice were developed by the American Nurses Association.

Nursing informatics supports the quality of nursing decisions by enhancing access to nursing knowledge and patient information using technology. This specialty practice promotes the development and use of tools compiled from a variety of sciences, including nursing and computer and technology sciences, to assist with managing and communicating information and knowledge between healthcare team members.

Nursing informatics is far more than understanding how to operate a computer. This growing field promotes access to current evidence-based nursing practice for integration into patient care. Nursing informatics specialists are involved in streamlining documentation, integrating safety measures online, and participating in new medication distribution systems, telemedicine, privacy protection programs, and wireless applications.

Simply knowing how to use a computer is no longer sufficient for providing safe and holistic patient care. Becoming an informatics consumer enables healthcare providers to provide high-quality care because of their ability to locate, evaluate, and apply scientific evidence from the cyberworld of healthcare databases to the real world of patients.

In today's healthcare environment clerical staff, clinical staff, and primary care providers must be familiar with the functionality of EHRs and have "hands-on" experience. Healthcare facilities find potential employees with this skill valuable. This textbook specifically covers the functionality and practical use of SpringCharts® EHR in the following chapters. While specific layouts and accessibility vary from other EHRs, the overall functions and capability are the same, allowing the student to transfer knowledge and experience from one system to another.

FOCAL POINT

Becoming an informatics consumer will enable healthcare providers to provide high-quality care because of their ability to locate, evaluate, and apply scientific evidence from the cyber world of healthcare databases to the real world of patients.

Concept Checkup 1.5

A. What year did President George W. Bush set as a goal for most Americans to have EHRs? _____

B List three mechanisms by which electronic prescribing promotes greater patient safety and efficiency

1. _____

2. _____

3. _____

C. What is the purpose of the HITECH Act?

_____

D. List three areas of interest for nursing informatics specialists.

1. _____

2. _____

3. _____

Using Terminology

Match the terms on the left with the definitions on the right.

_____ 1. EHR

_____ 2. ARRA

_____ 3. CCD

_____ 4. PHR

_____ 5. HL7

_____ 6. Encrypted

_____ 7. Interoperability

_____ 8. IOM

_____ 9. MIPPA

_____ 10. Telehealth

A. American Recovery and Reinvestment Act of 2009

B. The ability of a software program to accept, send, or communicate data from its database to other software programs from multiple vendors.

C. Compatibility language with other software programs.

D. Change of computer data from its original format so that it's secure and unintelligible to unauthorized parties and then "decrypted" back into its original form for use.

E. The use of electronic and communication technology to deliver health information and services over large and small distances through a standard telephone line.

F. The most commonly accepted and used term for storing and accessing patient health information electronically.

G. This institution gives advice and information about government policies that affect human health.

H. Allow the patient access via the Internet to store and update personal health information and make inquiries to the patient's healthcare provider about prescriptions, appointments, or concerns.

I. Medicare Improvements for Patients and Providers Act of 2008

J. Health provider oriented; defines a core set of data reflecting the most relevant and timely facts about a patient's healthcare and is accessible and readable by other electronic systems.

Checking Your Understanding

Write "T" or "F" in the blank to indicate whether the statement is true or false.

_____ 11. Voice recognition systems cannot be used with electronic health records systems.

_____ 12. LAN technology provides a wireless network for the tablet PC.

_____ 13. A high-speed Internet connection is necessary for an ASP.

_____ 14. The implementation of an EHR does not bring process changes to the inpatient healthcare setting.

_____ 15. The challenge and danger of handwritten prescriptions is nonexistent with an EHR.

_____ 16. Better patient care is a direct result of more thorough and detailed clinical information.

Answer the question below in the space provided.

17/18. List three main benefits of EHRs and provide an example of each benefit. (2 points)

a) _____

_____

b) _____

_____

c) _____

_____

19/20. List the three tasks that in September 2005 the U.S. Department of Health and Human Services awarded CCHIT a three-year contract to do. (2 points)

1. _____

2. _____

3. _____

Choose the best answer and circle the corresponding letter.

21. What organization created 20 standards to promote sharing of healthcare and health-related information by government agencies?
    a) HIPAA
    b) CHI
    c) AHIMA
    d) SNOMED

22. CCHIT specifically addressed the following:
    a) EHR costs
    b) Security issues
    c) Lack of industry standards
    d) The appropriation of government money

23. With an EHR, the healthcare practitioner provides more consistent care for the patient because the information is
    a) More accessible and better utilized with care plans and alerts
    b) Reviewed with the patient
    c) Neatly typed out by transcriptionists
    d) Backed up electronically on a regular basis

24. CCHIT is an acronym for
    a) Credentialing Certification for Healthcare Information Technology
    b) Certification Criteria for Health Impaired Technicians
    c) Certification Commission for Health Information Technology
    d) Certification Committee for Healthcare Informatics Technology

25. MIPPA is an acronym for
    a) Medical Improvements per Patient Annually
    b) Medicaid Improvement for Patients Act
    c) Medicare Improvement for Patients and Providers Act
    d) Medicare Installments for Patients Pay Act

26. The Stimulus Package of 2009 is officially known as the
    a) Centers for Medicare and Medicaid Services (CMS)
    b) American Recovery and Reinvestment Act (ARRA)
    c) Health Information Technology for Economic and Clinical Health (HITECH)
    d) Troubled Asset Relief Program (TARP)

27. Which of the following contribute to cost savings as a result of using an EHR? (Select all that apply.)
    a) Reduction in nursing workload
    b) Reduction in chart storage space
    c) Reduction in costs for paper
    d) Elimination of chart retrieval processes by clerks

28. For security, data on a wireless network are
    a) Encrypted
    b) Scrambled
    c) Broken
    d) Blocked

29. When was nursing informatics formally recognized as a nursing specialty?
    a) When nurses developed the initial set of NANDA diagnoses
    b) When Florence Nightingale recognized the need for standardization of nursing language
    c) When its scope and practice were developed by the American Nurses Association
    d) When Harriet Werley first provided nursing input for computer use in the healthcare arena

30. Which of the following is a benefit of using e-prescribing in an EHR program? (Select all that apply.)
    a) The elimination of handwritten prescriptions
    b) The ability to see a patient's total prescription history
    c) The improvement of quality and patient safety
    d) The automatic generation of prescriptions based on patient symptoms

References

Agency for Healthcare Research and Quality (AHRQ). (2010). *National Guideline Clearinghouse*. Retrieved July 13, 2010, from http://www.guideline.gov

Anderson, J.A., & Wilson, P. (2008). Clinical decision support systems in nursing: Synthesis of the science for evidence-based practice. *CIN: Computers, Informatics, Nursing, 26*(3), 151–156.

Associated Press. (2004, April 27). Bush proposes update to patient records. Retrieved from http://www.foxnews.com/story/0,2933,118330,00.html

Baker, V., & Copping, M. (2009). A pilot study exploring the clinical benefits when using a mobile clinical assistant, the Motion C5 in medical wards. In K. Saranto, P.F. Brennan, H.-A. Park, M. Tallberg, & A. Ensio (Eds.), *Proceedings of NI2009–The 10th International Congress on Nursing Informatics: Connecting health and human*. Fairfax, VA: IOS Press.

Board of Healthcare Services. (2003, July 31). *Key capabilities of an electronic health record system*. Retrieved from http://iom.edu/Reports/2003/Key-Capabilities-of-an-Electronic-Health-Record-System.aspx

CCHIT. (2009). *About the Certification Commission for Health Information Technology*. Retrieved from http://www.cchit.org/about

Certification Commission for Healthcare Information Technology. (n.d) Home page. Retrieved July 13, 2010, from http://www.cchit.org

Chin, T. (2004, February 9). Growth in electronic medical record. *AMNews*. Retrieved July 13, 2010, from http://www.amednews.com

CMS/Centers for Medicare & Medicaid Services. (2010). *EHR Incentive Programs*. Retrieved from http://www.cms.gov/EHRIncentivePrograms

Dassenko, D., & Slowinski, T. (1995). Using the CPR to benefit a business office. *Healthcare Financial Management 68*, 68–70, 72–73.

Fetter, M.S. (2009). Mastering the challenge of interoperability in nursing informatics. *Issues in Mental Health Nursing, 30*(9), 591–592.

Halley, E.C., Brokel, J.M., & Sensmeier, J. (2009). Nurses exchanging information: Understanding electronic health record standards and interoperability. *Urologic Nursing, 29*, 305–313.

Jamal, A., K. McKenzie, & M. Clark. (2009). The impact of health information technology on the quality of medical and health care: A systematic review. *Health Information Management Journal, 38*, 26–37.

Melczer, A.H., Berkeyheiser, L., Miller, S., & Yeager, M. (2005, January) *Background on electronic health records for small practices* (White paper, Illinois State Medical Society). Retrieved August 7, 2007, from http://www.providersedge.com/ehdocs/ehr_articles/Background_on_EHRs_for_Small_Practices.pdf

Mildon, J., & Cohen, T. (2001). Drivers in the electronics medical records market. *Health Management Technology, 22*, 14–16, 18.

Moody, L.E., Slocumb, E., Berg, B., & Jackson, D. (2004). Electronic health records documentation in nursing: Nurses' perceptions, attitudes, and preferences. *CIN: Computers, Informatics, Nursing, 22*, 337–344.

Obama, B. (2009, February 24). Transcript: Obama's Speech to Congress. Washington, D.C. Retrieved from http://www.cbsnews.com/stories/2009/02/24/politics/main4826494.shtml

Office of the National Coordinator for Health Information Technology. (2009). *About ONC*. Retrieved from http://healthit.hhs.gov/portal/server.pt/community/healthit_hhs_gov__onc/1200

Ozbolt, J.G., & Saba, V.K. (2008). A brief history of nursing informatics in the United States of America. *Nursing Outlook, 56*(5), 199–205.

Saleem, J.J., Russ, A.L., Justice, C.F., Hagg, H., Ebright, P.R., Woodbridge, P.A., et al. (2009). Exploring the persistence of paper with the electronic health record. *International Journal of Medical Informatics, 78*, 618–628.

Scott, J.T., Rundall, T.G., Vogt, T.M., & Hsu, J. (2005, December 3). Kaiser Permanente's experience of implementing an electronic medical record: a qualitative study. *BMJ, 331*, 1313–1316. Obtained from *The Commonwealth Fund*, February 24, 2006, 29. Retrieved July 13, 2010, from http://www.commonwealthfund.org

Sensmeier, J. (2007). Leveraging health information exchange to improve quality and efficiency. Retrieved May 16, 2010, from http://tigerstandards.pbworks.com/f/Leveraging+Health+Information+Exchange+to+Improve+Quality+and+Efficiency+-+TIGER.pdf

Stammer, L. (2001). Chart pulling brought to its knees. *Healthcare Informatics, 18*, 107–108.

The TIGER Initiative. (n.d.). *The TIGER Summit*. Retrieved May 16, 2010, from http://www.tigersummit.com/Summit.html

U.S. Department of Health & Human Services. (2010) *Incentive Program Made Simple*. Retrieved July 13,2010, from http://www.cms.hhs.gov/EPrescribing

U.S. Department of Health & Human Services. (2004, May 6). *Office of the National Coordinator for Health Information Technology (ONC): Presidential Initiatives*. Retrieved from http://www.hhs.gov/healthit/chiinitiative.html

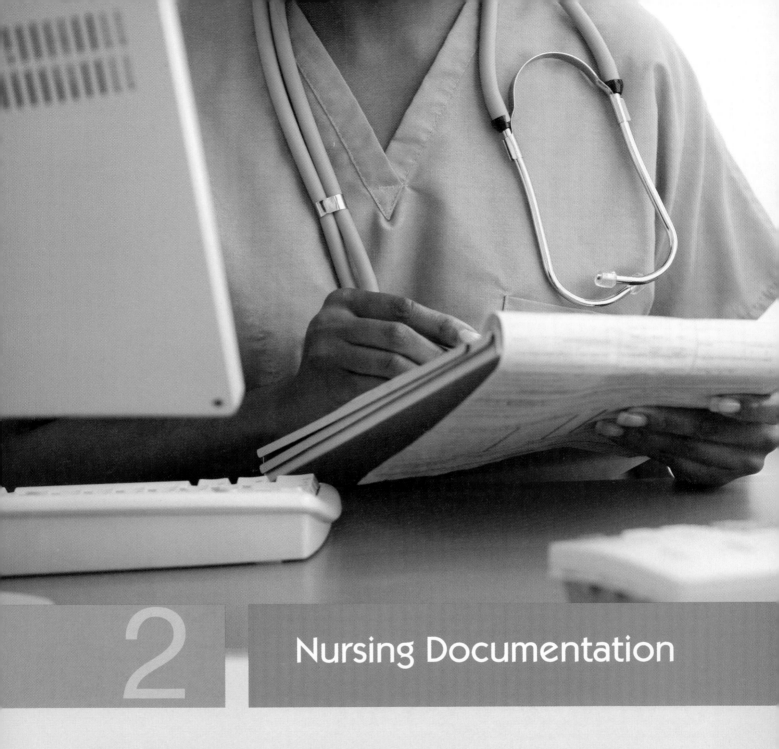

2 Nursing Documentation

Key Terms

Terms and abbreviations you will encounter in Chapter 2; they are defined in the end-of-book glossary:

Accreditation

Ambulatory Healthcare

Charting by Exception (CBE)

Computerized Charting

Critical Pathway/Care Map

Database

Diagnosis-Related Group (DRG)

Documentation

eMAR

Focus Charting/DAR

Inpatient Care

MAR

NANDA-I

Narrative Charting

NIC

NOC

Nursing Standards of Care

PIE

Problem-Oriented Medical Record (POMR)

Quality Improvement (QI)

Record

SOAP

SOAP(IE)

SOAP(IER)

Source-Oriented Charting/Source Records

The Joint Commission

Learning Outcomes

When you complete Chapter 2, you will be able to:

2.1   Describe the role of documentation in nursing practice.

2.2   Identify the purposes of documentation.

2.3   Identify and explain different types of documentation methods.

2.4   Explain documentation of medication administration using an electronic Medication Administration Record (eMAR).

2.5   Explain the importance and relevance of nursing diagnoses, NOC, and in nursing documentation.

Overview

What You Need to Know

To understand Chapter 2, you need to know:

- The importance of documenting patient care.

LO 2.1   Introduction to Documentation

Communication among healthcare professionals is an essential component of safe, quality patient care. Most healthcare errors are the result of poor communication. **Documentation** provides one mechanism for communication among healthcare professionals. Each member of the healthcare team is required to document contributions to patient care, such as assessments, diagnostic tests, therapeutic treatments, medications, and preparation of the patient and family for discharge. As indicated in Chapter 1, healthcare providers and organizations are increasingly implementing EHRs in order to enhance the quality of documentation and ultimately promote safe, effective patient care. In review, some benefits of the EHR include readily accessible information, elimination of illegible handwriting, automatic alert systems, decision support, and reduction in duplicate diagnostic testing. While the EHR has the potential to enhance quality of care, critics cite several concerns. A primary concern is confidentiality of patient records.

In April 2003, healthcare organizations became responsible for adherence to the Health Insurance Portability and Accountability Act (HIPAA) that was passed in 1996 to protect the privacy of patient health information (Potter & Perry, 2009). All healthcare members, teams, and systems are held accountable to this legislation, which gives greater control to patients for their care, provides patient education on privacy protection, ensures patient access to personal records, ensures patient consent prior to release of medical information, and provides recourse if privacy violations occur.

In addition to privacy concerns, opponents fear that EHRs may be subject to power outages, computer "crashes," and computer viruses that may corrupt patient data without the knowledge of the healthcare team or the patient. However, with the advent of increased Internet security systems, the acquisition of highly skilled informational technologists to monitor the patient system, and increased computer and documentation education for healthcare team members, these concerns are becoming less of a threat to the integration of EHRs into mainstream healthcare. The electronic format is fast becoming a dependable and flexible manner to document patient care.

 Concept Checkup 2.1

A. Several concerns have been raised by critics of electronic documentation. List four of these concerns.

1. _____
2. _____
3. _____
4. _____

B. What are some advantages of electronic documentation?

1. _____
2. _____
3. _____
4. _____
5. _____

C. What is the ultimate purpose for the implementation of EHRs?

_____
_____
_____

D. What are the primary purposes of HIPAA?

_____
_____
_____

LO 2.2   Purposes of Documentation

Documentation should be comprehensive, concise, and clear. All patient care must be documented in the patient's record in order to (1) prevent medical errors, (2) communicate with other healthcare providers, (3) demonstrate the delivery of care to ensure appropriate reimbursement, (4) adhere to accreditation standards, (5) provide a source of evidence in the event of legal proceedings, and (6) promote knowledge development through research. Accurate documentation is critical for patient safety.

To ensure patient safety, healthcare providers must avoid documentation errors, such as the failure to record pertinent health or drug information, nursing actions, medication administration, drug reactions, changes in a patient's condition, and discontinued medications (Nurses Service Organization, n.d.). Documentation omissions are a particular threat to patient safety. For example, failure to document a medication when administered may result in a duplicate dose being given to the patient.

As stated earlier, documentation is a method of communicating all the activities surrounding patient care. It is the primary means for all healthcare team members involved with a patient to remain current on the treatment regimen and progress of the patient throughout a hospital stay, during a visit to an **ambulatory healthcare** center, or in the home. Each discipline is responsible to document assessments; plan of care; patient care activities, including education; and the patient's response to those activities. In settings where little ongoing contact occurs among disciplines, accurate documentation is an integral component of care coordination and communication. Characteristics of good documentation are delineated in Figure 2.1.

In addition to being a method of communication, documentation serves as the evidence of the care administered to a patient. This evidence can be used to determine compliance with **nursing standards of care** or accrediting agencies such as **The Joint Commission**. The Joint Commission delineates criteria that must be met to demonstrate quality care in order for an organization to receive **accreditation** (The Joint Commission, 2010). Review of documentation in the patient's health record is commonly used to determine adherence to accreditation criteria.

Documentation, as evidence of care rendered, serves as a resource for auditing. Audits may be conducted in response to internal quality initiatives. The Joint Commission requires hospitals to create and maintain **quality improvement (QI)** programs to track the quality of patient care in an objective and ongoing fashion. Patient charts are selected randomly by an institution's QI department for auditing purposes and the documentation within these records is evaluated for adherence to facility policies and nursing standards. For example, a nursing unit that is actively engaged in reducing patient falls may conduct documentation audits to determine the percentage of patients who are assessed for fall risk on admission. The evidence of that assessment is found in the documentation. These audits allow nurses and other healthcare providers to remain informed of progress toward meeting QI goals.

FOCAL POINT

Documentation should be comprehensive, concise, and clear.

FOCAL POINT

Auditing programs enable nurses and other healthcare providers to be informed of adherence to current standards of practice.

Factual	Descriptive; objective; professional; no personal judgment of situation
Accurate	Measures exactly; adheres to The Joint Commission (formerly the Joint Commission on Accreditation of Healthcare Organizations; JCAHO) "do not use" abbreviation list
Complete	Includes all pertinent information; descriptive; factual; chart completed and signed by responsible party; never document for another person
Current	On time; uses military time
Organized	Cohesive and coherent flow of thought; entries opened with date and time and concluded with signature (physical or electronic)
Legible	Clearly legible, written in black ink, proper grammar and spelling. No erasures, scratch outs or use of correction fluid. Errors corrected per facility policy—usually using one line drawn through error
Security	Privacy of log-on and password maintained

Figure 2.1
Characteristics of Good Documentation

Appropriate documentation is critical for reimbursement purposes. **Diagnosis-related groups (DRGs)** are classifications used to establish the amount of payment a hospital, ambulatory care center, or home health agency receives. Healthcare organizations receive a standard DRG payment for Medicare and Medicaid claims regardless of duration or type of services rendered. DRG determination is dependent on documentation. Documentation omissions may result in the assignment of a DRG that results in lower reimbursement.

Reimbursement is also affected by new regulations related to certain hospital-acquired conditions (HAC) such as pressure ulcers and urinary tract infections. Hospitals may not be reimbursed for certain conditions that a patient contracts while hospitalized. The documentation of such conditions as present on admission is imperative if the organization is to be paid.

In addition to Medicare and Medicaid, private insurance companies require documentation to support claims for reimbursement. Proper documentation of services, supplies, and nursing education for the patient and the family during a patient's encounter with the organization enhances the likelihood the patient will receive maximum coverage for a medical claim, reducing the amount of out-of-pocket expense to the patient. Incomplete or inaccurate documentation may result in denial of insurance claims for services rendered by the organization.

Incomplete or inaccurate documentation may also be a source of liability in the event of legal proceedings against an organization or healthcare professional. Often, malpractice suits are not filed for months after the patient encounter. By the time care providers are subpoenaed to provide testimony, years may have elapsed and individual memory may not be reliable. The documentation recorded at the time of the event is likely to be the only evidence of the actions of the healthcare provider. Ideally, documentation provides the evidence to demonstrate that the healthcare professional adhered to current standards of care and facility policy.

Finally, documentation is pertinent in healthcare education and research. Patient records may be reviewed to identify patterns of an illness, the response of a patient to new therapies in clinical trials, or the reactions of patients to established treatment modalities. In addition, review of documentation helps identify nursing's contribution to patient outcomes through monitoring of nursing-sensitive indicators. Identifying new knowledge in each of these areas can bring about positive change in a treatment regimen for a particular disease or patient need and can lead to additional research funding. Education and research exist not only at a national or regional level but are also pursued actively in many hospital units, ambulatory care centers, and even home health agencies.

FOCAL POINT

Incomplete or inaccurate documentation increases the likelihood of non-reimbursement for services rendered.

FOCAL POINT

Documentation serves as legal evidence of care provided. It promotes patient safety by providing a record of care rendered.

Concept Checkup 2.2

A. Name three characteristics of good documentation.

1. _____
2. _____
3. _____

B. List five purposes of documentation.

1. _____
2. _____
3. _____
4. _____
5. _____
   _____

Concept Checkup 2.2 (Continued)

C. List three common errors in documentation.

1. _____

2. _____

3. _____

D. What is the purpose of a DRG?

_____

_____

_____

_____

LO 2.3 Documentation Methods

The key to thorough, legal, and ethical documentation is to follow the nursing process to ensure the accuracy and comprehensiveness of the patient health record. Approaching documentation of nursing care in a systematic manner minimizes the risk of missed or inaccurate information.

A variety of documentation formats are available for nursing documentation. Nurses must know the type of charting used in the healthcare setting in which they work. Each healthcare organization provides education to ensure that nurses document according to facility policy.

Regardless of the format of documentation used by an organization, flowsheets are often used to document routine care such as intake and output and vital signs. Intake refers to fluids that are introduced into the body such as oral fluids, tube feedings, intravenous fluids, blood, and blood products. Output includes fluids that are eliminated from the body and may include urine, vomitus, nasogastric tube drainage, diarrhea, chest tube drainage, and drainage from surgical drains. Accurate monitoring and documentation of intake and output allow evaluation of fluid volume status and guide treatment decisions. Documentation of vital signs on flowsheets, with concurrent graphing of values, allows for rapid visualization of trends. Flowsheets augment documentation in both the paper and electronic environments.

Narrative charting is a common documentation style and traditionally has been the primary method of recording data for nurses. Narrative charting requires that the nurse write all care provided in a paragraph format. Narrative charting (Figure 2.2) is

FOCAL POINT

The key to thorough, legal, and ethical documentation is to follow the nursing process when recording patient data.

DATE	TIME	NARRATIVE NOTE
5-13-10	1900	Patient 2 hours post-op. Awakens easily. Oriented × 3. Denies abdominal pain PERRLA. Grips strong and equal bilaterally. Heart tones regular. NSR per telemetry in the 80s. Lungs clear to auscultation anterior and posterior fields. Bowel sounds hypoactive × 4 quadrants. Abdomen nontender to light palpation. Abdominal drsg dry and intact. Urinary catheter in place with clear yellow urine. Skin color appropriate for race and is warm and dry. Extremity pulses 2+ and regular. Encouraged patient to cough, deep breathe, and use incentive spirometry. Provided ice chips to moisten mouth and placed call light within reach. Encouraged patient to notify RN PRN _____ M. Christy, RN
5-13-10	2030	Patient complains of nausea. Vomited 300 mL of clear emesis. Droperidol 0.25 mg administered IV push. See MAR. Cool cloth placed on forehead. Will continue to monitor. _____ M. Christy, RN
5-13-10	2110	Patient resting with eyes closed. No further nausea or vomiting reported. Will continue to monitor. _____ M. Christy, RN

Figure 2.2
Narrative Note

considered an open-form, freely flowing expression of thoughts about the care delivered to the patient. The primary advantages of narrative documentation include that it is easy to read and understand what has occurred. On the other hand, narrative documentation can be time-consuming, repetitious, and prone to error, especially omissions, if the documentation is not completed at the time of occurrence.

Source-oriented charting, or source records, is similar to narrative charting but separates the narrative note of each healthcare provider into a separate section of the chart, separate sheet of paper, or separate data entry. This type of charting often fragments care and promotes repetition of similar information in numerous sections within the patient record.

With the advent of the EHR, narrative nursing documentation has given way to **charting by exception (CBE)** in both inpatient and outpatient settings. While CBE is less time-consuming than other forms of documentation, important information may be omitted. CBE assumes all patient parameters are within normal limits unless otherwise stated. This requires that organizations define "within normal limits." Exceptions to normal parameters are documented in detail. Narrative charting is often used to record these exceptions, even in electronic documentation software.

In the **focus charting/DAR** documentation format, all documentation is related to a focus or problem. Often the focus is stated in terms of a nursing diagnosis, but the focus may also be symptoms or complaints. The healthcare professional documents assessment data (D) related to the focus, the actions (A) taken, and the response (R) to the interventions. Focus charting is often recorded in a columnar format with a separate column for assessment data, actions, and response.

One common format for interdisciplinary documentation is the **critical pathway/ caremap**, which reflects the day-to-day progression, including treatments and interventions, for a patient with a particular diagnosis. Each discipline focuses on patient problems, key interventions, and expected outcomes within an established time frame. This type of charting is ideal for stable patients who progress in an expected manner through the course of a disease or procedure. Variations from the anticipated pathway require additional documentation, often narrative. Complex or unstable patients are rarely placed on this type of pathway. (Potter & Perry, 2009)

This text focuses on the **problem-oriented medical record (POMR)**, documentation based on the patient's problem. This type of **record** is used in the SpringCharts EHR charting system, which is introduced later in this textbook. In the POMR, data are organized by problem or category and a plan of care emerges from this newly created problem **database**. Data can be recorded using the **PIE, SOAP, SOAP(IE)**, or **SOAP(IER)** format.

When using PIE for documentation purposes, the nurse focuses on the patient's problem (P), the interventions (I) to be executed to resolve the problem, and the evaluation (E) of the patient's response to those interventions. While this format simplifies documentation by combining the plan of care and progress notes, it contains no assessment information. Figure 2.3 provides a example of PIE charting.

SOAP, SOAP(IE), and SOAP(IER) are widely used among healthcare professionals, including nursing, because of the ability to chart assessment findings. However, the SOAP model is primarily a medical model and does not allow for nursing diagnosis and evaluation of interventions. Consequently, nurses often use the SOAP(IER) documentation format since this style allows for the entire nursing process to be addressed. SOAP(IER) represents:

S–subjective data (verbalizations of the patient)

O–objective data (measurable and observable data)

A–assessment (nursing diagnosis based upon data gathered)

P–plan (goals/outcomes to be achieved)

I–interventions (actions taken, involves verbs such as turn, inject, elevate, etc.)

E–evaluation (patient response to the intervention)

R–revision (modifications to the plan based on the evaluation)

The nursing process fits into the SOAP(IER) format, as seen in Figure 2.4 and Figure 2.5.

DATE	TIME	PIE NOTE
5-13-10	1300	P #1: Constipation r/t insufficient physical activity and low fiber diet. _____
		I #1: Provide high fiber diet. Ambulate as tolerated. Teach patient ways to increase fiber intake and physical activity. _____
		E #1: Patient verbalizes 3 high fiber foods he can incorporate into his diet; ambulated 100 feet x 4 this shift without difficulty. _____ M. Christy, RN
5-13-10	1300	P #2: Anxiety r/t absence of spouse prior to surgery. _____
		I #2: Offer to call spouse at home or on cell phone to notify of surgery time; provide outlet for patient to express fears or concerns regarding surgery. _____
		E #2: Unable to reach wife by phone. Notified patient of unsuccessful attempt to speak with spouse. Patient stated remembering wife had hair appointment and would come to hospital as soon as she was finished. Patient did not appear anxious or worried and apologized for "causing such a ruckus." ___ M. Christy, RN

Figure 2.3
PIE Note

SOAP(IER)	NURSING PROCESS
Subjective Data Objective Data	Assessment
Assessment	Nursing Diagnosis
Plan	Nursing Outcome (NOC)
Intervention	Nursing Intervention (NIC)
Evaluation	Evaluation
Revision	Revision

Figure 2.4
Alignment of Nursing Process and SOAP(IER) Charting

DATE	TIME	SOAP(IER) NOTE
5-13-10	1300	S #1: Patient c/o headache, severe low back pain, and feeling nauseated. _____
		O #1: Diaphoretic; face flushed. B/P = 186/110; Resp = 26 and shallow; HR = 82; T = 101.4° F. Reports pain level 8 on scale of 1–10. _____
		A #1: Pain related to low back surgery AEB pt. report of pain. _____
		P # 1: Pain control; Decreased pain level; Thermoregulation. _____M. Christy, RN
5-13-10	1310	I #1: Dilaudid 2 mg IV ; see MAR. Acetaminophen 1000 mg p.o. Coughed and used incentive spirometer to 500 mL × 10 breaths. Repositioned patient to side-lying position. Ice pack to low back. Offered shoulder massage, music, or television as a distraction. _____ M. Christy, RN
5-13-10	1340	E #1: Patient reports pain being "tolerable" and rates pain at "5" on scale of 1–10 after analgesic. States he has been using spirometry at least "once every 5 minutes or so" and feels better lying on his side. Apologizes for declining the "nice offer to rub my back" and inquires if he may still have his massage. Declined use of television or music saying, "It would have driven me nuts listening to it." VS: B/P = 148/80; Resp = 16, nonlabored; HR = 68; T = 99.8° F. _____
		R #1: Will add patient education to plan in order to include notification of the nurse regarding discomfort prior to pain level reports at high rating. Also add education regarding positioning and spirometry use. Continue to monitor. _____ M. Christy, RN

Figure 2.5
SOAP(IER) Note

Concept Checkup 2.3

A. What is the key to documenting in a thorough, legal, and ethical manner?

_____
_____
_____
_____

B. What is a problem-oriented medical record?

_____
_____
_____

C. What does SOAP(IER) stand for and why is it used frequently by nurses?

S. _____
O. _____
A. _____
P. _____
I. _____
E. _____
R. _____

_____
_____
_____

LO 2.4 ## Overview of MAR Documentation

A major nursing responsibility is medication administration. Standards of nursing care require that nurses adhere to the "rights" of medication administration: the right patient, the right medication, the right date/time, the right dose, the right route, the right assessment, the right education, the right evaluation, the patient's right to refuse the medication, and right documentation. Medication administration is documented on the patient's medication administration record (**MAR**). While healthcare organizations use a variety of methods to record administration of medications, the critical aspects of recording medication administration remain the same. These critical aspects include documentation of the medication name, dosage, route of administration, date and time of administration, and the signature of the nurse who administers the medication. Patient allergies are routinely recorded on the medication administration record for ease of reference and to prevent administration of a drug to which a patient is allergic.

In addition to documenting medication administration, nurses must document when a medication is not given as ordered to prevent the appearance of an error of omission. Withholding a medication may occur for various reasons. Nurses use clinical reasoning to determine if a medication should be withheld. For example, if a patient's pulse is very slow, the nurse may hold a dose of digoxin and notify the primary care provider. If a patient is nauseated and vomiting, the nurse may choose not to administer an oral medication. As noted earlier, patients have the right to refuse medication. Such refusal must be documented. Nurses must follow organizational policy for documentation of medications that are not given as ordered.

Current technology such as bar coding is available to ensure safe and accurate medication administration. Medications have bar codes that when scanned electronically register the name, dose, and concentration of the drug; the drug manufacturer; and the expiration date. Many hospitals also use bar code scanners for patient and nurse identification tags (Bowen, Guido, & Leone, 2006). When these personal identifier bar codes

---

Documentation Tip

Document a patient's refusal of medication or treatment. Notify the primary care provider and document the notification and provider response.

Documentation Tip

Document care as soon as possible to prevent errors of omission and to keep other healthcare team members up-to-date.

are used, a nurse scans the bar code on her name tag, which logs her on to the computer and subsequently the EHR. The nurse selects the MAR tab within the EHR to bring up a list of patients on the nursing unit. The next step is to scan the patient's bar code on the patient's identification armband. The list of medications for this patient appears on the computer screen and the nurse selects the desired medications to scan and administer to the patient. In addition to the medication information, the scanning procedure locks in an exact time and date stamp of medication administration into the hospital database along with the nurse's electronic signature.

Although a computer operating system can be quite costly to a large healthcare organization, the benefits are great. **Electronic MARs (eMARs)** reduce the number of medication errors, protecting the patient from harm and the nurse from liability. In addition, eMARs allow for more efficient tracking of medications within the healthcare system. EMARs are usually user-friendly and reduce the time spent searching for missing medications.

Some healthcare facilities have **computerized charting** but do not have eMARs. As patient advocates, nurses should collaborate with management and information technology to support the acquisition of eMARs to enhance quality, continuity of care, patient safety, and patient satisfaction (Potter & Perry, 2009).

Concept Checkup 2.4

A. What are the key components of documenting medication administration?

_____
_____
_____
_____

B. List three benefits of using an eMAR.

_____
_____
_____
_____

LO 2.5   Standardized Nursing Language

As EHRs have gained acceptance in an increasing number of healthcare organizations across the United States and throughout the world, the necessity for a unified language for documenting nursing care has become apparent. The need to communicate quality, effectiveness, and the value of nursing services led to the creation of databases accessible to all nurses to assist with accurate, legal, and reimbursable documentation criteria. In 1991, the National Center for Nursing Research of the National Institutes of Health recommended the development of standard terminology for nursing data. This led to the formation of standardized nursing diagnoses, nursing outcomes, and nursing interventions (Potter & Perry, 2009).

The **North American Nursing Diagnosis Association-International (NANDA-I)** is considered the primary force behind the development and universal acceptance of nursing diagnostic criteria. NANDA-I nursing diagnosis classifications are used to guide nursing decisions and plans of care for individual patients. Selection of diagnostic criteria enables the nurse to develop a plan of care in a variety of settings including hospitals, home healthcare, hospice, ambulatory care centers, schools, and nursing homes.

Every nurse's encounter with a patient begins with assessment and gathering subjective and objective data. Similar assessment data are grouped together in logical categories in order to select the priority nursing diagnoses. Once the nursing diagnoses

FOCAL POINT

Electronic MARs protect both the patient and the nurse by reducing the number of medication errors, and allowing for more efficient tracking of medications within the healthcare system.

FOCAL POINT

As patient advocates, nurses should collaborate with management and information technology to support the acquisition of eMARs to enhance quality, continuity of care, and patient safety and satisfaction.

FOCAL POINT

NANDA-I nursing diagnoses are used to reflect nursing needs of individual patients in standardized format.

have been made, the nurse identifies outcomes and interventions to meet those outcomes. This is the nursing process.

Nursing outcomes classification (NOC) and **nursing intervention classifications (NIC)** were developed at the University of Iowa College of Nursing to provide a standardized classification of outcomes and nursing interventions. NOC and NIC are linked to nursing diagnoses. This standardization reflects nursing practice and permits comparison of nursing care across settings. Although nursing diagnoses, NIC, and NOC have been used primarily in schools of nursing and hospitals where the focus is on **inpatient care**, they are comprehensive and can be used in any healthcare setting. They are research-based from patient encounters and are easy to use and apply to a variety of patient situations (University of Iowa, 2009). Using standardized nursing documentation criteria that reflect the nursing process facilitates nursing research. This research provides an evidence base for nursing practice to ensure optimal patient outcomes.

Concept Checkup 2.5

A. How are nursing diagnoses, NOC, and NIC relevant to nursing documentation?

_____

_____

_____

_____

B. In what settings can nursing diagnoses, NOC, and NIC be used by nurses?

_____

_____

_____

C. List three benefits of documenting the nursing plan of care using standardized nursing diagnoses, NOC, and NIC.

1. _____

_____

2. _____

_____

3. _____

_____

Using Terminology

Match the terms on the left with the definitions on the right.

_____ 1. NIC

_____ 2. eMAR

_____ 3. Computerized charting

_____ 4. Inpatient care

_____ 5. Quality improvement

_____ 6. Critical pathway

_____ 7. NOC

_____ 8. Ambulatory healthcare

_____ 9. Documentation

_____ 10. NANDA-I

A. Care provided to patients in a hospital involving overnight stays ordered by a primary care provider.

B. Use of electronic sources and databases to record data relating to patient care.

C. Provision of healthcare services to patients who are not admitted overnight to a hospital.

D. Act of recording patient information in written or electronic format; carries legal and ethical importance.

E. Electronic format for documentation of administering drugs.

F. Comprehensive preprinted interdisciplinary standardized plan of care for the average, stable patient experiencing a particular disease process or procedure with predictable outcomes.

G. Serves as an evaluative tool for the effectiveness of nursing interventions.

H. Responsible for developing diagnostic criteria for governing and guiding nursing care of the patient.

I. Provide nurses with standardized treatment options and activities for patients to assist the patients in attaining positive outcomes relating to their disease processes or medical interventions.

J. A formal process of collecting data about performance, comparing those data to accepted norms, and taking action to enhance performance.

Checking Your Understanding

Write "T" or "F" in the blank to indicate whether the statement is true or false.

_____ 11. Detailed and accurate nursing documentation within patient charts enables billing institutions to process claims in a timely manner.

_____ 12. Current Internet security systems are unable to handle the majority of issues surrounding confidentiality in electronic patient charting programs.

_____ 13. The nursing process fits with the SOAP(IER) charting method.

_____ 14. Documentation of general amounts of intake and output of fluid is sufficient to determine a patient's fluid balance.

_____ 15. Using eMARs allows the nurse to administer medications to a patient without the necessity of checking the five rights of medication administration.

_____ 16. Nursing documentation requirements for reimbursement do not change from payor to payor even though the paperwork may vary.

_____ 17. Precise and accurate documentation can be an effective mode of communication between healthcare providers.

_____ 18. Documentation should be comprehensive, concise, and clear.

Answer the question below in the space provided.

19/20. List three purposes of documentation and provide an example of each purpose. (2 points)

a. _____

_____

b. _____

_____

c. _____

_____

21/22. Create a sample nursing note using the SOAP(IER) format. (2 points)

DATE	TIME	SOAP(IER) NOTE

Choose the best answer and circle the corresponding letter.

23. Which of the following would be documented on the I&O flowsheet? (Select all that apply.)
    a) A 240-mL cup of coffee that the patient leaves on his breakfast tray
    b) 200 mL of clear fluid that the patient vomits
    c) Sheets wet from perspiration
    d) 525 mL that the patient voids into a urinal

24. Which of the following can be considered a documentation error by a nurse?
    a) Failure to record reported health information
    b) Writing down a change in patient condition
    c) Listing discontinued medications in the chart
    d) All of the above

25. A student nurse sits down to review a patient's chart. Which of the following purposes of documentation is being fulfilled?
    a) Legal and ethical
    b) Communication
    c) Reimbursement
    d) Education

26. During a routine dressing change, the nurse observes that an abdominal incision is reddened. The hospital adheres to charting by exception. After noting that the incision is abnormal, what method should the nurse use to document the wound appearance?
    a) Narrative charting
    b) DAR charting
    c) PIE charting
    d) Source-oriented charting

27. Nursing outcomes classification (NOC) best fit into which part of the SOAP(IER) charting method?
    a) Interventions
    b) Subjective data
    c) Plan
    d) Assessment

28. Standardized nursing documentation promotes
    a) Patient safety
    b) Use of the nursing process
    c) Research opportunities
    d) All of the above

29. A medication error caution screen appears on the computer when the nurse scans a medication before administering it to the patient. The nurse should
    a) Document a note on the eMAR about the screen and proceed with medication administration.
    b) Completely log out of the computer and return to the patient's room with a different computer cart.
    c) Review the exact nature of the error screen and make a determination based upon the additional information whether to hold the medication or administer it to the patient.
    d) Override the error screen and proceed with medication administration.

30. Every nurse's encounter with a patient begins with assessment and gathering _____ and _____ data.
    a) Legal, ethical
    b) Subjective, objective
    c) Logical, emotional
    d) Medical, nursing

References

Bowen, M., Guido, G., & Leone, C. (2006). *Mosby's surefire documentation: How, what, and when nurses need to document* (3rd ed.). St. Louis, MO: Mosby.

Nurses Service Organization. (n.d.). *Eight common charting mistakes to avoid.* Retrieved September 18, 2010, from http://www.nso.com/nursing-resources/article/16.jsp

Potter, P.A., & Perry, A.G. (2009). *Fundamentals of nursing* (7th ed.). St. Louis, MO: Mosby.

The Joint Commission. (2010). *About Us.* Retrieved September 18, 2010, from http://www.jointcommission.org/AboutUs/

University of Iowa College of Nursing. (2009). *Center for Nursing Classification & Clinical Effectiveness.* Retrieved July 20, 2010, from http://www.nursing.uiowa.edu/excellence/nursing_knowledge/clinical_effectiveness/index.htm

U.S. Department of Health and Human Services. (n.d.). *Summary of the HIPAA privacy rules.* Retrieved September 14, 2010, from http://www.hhs.gov/ocr/privacy/hipaa/understanding/summary/index.html

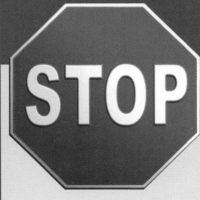

STOP

You need to download the SpringCharts EHR software before you begin working on the exercises in *Nursing Documentation Using Electronic Health Records.*

Important: SpringCharts EHR software is licensed for one-time single access use only.

ACCESS

Access the software on the text website at www.mhhe.com/nursingehr ·

DOWNLOAD

Download both the SpringCharts EHR software and the *EHR Material* folder (folder contains documents, files, and images to give you real scenarios for EHR documentation).

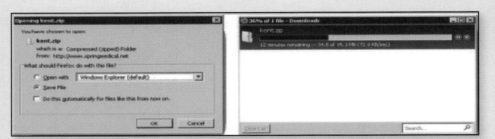

SpringCharts EHR is an electronic medical records software suite based on the latest industry standard Java technology. It requires a very modest network system for installation.

Follow the instructions below to download Java Runtime Environment, the SpringCharts EHR program, and the *EHR Material* folder to your computer.

If you encounter problems with the download, please contact one of our support teams below.

Support

- McGraw-Hill Higher Education technical support team: 1-800-331-5094
  8 a.m.–11 p.m. CST, Monday–Thursday
  8 a.m.–6 p.m. CST, Friday
  6 p.m.–11 p.m. CST, Sunday

- www.mhhe.com/support

- Med-Soft National Training Institute textbook support: questions@springmedical.com

SpringCharts is available in two different system configurations: single computer and network option.

For instructions on network installation, please refer to the Preface of this text, pages xvi–xxvii.

Single Computer Version

The single computer version of SpringCharts needs to be installed onto each student's computer in the classroom. We recommend that SpringCharts be installed to and run from a 2GB flash drive; refer to instructions that follow. This eliminates the need for the you to back up and restore your data on a daily basis.

The use of a flash drive enables a portable application of SpringCharts that can be used at home or with any other computer that accepts the flash drive and enables the students to continue their work outside the classroom. The single computer version of SpringCharts is not networked; therefore, the instructor is not able to view the students' exercises online. Exercises must be printed and turned in or the instructor must view the completed exercises from the desktop of the students' computers.

System Requirements

The minimum requirements for SpringCharts **single** computer version are

- An 800 MHz, or faster, processor

- 400 MB of available disk space

- 1 GB of memory

- A computer running one of the following operating systems: Windows 2000 or above, Mac OS 10.4 (Tiger) or above, or Linux Red Hat Version 7 or above

Note: You must have access to the Internet and a printer to complete the Exercises in this text.

Operating Environment Notice

SpringCharts is an online system that requires uninterrupted access to a minimum level of system resources. As a result, it is recommended that the SpringCharts server be located on a dedicated computer when possible. It is also recommended that highly resource-intensive programs and/or programs that may intermittently use up the majority of the system processing capacity or network bandwidth *not be run at the same time as SpringCharts.*

Examples of these types of programs are

- Virus scans of the entire hard drive (scans of individual files are acceptable).

- Music streaming programs.

- Certain backup programs (when activated).

Single Computer Installation
Installing Java Runtime Environment (JRE) 1.6

- JRE 1.6.0_11 must be installed on your computer before you run SpringCharts EHR.

- On your Internet browser, type in the following address: www.java.com.

- Click the *Do I have Java?* link to test your system for the correct version of Java.

- If your computer has JRE 1.6, you do not need to upgrade.

- If your system does not meet the requirements of JRE 1.6, you must download JRE 1.6.0_11 from the text website at www.mhhe.com/nursingehr.

Do not download the latest version of JRE from the Java website.

Running SpringCharts from a Flash Drive

If you are working in a computer environment that uses a product like Deep Freeze™ to return the computer to its baseline configurations each day, all your work in SpringCharts will be eradicated when the computer is reset to its original state. To bypass the need to back up and restore SpringCharts data on a daily basis, the SpringCharts program can be run from a flash drive that is placed into the computer's USB port daily.

A 2GB flash drive is needed. However, if your school requires an administrative password to run programs from a flash drive, you may not be able to use this method. Please consult with your IT department before proceeding.

A flash drive is a portable device for memory storage. It is also referred to as a jump drive or a thumb drive. Flash drives fit into any USB (universal serial bus) port on a computer.

- Simply install JRE 1.6.0_11, SpringCharts EHR, and the *EHR Material* folder as outlined in the next sections; however, **install the Java Runtime Environment (JRE) onto the computer** and the SpringCharts program and *EHR Material* folder to the flash drive.

- When installing SpringCharts, you are presented with an option to change the default location of installation. To install SpringCharts to your flash drive, select this option and locate *My Computer*, then choose the USB port where your flash drive is located. **Once installed, a SpringCharts icon appears on your desktop.**

- To access SpringCharts, place your flash drive into the computer's USB port and double-click on this icon. If this icon has been removed, you must locate the flash drive and double-click the SpringCharts icon in the SpringCharts folder.

- When you close down the SpringCharts program, you are given the option to back up. If you are using a flash drive, select **No** at this point. You will also be able to place your flash drive in any computer's USB port and continue to work on the exercises in this text.

Note: You do not need to back up and restore data when SpringCharts is operating from your flash drive.

Installing SpringCharts EHR on a Single Computer

The SpringCharts installation procedure has just a few easy steps. Remember, the JRE needs to be installed on your computer before SpringCharts EHR will run.

- On your Internet browser, type in the following address: www.mhhe.com/nursingehr
- Click the *SpringCharts* link in the left-hand menu.
- Locate the *Downloading and Installing Spring-Charts EHR* portion of the page.
- Click either the *SpringCharts PC Demo installer zip file* link or the *SpringCharts Mac Demo installer stuffed file* link depending on your operating system.
- Download the installer file to your computer desktop.
- Decompress the downloaded file (use a file program such as Winzip or StuffIt.)
- Double-click either the **SpringChartsDEMO-Setup.exe** or **SCDemoSetupMac** installation application (depending on your operating system).
- Follow the directions offered by the installer. You will see a screen similar to this one:

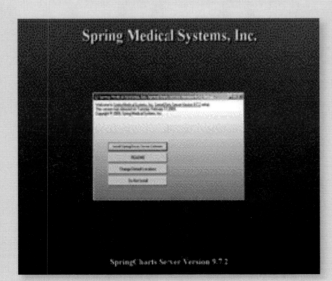

SpringCharts installation window

- SpringCharts program files are installed in the default location of C:\Program Files\SCDemo. This is the recommended installation location for a computer. To accept this default, simply click on the **Install SpringCharts Software** button. However, if you are installing Spring-Charts to a flash drive, select the **Change Default Locations** button and select the appropriate drive.
- Accept the license agreement and the installation begins.
- After the files have been successfully installed, the final installation completion screen appears.
- Click on the **Thanks!** button and the installation is complete.
- Close open windows to see the SpringCharts shortcut icon on your desktop. Double-click on the SpringCharts icon to open the program. A *Log On* window appears, illustrated below. The user name and password is hardcoded in. Simply select the **Log on** button.

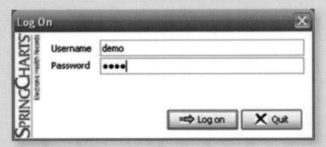

SpringCharts log on window

Note: There are several files you need to import into your SpringCharts program to complete many of the Exercises. You can access these files at the text website at www.mhhe.com/nursingehr.

Downloading *EHR Material* Folder

- Access this website, www.mhhe.com/nursingehr, via your browser.

- Click the *SpringCharts* link in the left-hand menu.

- Locate the *Downloading the EHR Material folder* portion of the page.

- Click the *EHR Material* link.

- Download the zip file to your computer desktop.

- Decompress the downloaded file (use a file decompression program such as Winzip or StuffIt.)

- Once the folder has been copied to your desktop or flash drive you may close the Web browser window.

For complete download instructions, see pages xvi–xxvii in the Preface of this text.

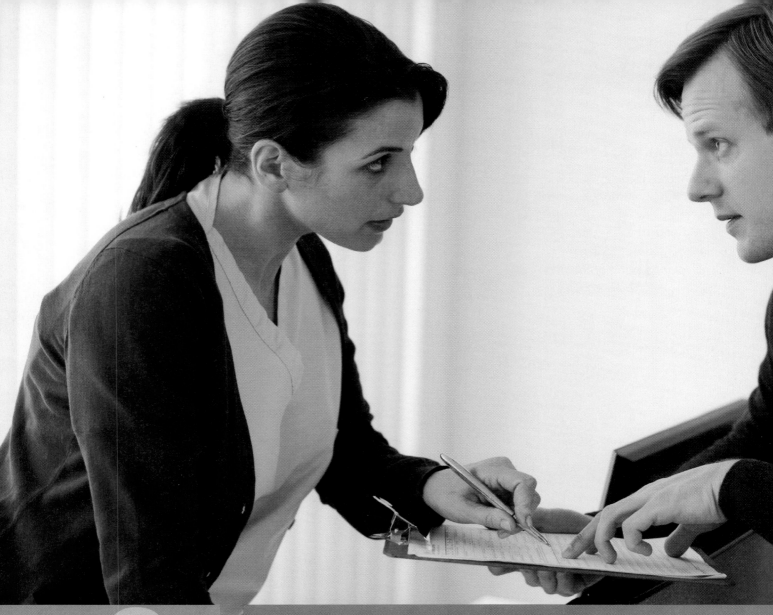

3 Essential EHR

Key Terms

Terms and abbreviations you will encounter in Chapter 3; they are defined in the end-of-book glossary:

Care Tree

Category Preferences

Chart Alert

Electronic Chart

Encounters

Face Sheet

Family Medical
History (FMHX)

Graphic User Interface

Imperial Units

Metric Units

Office Visit (OV)

Past Medical History
(PMHX)

Practice Management
Software (PMS)

User Preferences

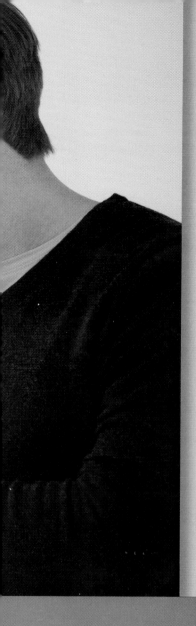

Learning Outcomes

When you complete Chapter 3, you will be able to:

3.1   Describe the basic features of SpringCharts EHR.

3.2   Describe the history of SpringCharts EHR.

3.3   Apply user preferences.

3.4   Carry out setting up and editing patients.

3.5   Use pop-up text.

3.6   Explain the concept of an electronic chart.

3.7   Use the electronic chart's face sheet.

3.8   Use the SpringCharts EHR care tree.

Documentation

What You Need to Know

To understand Chapter 3, you need to know:

- The purpose of a patient's chart in a healthcare encounter.
- The function of an EHR.
- The history and standards for an EHR.
- How to download, install, and log into SpringCharts EHR.

LO 3.1   SpringCharts Features

The *SpringCharts EHR™* software has been chosen as the training tool for this textbook because of its ease of use, its richness in features, and its ability to be customized to suit a wide range of healthcare specialties. SpringCharts is an international program and is used by over 1,500 physicians and thousands of nurses, medical assistants (MA), nursing assistants (NA), and other healthcare personnel.

SpringCharts EHR software was designed by practicing physicians and technology executives to introduce easy-to-use, yet functional, technology to practitioners who remain dependent on paper charting systems and traditional clinical work flows. The program is largely focused on streamlining communications and documentation and improving work flow in both administrative and clinical practice areas.

SpringCharts EHR was initially developed and implemented over a period of 10 years to provide primary care providers and healthcare staff with a powerful and intuitive software solution for the clinical side of the outpatient office. Later, it was expanded to include inpatient functions. The program is designed to manage all *nonfinancial* activities of a healthcare practice. It combines robust clinical tools to enhance patient care such as a template-based electronic health records system, a chart evaluation manager for proactive patient healthcare maintenance, an evaluation and management (E&M) coder for automatic and accurate E&M coding, plan-of-care practice guidelines, and real-time drug and allergy interaction. These clinical features are incorporated with integrated patient tracking, integrated e-mail, messaging, reminders, a time clock, and template-based clerical tools designed to streamline healthcare communication and documentation. SpringCharts EHR provides a one-click link to many powerful websites providing integrated access to evidence-based practice guidelines, industry-standard drug formularies (i.e., listings of pharmaceutical substances and formulas for making medicinal preparations), dosage information, patient education instructions, and electronic faxing.

LO 3.2   A Brief History

In 2004, National Data Corporation (NDC) Health Inc. and Spring Medical Systems Inc. (SMSI) launched a jointly developed software communication piece enabling the bidirectional flow of data between SpringCharts EHR and two popular **practice management software (PMS)** programs, Medisoft™ and Lytec™. This communication model provides data exchange of patient demographics, insurance information, and transaction details. Since that time, over 50 links have been developed to many other popular Windows-based and Macintosh PMS programs.

In 2006, SpringCharts was one of the earliest ambulatory EHR programs to be certified with the Certification Commission for Health Information Technology (CCHIT). In 2009, SpringCharts EHR Version 9.7 became SureScripts certified, enabling the delivery of electronic prescriptions and refills across the Internet and making use of real-time clinical decision support tools including drug and allergy interactions, formularies, and dosage checking. Patients benefit through faster service and the highest levels of safety and security available.

Version 10 of SpringCharts EHR was certified with the Office of the National Coordinator for Health Information Technology (ONC) in 2010 to qualify for financial rebates to physicians under the HITECH Act for ambulatory EHRs. That means that SpringCharts EHR has met a comprehensive set of criteria for

- Functionality—setting features and functions to meet a basic set of requirements.
- Interoperability—establishing basic functionality enabling standards-based data exchange with other sources of healthcare information in future versions of the product.
- Security—ensuring data privacy and robustness to prevent data loss.

FOCAL POINT

SpringCharts is an international, fully functional EHR program. SpringCharts EHR was initially certified in 2006.

Concept Checkup 3.1

A. List three features of SpringCharts EHR that promote its use as the instructional software for this textbook.

1. _____
   _____

2. _____
   _____

3. _____
   _____

B. List three areas in which SpringCharts EHR qualified for ONC certification.

1. _____
   _____

2. _____
   _____

3. _____
   _____

LO 3.3   User Preferences

The initial phase of using any software program involves establishment of personal user preferences. SpringCharts allows the creation of **user preferences** that determine the default **graphic user interface** of several key areas of the program specific for each user. To set the user preferences, each user accesses the main *File* menu and selects *Preferences>User Preferences* (see Figure 3.1).

In the *Set User Preferences* window, each user sets

- The primary provider's name that appears as the default on reports and letters. The list of providers is based upon those set up in the administration panel of the SpringCharts server.

- The practice name or healthcare facility that defaults for letterheads. Although the provider's and the practice's name are selected here as "default," they can be changed within the program during the creation of various letters and reports. An organization may have facilities in various locations but use the same database for SpringCharts across the Internet, enabling the complete patient health record to be viewed by any of the practices.

- The default appointment schedule in a stand-alone ambulatory SpringCharts system. Many appointment schedules can be set up in SpringCharts for different providers and therapy resources. Here the user selects which schedule to view as the main screen upon successful entry into the SpringCharts' *Practice View* screen in an ambulatory health location.

- The number of minutes of inactivity before SpringCharts closes down, displaying only the login window.

- The Tracker Group that displays the list of patients in the *Patient Tracker* window of the *Practice View* screen. Organizations that have several locations and work from the same patient database over the Internet are able to track patients separately for each location. The various tracker groups are set up in the administrative panel of the SpringCharts server. *Show All* displays all patients in the *Patient Tracker* window from all locations. If the healthcare facility has only one location, the *Tracker Group* field is left blank.

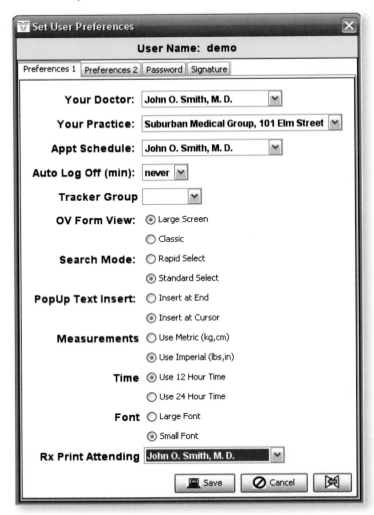

Figure 3.1
Set User Preferences window

OV Form View

The *Large Screen* view of the **office visit (OV)** window was an added feature to SpringCharts, revising the original *Classic* view. Its layout is more user-friendly and provides easier navigation. In addition, face sheet information added to a panel in the *Large Screen* view enables providers to view face sheet information while engaged in an encounter with the patient. Items from the face sheet can also be added to the encounter note. All new users should select the *Large Screen* view.

Search Mode

The *Rapid Select* function enables the user to immediately type a letter or series of letters in many search windows in the program. When the user pauses after typing the desired characters, the program automatically searches the database and displays the information relevant to the letters selected. Alternatively, with *Standard Select* activated, the user must type in the necessary letters and then click on the search icon to activate the program's search function. For new users to SpringCharts, the *Standard Select* feature option is recommended.

Pop-Up Text Insert

The user can determine where additional pop-up text is added to existing pop-up text throughout the program. It can be added at the end of existing sentences or wherever the cursor is positioned, for example, in the middle of a sentence. It is recommended that all users select *Insert at Cursor* for the pop-up text insert option.

Measurements

The measurements option allows the user to select the units of measure in which the vital signs will be recorded—either **metric units** or **imperial units**. Most countries of the world use the metric system of weights and measures. The United States continues to use the imperial measurements in most cases. However, because this is a user-defined option, the program adjusts to the desired measurement units according to the user's preferences. Ask your instructor what the appropriate selection will be for you.

Time

Time stamps are available in various places throughout the program. The user's selection here determines whether notes and other documents are stamped in a 12-hour time style with a.m./p.m. or a 24-hour military style time. Most inpatient facilities use a 24-hour clock for documentation.

Font

The user may select either an Arial 10 or Arial 12 font size to be used in the program.

Rx Print Attending

This feature determines the name that is printed as the attending provider on the pharmacy prescription forms. See Figure 3.2 for an illustration of a prescription form displaying an attending provider. Based on state laws, nurse practitioners and other support providers may be required to indicate the supervising physician when creating prescriptions.

Legal/Ethical Considerations

Prescriptive authority of nurse practitioners varies by state. The Nurse Practice Act of each state delineates the scope of practice for nurse practitioners in that state.

Preferences 2

The user has an option to choose either left or right orientation for the SpringCharts program. The point of reference determines the location of the navigation tabs in the nurse note screen. The program defaults to "right." If the user selects "left," then the navigation tab list appears on the left side of the screen. This allows for a greater ease of use on a portable computer; right-handed users may prefer having the navigation panel on the right side of the nurse note screen, whereas left-handed users may prefer the left side so that the user's arm does not block the screen when accessing the navigation tabs. Once the orientation preference has been chosen, the user selects the *Save* button.

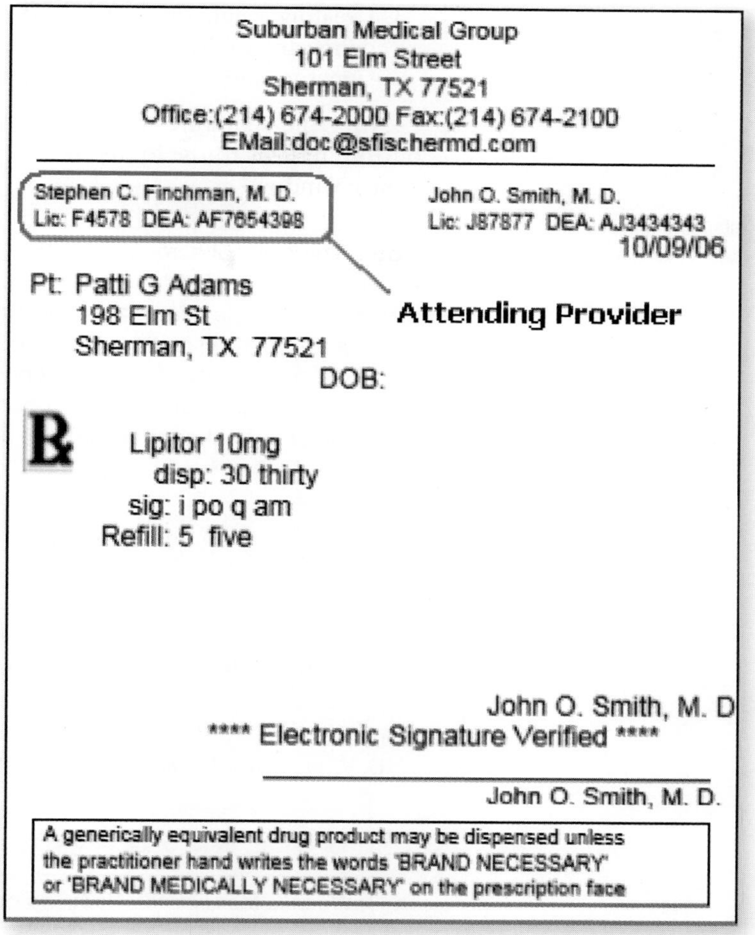

Password

Passwords can be changed under the third tab of the *Set User Preferences* window. The user simply adds a new password, verifies the password, and clicks *Change Password*. Figure 3.3 illustrates the *Password* tab in the *Set User Preferences* window. Passwords may be changed as often as needed when *Low Security* has been selected on the server administrator. However, when *High Security* has been selected on the SpringCharts server, the program enforces rigorous password rules, including minimum and maximum number of characters, and alphanumeric usage. Setting SpringCharts to high security is an administrative option. Hospitals typically require rigorous passwords that are routinely changed.

Signature

SpringCharts allows users to import a digital signature. This signature image may be used in various places throughout the program to stamp the user's actual signature image on documents such as letters, reports, and prescriptions. Users' signatures may be set up in three ways:

1. Creating a handwritten signature, scanning the image, and saving it to the computer. Then select the *Import* button to navigate to the file, and import it into the *Set User Preferences* window.
2. Using the stylus pen on a portable computer to create the digital signature directly in the signature box.

Suburban Medical Group
101 Elm Street
Sherman, TX 77521
Office:(214) 674-2000 Fax:(214) 674-2100
EMail:doc@sfischermd.com

Stephen C. Finchman, M. D.
Lic: F4578 DEA: AF7654398

John O. Smith, M. D.
Lic: J87877 DEA: AJ3434343
10/09/06

Pt: Patti G Adams
198 Elm St
Sherman, TX 77521

Attending Provider

DOB:

℞ Lipitor 10mg
disp: 30 thirty
sig: i po q am
Refill: 5 five

John O. Smith, M. D
**** Electronic Signature Verified ****

John O. Smith, M. D.

A generically equivalent drug product may be dispensed unless the practitioner hand writes the words 'BRAND NECESSARY' or 'BRAND MEDICALLY NECESSARY' on the prescription face

Figure 3.2

Prescription form with attending physician

Figure 3.3

Password tab in *Set User Preferences* window

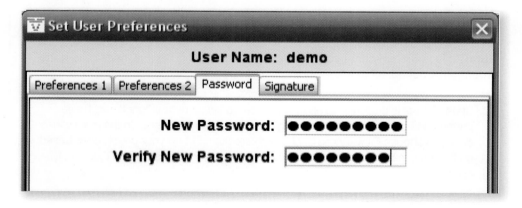

3. Creating a signature in the field by signing an electronic signature pad that is connected to the computer via the Universal Serial Bus (USB) port. The digital signature should be a maximum size of 2.3 inches by 0.75 inch.

   After the signature has been placed in SpringCharts, the user selects the *Save* button, returns to the Preferences 1 tab, and saves all changes to the Set User Preference window.

Note: The optimal screen resolution for SpringCharts is 1024 × 768 pixels. This can be modified on a Windows PC in the *Control Panel > Display > Settings* or by right-clicking on the desktop, selecting *Properties*, then choosing the *Settings* tab. If the monitor's screen resolution is less than this optimum setting, for example, 800 × 600 pixels, a large window display of SpringCharts, which requires the use of side scroll bars to view the program or windows that cannot be manipulated easily, will be viewed. This is a good time to change the screen resolution of your computer for optimal display.

Concept Checkup 3.2

A. What two default options may be selected for reports and letters?
_____
_____

B. When is the *Tracker Group* option used?
_____
_____
_____

C. When is the *Rx Print Attending* option used in SpringCharts?
_____
_____
_____
_____

Exercise 3.1

Setting Your User Preferences

Note: If you have not downloaded the SpringCharts program to your computer, please review the Preface of this text for downloading instructions, starting on page xvi, before commencing the following exercise.

1. Double-click on the SpringCharts icon on your desktop.

Note: This is the only time you double-click while using SpringCharts. Once the program is opened, all functions are activated by a single click of the mouse.

2. SpringCharts is designed to allow each user to select default functions. These preferences adjust when the user logs on. Select the *File* menu on the main window and choose *Preferences > User Preferences*. Set up your preferences based on the items selected in the *Set User Preferences* window (shown in Figure 3.1).

3. Click the *Save* button to save your material.

LO 3.4 Setting Up and Editing Patients

Adding a New Patient

The *New Patient* feature is used to create an electronic chart for a new patient. While nurses do not typically create charts for new patients, this process is required to set up a patient for your exercises.

When admitting personnel click on the *New* menu option in the main *Practice View* window, a *New Patient* window appears as seen in Figure 3.4. Fields marked in red are required fields for the patient record to be saved and a chart created. A patient's chart can be created rapidly by recording only the patient's first and last names and the date of birth. In an office clerical environment, this basic information can be received from the patient over the phone. The patient file can be saved and the patient added to the schedule. On the scheduled appointment or admission day, the remaining information can be added when the patient completes the intake forms. The *Patient ID* field is grayed out because the program assigns a unique consecutive ID number to the patient when the new patient information is saved. SpringCharts can store up to one million patient ID numbers.

Existing demographic information can be copied from a family member who is already set up in SpringCharts by selecting the *Copy Patient* button. In the *Choose Patient* window, the staff enters the first few letters of the patient's last name and clicks on the *Search* button, then selects the appropriate patient name. The last name, address, and phone number are copied automatically into the *New Patient* window.

Editing Patients

When editing a patient, clerical staff select *Patients* under the main *Edit* menu. Patients can be located by selecting one of the criteria in the *Search* drop-down list: last name, zip code, social security (SS) number, home phone number, work phone number, patient number, birth date, and e-mail. Demographic information can be modified once the desired patient is located.

From the *Edit Patient* window, shown in Figure 3.5, one may obtain the patient's chart, track the patient into the *Patient Tracker*, delete the selected patient, or create a new patient. A patient can be removed from the active list and

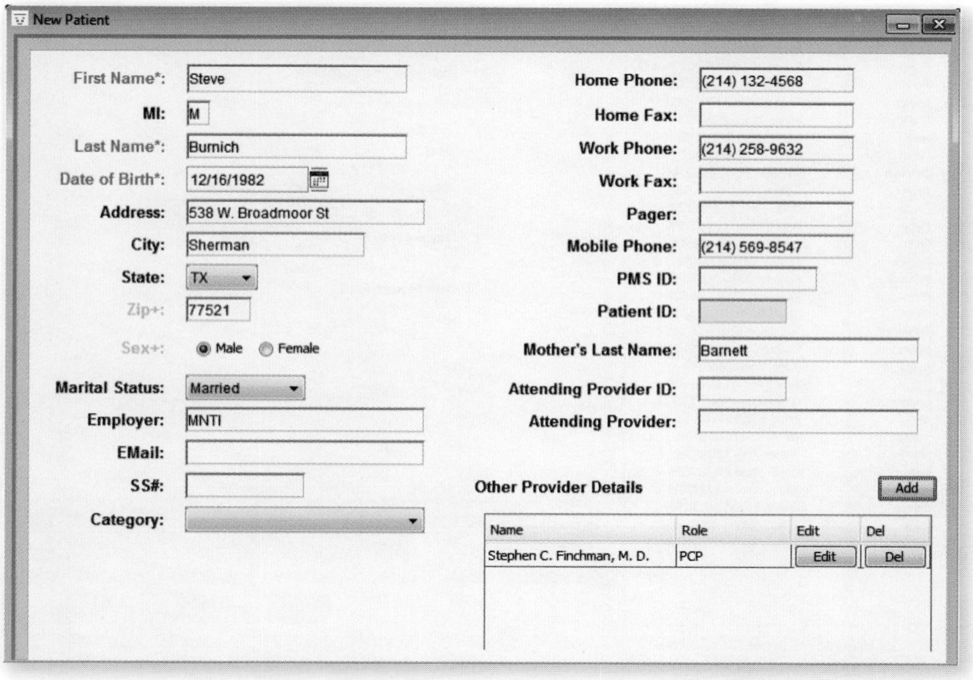

FOCAL POINT

Only the patient's first name, last name, and date of birth are necessary to create a new patient chart.

Figure 3.4

New Patient setup window

moved to an archived patient list by selecting the *Archive* button at the bottom of the screen.

The entire list of patients can be viewed by clicking the *Search* button without entering any data in the *Search* field, illustrated in Figure 3.5.

Figure 3.5
Edit Patient window

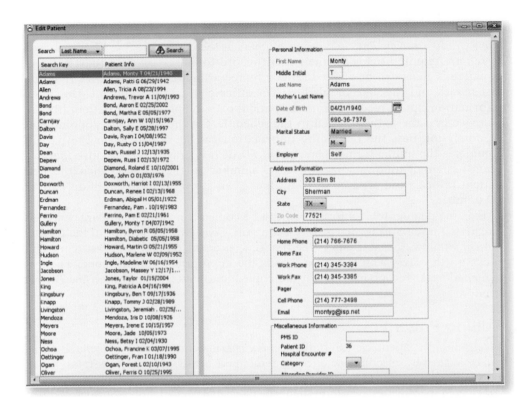

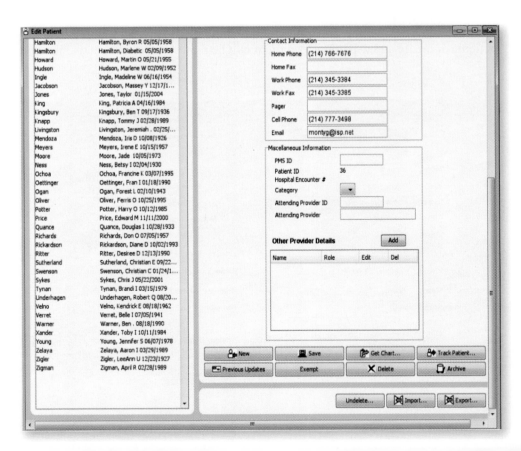

Exercise 3.2

Adding a New Patient

1. In the *New Patient* window of the *New* menu on the main screen, enter yourself as a patient. Note the first name is filled out first. Fill out as much information as you can. The PMS ID field can be left blank. This field automatically populates when patient data are transmitted from a practice management system program. Save the information.

Note: We will now add an additional 10 patients into SpringCharts. You will use these patients to complete the remaining exercises in the text.

2. Once again, open a *New Patient* window and record the patient's first name as *Diabetes*. **Record your date of birth**. Click the *Copy Patient* button and type your last name (or a portion of it) in the *Choose Patient* window. Click on the binocular icon to search. Click on your name. Note the family information that is copied from an existing patient. The new patient should have your last name, address, and home phone number. You do not need to complete any more information. The program uses the home phone number to link patients together from the same household. Save the information.

3. Repeat step 2 and set up nine more patients. Use the following list of diseases and assign a disease as the patient's first name. For each patient add the first name (disease process) and your date of birth, and then copy your own information into the record by accessing the *Copy Patient* button.
   Patients' First Names: **CHF, Pneumonia, COPD, Fractured Hip, Colon Cancer, Stroke, Cellulitis, Chest Pain, and Bipolar Affective Disorder.**

Note: If SpringCharts is used for simulation activities in the lab setting, the simulation name may be inserted as the first name. Using your last name identifies the patient chart as your work.

4. Open your own chart by clicking on the *Open a Chart* icon on the tool bar (see margin illustration). Type in your last name and click the binocular icon to search. Select your name from the list. (If there is another student in the same network who has the same name as you, the date of birth can be used to identify your chart.)

5. In your patient's chart, click on the *File* menu and select the *Household List* submenu. The ten patients that you added to SpringCharts are listed. The home phone number connects the patients together.

Open a Chart icon

Documentation Tip

When patients have the same name, healthcare facilities often validate identity by the middle initial and date of birth. Selection of the correct patient record is imperative to prevent documentation errors.

LO 3.5 Customizing Pop-Up Text

SpringCharts EHR is driven by templates and pop-up text. Pop-up text functions like pick lists that appear in numerous places throughout the program. They enable the user to select words, phrases, or paragraphs with the click of the mouse. This provides a speedy way to document verbiage without the need for cumbersome typing.

SpringCharts pop-up text can be edited from multiple locations. In any dialogue box within SpringCharts that displays pop-up text, the edit icon (seen in Figure 3.6) gives access to the *Edit PopUp Text* window where, text can be added, deleted, or modified. Pop-up text is stored in the SpringCharts database by user login name; therefore, each user has a personal set of pop-up texts that can be modified without affecting any other user's pop-up text.

If a user wants to spend some time modifying pop-up text, the *Edit PopUp Text* window (Figure 3.7) can be accessed without being in a specific area of the program. In this case, the user clicks on *File > Preferences > PopUp Text* on the main *Practice View* screen. To edit pop-up text, the user locates the appropriate category of text in the left column and then modifies, deletes, or adds to the existing text.

Figure 3.6
Edit PopUp Text icon.

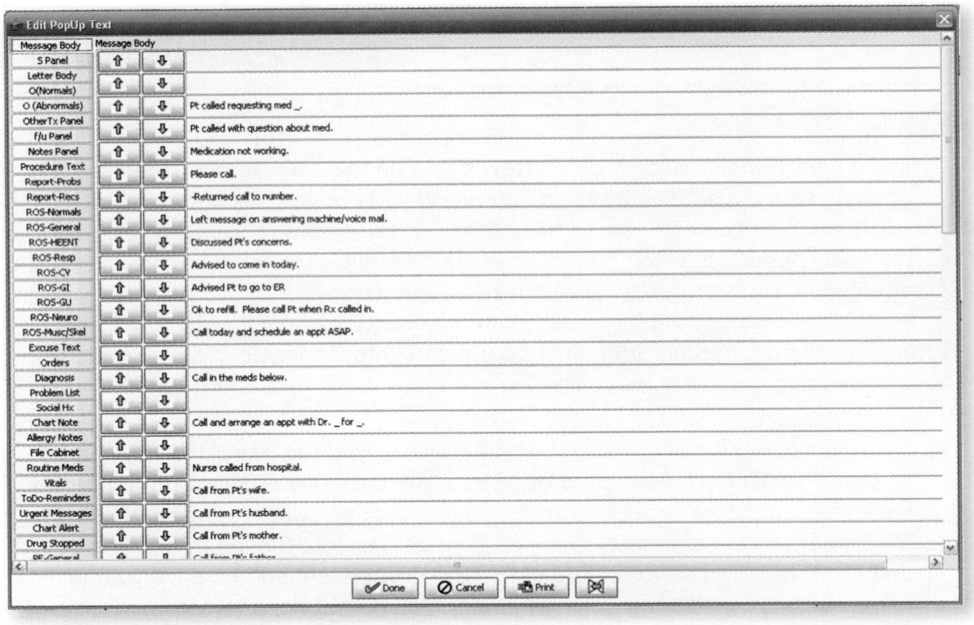

Figure 3.7

Edit PopUp Text window

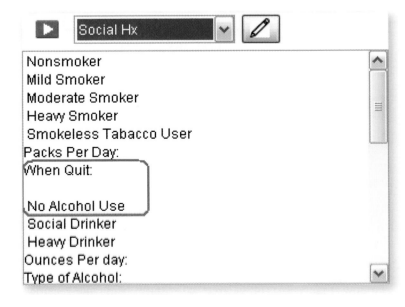

Additional categories can be added to the existing pop-up text list. The *Edit PopUp Text* window allows for 60 line items to be added to any pop-up text category displayed on the right. These text lines can be individual words, sentences, or complete paragraphs. In addition to the 34 preset category headings that come with the installed program (and therefore cannot be altered), 20 customizable categories are in the side menu.

The customizable category headings are edited from the main menu bar—*File > Preferences > My List Names*, seen in Figure 3.8. Once new text has been added in the *Edit PopUp Text* window to a new category, the corresponding category name must be created.

The "up" and "down" arrows to the left of the pop-up text enable the user to manipulate the text in any desired order, such as priority, topic, or alphabetized, for quick selection when working within SpringCharts. If an empty line is needed in the pop-up text listing to divide groups of text, the user moves an empty line between text by using the up and down arrows in the *Edit PopUp Text* window. Once an empty line has been positioned, the user places the cursor on the empty line and hits the space bar. This adds an invisible character to the line and activates the program to display a space between text items in the pop-up text list, as seen below in Figure 3.9.

Figure 3.8

Customizing pop-up
category headings

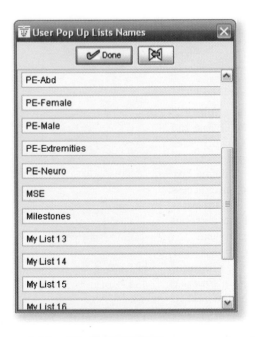

Figure 3.9

Placing lines between pop-up text

Concept Checkup 3.3

A. [pencil icon] What is the purpose of this icon?

_____

_____

_____

B. What does the following mean: the pop-up text is stored in SpringCharts "**by user**"?

_____

_____

_____

_____

Exercise 3.3

Adding Pop-Up Text

1. Let's add some pop-up text that facilitates documentation of your patient's recent admission to the hospital for elective knee surgery. Click on the *File* menu in the *Practice View* screen and select *Preferences > PopUp Text*.

2. Choose the *S Panel* and scroll down until you find an empty line. Type: *Knee Surgery*. Using the arrows to the left, move the text up until it is alphabetized.

3. We want to also make sure we have appropriate text in the *Nursing Outcomes Classification* panel. Locate this category. Scroll down in this panel and find an empty line at the bottom. Type: *Wound Healing: Primary Intention: Extent of regeneration of cells and tissue following intentional closure*. On the next line type: *Wound healing: Secondary Intention: Extent of regeneration of cells and tissue in an open wound*. Using the arrows to the left, move the text up and position it above PRIORITY OUTCOME:. Click on the *Done* button.

LO 3.6 Understanding The Electronic Chart

The **electronic chart** is the repository for patient health data created through computer automation in the healthcare setting. Similar to the traditional paper chart, it holds such static information as the patient's demographics, allergies, medical history, and medical problems as well as the dynamic information including encounter notes, nurse notes, tests, letters, and reports concerning the patient. In SpringCharts a patient's chart can be retrieved by clicking on the *Open a Chart* icon on the main menu bar. It can also be accessed from the *Actions* menu and then selecting *Open a Chart*. Figure 3.10 illustrates several options for accessing a patient's chart.

Open a Chart icon

Figure 3.10

Main menu displaying option for opening a chart

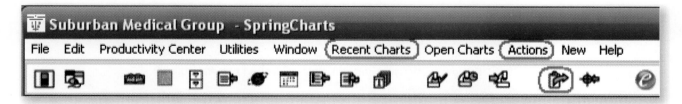

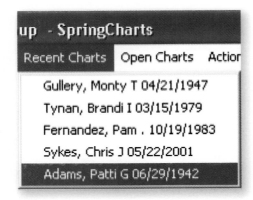

Figure 3.11

Recent charts opened during current logon session

The *Recent Charts* menu provides a drop-down window, as seen in Figure 3.11, that allows the user to access charts that have been opened during the current logon session.

The patient chart is composed of a series of panels on the left for displaying and editing the comprehensive **face sheet**. The face sheet contains more constant patient information such as allergies, problem list, and past health history (PMHX) and is used in both inpatient and outpatient settings. The dynamic **care tree** on the right side lists **encounters** (progress notes), tests, and other current records and documents.

SpringCharts EHR provides practitioners a unique view of the entire chart at a glance, as illustrated in Figure 3.12. It resembles having a paper chart open in front of you. The user does not have to navigate to other areas of the program to view various elements of the chart. A patient's chart can be opened by multiple users in SpringCharts at the same time. In fact, all users can be editing the same chart at the same time. However, because of data protection, the same *specific area* of the chart cannot be edited simultaneously by different users. Three different patient electronic charts can be opened simultaneously by the same user.

Figure 3.12

Patient chart screen

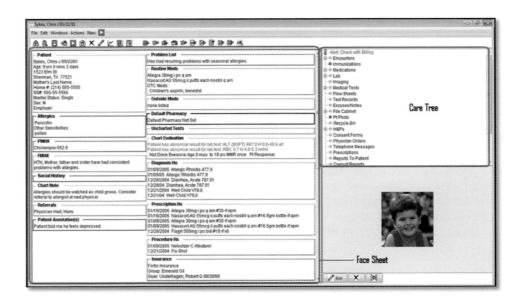

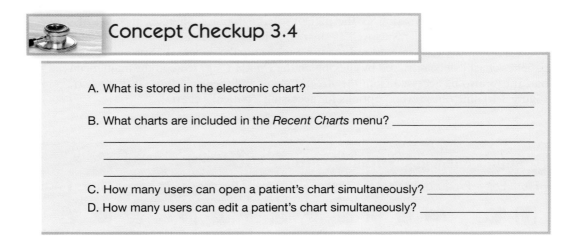

Concept Checkup 3.4

A. What is stored in the electronic chart? _____

_____

B. What charts are included in the *Recent Charts* menu? _____

_____

_____

_____

C. How many users can open a patient's chart simultaneously? _____

D. How many users can edit a patient's chart simultaneously? _____

LO 3.7   The Face Sheet

In a traditional paper chart, the face sheet contains the patient's demographic information and insurance data. In SpringCharts EHR, more categories, such as past health history and family health history, are also included in the face sheet. Face sheet categories can be edited by simply clicking on the *Open Face Sheet* icon on the chart menu bar (see margin illustration). The *Face Sheet Edit* window, shown in Figure 3.13, allows rapid entry of health information data by the healthcare staff. Most subdivisions of the face sheet have a search function to add information such as diagnoses and medications and a pop-up text area for additional clarification.

The social history, past medical (PMHX), and family medical history sections contain health history (FMHX) items that are set up in the **category preferences** table on the SpringCharts server (see Figure 3.14). The category preferences table enables the administrator to create predetermined customized lists of healthcare data. The lists are displayed in SpringCharts on each computer and facilitate selection of items from these checklists to build the face sheet. These server healthcare lists can be easily customized for each facility, displaying pertinent items. In the initial setup on the server, the administrator can add up to 30 items in each of these categories.

Information to complete the electronic face sheet is taken from paper intake forms or through interviews to obtain past health history, routine medications, and current health problems. Paper intake forms are used by some facilities and may be completed by patients in the waiting room while they wait to be seen or admitted. The paper intake forms may be designed to cover the same categories and data flow that appear in the SpringCharts face sheet. (See Appendix B, *Source Documents—Document 1: Admission Data Base*.)

Allergies

By clicking on the *Allergy* button at the top left of the screen, as shown in Figure 3.13, drug allergies and other sensitivities can be added or edited. Drug and non-drug allergies can be added by locating them through the *Search* window located on the right-hand side. For established patients with a prescription history, drugs can also be pulled from the *Previous Prescriptions* display window.

A link is available under both the *Allergies* and *Routine Meds* categories for direct access to the *Epocrates* website (see margin illustration). This popular website provides the user with a current web-based drug interaction and formulary reference, allowing the provider to make clinical decisions quickly and confidently. This optional

Open Face Sheet icon

FOCAL POINT

Pop-up text and customized lists allow rapid data entry when editing the face sheet.

FOCAL POINT

Healthcare lists and category preferences are set up on the server and are available on all client computers.

Epocrates link icon

FOCAL POINT

The patient's allergies and other sensitivities are displayed in SpringCharts whenever the user accesses the patient's routine medications or writes a prescription.

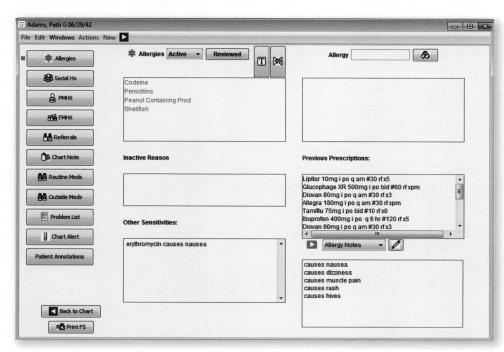

Figure 3.13
Face Sheet Edit window

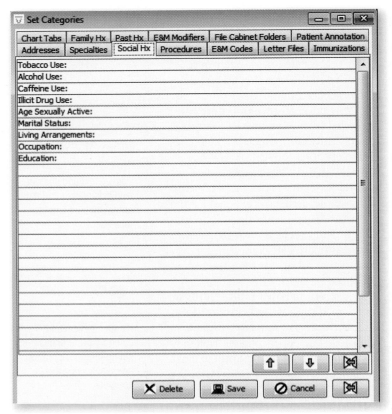

SpringCharts feature is accessed by pressing the *Epocrates* link button located in various screens throughout the program. Epocrates. com is a subscription-based website.

Other Sensitivities is a text field in the lower half of the *Allergies* window. The information displayed here is shown as a separate category on the face sheet. Pop-up text is available to choose the sensitivity or add descriptive text to the sensitivity, such as specific adverse reactions. Both allergies and the sensitivities can be removed from the patient's face sheet by highlighting and deleting the entry. If no allergies are entered into the patient's face sheet, the program automatically enters NKA (no known allergies) into the *Allergies* section of the face sheet.

Social History

Social History allows the patient's social history to be entered or edited. A checklist is provided for rapid entry. The *Preferences* checklist is defined under *Category Preferences* on the SpringCharts server or under the *Administration* menu on a single-user version (see Figure 3.14). Additional defining text can be added to the chosen preference categories by selecting text from the upper *PopUp Text* window, as seen in Figure 3.15.

Past Medical History (PMHX) and Family Medical History (FMHX)

Two sections in the face sheet allow the **past medical history (PMHX)** and **family medical history (FMHX)** to be added or edited, as seen in Figure 3.16. A medical diagnosis (Dx) may be chosen in a system-coded form or a description in the upper-right portion of the screen if the desired diagnosis is not located in the *Preferences* list. Again a *Preferences* checklist (lower right) is provided for rapid entry. The checklist

Figure 3.14

Customized lists in category preferences

Figure 3.15

Social History setup in *Edit Face Sheet* window

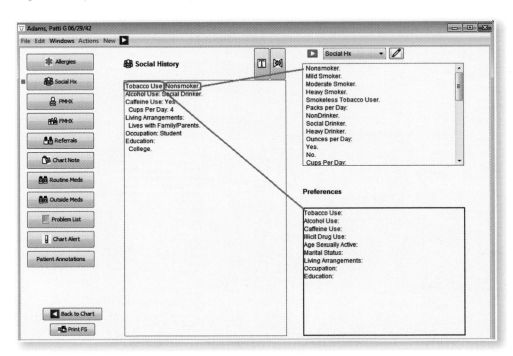

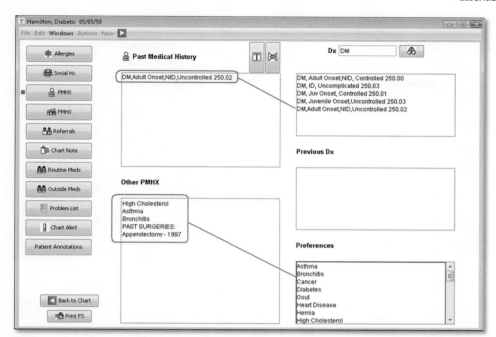

Figure 3.16

PMHX section of the *Face Sheet Edit* window

is defined on the SpringCharts server under the *Category Preferences* section. Items from the *Preferences* are added to the *Other PMHX* or *Other FMHX* windows once selected. They are stored in a free-text format. This window also allows free-typed text for further clarification. Whether the patient history has been added from the *Dx* field or the *Preferences* window, selected items can be deleted by highlighting the entry and deleting from within the *Edit Face Sheet* window.

Referrals

In the *Referrals* section of the face sheet, the user may select the referring healthcare provider or primary care provider. Referring practitioners must be first set up in the address book in order to be chosen in the face sheet. The user simply types in the healthcare provider's last name and conducts a search. The appropriate provider is selected from the list and the name is added to the face sheet.

Chart Note

The *Chart Note* section is a location for entering important information about a patient that needs to be seen when opening a patient's chart. Pop-up text is provided in this window to rapidly add predefined text. Many times this *Chart Note* section is used to record specific health history based on the specialty of the clinic. For example, an obstetrics and gynecology practice may use the area to document menstrual history, menopausal history, births, types of deliveries, and miscarriages. A psychologist may use the *Chart Note* to record information such as previous psychiatric treatment, substance abuse treatment, or history of harmful mood and behavior.

Routine Meds

Routine Meds allows the patient's current routine medications and over-the-counter (OTC) drugs to be modified. Routine medications are selected by searching for the desired medication. Again a direct link is available to the *Epocrates* website to investigate drug interactions and formulary references. Pop-up text is presented for *Routine Meds*, which allows easy listing of common medications and other OTC remedies. Medications can be edited by clicking once on the prescription in the *Routine Medication* window and adjusting any of the specifications in the *Edit Rx* window, illustrated in Figure 3.17.

Changes made in this section affect only the patient whose chart is open, not the entire database. *Allergies* and *Other Sensitivities* are displayed in red in the upper window each time routine medications are accessed in SpringCharts.

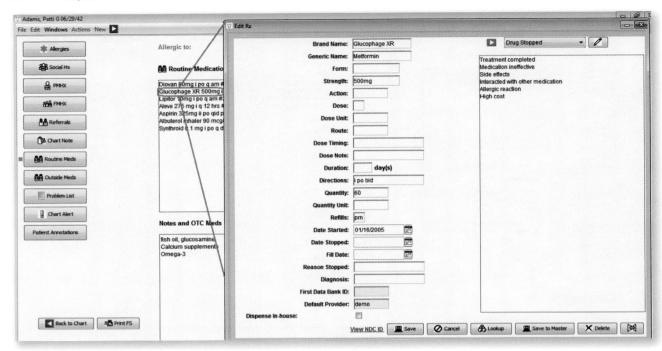

Figure 3.17

Editing drugs in *Routine Medication* window

Outside Meds

The *Outside Medication* section documents medications prescribed by other providers. This section of the face sheet automatically populates when SpringCharts makes an Internet connection through SpringScripts to conduct e-prescribing. A national clearinghouse for e-prescribing transfers data regarding prescribed medication for this patient from other providers. The information about outside meds can be viewed here but not altered.

Problem List

The *Problem List* allows the patient's chronic health problems to be added or edited. Entries can be either diagnoses or text. When a healthcare provider selects a medical diagnosis in the office visit screen, it also may be added to the *Problem List* at that time. For established patients who have been previously assigned a diagnosis in a Spring-Charts' office visit note, the diagnosis code and description are available to select when building the *Problem List* in the face sheet. Again, pop-up text is available to select items from predefined *Problem List* text. SpringCharts automatically stamps the user ID and date at the bottom of the problem list when exiting the *Edit Face Sheet* window.

Back to Chart button

Chart Alert

The **Chart Alert** allows the inclusion of important text that appears in red above the *Encounters* category on the chart's care tree, as seen in Figure 3.18. Text can be typed in the *Chart Alert* window or selected from predefined text in the *Chart Alert* pop-up text list.

Figure 3.18

Chart alert in patient's chart

Patient Annotations

Additional explanations or comments that a patient may state during admissions or an encounter can be displayed in the face sheet in the *Patient Annotations* section. Sometimes it is helpful to have important patient comments displayed in the face sheet rather than buried in an encounter note. Preset text may be chosen from the *Preferences* section on the right or typed into the upper-left window. When this section of the face sheet is subsequently accessed, previous annotations move to the lower *Previous Annotation(s)* window and cannot be edited.

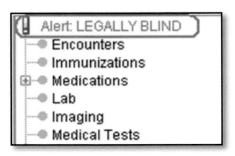

New and modified face sheet information is saved into the left-hand side of the chart when the *Back to Chart* button at the bottom left of the *Face Sheet Edit* window (see Figure 3.13) is selected. The newly completed face sheet can be printed for new patients to allow them to confirm the accuracy of their health information. The face sheet is printed by selecting the *Print FS* button pictured in the margin. All information in the *Edit Face Sheet* window is printed except the *Chart Alert*, preventing the Chart Alert information from being seen by the patient. The patient's demographics and primary insurance details are also printed on the face sheet form. (See Appendix A, *Sample Documents—Document 1: Patient's Face Sheet.*)

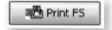

Print Face Sheet button

Diagnosis, Prescription, and Procedure History

Three additional windows in the face sheet portion of the chart provide for the automatic recording of diagnoses, prescriptions, and procedures. This information is extracted from the patient's various encounters. As diagnoses, prescriptions, and procedures are entered in the nurse note and/or office visit screen, they appear on these lists with the most recent item at the top. These lists can be opened and printed by accessing the *Actions* menu within the patient's chart and selecting the appropriate heading, seen in Figure 3.19. If any section of the face sheet requires amending at a later date, the user can simply right-click on the appropriate segment of the face sheet and select *Edit*. The *Face Sheet Edit* window opens at that specific section.

Figure 3.19

Diagnosis List display in patient's chart

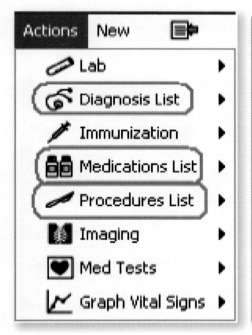

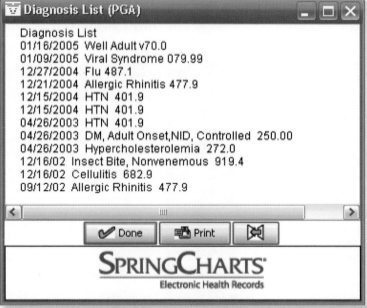

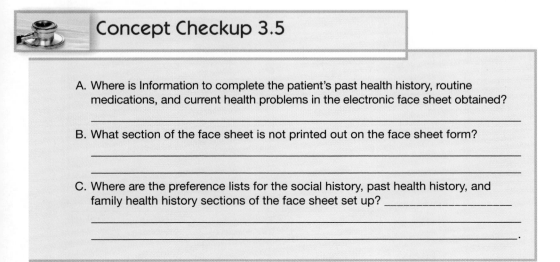

Concept Checkup 3.5

A. Where is Information to complete the patient's past health history, routine medications, and current health problems in the electronic face sheet obtained?

_____

B. What section of the face sheet is not printed out on the face sheet form?

_____

_____

C. Where are the preference lists for the social history, past health history, and family health history sections of the face sheet set up? _____

_____

_____ .

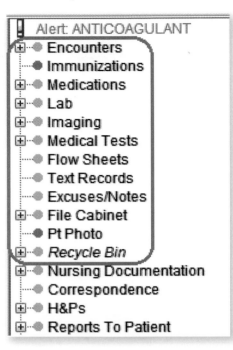

Figure 3.20

Permanent categories in the care tree

LO 3.8   The Care Tree

The care tree is where the different items of the patient's chart are accessed in SpringCharts. As seen in Figure 3.12, the care tree appears on the right side of the patient chart screen. To edit an item in the care tree, the user clicks on the "+" symbol to the left of the category to expand the list and then selects the specific item; the particular "branch" item is displayed in the bottom right window. (On a MacIntosh computer the + sign appears as an arrow.) To edit an item in the care tree, the user clicks the *Edit* button at the bottom of the screen; SpringCharts judges the screen size and displays as much information as possible to the user.

There are preset categories in the care tree that cannot be altered or edited. These current categories include all categories from *Encounters* through *Recycle Bin* as seen in Figure 3.20. When certain documents and tests are saved, they are automatically saved to the appropriate care tree category.

Up to 30 categories can be added to the care tree list, providing users the opportunity to store documents and imported files in customized categories. Figure 3.20 shows an additional four categories that have been added to the care tree: *Nursing Documentation, Correspondence, H&Ps,* and *Reports To Patient.*

FOCAL POINT

Up to 30 categories can be added to the preset categories in the care tree list. Additional categories are set up on the server.

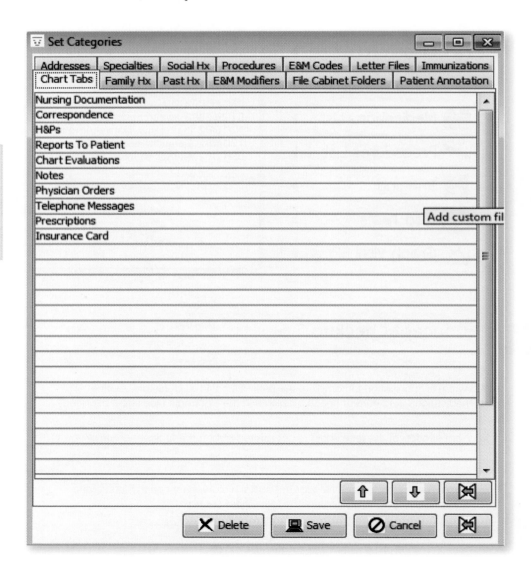

Figure 3.21

Customized chart tab categories in *Category Preferences* window

Many newly created documents provide the user with an option to choose a care tree category before saving. Users may find it more convenient to store certain documents in customized categories rather than under the default *Encounters* tab. Because many of the created forms are initiated from encounters with the patient, the *Encounters* tab is displayed as the default location to save these documents. However, with customized categories added to the care tree, the user has other options under which to store documents. Additional customized categories are added through the setup function of the SpringCharts server in the *Category Preferences*, seen in Figure 3.21. Once new items are added to the SpringCharts server, all SpringCharts clients must be refreshed by shutting down and rebooting the program in order for the changes to be seen.

After the documents have been saved into the care tree, the category may be changed by selecting the *Edit* button in the bottom window. Once the window is reopened, the user chooses the *Change Tab* button, illustrated in Figure 3.22, and selects another category. The program moves the document from the former category to the newly selected one.

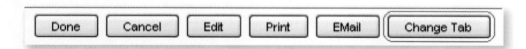

Figure 3.22
Change Tab button in
Document Edit window

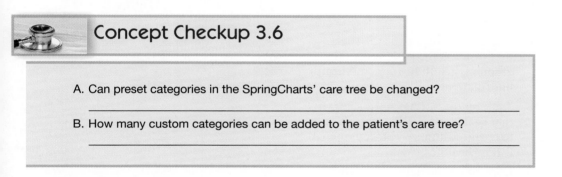

Concept Checkup 3.6

A. Can preset categories in the SpringCharts' care tree be changed?

_____

B. How many custom categories can be added to the patient's care tree?

_____

Using Terminology

Match the terms on the left with the definitions on the right.

_____ 1. Care tree

_____ 2. Category preferences

_____ 3. Chart alert

_____ 4. Electronic chart

_____ 5. Encounters

_____ 6. PMS

_____ 7. Face sheet

_____ 8. FMHX

_____ 9. Imperial units

_____ 10. User preferences

_____ 11. PMHX

_____ 12. Metric units

A. The patient's past health history.

B. Having to do with weights and measures that conform to the standards legally established in Great Britain.

C. *Setup* window in SpringCharts that enables each user to preset the default practice name, provider name, schedule, and various other features that are displayed when the user logs into the program.

D. The family health history records.

E. Also known as the International System of Units.

F. The portion of a patient's chart that displays the patient demographics, health history, and health information.

G. Table on the SpringCharts server that enables the EHR administrator to create customized predetermined lists of healthcare data.

H. Located on the right side of the patient's chart, it lists encounters (progress notes), tests, and other records.

I. Practice management software responsible for financial transactions and billing of insurance companies and patients.

J. Important text that appears in red above the *Encounters* category on the chart's care tree.

K. A category in the care tree where many of the documents that are created from encounters with the patient are stored by default.

L. The equivalent to a patient's paper chart containing face sheet information and ongoing healthcare encounter documentation.

Checking Your Understanding

Write "T" or "F" in the blank to indicate whether the statement is true or false.

_____ 13. SpringCharts EHR provides practitioners a unique electronic view of the patient's chart similar to a paper chart.

_____ 14. All of the preset categories in the care tree can be altered or edited.

_____ 15. Only 1,000 new patients can be added to SpringCharts.

_____ 16. Sixty lines of preset type can be added to each pop-up text category.

_____ 17. The *Category Preferences* window enables the EHR administrator to create a collections module for 30 to 60 days, 60 to 90 days, or 90+ days past due accounts.

_____ 18. Information to complete the electronic face sheet may be taken from the intake forms that the patient fills out regarding personal PMHX, routine meds, and current health problems.

Choose the best answer and circle the corresponding letter.

19. The care tree (Select all that apply)
    a) has preset categories that cannot be altered or edited.
    b) can be edited.
    c) allows the user to add up to 30 categories.

20. SpringCharts EHR was chosen as the training tool for this text because of its
    a) ease of use, full features, and customization.
    b) customization, cost, and bright colors.
    c) nurse note, office note, and MAR form.

21. *Set User Preferences* allows the nurse to choose (Select all that apply)
    a) customized popup text and font size.
    b) the default healthcare provider, default practice, and default measurement units.
    c) digital signature, password, and pop-up text.

22. When creating a new patient profile, the fields marked in red indicate
    a) information to be avoided.
    b) optional patient information.
    c) information required to create a chart.

23. When a user modifies personal pop-up text
    a) it is also modified for each other user at the same time.
    b) it only modifies that user's pop-up text.
    c) it changes the number of categories that can be added.

24. The *Face Sheet* contains a record of the patient's
    a) PMHX, FMHX, social history, and routine medications.
    b) allergies, routine meds, OTC meds, and current nurse note.
    c) problem lists, chart alert, chart note, and intake sheet.

25. A document saved under a category in the care tree can be moved to another category by selecting
    a) the *Encounter* category.
    b) a document cannot be moved to another category.
    c) the *Change Tab* button.

Reference

Cornish, P.L., Knowles, S.R., Marchesano, R., Tam, V., Shadowitz, S., Jurrlink D.N. et al. (2005). Unintended medication discrepancies at the time of hospital admission. *Archives of Internal Medicine, 165*(4), 424–429.

Nurse Note

Key Terms

Terms and abbreviations you will encounter in Chapter 4; they are defined in the end-of-book glossary:

Body Mass Index (BMI)

Nurse Note

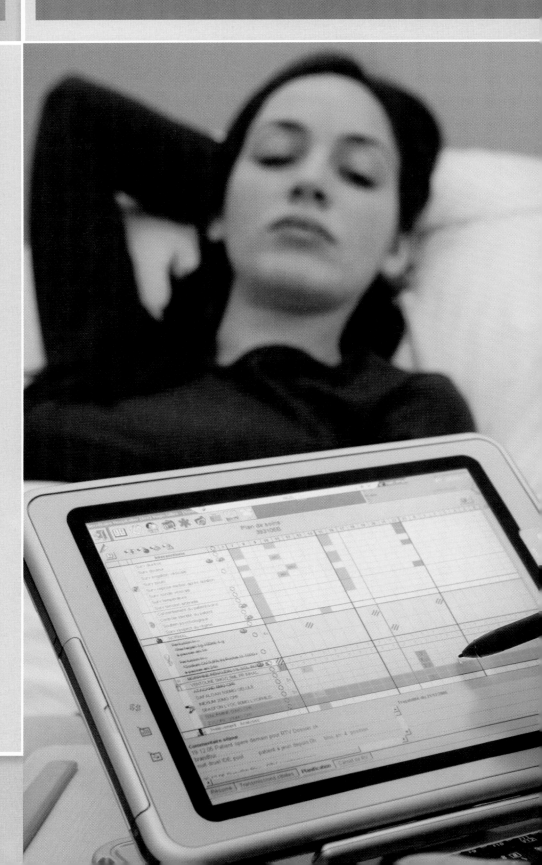

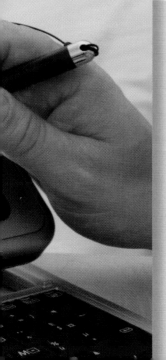

Documentation—Level 1

Learning Outcomes

When you complete Chapter 4, you will be able to:

4.1   Describe the components of a *Nurse Note*.

4.2   Carry out documentation of a *Nurse Note*.

4.3   Use *Chief Complaints*.

4.4   Carry out documentation of *Vitals* (Vital Signs).

4.5   Carry out documentation of an *Exam* (Physical Assessment).

What You Need to Know

To understand Chapter 4, you need to know how to:

- Start SpringCharts EHR.
- Enter new patient demographics.
- Create your own electronic patient chart.
- Create and edit electronic pop-up text.
- Explain the concept of an electronic chart.
- Identify the patient's chart screen and icons.
- Build and print a face sheet for a new patient.

LO 4.1 # Nurse Note Components

A large percentage of nurses are employed in an acute care inpatient setting (Bureau of Labor Statistics, 2010). In this milieu nurses provide care for 2 to 12 patients depending on the shift, the acuity level of the patients, and the staffing ratio of the nursing unit. Since nurses have a heavy workload, facilitation of patient information retrieval and documentation is important. EHRs allow nurses to have access to patient information at the click of a mouse, in many cases at the bedside, instead of searching a paper chart in the nurse's station. Documentation in EHRs is often streamlined by using *charting by exception* as described in Chapter 2.

Nurses typically document in a nurse's note section of the patient's record. In SpringCharts, a new **Nurse Note** is created by selecting the *New* menu within the patient's chart and clicking *New Nurse Note*. The *Nurse Note* displays, as seen in Figure 4.1.

The *Nurse Note* screen is in the SOAPIER format displaying the subjective (*S*), objective (*O*), assessment (*A*), plan (*P*), intervention (*I*), evaluation (*E*), and Revision (*R*) in the left panel. The information documented by the nurse populates the appropriate section of the format as the nurse completes documentation. All of the text items

---

THE SOAPIER FORMAT

The *Subjective* component consists of the patient's description of the current health condition. It generally includes the symptoms, the history of the present illness, and a review of the patient's body systems as stated by the patient.

The *Objective* component contains the nurse's observations and generally includes vital signs and findings from the physical assessment.

The *Assessment* component details the nursing diagnosis(es) based on the examination, listed in order of priority.

The *Plan* component includes the nursing goals applicable to the patient stated in Nursing Outcomes Classification (NOC) (St. Louis: Mosby 2008) format. In the planning phase, the nurse sets the anticipated time frame for goal attainment. Outcomes are reviewed periodically, typically every shift to determine patient progress.

The *Intervention* component is made up of the list of patient-specific actions that the nurse takes stated in Nursing Intervention Classification (NIC) (St. Louis: Mosby 2008) format. These interventions, including patient education, are designed to positively impact the patient and move the patient toward achieving the planned goals (NOC).

The *Evaluation* component involves reviewing the outcomes that have been set and the patient's progress toward achieving these goals.

The *Revision* component, based on the evaluation, involves streamlining, adding, and reassessing goals.

Figure 4.1
Nurse Note view

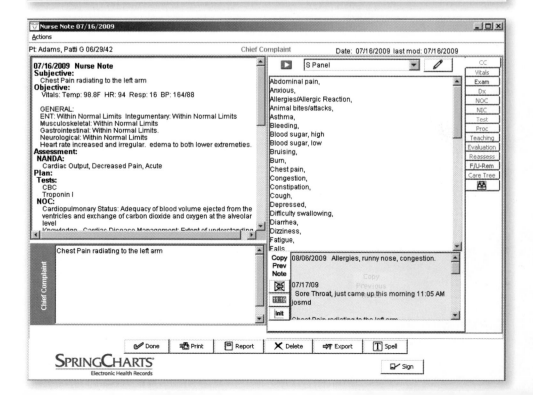

selected in the *Nurse Note* pop-up text categories or text manually added to the text fields automatically save into the appropriate SOAPIER category in the Nurse Note.

Upon opening a new *Nurse Note* window, the *Show Chart Summary* icon (see margin illustration) located at the bottom right of the Nurse Note screen, provides access to the *Face Sheet Overview* panel. This panel allows the nurse to access the face sheet information without having to exit the *Nurse Note* window. Double-clicking on any of the *Face Sheet* categories enables the user to edit that specific *Face Sheet* area, a useful feature if the nurse needs to add information to the face sheet.

Show Chart Summary icon

FOCAL POINT

The *Facesheet Panel* is available throughout the *Nurse Note* for retrieval of information and editing.

Concept Checkup 4.1

A. The SOAPIER acronym stands for:

S. _____

O. _____

A. _____

P. _____

I. _____

E. _____

R. _____

B. What icon allows the nurse to view the patient's face sheet from the *Nurse Note* screen? _____

LO 4.2   Documenting a Nurse Note—Level 1

This section of the chapter focuses on initiating a *Nurse Note* and documenting the chief complaint, vital signs, and an assessment. The Navigation tabs along the right side of the screen, seen in Figure 4.2, enable the nurse to proceed through the *Nurse Note* in a logical flow; however, the various panels may be selected in any order. Navigation tabs include *CC (Chief Complaint), Vitals, Exam (Physical Assessment), Dx (NANDA-I/ Diagnosis), NOC (Nursing Outcomes Classification), NIC (Nursing Interventions Classification), Test (Tests), Proc (Procedures), Teaching, Evaluation, Reassess (Reassessment), F/U-Rem (Follow-up-Reminders), Care Tree*, and the *Show Chart Summary* icon.

Once a tab has been selected, a list of pop-up text relevant to that tab of the Navigation panel appears on the right side of the screen, also seen in Figure 4.2. Data can be entered by (1) tapping with a stylus tool (as with a portable computer), (2) clicking on pop-up text items with a mouse, or (3) typing directly into the text box. On a tablet PC or iPad™ with handwriting recognition software, hand script is recognized and automatically typed into the text box. Also, through voice recognition software the user can dictate and have the text automatically entered into the text field. However, it is recommended that pop-up text be used rather than these other methods of data entry because pop-up text is the most rapid way to build documentation for a *Nurse Note*.

Figure 4.2

Navigation panel

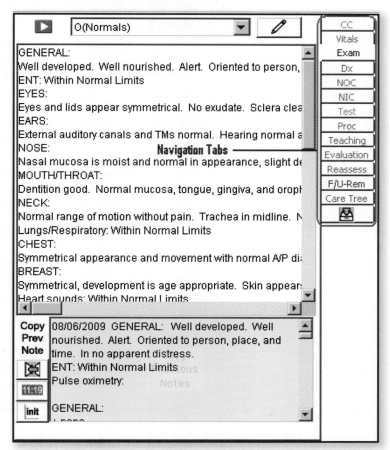

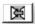

Figure 4.3
Copy Note icon

The *Chief Complaint, Exam, NOC, NIC, Teaching, Evaluation, Reassess,* and *Follow-up* tabs allow notes from previous encounters to be viewed in the bottom right window. A clinician can highlight previous note text and copy it to the present note by clicking on the *Copy Note* icon, displayed in Figure 4.3. These previous notes are dated and organized by most recent first. *Past encounter* notes enable clinicians to compare their findings with those of nurses from previous shifts and copy similar notes quickly into the current *Nurse Note*. This is particularly useful with shift to shift documentation when assessments and interventions are similar. The previous note panel only displays the portion of the previous *Nurse Note* documentation specific to the tab selected on the Navigation panel.

Although the program defaults to the appropriate pop-up text category when a specific navigation tab is selected, additional lists of pop-up text are located by category in the pop-up text header field, seen in Figure 4.4. By accessing this list, the practitioner has multiple categories of text available from which to choose. Text selected from other categories are added to existing text in the panel section that the nurse has currently opened. For example, a practitioner may create specific categories of text for procedures, review of systems, or chief complaints. Pop-up text that is selected from another category will be saved in the *SOAPIER* category tab that is open. The program offers an additional 20 user-defined categories that can be added to the pop-up text feature.

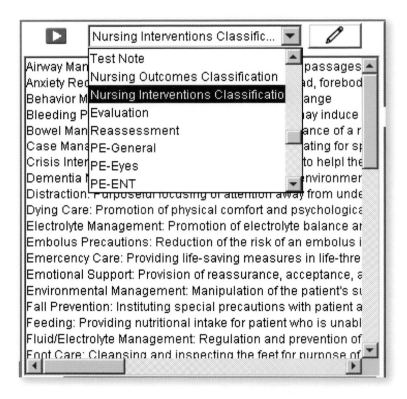

Figure 4.4
Pop-up text header field

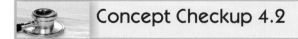

Concept Checkup 4.2

A. True or False: When documenting patient care, the nurse must select tabs from the Navigation panel in the order listed. _____

B. Which icon allows nurses to copy highlighted text from a previous *Nurse Note* into the current *Nurse Note*? _____

LO 4.3   CC (Chief Complaint)

In the *CC (Chief Complaint)* field, the *S Panel* pop-up text defaults with a list of chief complaints as shown in Figure 4.5. After discussing the patient's symptoms, the nurse documents these in the *Chief Complaint* area by clicking on the applicable items, sending the documentation to the *Chief Complaint* box on the lower left side of the window. The nurse can describe these complaints in more detail or add something not in the *S Panel list* by simply clicking into the *Chief Complaint* box on the left and typing the information directly into the field. The selected text is moved into the body of the SOAPIER format by clicking on any other navigational tab. *CC (Chief Complaint), Vitals, Exam (Physical Assessment), Dx (NANDA-I/ Diagnosis), NOC (Nursing Outcomes Classification), NIC (Nursing Interventions Classification), Teaching, Evaluation, Reassess (Reassessment),* and *F/U-Rem (Follow Up-Reminders)* all operate in a similar manner with the appropriate pop-up text appearing on the right side once a different tab in the note is selected.

The *Chief Complaint* pop-up text area can also be individualized to allow for symptoms that are specific to a certain area, for example, orthopedics or neurology. In order to individualize pop-up text, the user selects the pencil icon to open the *Edit PopUp Text* window (see margin illustration). The nurse can add any text that is useful into one of the open fields. The nurse may also modify the order of the list by using the up and down arrows on the left side of the screen (see margin illustration). The user clicks *Done* when the changes are complete.

Documentation Tip

Chief complaints should be documented in the patient's words using direct quotes when possible.

FOCAL POINT

Users can individualize the pop-up text in any of the categories that are available using the pencil icon.

Edit PopUp Text Icon

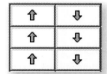

Text order arrows in *Edit PopUp Text* window

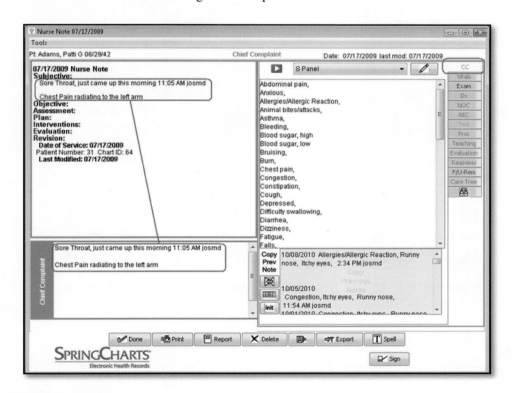

Figure 4.5

System text and free text in the *Chief Complaint* section

Concept Checkup 4.3

A. How does the nurse move chief complaints that are documented to the body of the SOAPIER format? _____

B. True or False: The *Chief Complaint* pop-up text can be individualized for a specialty area of nursing practice.

LO 4.4   Vitals (Vital Signs)

Although vital signs typically consist of blood pressure, pulse, respirations, and temperature, SpringCharts lists nine measurements in the *Vitals* section. In addition to the typical vital sign measurements, height, weight, head circumference (HC), **body mass index (BMI)**, and body fat percentage can be documented on the left bottom corner of this screen. These appear in the *Objective* area of the *SOAPIER* note once the clinician clicks on any other navigation tab on the right side of the *Nurse Note*. Along with all nine basic vitals, three additional custom measurements, such as pain and oxygen saturation (SaO2), can be added to the program. These are added to the SpringCharts server and appear in the *Vitals* section of the *Nurse Note* screen and in the *New Vitals Only* screen of the patient's chart.

The BMI is automatically calculated for the user based upon the patient's height and weight. Height and weight will be documented in either metric or imperial units depending on the measurement choice selected in the User Preferences window, mentioned in chapter 3. See Table 4.1 to see how disease risk is affected by BMI.

SpringCharts displays four vital charts (Height, Weight, Blood Pressure, and BMI) by accessing the *Height/Weight Graph* or *BP/BMI Graph* icon at the top right in the *Vitals* panel (see margin illustration).

As an additional tool for pediatric patients, the system displays age-appropriate growth charts and vital sign ranges for pediatric patients. The program automatically adjusts the display of the growth charts when the patient reaches 19 years of age after which the vitals are presented on adult graphs without national percentiles. Figure 4.6 displays weight, height, BMI, and head circumference for a boy between the ages of 3 and 18 years.

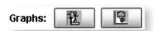

Documentation Tip

Pain is considered to be the fifth vital sign and should be assessed and documented whenever vital signs are monitored.

Graphs:

Height/Weight/BP/BMI Graphs

Table 4.1

BMI disease risk table

RISK OF ASSOCIATED DISEASE ACCORDING TO BMI AND WAIST SIZE			
BMI	OBESITY LEVEL	WAIST LESS THAN OR EQUAL TO 40 IN. (MEN) OR 35 IN. (WOMEN)	WAIST GREATER THAN 40 IN. (MEN) OR 35 IN. (WOMEN)
18.5 or less	Underweight	N/A	N/A
18.5–24.9	Normal	N/A	N/A
25.0–29.9	Overweight	Increased	High
30.0–34.9	Obese	High	Very High
35.0–39.9	Obese	Very High	Very High
40 or greater	Extremely Obese	Extremely High	Extremely High

Concept Checkup 4.4

A. What two measurements are needed for the BMI to be automatically calculated? _____

_____.

B. What are the four standard measurement graphs in SpringCharts?

1. _____

2. _____

3. _____

4. _____

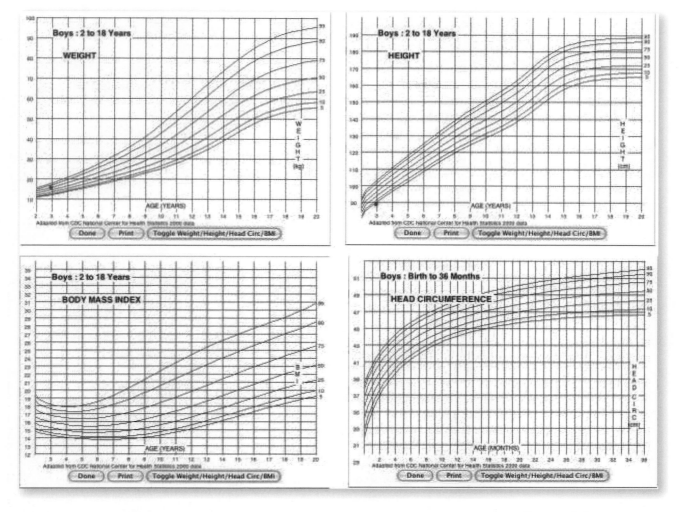

Figure 4.6
Age-appropriate measurements

LO 4.5   Exam (Physical Assessment)

The nurse assesses the patient and documents that assessment using the *Exam* panel. As mentioned previously, charting by exception is commonly used in the inpatient care setting and SpringCharts pop-up text lends itself to this type of documentation. Using the defaulted text, *O (Normals)*, the nurse clicks on systems that are within normal limits upon examination to send that text to the *Examination* text field in the lower-left section of the window. Using the *O (Abnormals)* drop-down selection box the nurse can easily choose the applicable text and modify it as necessary. The user also has the ability to type text if the desired text is not available by clicking directly into the *Examination* text field.

The *Exam* pop-up text area can be individualized to allow for assessment items that are specific to a certain specialty area, such as cardiology or urology. In order to individualize pop-up text, the user selects the pencil icon to open the *Edit Pop-Up Text* window. The nurse can add useful text into one of the open fields. The nurse can modify the order of the list by using the up and down arrows on the left side of the screen. The user clicks the *Done* button when the changes are completed.

The *Nurse Note* is placed in the patient's chart by selecting the *Done* button. The *Nurse Note* can be recalled for further edits by anyone with chart-editing privileges. However, once the *Nurse Note* is locked, which is accomplished by clicking the *Sign* button, then *Permanent Sign and Lock*, it cannot be unlocked or edited, even by the user who permanently locked it. Nurses should sign and lock each entry as completed to prevent editing of entries by other users.

Legal/Ethical Considerations

Charting by exception requires that the nurse know how the organization defines "normal" parameters in order to document exceptions to these parameters.

Edit PopUp Text icon

⇧	⇩
⇧	⇩
⇧	⇩

Text order arrows in *Edit PopUp Text* window

Concept Checkup 4.5

A. True or False: If the nurse is unable to find the appropriate pop-up text to describe an assessment, the nurse can type directly into the *Examination* field itself. _____

B. What is the purpose of *Permanent Sign and Lock*? When should it be used?

_____

_____

_____

Exercise 4.1

Diabetes

1. After launching SpringCharts, from the top horizontal toolbar click on *Actions, Open a Chart*. Type in your last name and click the *Search* button. Select your "diabetes" patient and the chart opens.

2. Your patient tells you she discovered she has an allergy to shellfish this past week. In the second section of the left side of the chart, click on *Allergies* and it populates the right corner box. Click the *Edit* button below the red *Allergies* box and a new window opens.

   - On the right side of the screen in the *Allergy* field, type: *shellfish* and click the *Search* button. *Shellfish* appears in the box below the *Search* button. Click on *Shellfish* and it moves over to the patient's chart on the left.

   - Click on the word *Shellfish* on the left and the *Edit Shellfish* window opens. In the *Adverse Reaction* field, type: *difficulty breathing*. Click *Save*. In the lower-left corner of the window, click *Back to Chart*.

   - Click on the *Allergies* field on the left and when it populates the right corner box, you can see the note "difficulty breathing" that you entered.

3. You ask your patient about her smoking history and the patient says she smokes a pack a day and has done so for 20 years. Click on the *Social History* field on the left and it populates the box on the right side of the screen.

   - Click the *Edit* button below the *Social History* box on the right side of the screen and a new window opens.

   - On the right in the list below the *Social History* pop-up text click on *Packs per Day*. This text is added to the text in the *Social History* box on the left.

   - In the *Social History* box on the left, click after "Packs per Day" and type: *1 for 20 years*.

   - In lower-left corner of the window, click *Back to Chart*. Your new entry appears in the *Social History* field.

4. Open your *Nurse Note*. On the top menu bar, click *New, New Nurse Note*. The *Nurse Note* opens to the *Chief Complaint* tab at the top of the vertical navigation bar on the right side of the window.

5. Your patient complains of a headache and high blood sugar. Under the *S Panel* (for *Subjective*) in the text box on the right side, click on *blood sugar, high* and *headache*. The text populates the *Chief Complaint* box on the

Exercises

bottom left of the screen. Click before "headache" in the *Chief Complaint* box on the left bottom of the screen to place the cursor and click the Enter key on your keyboard. This places the two complaints on separate lines.

6. Click on the *Vitals* button located below the *CC* button in the navigation bar on the right side of the screen. Note that your *Chief Complaints* now appear in the *Subjective* section of the *Nurse Note.*

   - You take your patient's vital signs. Document the following in the boxes on the lower-left section of the window: Temp *100.4*, Resp *18*, Pulse *98*, BP *154/84*, Ht *64 inches*, Wt *200 lbs*, SaO2 *94%*.

   - Under the *Vitals* text box on the lower right click: *BP right arm*, *Pt position—supine*, *Temp source—Oral*, and *Room Air*. This sends this text to the *Notes* box on the left. You can separate the "Temp source—Oral" and then "Room Air" from the other text by clicking in front of it and striking the Enter key on the keyboard.

   - Under the *Vitals* text box on the right, scroll down to click: *Pt complains of pain*, *Pain location*, *Pain rating 0–10 scale*, *Pain Description*, *Factors affecting pain*, and *Factors relieving pain*. This sends the text to the *Notes* box on the left.

   - You question your patient to determine the characteristics of her pain. Type in the following information in the *Notes* box following the appropriate labels. Pain location: *Headache right above eyes*, Pain rating 0–10 scale: *8*, Pain Description: *throbbing*, Factors affecting pain: *noise*, Factors relieving pain: *medication*. If you make a mistake, you may place your cursor in the lower left *Examination* box and delete unwanted text.

   - When you select another tab on the horizontal navigation bar on the right side of the window, the *Vitals*, including the pain assessment, populate under the *Objective* heading in the upper-left box.

7. You complete your admission physical assessment. To document your findings, click on the *Exam* button located below *Vitals*. The *O (Normals)* defaults in the text box in the upper-right box of the window. In this area select the following systems that are within normal limits when you assess your patient: *HEENT (Head, Eyes, Ears, Nose, and Throat)*, *Lungs/Respiratory*, *Gastrointestinal*, *Musculoskeletal*, *Heart Sounds*, *Integumentary*, and *GU/GYN (Genitourinary/Gynecologic) (female)*. As you click on each system, the text populates the *Examination* box on the lower-left side of the window. Use the Enter key to put these items on separate lines to streamline your documentation.

   - Click the drop-down arrow next to *O (Normals)* and select *O (Abnormals)*. Select the *General* category followed by: *overweight*. Select the *Neuro* category followed by: *numbness and tingling*. If you make a mistake, you may place your cursor in the lower-left *Examination* box and delete unwanted text.

   - Click in the *Examination* box after "numbness and tingling" and type: i*n fingers and toes, worse over the last year.*

8. Click *Done*. The *Save As* screen populates. Accept the default entries of *Save to Tab: Encounters* and *Save As: Nurse Note*. Click *Save*.

9. A pop-up appears asking if you want to create a routing slip. Click *No*.

10. In the *Care Tree,* in the upper-right corner of the chart window, click the + next to *Encounters*. Click on the date of your *Nurse Note* to view it in the bottom-right corner box.

11. Click *Edit* below the bottom-right box. Click *Sign*. Select *Permanent Sign and Lock* when finished with your *Nurse Note*.

Exercises

Congestive Heart Failure

1. After launching SpringCharts, from the top menu toolbar click on *Actions, Open a Chart*. Type in your last name and click the *Search* button. Select your "CHF" patient and the chart opens.

2. Your patient tells you he was diagnosed with congestive heart failure while on vacation last month in Florida. Click on *PMHX* on the left and the past medical history populates the box on the right-lower side of the screen. Click *Edit* below that box.

   • The *Past Medical History* screen opens and populates in a new window. In the field after *Dx* in the upper right of the window, type: *CHF* and click the *Search* icon. Options appear in the box below. Click on *CHF, Acute 428.0*, which sends this to the *Past Medical History* list on the upper-left side of the window.

   • Click *Back to Chart* in the lower-left corner of the window. The information you added appears in the *PMHX* box.

3. Your patient also informs you the physician in Florida started him on Maxzide 75/50 mg one pill by mouth daily (every AM) at the time of his CHF diagnosis. Click on the *Routine Meds* box and it populates in the bottom-right corner. Click *Edit* and a new window opens.

   • Click in the field after *Brand Name* on the upper-right side of the window and type: *Maxzide*. Click *Search*. Click on the correct dosage. This adds the medication to the *Routine Medications* list in the upper-left box of the window.

   • Click on the *Maxzide* that is in the *Routine Medications* list in the upper left. The *Edit Rx* window opens. Click on the calendar to the right of *Date Started* in the left column and choose a date one month ago. Click *Save*.

   • Click *Back to Chart* at the lower-left side of the window. Maxzide is now listed in the *Routine Meds*.

4. Open your *Nurse Note*. Click *New, New Nurse Note*.

5. Your patient complains of shortness of breath and says he has swelling in his legs. Select these two items in the *S Panel* text and they populate the *Chief Complaint* box on the bottom left of the screen.

6. Click on the *Vitals* button located below the *CC* button on the right side of the screen. The *Chief Complaints* now appear in the *Subjective* section of the *Nurse Note*.

   • You take your patient's vital signs. Document the following in the boxes on the lower-left section of the window: Temp *98.4*, Resp *24*, Pulse *104*, BP *162/84*, Ht *72 inches*, Wt *210 lbs*.

   • When you take the pulse oximetry reading, your patient's oxygen saturation is 88%. Enter this value in the *O2SAT* (SaO2) field. You start oxygen at 2 liters/min per nasal cannula and direct him to breathe in through his nose and out through his mouth. His O2 saturation increases to 94%. Under the *Vitals* text box on the right click *O2 Saturation*. Click into the *Notes* box and type the text explaining your assessment and intervention.

   • From the *Vitals* box on the lower right side of the window, also select *BP left arm*, *Pt position—Supine*, *Temp source—Tympanic*, and *No complaints of pain*.

7. You complete your admission physical assessment. To document your findings, click on the *Exam* button located below *Vitals*. Notice the *O (Normals)* defaults in the text box in the upper-right box of the window. In this area select the following systems that are within normal limits when you assess your patient: *HEENT*, *Integumentary*, *Musculoskeletal*, *GU (male)*, and

Neurological. As you click on each system, the text populates the *Examination* box on the lower-left side of the window. Use the Enter key to put these items on separate lines to streamline your documentation.

- Click the drop-down arrow next to *O (Normals)* and select *O (Abnormals)*. Select *Chest/ABD* followed by *tachypneic, Posterior Left UL/LL Right UL/ ML/LL crackles.*

- Click into the *Examination* box on the lower left and delete the *UL* on the left and the *UL/ML* on the right so that it reads "Posterior Left LL Right LL crackles". Click your Enter key on your keyboard to put the cursor on the next line.

- Type: *Cardiac: heart sounds—S3.*

- From the *O (Abnormals)* select *Extremities* followed by *edema.* Click into the *Examination* box and type: *bilateral LE +2 pitting on left, +1 pitting on right.*

8. Click *Done.* The *Save As* screen populates. Accept the default entries of *Save to Tab: Encounters* and *Save As: Nurse Note.* Click *Save.*

9. A pop-up appears asking if you want to create a routing slip. Click *No.*

10. In the *Care Tree* in the upper-right corner of the chart window, click the + next to *Encounters.* Click on the date of your *Nurse Note* to view it in the bottom-right corner box.

- Click *Edit.* Click *Sign.* Select *Permanent Sign and Lock* when finished with your *Nurse Note.*

Exercise 4.3

Pneumonia

1. After launching SpringCharts, from the top menu toolbar click on *Actions, Open a Chart.* Type in your last name and click the *Search* button. Select your "pneumonia" patient and the chart opens.

2. Your patient tells you her mother was recently diagnosed with breast cancer. Click on *FMHX* on the left and the *FMHX* populates the box on the right lower side of the screen. Click *Edit* below that box.

- The *Family Medical History* window opens. In the space after *Dx* at the top right type: *breast cancer* and click the *Search* button. *Breast Cancer 174.9* appears in the box below. Click on the listing, which sends this to the *Family Medical History* list on the left-upper box in the window.

- Click *Mother* under the *Preference* section in the lower-right box.

- Click *Back to Chart* at the lower-left side of the window. The information you added appears in the *FMHX* box.

3. Your patient also informs you she takes the over-the-counter medication Zyrtec® 10 mg by mouth daily for allergies she has been having for the last 2 weeks. Click on the *Routine Meds* box and it populates in the bottom right corner. Click *Edit* below that box.

- Click in the space after *Brand Name* at the upper right and type: *Zyrtec.* Click *Search.* Click on the correct dosage/frequency. This sends the medication to the *Routine Medications* list at the upper left.

- Click on the *Zyrtec* that is in the *Routine Medications* list at the upper left. The *Edit Rx* window opens. Click in the calendar to the right of *Date Started* in the left column and choose a date 2 weeks ago. Click *Save.*

- Click *Back to Chart* at the lower-left side of the window. Zyrtec is now listed in the *Routine Meds*.

4. Open your *Nurse Note*. Click *New, New Nurse Note*.

5. Your patient complains of chest congestion, a terrible cough, and shortness of breath. Select these three items in the *S Panel* list at the upper right and they populate the *Chief Complaint* box on the bottom left of the screen.

6. Click on the *Vitals* button located below the *CC* button on the vertical navigation bar on right side of the screen. The *Chief Complaints* now appear in the *Subjective* section of the *Nurse Note*.

   - You take your patient's vital signs. Document the following in the boxes on the lower-left section of the window: Temp *101.4*, Resp *24*, Pulse *110*, BP *120/72*, Ht *68 inches*, Wt *140 lbs*, SaO2 *92%*.

   - Also select *BP left arm*, *Pt position—Supine*, *Temp source—Oral*, *No complaints of pain*, and *Room Air*.

7. You complete your admission physical assessment. To document your findings click on the *Exam* button located below *Vitals*. The *O (Normals)* defaults in the text box in the upper-right box of the window. In this area select the following systems that are within normal limits when you assess your patient: *HEENT*, *Heart Sounds*, *Integumentary*, *Musculoskeletal*, *GU/GYN (female)*, and *Neurological*. As you click on each system, the text populates the *Examination* box on the lower-left side of the window. Use the Enter key to put these items on separate lines to streamline your documentation.

   - Click the drop-down arrow next to *O (Normals)* and select *O (Abnormals)*. Select the *General* section followed by *tachypneic*. Select the *Chest/ABD* section followed by *Anterior wheezes Left UL/LL Posterior Left UL/LL crackles*.

   - Click into the *Examination* box on the left. Delete the *LL* on the anterior left and delete the *UL* after the posterior left so that it reads: "Anterior wheezes Left UL Posterior Left LL crackles".

   - In the same area, click after *crackles* and select Enter on the keyboard. Type in: *Productive cough, moderate amount of thick yellow sputum*.

8. Click *Done*. The *Save As* screen populates. Accept the default entries of *Save to Tab: Encounters* and *Save As: Nurse Note*. Click *Save*.

9. A pop-up appears asking if you want to create a routing slip. Click *No*.

10. In the *Care Tree*, click the + next to *Encounters*. Click on the date of your *Nurse Note* to view it in the bottom-right corner box.

    - Click *Edit*. Click *Sign*. Select *Permanent Sign and Lock* when finished with your *Nurse Note*.

References

Bureau of Labor Statistics. (2010). *Occupational outlook handbook, 2010–11 edition*. Retrieved July 27, 2010, from http://www.bls.gov/oco/ocos083.htm

McCloskey, J.C., Bulechek, G.M & Butcher H. (2008). *Nursing interventions classification (NIC)*(5th ed). St. Louis: Mosby.

Moorhead, S., Johnson, M., Mass, M & Swanson, E. (2008). *Nursing outcomes classification (NOC)*(4th ed). St. Louis: Mosby.

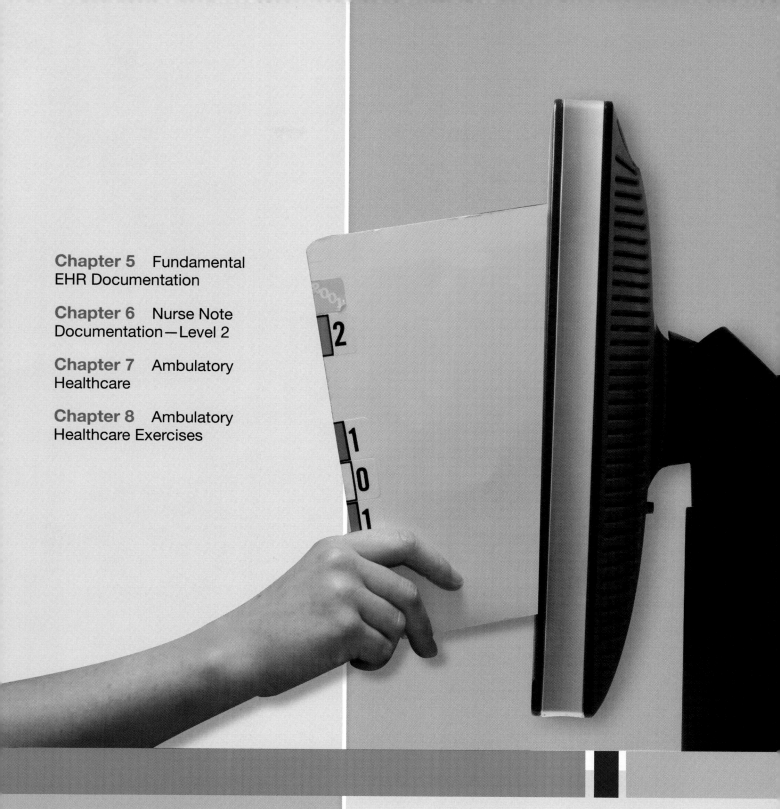

Level Two

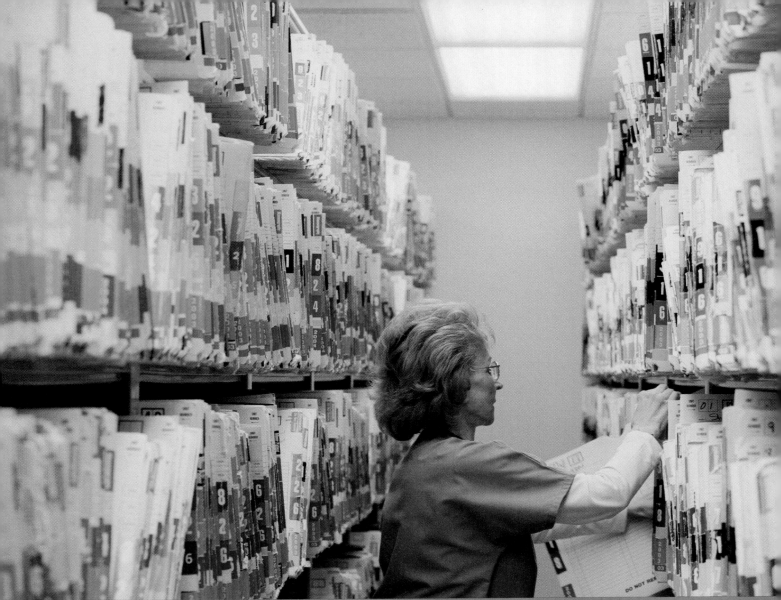

5 Fundamental

Key Term

Terms and abbreviations you will encounter in Chapter 5; they are defined in the end-of-book glossary:

Clinical Practice
Guidelines

Estimated Date of
Delivery (EDD)

Licensed Independent
Practitioner

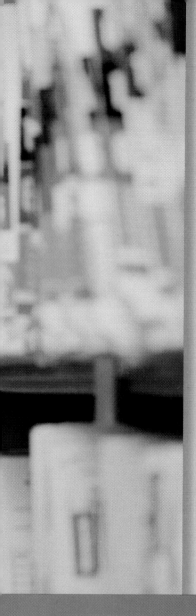

Learning Outcomes

When you complete Chapter 5, you will be able to:

5.1	Use SpringCharts to record vitals.
5.2	Carry out documentation for telephone calls.
5.3	Use SpringCharts to create a letter to a patient and about a patient.
5.4	Use SpringCharts to create a letter unrelated to a patient.
5.5	Carry out sending a test report to a patient.
5.6	Use SpringCharts to create an excuse note and an order form for a patient.
5.7	Use the Plan of Care Manager.
5.8	Use *My Websites*.
5.9	Use the calculator utilities.

EHR Documentation

What You Need to Know

To understand Chapter 5, you need to know how to:

- Start SpringCharts EHR.
- Set user preferences.
- Set up new patients and demographic information.
- Complete face sheets for patients.

LO 5.1   Recording Vital Signs

Typically, vital signs are recorded as part of a regular nurse note or on a flowsheet in an acute care setting or as part of a provider note in an ambulatory setting. Spring-Charts EHR has a feature that allows vital signs to be recorded outside of a regular note. This feature in SpringCharts is primarily used when patients need frequent vital sign monitoring in either the inpatient or outpatient setting. For example, hypertensive patients may come to an outpatient healthcare clinic for the sole purpose of having their blood pressure monitored. In the inpatient setting, patients may have vital signs monitored frequently following procedures or if their condition is unstable. The *Vitals* window contains alert settings that warn the user if the vitals deviate from the accepted minimum and maximum values as illustrated in Figure 5.1. The nurse uses clinical judgment to determine which vital signs to monitor and record based on the patient's condition. It is not necessary to record all vital signs listed.

Note to reader: The following information is intended to be interactive. Take a moment to open SpringCharts on your computer and follow along with the text, performing the actions as instructed.

The *New Vitals Only* section is found under the *New* menu in the patient chart and allows the nurse to document vital signs as needed. A *New Vitals Only* note can be opened while the *Nurse Note* is open. Within the *New Vitals Only* screen a *Note* section can be used for free text documentation or the selection of pop-up text. In addition, previous notes may be copied and pasted here. New vitals are considered *Encounters* and may be viewed once completed.

The *HC* field is for recording the head circumference for infants. The body mass index is grayed out; the program calculates this item from the patient's height and weight. The clinician has the option of right-clicking in any vitals box and selecting a vital from the displayed drop-down lists. This feature is particularly useful when healthcare personnel are using a PC tablet, an iPad™, or other portable computers without a keyboard.

A *Notes* navigation button is available on the right side of the *Vitals* window providing pop-up text to record details about the vital signs (see margin illustration). A *Previous Notes* section is displayed in the lower-right quadrant where notes

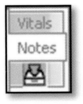

Notes tab in *Vitals* window

Figure 5.1
New Vitals Only window

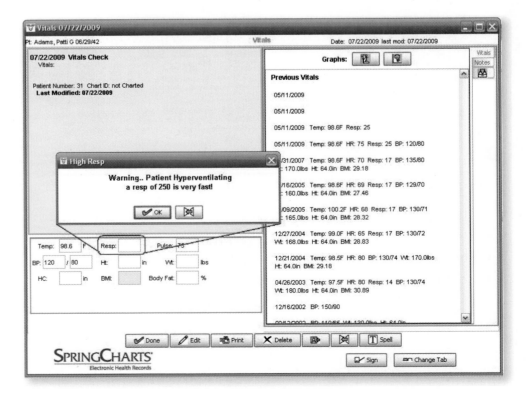

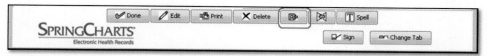

Figure 5.2
Convert Note button

recorded in prior encounters can be viewed and copied as current notes. A time and initial stamp in the *Notes* panel enables the nurse to record when the vital signs were measured.

Three additional customized fields can be created within the *Vitals* window to record other frequently monitored health measures. For example, in an intensive care setting, nurses may frequently measure and record pressures in the heart, lungs, and brain. In an outpatient setting, nurses may measure and record the height of a pregnant woman's uterus at each visit. Additional fields for such specialized measures are added in the *Administration* panel under the *Vitals* section. In the *Custom Vitals Editor* the label, units, and minimum and maximum values are added. Once "enabled," the newly created measurements are displayed in the *Vitals* window as an additional field. SpringCharts client programs must be shut down and rebooted to see these additional items added to the SpringCharts server.

In the outpatient setting, vital signs and notes can be transposed into a regular office visit note by selecting the *Convert Note* button at the bottom of the screen (see Figure 5.2). This action places the vital signs into an *Office Visit* note where they appear in the *Objective* portion of the SOAP note. Here, the provider may enhance the entry to include diagnoses and procedures. Once changed to an office visit note, the original *New Vitals Only* note cannot be filed separately. A nurse may change the vitals and notes into an office visit note if it is determined that the patient should be seen by the primary care provider during the same encounter. This may occur if the patient's vital signs are abnormal and require prompt attention. The ability to convert any kind of patient encounter note into an office visit note reduces documentation time and increases efficiency.

Before saving the vitals note, the nurse may initial or sign and permanently lock the note by choosing the *Sign* button. When the *Sign* window is displayed, the *Initial Only* option stamps the user's initials and time at the end of the note. The *Permanently Sign and Lock* option places the user's full name along with the date and time at the bottom of the note, then locks the note. After this point no modifications can be made to the vital signs or note. *Vitals* records are filed in the care tree under *Encounters*.

Graph Vital Signs: This feature is accessed by selecting one of the two *Graph Vital Signs* buttons (see margin illustration) located in the upper right area of the *Vitals* window, also shown in Figure 5.1. It is similar to vital sign graphs that can be viewed within the *Nurse Note* (discussed in Chapter 4) and provides graphic representation of blood pressure (BP), height/weight, body mass index (BMI), and body fat percentage for adults. Head circumference is also graphed for infants. For children between the ages of 2 and 18 years, data are viewed on a standard, gender-based growth chart, allowing a comparison of the child's height and weight to national percentiles. Height and weight for infants younger than 36 months of age are graphed against a backdrop showing the appropriate national percentiles. The graph type is automatically adjusted by the program based on the patient's age and gender. At the bottom of the *Graph* window the *[Print]* button may be used to print the graph that is currently being viewed. An adult graph is illustrated in Figure 5.3.

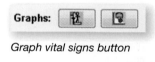

Graph vital signs button

Figure 5.3
Height/Weight graph for adult

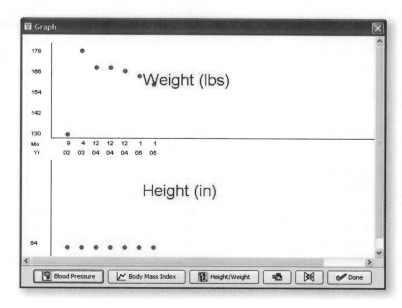

Concept Checkup 5.1

A. When is the *New Vitals Only* feature used in SpringCharts? _____
_____

B. *True or False.* A user must manually calculate a patient's BMI once the height and weight are recorded. _____

Legal/Ethical Considerations

Leaving messages on an answering machine or with anyone other than the patient may allow unauthorized persons to access private health information and may be a violation of HIPAA. Healthcare facilities have policies that determine how and to whom information may be given over the phone. Nurses should adhere to facility policy to protect themselves against liability.

Legal/Ethical Considerations

Hospitals have policies governing the release of information to a patient's significant others. For example, some hospitals provide a personal identification number to individuals who may receive information about a patient. Strict adherence to facility policy is necessary to prevent release of private health information to unauthorized individuals.

Documentation Tip

Record all phone calls to or from a primary care provider. Document the time the call was made, specific details of the message, and the response of the primary care provider.

Exercise 5.1

Recording and Viewing Vital Signs

1. Open your chart. Under the *New* menu select *New Vitals Only*.
2. Record a set of vital signs. Select verbiage from the pop-up text. Click the *Done* button and *Save* and *Skip Billing*.
3. Close and reopen your chart by selecting your name from the *Recent Charts* menu on the *Main* menu bar.
4. Open the *Actions* menu within the patient's chart. Select *Graph Vital Signs* and view the various graphed vital signs.
5. Open the *Body Mass Index* graph and print a copy. Write your name on the sheet and submit to your instructor. (See *Submitting Assignments Electronically* on page xxvii of the Preface for electronic submission instructions).

LO 5.2   ## Documenting Telephone Calls

Nurses often make telephone calls that require documentation. In the outpatient setting, the nurse may call to give a patient instructions, check on the patient's status after a procedure, or notify the patient of the date and time for a diagnostic test. In addition, the nurse may call in a prescription to the patient's pharmacy. In the inpatient setting, nurses call healthcare providers and patient families to inform them of changes in the patient's condition or to receive clarification of orders. While nurses make telephone calls for multiple reasons, documentation of these calls is important to demonstrate that standards of care have been followed. SpringCharts provides a mechanism for quick and easy documentation of telephone calls.

New TC Note creates a new telephone call encounter form. A user may create a *New TC Note* by selecting *New > New TC Note* from the patient's chart screen. Text can be chosen from predefined pop-up text in the displayed window (see Figure 5.4). Text from previous telephone call notes appears in the lower-right quadrant. This text can be highlighted and copied into the existing note using the *Copy Note* icon. The date stamp and initial stamp are also available in this window enabling the user to initial the note. The *Rx* navigation tab is displayed on the right side to access the patient's routine medications and a list of previous prescriptions. This function is useful in the outpatient setting, particularly if a medication needs to be prescribed or renewed as a result of the conversation. The provider may document and print the patient's prescription by selecting from these lists or adding the medication after searching the database. While a nurse practitioner may prescribe medications, an office nurse may print a prescription for a medication renewal for the **licensed independent practitioner** to sign.

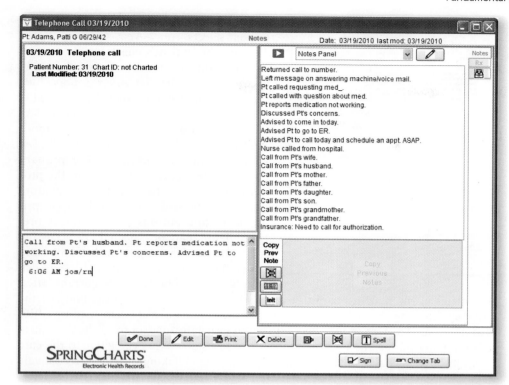

Figure 5.4
Telephone Call window

Chart Summary icon

Figure 5.5
Saving telephone call note to *Care Tree* window

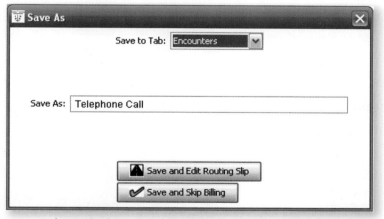

The *Chart Summary* icon is available in the navigation tabs below the *Rx* tab (see margin illustration). This tab is used to view the entire face sheet.

A *telephone call* note may be converted into an *office visit* note in this window. Once the *Convert Note* icon is selected (see Figure 5.4), text from the *TC note* appears in the *Objective* portion of the office visit note and prescribed medications appear in the *Plan* section on the SOAP note.

When the *TC note* is completed and the nurse selects the *Done* button, the program allows the option of billing for the phone consultation, as seen in Figure 5.5. In several states, patient telephone consultations are a billable encounter.

LO 5.3 Creating a Letter to a Patient or About a Patient

In the inpatient setting, nurses rarely create letters to patients. In the outpatient setting, however, the nurse may prepare letters to inform patients of scheduled diagnostic tests and the necessary preparation, lab results, or specific provider instructions. Creating patient letters is supported by SpringCharts.

New Letter to Pt creates a new letter addressed to the patient. To create a new letter to a patient, a user selects *New > New Letter to Pt* from the patient's chart screen. The program automatically inserts the patient's name, address, greeting, and close. The user completes the body of the letter by typing in the text field or by choosing appropriate pop-up text.

Typically, letters *about* patients are written from one primary care provider to another, usually regarding a consultation. *New Letter ABOUT Pt* creates a new letter concerning the patient, as illustrated in Figure 5.6.

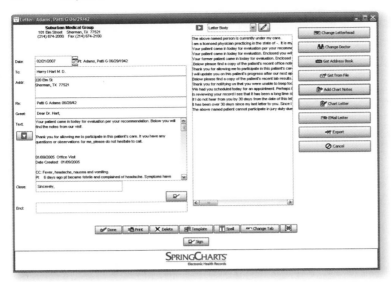

Figure 5.6

New Letter ABOUT Patient window

FOCAL POINT

Letters to or about the patient can be quickly created by using drop-in addresses and pop-up text and adding chart notes.

Signature icon button

Figure 5.7

New Letter option on the main menu

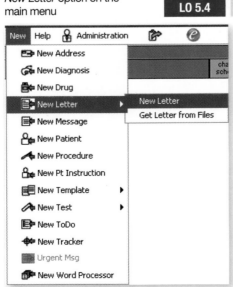

To create a new letter about a patient, a user selects *New>New Letter ABOUT Pt* from the patient's chart screen. Recipient and address information can be easily retrieved from the *Get Address Book* button in the right-hand panel. Pop-up text is available in the *Letter Body* category. As with all pop-up windows, text may be modified and added by selecting the *Edit Pen* icon. If multiple practices and/or primary care providers have been set up in the program, alternate letterheads and signature names can be selected using the appropriate navigation buttons to the right. A pretyped letter can be selected by accessing the *Get from File* button in the right-hand panel. These previously created letters can be added to the body of the current letter.

All entries in the patient's care tree are also available to add into the body of the letter by selecting the *Add Chart Notes* button. This is useful when sending office visit notes such as test results, encounter notes, or information from the face sheet to a referring physician. The *Chart It* button saves a copy of the letter to the care tree, although this also automatically happens when clicking on *Done*. To activate the spell checker for letter content, the user clicks on the *Spell* button. The letter can be printed or e-mailed to a recipient. The *Export* button enables the user to export the letter to another word processing program, where it can be reformatted, if necessary. The *Signature* icon, as seen in the margin reference, located at the bottom of the letter enables the user to choose the signature to be placed on the letter. The options are the user's name or the default practitioner's name that was chosen in the *User Preferences* window during setup. If a user wants to permanently lock a letter so that no changes can be made to it after it is sent, then the *Sign* button must be accessed and the *Permanently Sign and Lock* button activated. Once a letter has been signed and locked, then saved, it can be viewed but not edited, even by the author.

(See Appendix A, *Sample Documents*—Document 2: *Letter to a Patient*.)
(See Appendix A, *Sample Documents*—Document 3: *Letter About a Patient*.)

LO 5.4   Creating a Letter Unrelated to a Patient

Users can also produce correspondence in SpringCharts for recipients such as attorneys, hospitals, and accountants. Letter categories are set up in the *Administration* menu under the *Category Preferences* window. Letters unrelated to a patient are created in the SpringCharts client under *New > New Letter* on the main menu bar, illustrated in Figure 5.7.

Letters can be written by selecting pop-up text, by typing in the specific fields, by handwriting on a portable computer, or through voice recognition software. The template layout looks similar to the one used when creating *New Letter to Pt* and *New Letter ABOUT Pt* in the patient's chart; however, these letters cannot be placed in a patient's record. Once the letter is created, the user selects *File it* and chooses a category file under which to save the letter. Letters are retrieved by selecting *New > New Letter > Get Letter from Files*. A filed letter can also be incorporated into a letter to or about a patient by selecting the *Get from File* button in the *New Letter* window in the patient's chart.

LO 5.5 | Sending a Test Report to a Patient

Normal diagnostic test results may be posted or e-mailed to a patient, particularly from the primary care provider's office. *New Test Report* creates a blank test reporting form. A user may create a new test report by selecting *New > New Test Report* from the patient's chart screen. Completed tests for the patient can be added to the report from the selection list, shown in Figure 5.8. Identified *problem* areas and *recommendations* can be added from the pop-up list by selecting the appropriate categories. Test descriptions for *New Test Reports* are created and edited by selecting *Edit > Tests Explanations* from the main screen. When the specific test is selected from the patient's *Select Test* list, a report explanation, in layman's terms, is automatically added. Multiple tests can be selected and added to a single test report. The completed test report can be either printed or e-mailed to the recipient.

(See Appendix A, *Sample Documents*—Document 4: *Test Report to Patient.*)

FOCAL POINT

Test reports that contain the test result and test description can be created for patients. Text can be added to the report that identifies problem areas and recommendations.

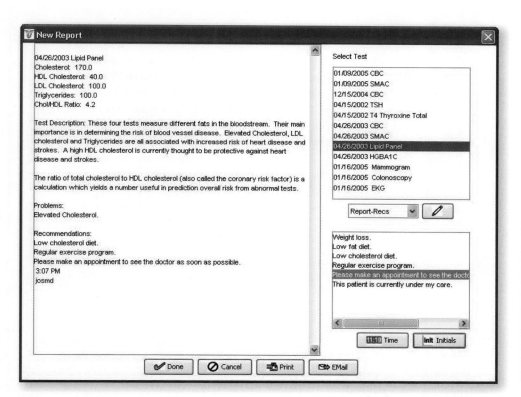

Figure 5.8
New Test Report window

Legal/Ethical Considerations

Transmitting private health information via e-mail risks disclosure to unauthorized individuals since it travels over the internet or may be accidentally sent to the wrong e-mail address. Nurses should adhere to facility policy to protect themselves against liability.

Concept Checkup 5.2

A. What is documented using *New TC Note*? _____

B. What navigation button is used in the *New Letter ABOUT Pt* window to include test results, encounter notes, or information from the face sheet when writing to a referring practitioner? _____

C. What is selected from the main screen to create and edit test descriptions for test reports? _____.

Exercise 5.2

Creating a New Letter About a Patient

1. Click Actions, Open a Chart. Type an "a" in the blank and click in the binocular icon to search. Click on Adams, Patti G. Under the *New* menu select *New Letter ABOUT Pt.*

2. Select the referring physician, Dr. Harry Hart, from the *Get Address Book* button.

3. Choose the pop-up text that begins with: *Thank you for allowing me to participate . . .*

4. Click on the *Edit PopUp Text* icon. Select the *Letter Body* category on the left-hand side of the *Edit PopUp Text* window.

5. Add the following sentence on an empty line: *Below please find a copy of the patient's recent lab results.* Click on the *Done* button.

6. Back in the *Letter* window, place the cursor in the letter body on a new line and select the newly added pop-up text sentence. Also, click on the sentence: *I will update you on this patient's progress after our next appointment.*

7. Click on the *Add Chart Notes* button and select the lipid panel results from the *Chart Entry* window. The lab test results are added to the body of the letter. Select the *Signature* icon and select a signature.

8. Print or electronically create the letter, including letterhead, and submit to your instructor. (See page xxvii in the Preface for instructions on submitting an electronic document.)

9. Click on the *Done* button and select *Correspondence* as the category to which the letter will be stored in the patient's care tree.

10. In your chart, click on the "+" expand symbol beside the *Correspondence* category in the care tree to see the saved copy of the letter.

Exercise 5.3

Creating a Test Report for a Patient

1. Click Actions, Open a Chart. Type an "a" in the blank and click in the binocular icon to search. Click on Adams, Patti G. Under the *New* menu select *New Test Report.*

2. Highlight the lipid panel in the *Select Test* window. The program automatically adds the test description to the bottom of the test results.

3. Place the cursor in the body of the report under the section heading *Problems.* Select *Elevated Cholesterol* from the pop-up text in the lower-right panel.

4. Click on the down arrow in the pop-up text category window to reveal the list of pop-up text categories. Select *Report-Recs.* Place your cursor under the section heading *Recommendations.* Now select the following pop-up text line items: *Low cholesterol diet. Regular exercise program. Please make an appointment to see your primary care provider as soon as possible.*

5. Print or electronically create the test report and submit to your instructor.

6. Click on the *Done* button and store a copy of the report under the *Reports to Patient* category in the care tree. A "+" expand symbol is placed beside the *Reports to Patients* header in the care tree. Click the "+" symbol to see the saved report.

LO 5.6 Creating an Excuse Note and Order Form for a Patient

In both the inpatient and outpatient setting, nurses may be asked to provide a work or school excuse for time missed due to illness. In addition, diagnostic testing may be ordered for a future date and the patient must have the provider's written order to have the test completed. All of these functions are available in SpringCharts.

New Excuse/Note/Order creates printable forms for work or school excuses, notes, and provider orders for tests or procedures. To create a new excuse for a patient, select *New > New Excuse/Note/Order > New Excuse/Note* from the patient's chart screen. Pop-up text is available to avoid typing a note each time. Excuse notes are automatically saved under the *Excuses/Notes* category of the care tree.

To create an order form for a patient, select *New > New Excuse/Note/Order > New Order* from the patient's chart screen. When completing an order form, the user is given the option to chart the order in the patient's care tree. Order forms are used to record orders for lab, imaging, and medical tests that are conducted at a third-party facility. Within the *Orders* window the user selects a medical diagnosis from the patient's *Previous Dx* window to associate a relevant diagnosis with the test that is ordered. The program automatically prints the ordering provider's name on the order form. The user is given the option to have the order form signed electronically by adding the phrase "Electronic Signature Verified" to the form. Many outside testing facilities require that the patient's insurance information be included on the order form. If the patient's primary insurance has been recorded in the face sheet, the user selects the *Add Patient Ins* button in the lower portion of the window and the insurance information is added to the bottom of the order form.

Figure 5.9

Selecting *Care Plan* from the *Tools* menu

LO 5.7 Using Practice Guidelines

As discussed in Chapter 1, healthcare professionals integrate research-based clinical guidelines into patient care planning. Retrieval of these guidelines is often difficult and time-consuming. To meet this need, SpringCharts provides access to the National Guideline Clearinghouse™ (NGC). The NGC is a comprehensive database of evidence-based **clinical practice guidelines** and related documents. The NGC website contains numerous healthcare treatment plans containing objective, detailed clinical information for physicians, nurses, and other healthcare professionals.

In order to keep evidence-based guidelines readily available for a patient's condition, a nurse may attach a text document with *Plan of Care* or *Practice Guidelines* to a patient's *Nurse Note* so it remains a permanent record associated with that nurse note. To access a practice guideline, the nurse selects the *Tools* menu from within the *Nurse Note* screen and chooses *Care Plan*, as seen in Figure 5.9. Once selected, an interface window opens that enables the user to import a *Plan of Care* document. This document may be a site-specific care plan document or a document accessed through the NGC. The user simply searches for and highlights the specific document, copies it using the [Ctrl]+[C] keys, then pastes it into the patient's *Care Plan/Guideline* window using the [Ctrl]+[V] keys. A saved plan of care guideline is displayed in Figure 5.10. After saving the *Nurse Note*, the *Care Plan* may be viewed at the bottom of the *Nurse Note* when selected in the patient's chart care tree, illustrated in Figure 5.11.

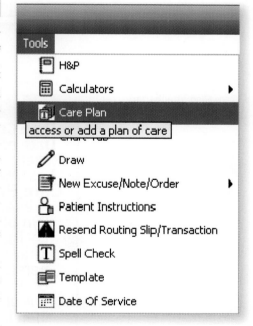

LO 5.8 Using "My Websites"

In addition to the National Guidelines Clearinghouse™, SpringCharts offers access to other Internet resources. *My Websites* is a feature found in the *Productivity Center* menu, illustrated in Figure 5.12. This window lists websites for rapid access. Figure 5.13 shows web addresses of several highly rated knowledge bases that are included with the SpringCharts setup. This feature is user-defined so all users can have their own unique

FOCAL POINT

The *My Websites* feature is a user-defined function of SpringCharts that contains websites commonly accessed by the user.

Figure 5.10

Care plan selected from
either the computer or the
NGC website

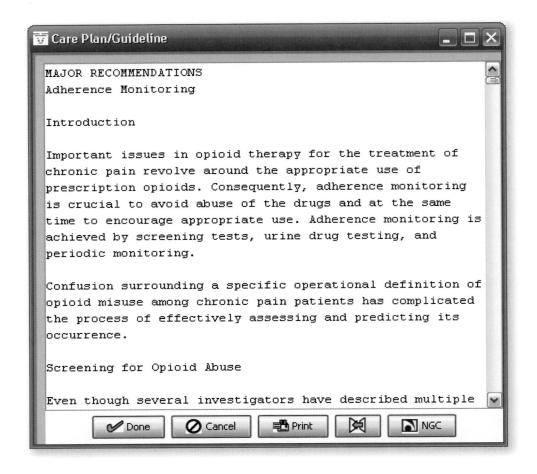

Figure 5.11

Care Plan attached to
Nurse Note

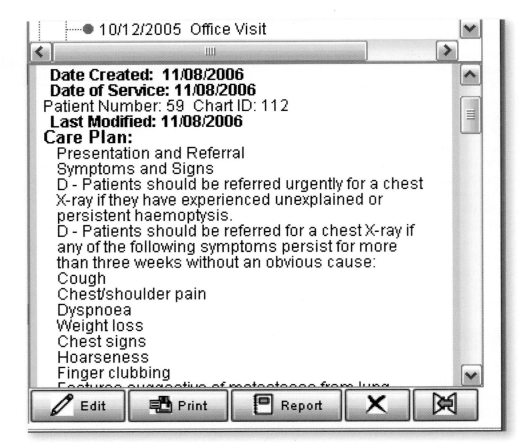

list of website links. The user simply clicks on an item to activate the browser to go to the website from within SpringCharts. The list can be edited by clicking the *Edit* button. The *My Websites* edit window, shown in Figure 5.14, is displayed. Here the user enters the website name and the URL address in the format indicated. The new website is added to the list in the *My Websites* window. Nurses may choose to add websites that contain nursing-specific best practice guidelines such as the Joanna Briggs Institute Best Practice Series at http://www.joannabriggs.edu.au/pubs/best_practice.php or the "How To *try this*" web site at http://www.nursingcenter.com/library/static.asp?pageid=730390 that provides evidence-based tools for the care of geriatric patients. The *My Websites* function may also be useful for acquiring patient education materials, but care must be taken to ensure that reputable websites providing accurate instructions are used. Ultimately, the nurse is responsible for the information given to patients.

LO 5.9 | Using the Calculator Utilities

Nurses perform multiple calculations in their practice. SpringCharts contains three types of calculators: a conversion calculator, a pregnancy expected date of delivery (EDD) calculator, and a simple calculator. The three types of calculators may be selected either from the *Utilities* menu from the main screen or from the *Tools* menu in the *Nurse Note* screen and the *Office Visit* screen.

Conversion Calculator

The SpringCharts conversion calculator, displayed in Figure 5.15, converts imperial units to metric measurements and vice versa. To activate the conversion calculator, the user clicks on the *Utilities* menu and selects *Calculator > Conversion Calculator*. The user adds the measurement in the weight, length, or temperature field; selects the originating units of measure; and then clicks on the *Convert* button to translate the units to the alternate measurements.

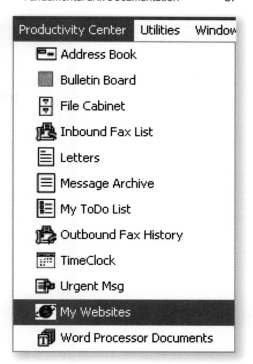

Figure 5.12

Accessing *My Websites* from the *Productivity Center* menu

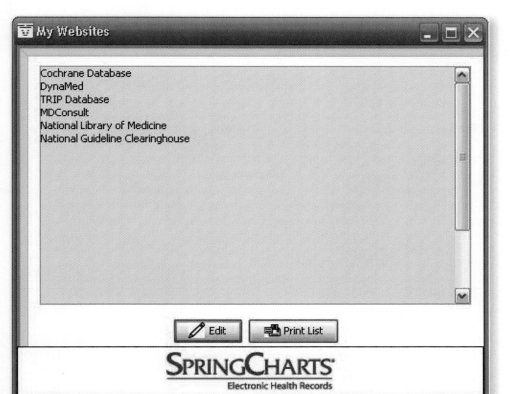

Figure 5.13

List of user-defined websites

FOCAL POINT

SpringCharts contains three types of calculators: conversion, pregnancy, and simple calculators.

Figure 5.14
My Websites edit window

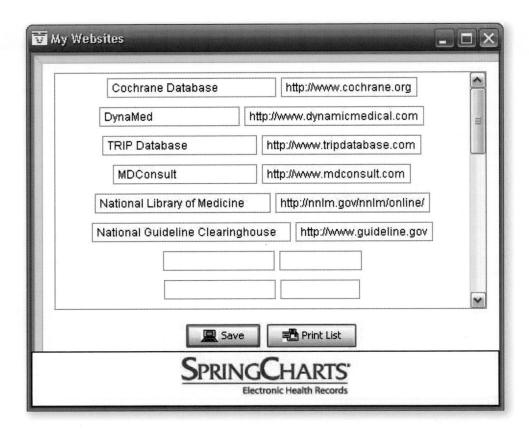

Figure 5.15
Conversion Calculator
window

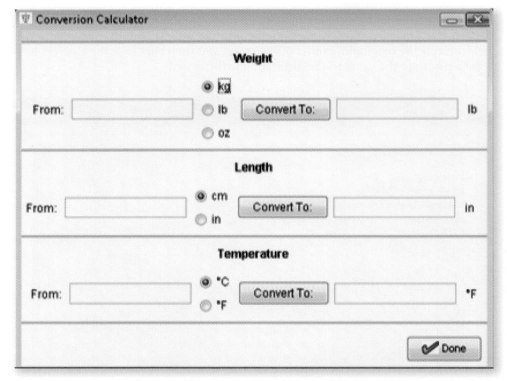

Delivery Date Calculator

The *Delivery Date Calculator*, seen in Figure 5.16, is useful for determining the **estimated date of delivery (EDD)** for a pregnancy. The nurse selects the last menstrual period (LMP) date from the calendar and the calculator extrapolates the approximate fetal age and delivery date. The EDD can be captured and pasted into the nurse note by selecting the *Copy EDD* button and pasting into a *Nurse Note* or note.

Simple Calculator

SpringCharts also provides a basic calculator to process simple algorithms.

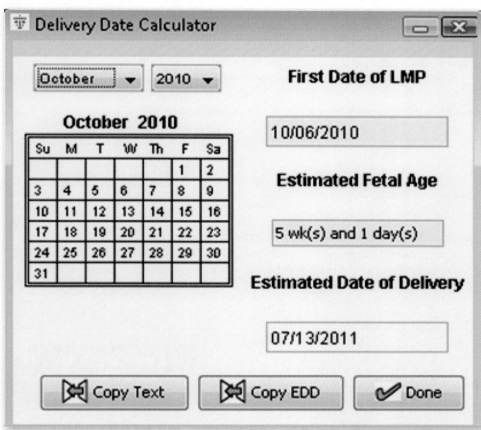

Figure 5.16
Delivery Date Calculator window

Concept Checkup 5.3

A. What items are ordered using order forms?

1. _____

2. _____

3. _____

B. Which menu item would a nurse select within the nurse note to document a plan of care guideline?

_____

C. What are the three types of calculators available in SpringCharts?

1. _____

2. _____

3. _____

Adding a New My Website Link

1. Under the *Productivity Center*, open the *My Websites* option. In the *My Websites* window, click on the *Edit* button.
2. In the next available field, place the cursor to the far left and type in the subject: *Patient Instructions.* In the right-side field, place the cursor to the far left of the field and type in the URL address: *http://www.familydoctor.org*. Follow the same format as the other links. Save your website addition.
3. In the *My Websites* window, click on the newly added *Patient Instructions* link. The Internet browser is activated and the website is accessed directly from SpringCharts. This website has a wealth of patient instruction sheets that can be copied into SpringCharts as patient instructions or printed directly from this website. The nurse is responsible to ensure that the instructions obtained from any website are accurate.
4. Close the Internet browser and the *My Websites* window.

Calculating an Estimated Delivery Date

1. Open the *Delivery Date* calculator under the *Utility* menu.
2. Your patient's last menstrual period was 6 weeks ago. Select that date from the calendar. The date is automatically entered into the LMP field and the estimated gestational age of your patient's fetus is calculated along with the estimated date of delivery.

Adding a Practice Guideline

1. Add a practice guideline to a patient's chart. Open the chart for your patient with diabetes. Select the *Nurse Note* in the care tree that dealt with the diabetes symptoms. Edit the *Nurse Note*.
2. In the *Nurse Note* screen, select the *Tools* menu and choose *Care Plan.* In the *Care Plan/Guideline* window, click on the *NGC* button. (Care plan guidelines can be attached from a location stored on the computer, stored on a computer on the network, or downloaded from the National Guidelines Clearinghouse.)
3. On the NGC website type: *diabetes* in the search field and search for the guidelines. Locate and open the *Basic guidelines for diabetes care* plan. Highlight the recommendations section, copy the information using the [Ctrl]+[C] keys, and close the web browser. Paste the material into the *Care Plan/Guideline* window by using the [Ctrl]+[V] keys. Click the *Done* button, close the *Nurse Note* screen, and skip billing.
4. Notice the practice guideline added to the bottom of the *Nurse Note* in the lower-right corner on the patient's chart.
5. Print or electronically create the *Nurse Note* by clicking on the *Print* button in the lower right. Submit the document to your instructor. (See page xxvii in the Preface for instructions on submitting an electronic document.)
6. Close the patient chart.

Checking Your Understanding

Write "T" or "F" in the blank to indicate whether the statement is true or false.

_____ 1. SpringCharts automatically calculates the BMI in the *Vitals* window once the blood pressure values are saved.

_____ 2. To graph vital signs in SpringCharts, a user must input the vital signs into a Microsoft Excel document and use the graphing feature that is available in the Excel document.

_____ 3. A user may add a patient's chart notes to a letter created in SpringCharts.

_____ 4. A user may add a practice guideline document to a *Nurse Note*.

_____ 5. *My Websites* is a feature that allows a nurse to create new practice guidelines.

_____ 6. A user may convert pounds to inches using the *Conversion Calculator.*

_____ 7. A nurse may create a *New Test Report* for a patient from the *New* menu within a patient's chart.

_____ 8. Order forms are used to record the ordering of lab, imaging, and medical tests.

Answer the questions below in the space provided.

9. List the three calculators that are available in SpringCharts.

   1. _____

   2. _____

   3. _____

10. Which vital sign text box is used to record the head circumference for infants?

   _____

11. What three items are automatically populated when creating a new letter to a patient in SpringCharts?

   1. _____

   2. _____

   3. _____

Choose the best answer and circle the corresponding letter.

12. Which of the following communication methods may present a risk of HIPAA violation? (Select all that apply.)

   a) Leaving a voice mail with a patient's lab results, which may allow unauthorized persons to access the information

   b) Leaving a voice mail for a patient to call the primary care provider against hospital policy

   c) E-mailing a patient report to another primary care provider outside the health system

13. One way to access *My Websites* is by

   a) accessing the *New* menu in a patient's chart

   b) accessing the *Productivity Center* menu from the main screen

   c) accessing the *Nurse Note* screen

14. The National Guideline Clearinghouse is a database of clinical practice guidelines that are
    a) Physician opinion articles
    b) Nursing theory
    c) Evidence-based

15. When a nurse uses practice guidelines in SpringCharts, which website is accessible from SpringCharts for importing recommended guidelines?
    a) Family Doctor
    b) American Medical Association
    c) National Guideline Clearinghouse

16. The nurse calls a patient to give instructions for upcoming diagnostic tests. Where should this information be documented?
    a) *New TC Note*
    b) *New Nurse Note*
    c) *New Phone Call*

17. A nurse on the medical-surgical unit often refers to the Joanna Briggs Institute Best Practice Series online to guide practice. Where can the nurse store this website in SpringCharts?
    a) *New Websites*
    b) *My Websites*
    c) *Website Archives*

18. The nurse practitioner determines that the patient needs a chest x-ray. How does the nurse practitioner access a *New Order Form* to order the chest x-ray?
    a) By selecting *New > New Excuse/Note/Order* from within the patient's chart
    b) By selecting *New > New Excuse/Note/Order* from within a *Nurse Note*
    c) From the *Productivity Center* menu in the main screen

19. What are the two types of letters that can be created from within a patient's chart?
    a) *Letter for Pt, Letter ABOUT Pt*
    b) *Letter to Pt, Letter ABOUT Pt*
    c) *Non-patient letter, Letter ABOUT Pt*

20. Which vital sign is automatically calculated in SpringCharts?
    a) Body fat percentage
    b) Body mass index
    c) O2 saturation

21. How many additional customized vital sign fields may be added from the *Administration* panel of SpringCharts?
    a) None
    b) 4
    c) 3

22. The nurse needs to communicate the results of a normal chest x-ray to a patient who has gone home. Which feature would the nurse use?
    a) *New Test Report*
    b) *New TC Note*
    c) *New Nurse Note*

23. Which additional navigation button appears in a *New TC Note* window?

    a) *[Other Tx]*

    b) *[Rx]*

    c) *[Dx]*

24. When graphing vital signs in SpringCharts, what age must a patient be in order to see height and weight graphed against a backdrop showing the appropriate national percentiles?

    a) Younger than 65 years

    b) Older than 36 months

    c) Younger than 36 months

25. Which menu in the *Nurse Note* screen does a user select to access the *Care Plan* feature?

    a) *Tools* menu

    b) *Actions* menu

    c) *New* menu

Reference

Institute of Medicine. (1990). *Clinical practice guidelines: Directions for a new program.* M.J. Field and K.N. Lohr (eds.) Washington, DC: National Academy Press.

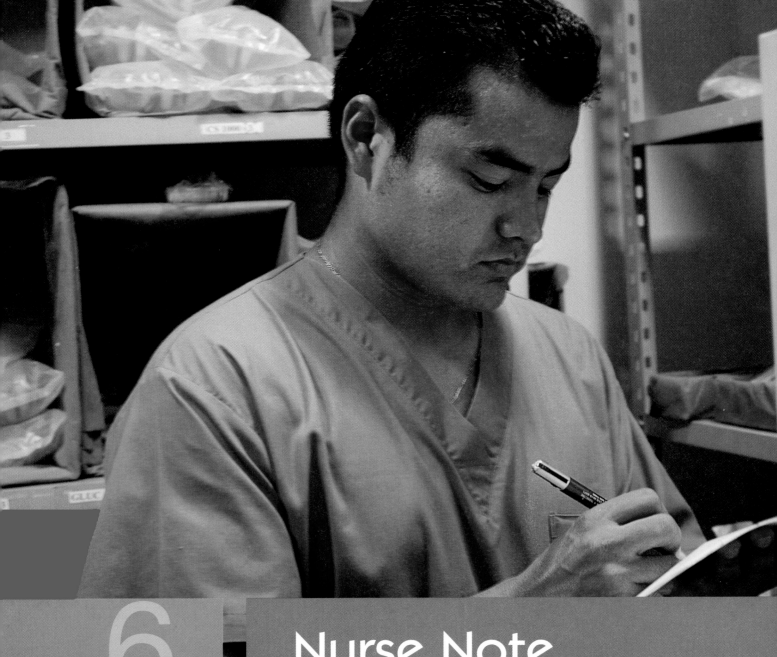

6 | Nurse Note

Key Terms

Terms and abbreviations you will encounter in Chapter 6; they are defined in the end-of-book glossary:

Medical Diagnosis

Nursing Diagnosis

Objective Data

Subjective Data

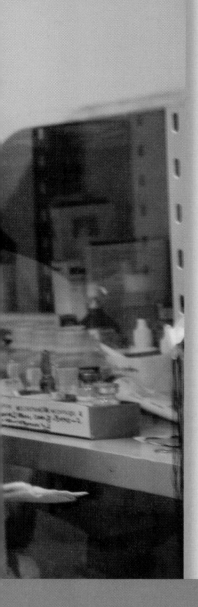

Learning Outcomes

When you complete Chapter 6, you will be able to:

6.1 Use NANDA-International (NANDA-I) approved nursing diagnoses to reflect patient needs.

6.2 Identify patient-specific goals using nursing outcomes classifications (NOC).

6.3 Identify and document nursing interventions using nursing intervention classifications (NIC).

6.4 Carry out documentation of medication administration.

6.5 Carry out documentation of intake and output (I&O).

Documentation—Level 2

What You Need to Know

To understand Chapter 6, you need to know how to:

- Create a new *Nurse Note* record.
- Navigate through the basic elements of a *Nurse Note*.
- Update *Face Sheet* information from the *Nurse Note*.
- Select applicable *Chief Complaints*.
- Document *Vital Signs*.
- Select/document an assessment.

Overview

Standardized language provides a mechanism by which a profession communicates. It promotes "shared understanding and continuity of care" (Thoroddsen and Ehnfors, 2007). In nursing, standard language reflects the nursing process: nursing diagnoses, nursing outcomes, and nursing interventions. In addition to facilitating the use of technology, standard language allows for comparison of nursing activities and outcomes in diverse settings and locations, thereby enabling nursing research to demonstrate the value of nursing in promoting positive patient outcomes. Another benefit of standardized terminology is enhanced quality of patient care through promotion of compliance to standards of care (Rutherford, 2008). The American Nurses Association (ANA) (2007) recognizes 12 current standard terminology systems. One of these systems, the NANDA-I nursing diagnosis classification, is widely used and researched internationally (Muller-Staub, 2009). Nursing outcomes classification (NOC) and nursing intervention classification (NIC) are research-based and comprehensive, and link to NANDA-I nursing diagnoses. Their widespread acceptance makes them ideal for use in an electronic health record (EHR) (University of Iowa College of Nursing, n.d.).

LO 6.1 Dx (Nursing Diagnosis)

Nursing care is guided by the nursing process. A nurse initiates the nursing process by assessing the patient's needs through the collection of subjective and objective data. **Subjective data** are the descriptions given by the patient or family about the patient's condition. **Objective data** are collected by the nurse through observation, auscultation or hearing, palpation or touch, and smell. Other sources of objective data include information obtained from the health record such as diagnostic results and medical diagnoses. These data allow the nurse to identify the patient's problems and potential problems that are communicated as **nursing diagnoses**. Nursing diagnoses differ from medical diagnoses. **Medical diagnoses** relate to a disease process while nursing diagnoses are concerned with a patient's response to illness. NANDA-I (n.d.) defines nursing diagnosis as "a clinical judgment about individual, family, or community experiences and responses to actual or potential health problems and life processes."

Once nursing diagnoses are identified, they must be prioritized. Maslow's hierarchy of needs may be used as a good, basic framework for setting priorities. High priority is assigned to nursing diagnoses that relate to vital physiologic functions such as airway, breathing, and circulation. The next level of priority is those problems that are a threat to the individual's health or ability to cope. Low-priority nursing diagnoses are those for which a delayed intervention will not cause significant harm to the patient.

The next step in the nursing process is planning. The nurse identifies the desired outcomes for the patient, which may be expressed using the nursing outcomes classification (NOC) statements. These outcomes describe the goals of nursing care and should be developed in collaboration with the patient. After establishing outcomes, the nurse plans actions to be taken to help the patient achieve these outcomes. These actions are stated using nursing intervention classifications (NIC).

In the subsequent phase of the nursing process, the nurse implements the interventions and determines the patient's response to each. Finally, the patient's progress toward meeting the outcomes is evaluated and nursing diagnoses are either resolved, continued, or modified.

SpringCharts uses NANDA-I nursing diagnoses, NOC, and NIC to facilitate documentation of the nursing process. Once the patient assessment is complete and subjective and objective data are collected and recorded as delineated in Chapter 4, the nurse is ready to analyze these data to identify patient problems or potential problems and assign nursing diagnoses. Nursing diagnoses are entered from the *Nurse Note* screen. (Reminder: A new *Nurse Note* is created by selecting the *New* menu within the patient's chart and clicking *New Nurse Note*.) The *Dx* tab on the navigation bar at the right, as seen in Figure 6.1, offers the user a view of medical diagnoses logged by providers from previous patient encounters. The nurse can see diagnoses from the *PMHX + Problem List* window or the *Previous Diagnoses* window, also seen in

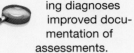

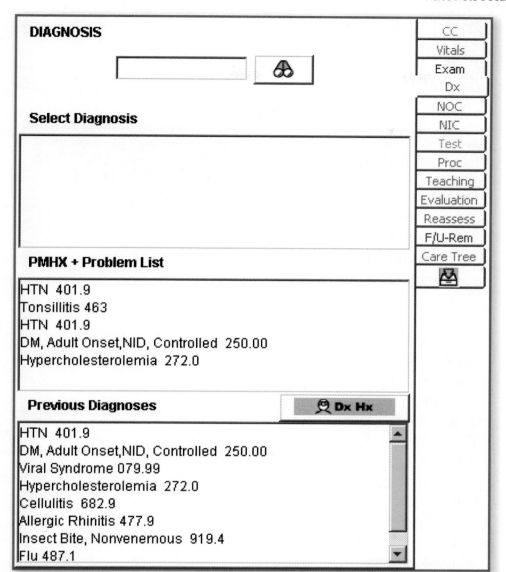

Figure 6.1
Previous Diagnoses
window in the *Dx* tab

Figure 6.1. The *PMHX + Problem List* window displays diagnoses from these two areas of the patient's *Face Sheet* and the *Previous Diagnoses* window displays all the medical diagnoses from previous physician encounters with this patient. This feature provides ambulatory nurses with a quick overview of the patient's past medical problems and allows a nurse practitioner to rapidly select a medical diagnosis previously assigned to the patient.

To document nursing diagnoses, the user clicks the red *NANDA* box on the far lower-left corner of the screen, as seen in Figure 6.2. The *Dx Text* window displays. The text at the top of the list encourages the user to enter the diagnoses in order of priority for the patient. High-priority nursing diagnoses should be selected first. When the user clicks on a nursing diagnosis, it is entered into the field at the bottom of the window. Notice the *[Date], [Time], [D & T]* (Date and Time), and *[Initials]* buttons. The user clicks into the free text field after the *NANDA* Dx is selected, enters the date and time, and initials the entry by using these icon buttons. The user clicks *Done* to add the nursing diagnosis to the red *NANDA* window.

The *NANDA* nursing diagnosis can be individualized from inside the *Dx Text* window. A well-formulated diagnostic statement includes an etiology that indicates the cause of the patient's problem or potential problem, thereby making the diagnosis specific to the patient. This is commonly referred to as the "related to" (R/T) component of the nursing diagnosis. Identification of the etiology helps to identify the interventions to address the patient's need. In addition to an etiology statement, the nurse may further individualize

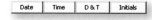

Date, *Time*, *D & T*, and
Initials stamp buttons

Figure 6.2
NANDA (*a*) selection window and (*b*) *Dx text*

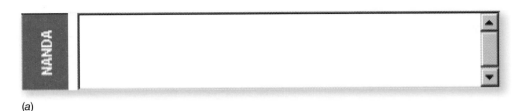

(*a*)

Dx Text

ENTER IN ORDER OF IMPORTANCE/PRIORITIZE FOR OUT
Anxiety,
Aspiration - Risk for,
Breathing Pattern, Ineffective
Cardiac Output, Decreased (ADD RELATED FACTOR)
Communication: Impaired, Verbal
Confusion, Acute
Constipation
Coping, Ineffective
Diarrhea
Falls, Risk for
Fatigue
Fluid Volume, Deficient
Fluid Volume, Excess
Fluid Volume, Imbalanced, Risk for
Gas Exchange, Impaired
Grieving
Grieving, Complicated
Health Maintenance, Ineffective
Hopelessness
Hyperthermia

(*b*)

Evidence-Based Practice 6.2

A systematic review of 36 research studies conducted by Muller-Staub (2009) found that when an etiology was included in the nursing diagnostic statement, both interventions and outcomes improved.

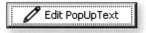

Edit PopUp Text icon

the nursing diagnosis by adding specific signs or symptoms of the problem by including an "as evidenced by" (AEB) component to the nursing diagnosis. For example, a priority nursing diagnosis for a surgical patient may be "Ineffective airway clearance r/t incisional pain AEB subjective report of pain when coughing and deep breathing."

The *DX Text* window may also be used to add nursing diagnoses that may not be available in the prebuilt text. These nursing diagnoses may be typed in or pop-up text may be inserted. In order to individualize pop-up text, select the pencil icon, labeled *Edit PopUp Text*. This opens the *Edit PopUp Text* window where the nurse can add frequently used text into the open fields. The order of the nursing diagnoses may be modified to reflect priorities of care by using the up and down arrows on the left side of the screen. High-level priority nursing diagnoses should be listed first. The user clicks *Done* when changes are complete.

While SpringCharts contains 60 pop-up text fields that can be modified, this is not sufficient for listing the over 200 NANDA-I nursing diagnoses. Therefore, individualizing the pop-up text to list frequently used nursing diagnoses for a particular nursing unit can be extremely useful.

Concept Checkup 6.1

A. List three purposes of standardized nursing language.

1. _____

2. _____

3. _____

B. True or False: The nurse develops nursing diagnoses based on critical thinking about a patient's assessment, past health history, and social history. _____

Text Order Arrows in *Edit PopUp Text* window

LO 6.2   NOC (Nursing Outcomes)

After the nurse develops and prioritizes the patient's nursing diagnoses based on problems or potential problems, the planning phase of the nursing process begins. The initial step in the planning phase is to identify desired goals for the patient. SpringCharts uses nursing outcomes classification (NOC) statements to document these goals. By clicking on the *NOC* tab on the right side of the *Nurse Note* window, the nurse has access to pop-up text that allows entering patient-specific outcomes, as seen in Figure 6.3. The user clicks on the desired text and it populates in the box on the lower-left side. The text can be modified at that time. Once an outcome is selected, the nurse designates a specific time frame for achievement of the goal. Nursing outcomes may be either short-term or long-term goals. Short-term goals may be goals that can be met during the course of an inpatient stay or on an outpatient basis, in the near future. Long-term goals may be goals that are not intended to be achieved during the hospitalization or in the immediate future, such as weight loss. In the example from the previous section, an appropriate NOC statement for the postoperative patient with ineffective airway clearance is "Respiratory Status: Ventilation." To individualize this outcome, the nurse may further state: "Lungs clear to auscultation at discharge." After entering

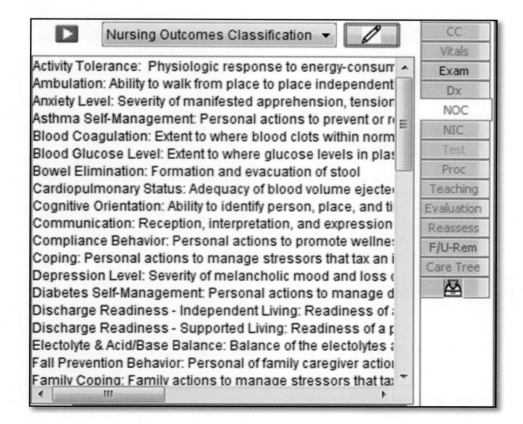

Figure 6.3
NOC pop-up text

the time component for the outcome, the nurse leaves the *NOC* panel and the NOC is entered into the *Plan* section of the SOAPIER documentation.

The *NOC* area can also be individualized from inside the *NOC* window to allow for nursing outcome classifications that may not be available in the prebuilt text. While 60 modifiable prebuilt text fields are available, this is not enough to include all 385 nursing outcomes. Therefore, modifying this area to list applicable outcomes for a particular nursing unit can be extremely useful. In order to individualize pop-up text, the user selects the pencil icon. This opens the *Edit PopUp Text* window where the nurse can add useful text into the open fields. The order of items may be modified by using the up and down arrows on the left side of the screen. The user clicks *Done* when changes are complete.

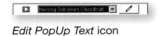

Edit PopUp Text icon

Concept Checkup 6.2

A. Nursing outcomes may be either _____ or _____ term, and should include a specific _____.

B. True or False: NOC statements cannot be individualized in SpringCharts. _____

LO 6.3   NIC (Nursing Interventions)

Once goals have been set for the patient, the nurse outlines the nursing interventions that are necessary to achieve the goals. Interventions are the activities the nurse provides in order to facilitate wellness or movement toward wellness. To select nursing interventions, the user clicks on the *NIC* tab on the right. A list of NIC interventions appears. The nurse uses the pop-up text as previously described to select interventions. In addition, the nurse may click into the *Nursing Interventions Classification* field on the lower left of the window to type interventions. For the postoperative patient with ineffective airway clearance, the nurse may select *Pain Management (alleviation of pain or reduction in pain to a level of comfort that is acceptable to the patient)*, *Airway Management (facilitation of patency of air passages)*, and *Respiratory Monitoring: (collection and analysis of patient data to ensure airway patency and adequate gas exchange)*. Specific pain management interventions may include analgesic administration, positioning, and splinting the incision during coughing and deep breathing. Specific airway management interventions may include use of incentive spirometer every two hours, coughing every two hours, and turning every two hours. Respiratory monitoring activities include auscultation of lungs and measurement of temperature, respirations, and pulse oximetry. Specific interventions are documented when completed.

The *NIC* area can also be individualized from inside the *NIC* window to allow for nursing interventions classifications that may not be available in the prebuilt text. While 60 modifiable prebuilt text fields are available, this not sufficient to include all 542 nursing interventions. Therefore, modifying this area to list applicable interventions for a particular nursing unit can be extremely useful. In order to individualize pop-up text, the user selects the pencil icon. This opens the *Edit PopUp Text* window where the nurse can add useful text into the open fields. The order of the intervention list may be modified by using the up and down arrows on the left side of the screen. The user clicks *Done* when changes are completed.

Edit PopUp Text icon

Concept Checkup 6.3

A. What is the purpose of nursing interventions? _____

_____

B. True or False: In the *Edit PopUp Text* area, the nurse can modify the intervention list including the order of items in the list. _____

LO 6.4   MAR (Medication Administration Record)

The *Nursing Documentation* area, which is outside the *Nurse Note* in the *Care Tree* section of the patient's chart, provides a rapid access area for documenting specialized assessments such as a fall risk assessment and a sedation scale, medication administration, and intake and output (I&O).

Medication administration is an important intervention that the nurses perform frequently. To access the medication administration record *(MAR)*, the user clicks the *Care Tree* navigation tab, seen in Figure 6.4.

The nurse clicks the "+" sign to the left of the *Nursing Documentation* heading, then clicks the *MAR*, as seen in Figure 6.5. Documents, like the *MAR* form, are imported into patients' charts via the *Import Items* feature in the *New* menu of the patient's chart. Original documents can be created in any format such as .pdf (scanned into the program and opened in Acrobat Reader), .xls (created in Microsoft Excel), and .doc (created in Microsoft Word). These original documents are typically stored in a common folder on the computer network. As specific documents are needed for specific patients, the documents are imported into the patient's chart. To document on the *MAR*, the user clicks on the *Doc* button in the lower-right corner of the window and the *MAR* form opens in Microsoft Excel, as seen in Figure 6.6. New medications are typed into the *MAR*, including the drug name, dosage, route, frequency, and scheduled time for administration. Administration of medications is documented when the user's initials, full name, and credentials are typed in the correct time box. The modifications to the *MAR* are saved and the nurse closes the *MAR* to return to the *Nurse Note*.

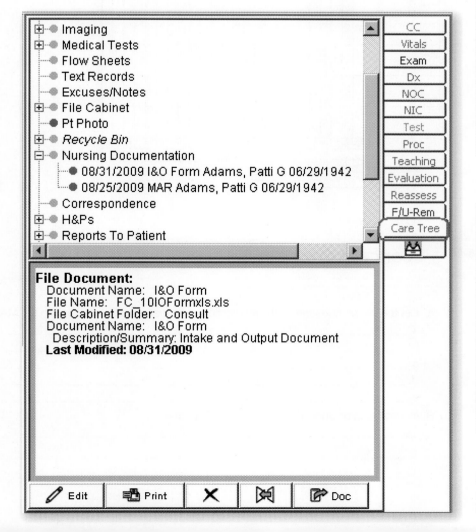

Figure 6.4

Care Tree navigation tab in *Nurse Note*

Legal/Ethical Considerations

Medication errors injure an estimated 1.5 million people annually, costing a projected $3.5 million. The IOM recommends electronic prescriptions to reduce errors attributed to illegible handwriting and to provide decision-support tools and automatic alerts to minimize interactions and prescription of drugs to which the patient is allergic (Office of News and Public Information, 2006).

Legal/Ethical Considerations

Nurses are responsible for their own actions. Medication orders that are not consistent with prescribing guidelines should be clarified before administration. Nurses have the right to refuse to administer a medication if the orders are not clear or consistent with prescribing guidelines.

Documentation Tip

At times, medications are not given as ordered. A patient may be NPO (nothing by mouth), may refuse the medication, or may have contraindications for administration. When medications are not given, the reason should be documented according to facility policy and the licensed practitioner who ordered the medication should be notified.

Figure 6.5

Accessing the *Medication Administration Record (MAR)*

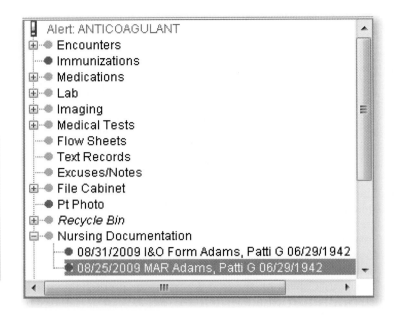

Figure 6.6

MAR form opened from the patient's chart

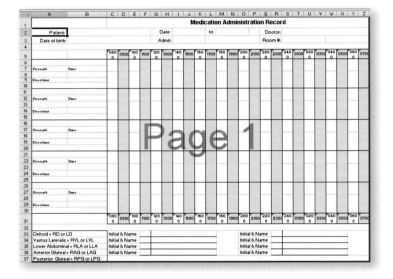

Concept Checkup 6.4

A. List the five components of the medication order that must be entered into the *MAR*.

a. _____

b. _____

c. _____

d. _____

e. _____

B. In what area of SpringCharts is the *MAR* located?

_____

LO 6.5 | I & O (Intake and Output)

Intake and output (*I&O*) documentation is another important function of nursing as it facilitates assessment of the patient's fluid balance. Like the *MAR*, in SpringCharts, *I&O* documentation is in the *Nursing Documentation* area, which is accessed via the *Care Tree* tab in the *Nurse Note*. The user selects the *I&O* form located in the *Nursing Documentation* heading of the *Care Tree*, as seen in Figure 6.7. *I&O* may be documented hourly and shift totals are calculated by the user each shift on the *I&O* form as seen in Figure 6.8. Intake such as oral fluids, blood products, and intravenous medications and output such as urine, chest tube drainage, and nasogastric tube drainage are a few of the items defaulted in the document. Additional intake and output categories, such as emesis, may be typed in at the top of an *I&O* column as needed.

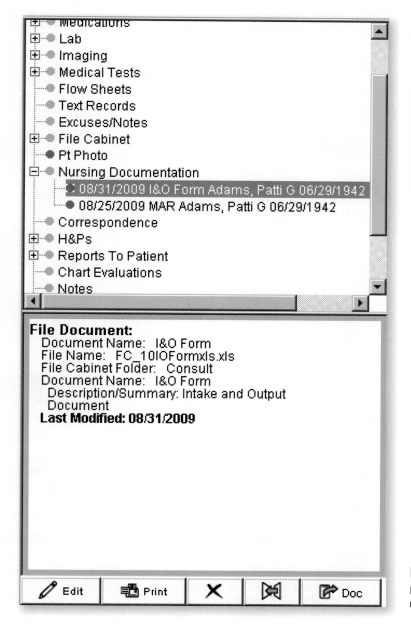

Figure 6.7

Intake and output *(I&O)* record

Figure 6.8
I&O form

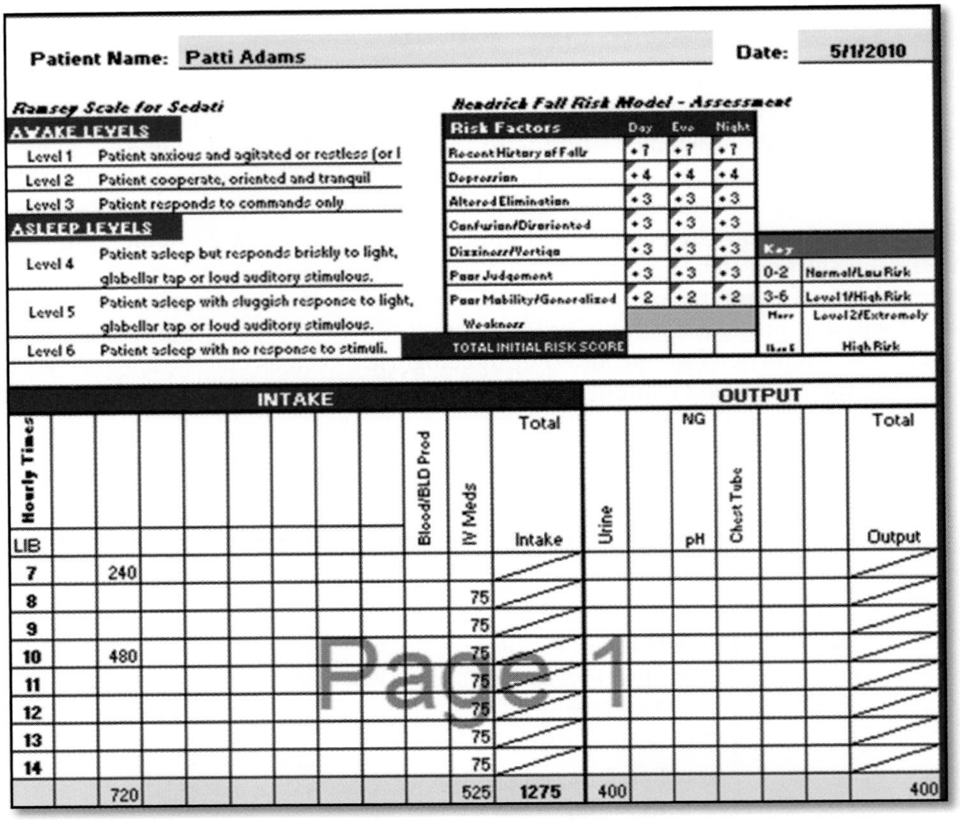

Patient Name: Patti Adams Date: 5/1/2010

Ramsey Scale for Sedati

AWAKE LEVELS	
Level 1	Patient anxious and agitated or restless (or l
Level 2	Patient cooperate, oriented and tranquil
Level 3	Patient responds to commands only
ASLEEP LEVELS	
Level 4	Patient asleep but responds briskly to light, glabellar tap or loud auditory stimulous.
Level 5	Patient asleep with sluggish response to light, glabellar tap or loud auditory stimulous.
Level 6	Patient asleep with no response to stimuli.

Hendrick Fall Risk Model - Assessment

Risk Factors	Day	Eve	Night
Recent History of Falls	+7	+7	+7
Depression	+4	+4	+4
Altered Elimination	+3	+3	+3
Confusion/Disoriented	+3	+3	+3
Dizziness/Vertigo	+3	+3	+3
Poor Judgement	+3	+3	+3
Poor Mobility/Generalized Weakness	+2	+2	+2
TOTAL INITIAL RISK SCORE			

Key	
0-2	Normal/Low Risk
3-6	Level 1/High Risk
More than 5	Level 2/Extremely High Risk

INTAKE												OUTPUT						
Hourly Times									Blood/BLD Prod	IV Meds	Total Intake	Urine		NG pH	Chest Tube			Total Output
LIB																		
7		240																
8										75								
9										75								
10		480								75								
11										75								
12										75								
13										75								
14										75								
		720								525	1275	400						400

Page 1

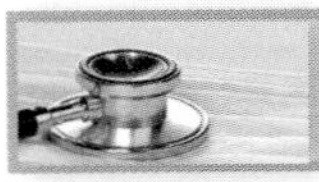

Concept Checkup 6.5

A. What tab is used to access the *Nursing Documentation* area from within the *Nurse Note*? ____________________

B. When are I&O (intake and output) totals routinely calculated? ____________________

____

Exercises

Exercise 6.1

Chronic Obstructive Pulmonary Disease

Note: (The MAR document is housed in the EHR Materials folder that was installed with the SpringCharts program. Your instructor or IT staff may need to inform you where this folder is kept.)

1. After launching SpringCharts, from the top horizontal toolbar, click on *Actions > Open a Chart*. Type in your last name and click the *Search* button. Select your "COPD" patient and the chart opens.
2. Your patient tells you he has been diagnosed with Chronic Obstructive Pulmonary Disease (COPD) this past week. Click on *PMHX* and it populates the right corner box. Click the *Edit* button below the right corner box and a new window opens.

- In the space after *Dx* at the upper-right portion of the window, type *COPD* and click the *Search* icon. COPD 496 appears in the box below the *Search* button. Click on *COPD* and it moves to the *Past Medical History* box on the left.

- In the lower-left corner of the window, click *Back to Chart*. Your new entry appears in the *PMHX* field.

3. You ask your patient about his smoking history and he says he smokes two packs a day and has done so for 24 years. Click on the *Social History* field on the left and it populates the box on the right side of the screen.

   - Click the [Edit] button below the *Social History* box on the right side of the screen and a new window opens.

   - On the right in the list below *Social History* click on: *Tobacco Use* and *Packs per Day*.

   - In the *Social History* box on the left, click after Packs per Day and enter *2 for 24 years*.

   - In lower-left corner of the window, click *Back to Chart*. Your new entry appears in the *Social History* field.

4. Open your *Nurse Note*. On the top horizontal toolbar, click *New > New Nurse Note*. The *Nurse Note* opens to the *Chief Complaint* tab at the top of the vertical navigation bar on the right side of the window.

5. Your patient complains of a cough and shortness of breath. Under the *S Panel* (for subjective) in the text box on the right side, click on these two items. The text populates in the *Chief Complaint* box on the bottom left of the screen.

6. Click on the *Vitals* tab located below the *CC* tab in the vertical navigation bar on the right side of the screen. Note your *Chief Complaints* now appear in the *Subjective* section of the *Nurse Note*.

   - You take your patient's vital signs, height, and weight. Document the following in the boxes on the lower left section of the window: Temp 99.4, Resp 26, Pulse 102, BP 144/80, Ht 66 inches, Wt 200 lbs.

   - You measure your patient's oxygen saturation on room air and find it to be 87%. Document this in the *O2Sat* field. You start oxygen at 2L/minute per nasal cannula and 5 minutes later his oxygen saturation has increased to 91%. To document this, under the *Vitals* text box on the bottom right side of the window, click *Oxygen via* and *O2 Saturation*. To document this, click into the *Notes* box on the left and document your intervention (O2 initiated at 2 L/minute per nasal cannula) as well as the reassessment (O2 sat increased to 91%).

   - Under the *Vitals* text box on the right click: *BP right arm, Pt position—supine* and *Temp source—Oral* to send this text to the *Notes* box on the left. The Temp source —Oral can be separated from the other text by clicking in front of it and striking the [Enter] key on the keyboard.

   - Under the *Vitals* text box on the right, click: *Pt Complains of pain, Pain location, Pain rating 0–10 scale, Pain Description, Factors affecting pain,* and *Factors relieving pain* to send the text to the *Notes* box on the left. Again, place each on a separate line using the [Enter] key.

   - Fill in the following information in the *Notes* box that your patient conveys to you: Pain location: *Right lower chest pain from coughing*, Pain rating 0–10 scale: *5 on 0–10 scale*, Pain description: *aches*, Factors affecting pain: *coughing*, Factors relieving pain: *medication*.

7. Click on the *Exam* button located below the *Vitals*. Notice the *O (Normals)* defaults. In this area select the following systems that are within normal limits when you assess your patient: *HEENT, Gastrointestinal, Musculoskeletal, Heart sounds, Integumentary,* and *GU (male)*. Use the [Enter] key to put these items on separate lines to streamline your documentation.

   - Click the drop-down arrow next to *O (Normals)* and select *O (Abnormals)*. Select the *General* section followed by: *overweight, restless,* and *tachypneic*. Select the *Chest/ABD* section followed by: *Respiratory Effort*, *diminished*, and *wheezes*.

- Click in the *Examination* box after Respiratory Effort and delete: *increased*, *intercostal retractions*, *accessory muscle use*, and *abdominal retraction* so that it reads simply "Respiratory Effort, diminished".
- Click after diminished and type: *with wheezes*.
- Click after wheezes and type: *throughout*. It now reads "diminished with wheezes throughout".

8. Click the *Dx* button below the *Exam* button in the vertical navigation bar on the right. Click on the red *NANDA* on the left bottom of the screen. The *Dx* **Text** window populates.
   - Click *Breathing Pattern, Ineffective* and *Gas Exchange, Impaired*. Click the [D&T] button to date and time the entry. Click *Done*.
   - Add the related factor (r/t) and as evidenced by (AEB) typing them into the field after each *NANDA* diagnosis. Remember to place each nursing diagnosis on a separate line using the [Enter] key.

9. Click the *NOC* tab in the vertical navigation bar on the right located below the *Dx* button. Notice that your *NANDA* documentation populates the *Nurse Note*.
   - Below the *Nursing Outcomes Classification* in the upper-right box select the following:
     - *Knowledge—Disease Process: Extent of understanding conveyed about a specific disease process and prevention of complications.*
     - *Respiratory Status: Movement of air in and out of the lungs and exchange of carbon dioxide and oxygen at the alveolar level.*
     - *Respiratory Status—Gas Exchange: Alveolar exchange of carbon dioxide and oxygen to maintain arterial gas concentrations.*
     - *Smoking Cessation Behavior: Personal actions to eliminate tobacco use.*
   - Use the [Enter] key on the keyboard to place each outcome on separate lines to streamline your documentation.
   - Use the up and down arrows to place the nursing diagnoses in order of priority.
   - Individualize the outcome statements for the client by indicating measureable goals and time frames.

10. Click the *NIC* button in the vertical navigation bar on the right below the *NOC* button. Notice that your outcomes populate the *Nurse Note*.
    - Select the following interventions:
      - *Medication Administration: Preparing, giving, and evaluating the effectiveness of prescription and nonprescription drugs.*
      - *Oxygen Therapy: Administration of oxygen and monitoring of its effectiveness.*
      - *Respiratory Monitoring: Collection and analysis of patient data to ensure airway patency and adequate gas exchange.*
      - *Teaching—Disease Process: Assisting the patient to understand information related to a specific disease process.*
      - *Vital Signs Monitoring: Collection and analysis of cardiovascular, respiratory, and body temperature data to determine and prevent complications.*
    - Click in the *Nursing Interventions Classification* box on the bottom-left side of the window, after the Oxygen Therapy line and type: *See Vitals documentation*.
    - Still in the *Nursing Interventions Classification* box click after Teaching: Disease Process and type: *Taught pursed lip breathing to patient and significant other. Verbalized understanding and demonstrated technique with verbal cues. Continue to reinforce.*

11. Move the *Nurse Note* by clicking the minimize icon in the upper right corner. This will bring you back to the patient's chart.

   - Click the *New* menu and *Import Items* at the bottom of the list. Select *Import File Cabinet Document* and the *File Cabinet* window appears. Type *MAR* into the *Document name*. In the *Chart* tab select the drop-down box on the right and choose *Nursing Documentation*. In the *Description* field type *MAR*. Click the [Attach] button. Select *Existing*. Click *OK*. Click *Done*. The document appears in the *Care Tree* on the right in the *Nursing Documentation* tab.

   - Click on the + in front of *Nursing Documentation*. Highlight the *MAR* and click [Doc] button at the bottom right-hand side of the screen. The *MAR* document opens. Enter the Patient, Date of Birth, Date, Admit date, Doctor, and Room #. Initial and sign at the bottom of the *MAR*. Include your credentials.

   - The primary care provider writes an order to continue the patient's Allegra 180 mg by mouth daily and Aspirin 325 mg by mouth daily. Add the medications to the *MAR* by typing the name of the medication, strength, dose, and directions into the form. Document that you gave the Allegra and Aspirin as ordered by typing your initials into the correct time box on the form.

   - Your patient requests Aleve for the pain he is having in his chest due to his cough. You confirm that the physician has ordered Aleve 550 milligrams by mouth every 12 hours as needed for pain. Add this medication to the *MAR* and document administration. Close the *MAR* by clicking the *X* on the top right corner of the form. A pop-up will ask you if you want to save the changes you have made, select yes. The *Update Document* window appears. Answer yes to the question, "Do you want to send a new version to the server?"

12. You are still in the *Nursing Documentation* area.

   - Click the *New* menu, select *Import File Cabinet Document* and the *File Cabinet* window appears. Type *Intake and Output* into the *Document name*. In the *Chart* tab, select the drop-down box on the right and choose *Nursing Documentation*. In the *Description* field type *Intake and Output*. Click the [Attach] button. Select *Existing*. Use the search mechanism to select the blank *Intake and Output* document from the *EHR Materials* folder. Click *OK*. Click *Done*. The document appears in the *Care Tree* on the right in the *Nursing Documentation* tab.

   - Click on the + in front of *Nursing Documentation*. Highlight the *Intake and Output* and click *Edit* at the bottom right-hand side of the screen. The *File Cabinet* window appears. Click on the blue hyperlink next to the word *File*. The *Intake and Output* document opens. Type in the Patient Name and Date.

   - Your patient has taken in 1000 milliliters (mL) of fluid orally: 400 mL at 0800, 300 mL at 1100, and 300 mL at 1300. He voided 500 mL: 250 mL at 0930 and 250 mL at 1230. Document your shift totals. Document the number of milliliters only; you do not need to type in *mls*. Close the I&O form by clicking the *X* on the top-right corner of the form. A pop-up will ask you if you want to save the changes you have made, select yes. The *File Cabinet Document* window appears. Click *Done*. The *Update Document* window appears. Answer yes to the question, "Do you want to send a new version to the server?"

13. The *Nurse Note* may be located at the bottom of the screen due to minimizing it earlier. Return to the *Nurse Note* by clicking the maximize icon on the upper right side of the *Nurse Note*. In the *Nurse Note* click *Done*. The *Save As* screen populates. Click *Save*.

14. A pop-up appears asking if you want to create a routing slip. Click *No*.

15. In the *Care Tree*, click the + next to *Encounters*. Click on the date of your *Nurse Note* and it appears in the bottom-right-corner box.

   - Click *Edit* below the bottom-right-corner box. The *Nurse Note* window opens. Click *Sign* at the lower right side of the window. The *Sign* window opens. Select *Permanent Sign and Lock* when finished with your *Nurse Note*.

Fractured Hip

1. After launching SpringCharts, click on *Actions > Open a Chart*. Type in your last name and click the *Search* button. Select your "fractured hip" patient and the chart opens.

2. Your patient has been admitted for a broken right hip. She tells you she has a history of osteoporosis. Click on *PMHX* on the left and the past medical history populates the box on the right lower side of the screen. Click *Edit*.

   - The *Past Medical History* screen populates. In the space after *Dx* type: *osteo* and click the *Search* icon. Options appear in the box below. Click on *osteoporosis 733.0*, which sends this to the *Past Medical History* list.

   - Click *Back to Chart*. The information you added appears in the *PMHX* box.

3. Open your *Nurse Note*. Click *New > New Nurse Note*.

4. Your patient complains of pain in her right hip. Select *Pain* in the *S Panel* text and it populates the *Chief Complaint* box on the bottom left of the screen. Click in the *Chief Complaint* box after Pain, and type: *right hip*.

5. Click on the *Vitals* button located below the *CC* button in the navigation bar on the right side of the screen. Note that your chief complaint now appears in the *Subjective* section of the *Nurse Note*.

   - You take your patient's vital signs. Document the following: Temp 98.4, Resp 16, Pulse 114, BP 162/94, Ht 60 inches, Wt 130 lbs, O2SAT% 94.

   - Also select: *BP left arm*, *Pt position—supine*, and *Temp source—Tympanic*.

   - Under the *Vitals* text box on the lower right click: *Pt Complains of pain*, *Pain location*, *Pain rating 0–10 scale*, *Pain Description*, *Factors affecting pain*, and *Factors relieving pain* to send the text to the *Notes* box on the left.

   - Fill in the following information in the *Notes* box that your patient conveys to you: *Right hip pain*, *4 on 0–10 scale* (she received morphine 4 mg IV in the ED one hour ago), Description: *stabbing*, Factors affecting: *movement*, Factors relieving: *medication*.

6. Click on the *Exam* button located below the *Vitals*. The *O (Normals)* defaults in the right upper box. Select the following systems that are within normal limits when you assess your patient: *HEENT*, *Heart sounds*, *Lungs/Respiratory*, *Integumentary*, and *Neurological*.

   - Click the drop-down arrow next to *O (Normals)* and select *O (Abnormals)*. Select the *General* section followed by: *avoiding movement*. Select the *GI/ GU* section followed by: *indwelling urinary catheter*. Select the *Extremities* section followed by: *edema*.

   - Click into the *Examination* box on the lower left after indwelling urinary catheter and type: *inserted in ED*. Click after edema and type: *right hip. Right leg shortened*.

7. Click the *Dx* button below the *Exam* button on the right. Click on the red *NANDA* on the left bottom of the screen. The *Dx Text* window populates.

   - Click *Falls, risk for*; *Pain, acute*; *Urinary elimination, altered*; *Physical mobility, impaired*. Click the *D&T* icon to date and time the entry. Click *Done*.

   - Add the related factor (r/t) and as evidenced (AEB) statement by typing them into the field after the *NANDA* diagnosis.

   - Place the nursing diagnoses in order of priority.

8. Click the *NOC* button on the right located below the *Dx* button. The *NANDA* documentation populates the *Nurse Note*.

- Below the *Nursing Outcomes Classification* select the following:
  - *Fall Prevention Behavior: Personal or family caregiver actions to minimize risk factors that might precipitate falls in the personal environment.*
  - *Knowledge—Treatment Procedure: Extent of understanding conveyed about a procedure required as part of a treatment regimen.*
  - *Mobility: Ability to move purposefully in own environment independently with or without assistive device.*
  - *Pain Control: Personal actions to control pain.*
  - *Urinary Elimination: Collection and discharge of urine.*
- Use the [Enter] key on the keyboard to place text on separate lines to streamline your documentation.

9. Click the *NIC* button on the right below the *NOC* button. Notice that your outcomes populate the *Nurse Note*.
  - Select the following interventions:
    - *Fall Prevention: Instituting special precautions with patient at risk for injury from falling.*
    - *Pain Management: Alleviation of pain or a reduction in pain to a level of comfort that is acceptable to the patient.*
    - *Surgical Preparation: Providing care to a patient immediately prior to surgery and verifying required procedures/tests and documentation in the clinical record.*
    - *Teaching: Procedure/Treatment: Preparing a patient to understand and mentally prepare for a prescribed procedure or treatment.*
    - *Urinary Catheterization: Insertion of a catheter into the bladder for temporary or permanent drainage of urine.*
    - *Vital Signs Monitoring: Collection and analysis of cardiovascular, respiratory, and body temperature data to determine and prevent complications.*
  - Click in to the Fall Prevention line and type: *Patient instructed that she is on bed rest and should not attempt to get out of bed, verbalizes understanding. Call light within reach.*
  - Click in to the Surgical Preparation line and type: *Glasses and jewelry removed. Hibiclens scrub to right side completed.*

10. Move the *Nurse Note* by clicking the minimize icon in the upper right corner. This will bring you back to the patient's chart.
  - Click the *New* menu and *Import Items* at the bottom of the list. Select *Import File Cabinet Document* and the *File Cabinet* window appears. Type *MAR* into the *Document name*. In the *Chart* tab select the drop-down box on the right and choose *Nursing Documentation*. In the *Description* field type *MAR*. Click *Attach*. Select *Existing*. Click *OK*. Click *Done*. The document appears in the *Care Tree* on the right in the *Nursing Documentation* tab.
    - Click on the + in front of *Nursing Documentation*. Highlight the *MAR* and click *Edit* at the bottom right-hand side of the screen. The *File Cabinet* window appears. Click on the blue hyperlink next to the word *File*. The *MAR* document opens. Enter the Patient, Date of Birth, Date, Admit date, Doctor, and Room #.
    - Add the medications to the *MAR* by typing the name of the medication, dosage, route, frequency, and scheduled administration time into the form. Document that you did not give the patient's routine medications by typing *NPO* and your initials in the correct time box for each medication. Close the *MAR* by clicking the *X* on the top right corner of the form. A pop-up will ask you if you want to save the changes you have made, select yes. The *File Cabinet Document* window appears. Click *Done*. The *Update Document* window appears. Answer yes to the question, "Do you want to send a new version to the server?"

11. You are still in the *Nursing Documentation* area.

- Click the New menu, select *Import File Cabinet Document* and the *File Cabinet* window appears. Type *Intake and Output* into the *Document name*. In the *Chart* tab select the drop-down box on the right and choose *Nursing Documentation*. In the *Description* field type *Intake and Output*. Click *Attach*. Select *Existing*. Use the search mechanism to select the blank *Intake and Output* document. The I&O document is found in the *EHR Materials* folder. Click *OK*. Click *Done*. The document appears in the *Care Tree* on the right in the *Nursing Documentation* tab.

- Click on the + in front of *Nursing Documentation*. Highlight *Intake and Output* and click *Edit* at the bottom right-hand side of the screen. The *File Cabinet* window appears. Click on the blue hyperlink next to the word *File*. The *Intake and Output* document opens. Type in the Patient Name and Date.

  - Your patient has been NPO. It is the end of the shift; you empty her indwelling urinary catheter drainage bag of 400 mL of clear, yellow urine. Document your patient's I&O including shift totals. Close the I&O form by clicking the *X* on the top-right-corner of the form. A pop-up will ask you if you want to save the changes you have made, select yes. The *File Cabinet Document* window appears. Click *Done*. The *Update Document* window appears. Answer yes to the question, "Do you want to send a new version to the server?"

12. The *Nurse Note* may be located at the bottom of the screen due to minimizing it earlier. Return to the *Nurse Note* by clicking the maximize icon on the upper right side of the nurse note. In the *Nurse Note* click *Done*. The *Save As* screen populates. Click *Save*.

13. A pop-up appears asking if you want to create a routing slip. Click *No*.

14. In the *Care Tree*, click the + next to *Encounters*. Click on the date of your *Nurse Note* and it appears in the bottom right corner box.

- Click *Edit*. Click *Sign*. Select *Permanent Sign and Lock* when finished with your *Nurse Note*.

Exercise 6.3

Colon Cancer

1. After launching SpringCharts, click on *Actions > Open a Chart*. Type in your last name and click the *Search* button. Select your "colon cancer" patient and the chart opens.

2. Your patient tells you he recently discovered he was allergic to Dilaudid after his colectomy. He tells you he broke out in hives all over his body. Click on *Allergies* in the red box on the left side of the screen and a red *Allergies* box opens in the lower-right corner of the window. Click *Edit* below this box. A new window opens.

- Click into the space after *Allergy* in the text box in the upper-right side of the window and enter *Dilaudid*. Click the *Search* icon. Options appear in the box below. Click on *Dilaudid* and it moves to the *Allergies* field to the left.

- Click on *Dilaudid* in the *Allergies* field. The *Edit Dilaudid* window opens. Enter *Hives* in the *Adverse Reaction* field. Click *Save* at the bottom of the window.

- Click *Back to Chart* at the lower-left corner of the window. The information you added appears in the *Allergies* box.

3. Your patient had a colectomy six months ago for colon cancer. Click on the *PMHX* box and it populates in the bottom-right corner. Click *Edit* below the box.

- Click in the space after *Dx* at the upper right of the screen and type: *colon*. Click the *Search* icon. Colon CA 153.9 appears in the box below.
- Click on *Colon CA 153.9* and it moves to the *Past Medical History* field to the left.
- Click into the *Other PMHX* box on the bottom left of the screen. Type: *Colectomy 2009*.
- Click *Back to Chart*. The colon CA and colectomy are now listed in the *PMHX*.

4. Your patient tells you he takes Zofran 8 mg po prn for nausea related to his chemotherapy. Click on the *Routine Meds* box and it populates in the bottom-right corner. Click *Edit*.
   - Click in the space after *Brand Name* and type: *Zofran*. Click the *Search* icon.
   - Click on *Zofran 8 mg* to send the medication to the *Routine Medications* list.
   - Click on *Zofran 8 mg*. The *Edit Rx* window opens. Click into the *Directions* field and type: *po prn nausea b.i.d.* Click in the calendar to the right of *Date Started* and choose a date six months ago. Click *Save*.
   - Click *Back to Chart*. Zofran is now listed in the *Routine Meds*.

5. Open your *Nurse Note*. Click *New > New Nurse Note*.

6. Your patient complains of nausea and vomiting. He had a chemotherapy treatment earlier this week. Select *nausea* and *vomiting* from the *S Panel* text and they populate the *Chief Complaint* box on the bottom left of the screen.

7. Click on the *Vitals* button located below the *CC* button on the right side of the screen. The chief complaints now appear in the *Subjective* section of the *Nurse Note*.
   - You take your patient's vital signs. Document the following: Temp 100.2, Resp 20, Pulse 114, BP 110/72, Ht 70 inches, Wt 170 lbs, O2SAT% 98.
   - Under the *Vitals* text box on the right click: *BP left arm*, *Pt position—supine*, *Temp source—Oral*, and *No complaints of pain*.

8. Click on the *Exam* button located below the *Vitals*. The *O (Normals)* defaults. Select the following systems that are within normal limits when you assess your patient: *Heart sounds*, *Musculoskeletal*, *GU (male)*, *Lungs/Respiratory*, and *Neurological*.
   - Click the drop-down arrow next to *O (Normals)* and select *O (Abnormals)*. Select *HEENT* followed by: *Dry mucous membranes*.
   - Click into the *Examination* field and type: *pt vomited 200 ml green emesis. Bowel sounds hyperactive*. Click after Dry mucous membranes and type: *tenting of skin*.

9. Click the *Dx* button below the *Exam* button on the right. Click on the red *NANDA* on the left bottom of the screen. The *Dx Text* window populates.
   - Click *Fluid Volume, Deficient* and *Infection, Risk for*. Click the *D&T* icon to date and time the entry. Click *Done*.
   - Add the related factor (r/t) and as evidenced (AEB) statement by typing it into the field after each *NANDA* diagnosis.
   - Use the [Enter] key on the keyboard to place text on separate lines to streamline your documentation.

10. Click the *NOC* button on the right located below the *Dx* button. The *NANDA* documentation populates the *Nurse Note*.
    - Below the *Nursing Outcomes Classification* select the following:
      - *Fluid Balance: Water balance in the intracellular and extracellular components of the body.*

- *Knowledge—Disease Process: Extent of understanding conveyed about a specific disease process and prevention of complications.*
- *Nausea and Vomiting Control: Personal actions to control nausea, retching, and vomiting symptoms.*
- *Vital Signs: Extent to which temperature, pulse, respiration, and blood pressure are within normal range.*
  - Use the [Enter] key on the keyboard to place text on separate lines to streamline your documentation.

11. Click the *NIC* button on the right below the *NOC* button. The outcomes populate the *Nurse Note*.
    - Select the following interventions:
      - *Fluid/Electrolyte Management: Regulation and prevention of complications from altered fluid and/or electrolyte levels.*
      - *Medication Administration: Preparing, giving, and evaluating the effectiveness of prescription and nonprescription drugs.*
      - *Vital Signs Monitoring: Collection and analysis of cardiovascular, respiratory, and body temperature data to determine and prevent complications.*

12. The physician orders Zofran 4mg IV x 1 dose for nausea. Move the nurse note by clicking the minimize icon in the upper right corner. This will bring you back to the patient's chart.
    - Click the *New* menu and *Import Items* at the bottom of the list. Select *Import File Cabinet Document* and the *File Cabinet* window appears. Type *MAR* into the Document name. In the *Chart* tab select the drop-down box on the right and choose *Nursing Documentation*. In the *Description* field type *MAR*. Click *Attach*. Select *Existing*. Click *OK*. Click *Done*. The document appears in the *Care Tree* on the right in the *Nursing Documentation* tab.
    - Click on the + in front of *Nursing Documentation*. Highlight the *MAR* and click *Edit* at the bottom right-hand side of the screen. The *File Cabinet* window appears. Click on the blue hyperlink next to the word *File*. The *MAR* document opens. Enter the Patient, Date of Birth, Date, Admit date, Doctor, and Room #. Add the Zofran on the left in the first open medication slot. Complete the strength, dose, and directions fields. Document that you gave the Zofran by typing your initials in the correct time box for the medication. Close the *MAR* by clicking the *X* on the top right corner of the form. The *File Cabinet Document* window appears. Click *Done*. The *Update Document* window appears. Answer yes to the question, "Do you want to send a new version to the server?"

13. You are still in the *Nursing Documentation* area.
    - Click the New menu, select *Import File Cabinet Document* and the *File Cabinet* window appears. Type *Intake and Output* into the *Document name*. In the *Chart* tab select the drop-down box on the right and choose *Nursing Documentation*. In the *Description* field type *Intake and Output*. Click *Attach*. Select *Existing*. Use the search mechanism to select the blank *Intake and Output* document. The I&O document is found in the *EHR Materials* folder. Click *OK*. Click *Done*. The document appears in the *Care Tree* on the right in the *Nursing Documentation* tab.
      - Click on the + in front of *Nursing Documentation*. Highlight *Intake and Output* and click *Edit* at the bottom right-hand side of the screen. The *File Cabinet* window appears. Click on the blue hyperlink next to the word *File*. The *Intake and Output* document opens. Type in the Patient Name and Date.
    - Your patient has vomited 240 mL of emesis this shift: 120 mL at 1500 and 120 mL at 1700. Add emesis to one of the columns at the top of the form and enter the emesis as output. Your patient has been NPO due to his nausea and vomiting. He has received 1000 mL of IV fluid since admission.

Make sure you document your shift totals. Close the I&O form by clicking the *X* on the top right corner of the form. The *File Cabinet Document* window appears. Click *Done*. The *Update Document* window appears. Answer yes to the question, "Do you want to send a new version to the server?"

14. The *Nurse Note* may be located at the bottom of the screen due to minimizing it earlier. Return to the *Nurse Note* by clicking the maximize icon on the upper right side of the *Nurse Note*. In the *Nurse Note* click *Done*. The *Save As* screen populates. Click *Save*.

15. A pop-up appears asking if you want to create a routing slip. Click *No*.

16. In the *Care Tree*, click the + next to *Encounters*. Click on the date of your *Nurse Note* and it appears in the bottom right corner box.

- Click *Edit*. Click *Sign*. Select *Permanent Sign and Lock* when finished with your *Nurse Note*.

References

American Nurses Association. (2007). Relationships among ANA recognized data element sets and terminologies. Retrieved June 14, 2010, from http://www.nursingworld.org/npii/relationship.htm

Continuous bladder irrigation: court faults nurses. *Legal Eagle Eye Newsletter for the Nursing Profession, 15*(6), 5.

McCloskey, J.C., Bulechek, G.M & Butcher H. (2008). *Nursing interventions classification (NIC)*(5th ed). St. Louis: Mosby.

Moorhead, S., Johnson, M., Mass, M & Swanson, E. (2008). *Nursing outcomes classification (NOC)*(4th ed). St. Louis: Mosby.

Muller-Staub, M. (2009). Evaluation of the implementation of nursing diagnoses, outcomes and interventions. *International Journal of Nursing Terminologies and Classifications, 20*(1), 9–15.

NANDA-International. (n.d.). Nursing diagnosis frequently asked questions. Retrieved September 22, 2010, from http://www.nanda.org/NursingDiagnosisFAQ.aspx

Office of News and Public Information. (2006). Medication errors injure 1.5 million people and cost billions of dollars annually; report offers comprehensive strategies for reducing drug-related mistakes. Retrieved June 16, 2010, from http://www8.nationalacademies.org/onpinews/newsitem.aspx?RecordID=11623

Rutherford, M. (2008, January 31). Standardized nursing language: What does it mean for nursing practice? *OJIN: The Online Journal of Issues in Nursing, 13*(1), Retrieved June 14, 2010, from http://www.nursingworld.org/MainMenuCategories/ANAMarketplace/ANAPeriodicals/OJIN/TableofContents/vol132008/No1Jan08/ArticlePreviousTopic/StandardizedNursingLanguage.aspx

Thoroddsen, A., & Ehnfors, M. (2007). Putting policy into practice: Pre- and post-tests of implementing standardized languages for nursing documentation. *Journal of Clinical Nursing, 16*, 1826–1838.

University of Iowa College of Nursing. (n.d.). Center for Nursing Classification & Clinical Effectiveness. Retrieved June 14, 2010, from http://www.nursing.uiowa.edu/excellence/nursing_knowledge/clinical_effectiveness/index.htm

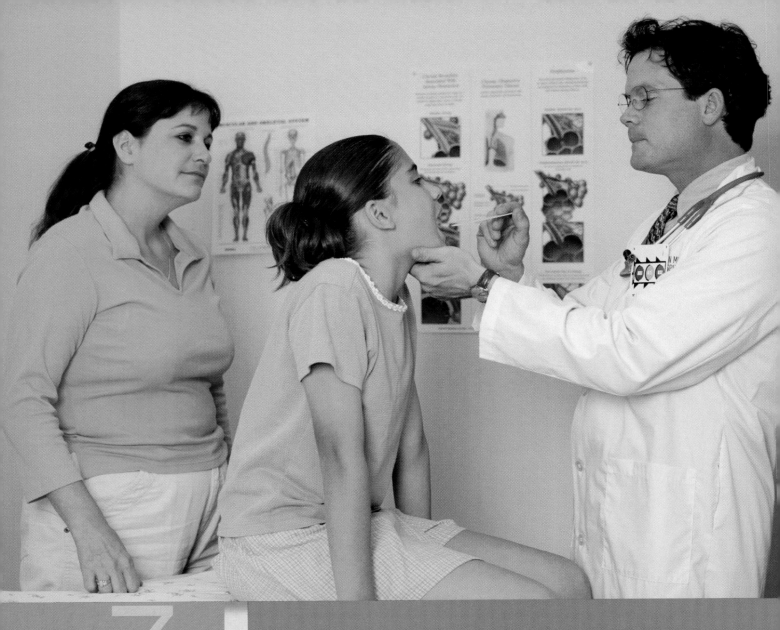

7 Ambulatory

Key Terms

Terms and abbreviations you will encounter in Chapter 7; they are defined in the end-of-book glossary:

AAACN

AANP

Addendum

American Medical
   Association (AMA)

CPT Codes

Drug Formulary

ICD-9 Codes

Lab Analyte

NDC

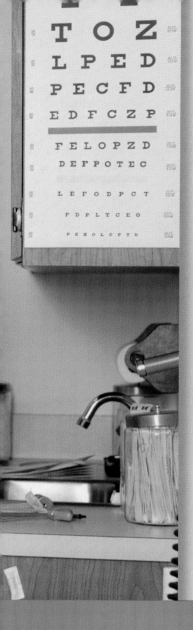

Learning Outcomes

When you complete Chapter 7, you will be able to:

7.1   Describe the role of an ambulatory nurse.

7.2   Use SpringCharts to create an office visit note.

7.3   Use SpringCharts to modify an office visit note.

7.4   Carry out preparing an addendum to the office visit note.

Healthcare

What You Need to Know

To understand Chapter 7, you need to know how to:

- Open an electronic patient chart.
- Add pop-up text.
- Distinguish the various components of the face sheet.

LO 7.1   The Ambulatory Nurse

While the majority of nurses work in the hospital setting, patient care is increasingly moving to the outpatient, or ambulatory, setting. This movement of patient care to the outpatient setting is creating a demand for ambulatory care nurses (Haas, 2010). Ambulatory nursing is a nursing specialty that requires unique nursing skills to care for a variety of patients across the lifespan often during multiple episodes that generally last less than 24 hours (AAACN, n.d.). Ambulatory care nurses may work in same-day surgery centers providing pre-, intra-, and postoperative care to patients. They may work in oncology clinics administering chemotherapy and helping patients and families cope with a diagnosis of cancer. Ambulatory care nurses may also work in call centers, telehealth, public health clinics, primary care practices, hospital-based clinics, or occupational health settings. In the ambulatory care setting, nurses work with a variety of interdisciplinary team members including physicians, nurse practitioners, radiology technicians, lab technicians, case managers, physical therapists, and respiratory therapists. Ambulatory care nurses are skilled in assessment, health promotion, health maintenance, patient education, patient advocacy, and collaboration. They may be highly involved in the financial aspects of care, ensuring optimal payor reimbursement, helping patients decipher insurance requirements, and promoting cost-effective care. Like nurses in the inpatient setting, ambulatory care nurses are challenged to demonstrate their contributions to patient care through the use of standardized languages in EHRs. Ambulatory care nurses may belong to the **American Association of Ambulatory Care Nurses (AAACN)**, a professional organization with a mission to advance the specialty of ambulatory nursing.

Nurse practitioners are advanced practice nurses who are licensed, independent healthcare providers (AANP, n.d.) They typically have advanced education, such as a master's degree or doctorate. The scope of practice of nurse practitioners is regulated by individual states' nurse practice acts, but generally nurse practitioners may assign medical diagnoses and prescribe medications and treatments. Nurse practitioners bring a unique perspective to primary care through their holistic focus on the patient with an emphasis on counseling and education. The professional organization for nurse practitioners, regardless of specialty, is the **American Association of Nurse Practitioners (AANP)**. Throughout this chapter, primary care provider and practitioner are used to refer to independent licensed practitioners such as physicians and nurse practitioners.

LO 7.2   Building an Office Visit Note

Perhaps the most common encounter with the patient in an ambulatory setting is the office visit. A new office visit encounter is created by selecting the *New* menu within the patient's chart and clicking *New OV*. Depending on the user preferences, one of two different formats, large screen or classic, appears. Figure 7.1 shows the "Large Screen" view. An *OV* window has three main sections. Typically, the left side panel displays the patient's face sheet overview. This panel allows the practitioner to view the face sheet items without having to exit the *Office Visit* display. Any of the face sheet categories can be added into the office visit note to document that the provider discussed these issues with the patient. The middle panel is the portion where the notes are stored in the *SOAP* format, containing subjective, objective, assessment, and plan categories. All text selected from the pop-up text categories or manually added to the text fields automatically saves into one of these areas. Below the *OV* note section is the text box. This functions as a work area where text can be created and modified. The right side of the *OV* screen contains the pop-up text window along with the navigation panel tabs used to access different information that is selected for the *Office Visit* note.

The left and right panels in the *Office Visit* can be reversed. Left-handed users typically like to have the navigation buttons on the left side of the screen so their hand is not covering the *OV* note when selecting pop-up text. This is especially true when

Evidence-Based Practice 7.1

Dozens of research studies demonstrate that nurse practitioners (NPs) produce patient outcomes that are at least comparable to those of physicians. In fact, in a review of over 100 studies, no evidence was found that suggested that NPs provide inferior care to physicians. Care provided by NPs is more cost-effective, in some cases only one-third the cost of care provided by phsyicians. NPs also rank higher than physicians in patient satisfaction (AANP, 2010a, 2010b; Bauer, 2010).

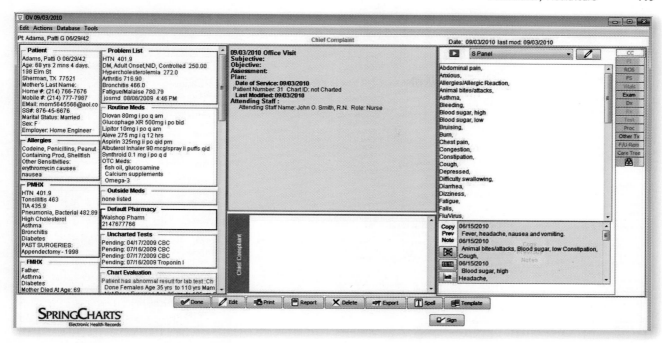

Figure 7.1

New OV window with face sheet panel

using a portable device like a tablet PC or an iPad™. The office visit orientation is determined by selecting either the right or left options under the *Preference 2* tab in the *Set User Preferences* window as described in Chapter 3.

The navigation tabs along the right side of the screen, seen in Figure 7.2, enable the provider to proceed through the office visit in a logical manner; however, the various tabs may be selected in any order. Tabs include chief complaint (*CC*), history of present illness (*PI*), review of systems (*ROS*), face sheet (*FS*), *Vitals*, *Exam*, diagnosis (*Dx*), prescriptions (*Rx*), tests (*Test*), procedures (*Proc*), other treatment (*Other Tx*), and follow-up and reminders (*F/U-Rem*). In the outpatient setting, the office nurse may be responsible for documenting the chief complaint, history of present illness, review of systems, the face sheet, and the vital signs. The primary care provider documents the examination, assigns the medical diagnosis(es), prescribes medication, orders tests and procedures, conducts counseling/coordination of care, and determines the follow-up time. On many occasions the office nurse closes out the visit, implementing the primary care provider's orders, coordinating follow-up, providing and documenting patient education, and performing a final patient assessment before the visit is completed.

Once a tab has been selected from the navigation panel, a list of pop-up text relevant to that topic appears in the third panel of the screen, as seen in Figure 7.2. Data can be entered by (1) tapping with a stylus tool (as with a tablet PC), (2) clicking on pop-up text items with a mouse, (3) typing directly into the text box, or (4) using a third-party voice recognition program to dictate and have the text automatically entered into the text field. In addition, a portable computer with handwriting recognition software may be used so that handwritten script is recognized and automatically typed into the text box. Use of pop-up text is recommended as the quickest method of building documentation for an office visit note.

Chief Complaint

The chief complaint is the significant or cardinal symptom or group of symptoms that prompt the patient to seek healthcare. It is the first part of the *Subjective* area of the *SOAP* note and should be recorded in the patient's own words. The chief complaint is often recorded by a medical assistant or the ambulatory care nurse.

The *Chief Complaint*, *Present Illness*, *Review of Systems*, *Examination*, *Procedure*, *Other Treatment*, and *Follow-up/Reminder* areas have notes from previous encounters visible in the bottom right window, with the most recent note appearing first. Past

---

Documentation Tip

The chief complaint is a subjective component of the assessment and is documented in the patient's words, often as a quote.

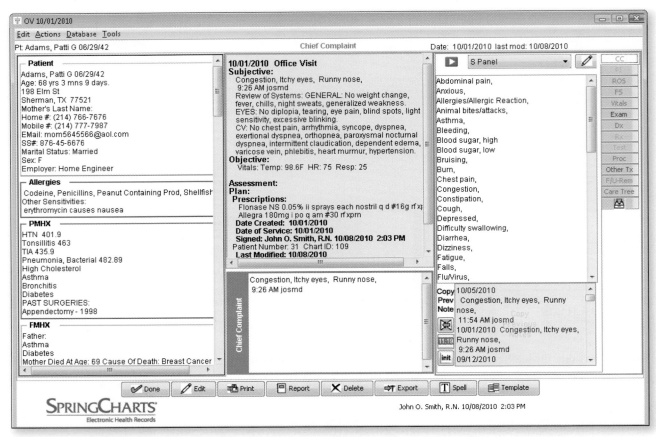

Figure 7.2

Office Visit screen with pop-up text

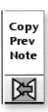

Figure 7.3

Copy Previous Note button

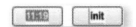

Time-Stamp and *Initial* buttons

encounter notes enable clinicians to refresh their memory of past visits and copy similar notes quickly into the current office visit if necessary. A clinician can highlight previous note text and copy it to the present note by clicking on the [Copy Previous Note] button, displayed in Figure 7.3. The *Previous Note* panel displays only that portion of the previous office visit documentation specific to the tab selected on the navigation panel.

Below the *Previous Note* panel are *Time-Stamp* and *Initial* buttons, shown in the marginal illustration, that enable the user to time-stamp and initial that portion of the office visit note. This feature allows various healthcare providers to document their actions in the same patient encounter. For example, a medical assistant may record the chief complaint when first admitting the patient to the exam room. The user identification and time can be recorded in the *Chief Complaint* portion of the *OV* note. The primary care provider who conducts the physical examination also applies personal identification and time. Similarly, the office nurse may administer an injection and document, initial, and time-stamp that procedure as well as the assessment of the patient's response to the medication. Thus, one *OV* note can reflect the interventions of each member of the healthcare team.

Present Illness

The history of the present illness is an account of the onset, duration, severity, and associated characteristics of the presenting illness. It may include aggravating and alleviating factors. This portion of the interview may be conducted by the ambulatory care nurse or the primary care provider. During this phase of the assessment, the healthcare professional verbally probes for causes, aggravating factors, relieving factors, and past similar conditions. Because the present illness information is obtained during the interview with the patient, the notation is stored as part of the *Subjective* area of the *SOAP* note.

The *Present Illness* panel navigation tab accesses the same *S Panel* pop-up text as the *Chief Complaint* panel tab, since both sections of text are placed in the *Subjective* area of the *SOAP* note, seen in Figure 7.4. However, in a **History & Physical (H&P) report**, the chief complaint and the present illness are separate categories.

Although the program defaults to the appropriate pop-up text category when a specific navigation tab is selected, additional lists of pop-up text are located in the pop-up text header field by category, as seen in Figure 7.5. By accessing this list, the practitioner has multiple categories of text available to choose from. Text selected from categories other than the default category can also be added to existing text in the currently opened section. For example, a practitioner may create a new category of text specific to a certain procedure, a unique review of systems, or chief complaints. Regardless of the category of pop-up text selected, the text is saved in the appropriate *SOAP* category based upon the navigation tab that is open at the time of text selection. The program offers an additional 20 user-defined categories that can be added to the pop-up text feature.

To add the highlighted text into the body of the *SOAP* format, the user simply clicks the *In Box* (see margin illustration) or selects any other navigation panel tab. By clicking on the *In Box*, the user can view the entire *OV Note* in the upper middle section. The *Chief Complaint*, *Present Illness (History)*, *Review of Systems*, *Examination*, *Other Treatment*, and *Follow-Up/Reminder* all operate in similar manner with the appropriate pop-up text appearing on the right side of the screen.

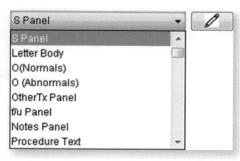

Figure 7.4
S panel category in pop-up text window

In Box button

Review of Systems (ROS)

The review of systems is a critical element of the health history and is conducted during the patient interview. During the review of systems, the nurse questions the patient about each body system to identify a history of abnormal conditions. At this time, the nurse has the opportunity to ask focused questions regarding issues that the patient may not have voluntarily provided. The *ROS* begins with the patient's general health, and then moves to specific body systems. As with the *Chief Complaint* and *Present Illness* sections of the *Nurse Note*, pop-up text can be chosen from the default *ROS-Normals* pop-up text category. The healthcare professional may also select another pop-up text heading and drill down further to more specific ROS categories like *ROS-HEENT* or *ROS-Resp*. In these sections the nurse finds specific text that deals with abnormal conditions that address the patient's chief complaints. The *ROS* is part of the *Subjective* area of the *SOAP* note.

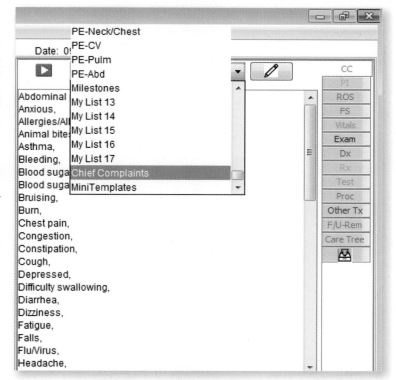

Figure 7.5
Pop-up text category list showing chief complaints

Face Sheet/Medical History

Although the health history is always gained during the initial patient encounter, it is reviewed and amended as needed with each subsequent visit. Obtaining a concise yet thorough history promotes effective diagnosis and treatment. The various components of the health history are discussed in detail in Chapter 3.

Face sheet information is displayed in the *OV Note* screen and can be selected and documented as part of the current *OV Note*. The *FS* navigation tab allows the healthcare professional to add components of the face sheet to the encounter documentation by simply clicking on one or more of the category icons. The selected face sheet items are placed in the *Subjective* area of the *OV Note*. Clicking on the icon at the top of the screen beside *Face Sheet—Add All to this Note* adds the entire face sheet to the current office visit documentation.

Note: To change information in the face sheet, the user must edit the face sheet itself. Changes made in the *Office Visit* note do not modify the information in the patient's face sheet, even if the original information was copied from the face sheet.

Vitals

Along with the nine vital signs defined by SpringCharts, three additional custom measurements can be added to the program, such as peak flow rate or oxygen saturation. These are added to SpringCharts' server and appear in the *Vitals* section of the *Office Visit* screen and in the *New Vitals Only* window of the patient's chart. Vital sign measurements are automatically recorded under the *Objective* element of the *SOAP* note.

SpringCharts displays four graphs (height, weight, blood pressure, and BMI) by accessing the [Growth Chart] buttons at the top right in the *Vitals* panel (see margin illustration). Figure 7.6 displays an adult vitals graph. From this window clinicians are able to view weight/height, blood pressure, and BMI graphs. For children, growth chart backgrounds are specific to age and gender of the patient for comparison with national percentiles.

Examination

During the physical examination, the practitioner obtains objective data about the patient using inspection, palpation, percussion, and auscultation. Documentation of the physical assessment in SpringCharts begins with documenting systems that are within normal limits and progresses to the documentation of systems with abnormal findings. Pop-up text is available for rapid documentation of the physical assessment. SpringCharts defaults to the normal verbiage in each body system. Pop-up text

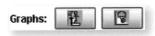

FOCAL POINT

Body Mass Index (BMI) is the measurement of choice for studying obesity.

Graphs: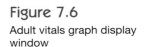

Growth Chart butttons

Figure 7.6

Adult vitals graph display window

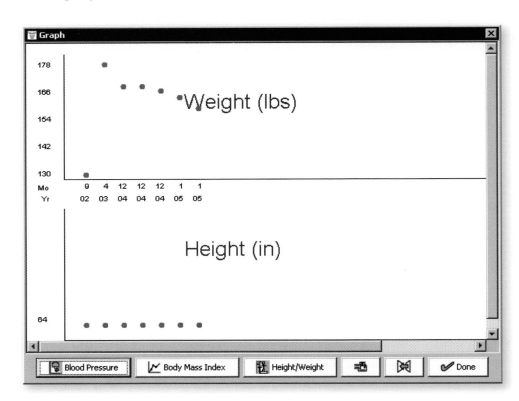

categories are available for documenting specific abnormal conditions.

Diagnosis (Dx)

SpringCharts comes equipped with the complete **American Medical Society (AMA)** library of **International Classification of Diseases, Volume 9 (ICD-9)** codes, the international standard diagnostic classification for all health data. However, each outpatient clinic must activate specific codes for use based on its speciality. Restricting the number of ICD codes shortens the selection time for the end user. Although nurses rely on NANDA-I nursing diagnoses to reflect nursing care, nurse practitioners are required to document medical diagnoses for reimbursement of insurance claims from Medicare, Medicaid, and commercial insurance carriers. Medical diagnoses are selected from the ICD codes.

The diagnosis (*Dx*), prescription (*Rx*), *Test*, and procedure (*Proc*) navigation tabs operate the same by offering a search feature of the database rather than using pop-up text. The diagnosis, prescription, and procedure panels also offer the clinician a choice from items logged from previous patient chart entries. Selecting the *Dx* navigation tab produces a dialog window enabling the practitioner to choose medical diagnoses from the *PMHX + Problem List* window or the *Previous Diagnoses* window, seen in Figure 7.7. The *PMHX − Problem List* displays diagnoses from these corresponding areas of the patient's face sheet and the *Previous Diagnoses* window displays all the diagnoses from previous encounters with this patient in the clinic. These features facilitate selection of previous diagnoses, drugs, and procedures within the office visit.

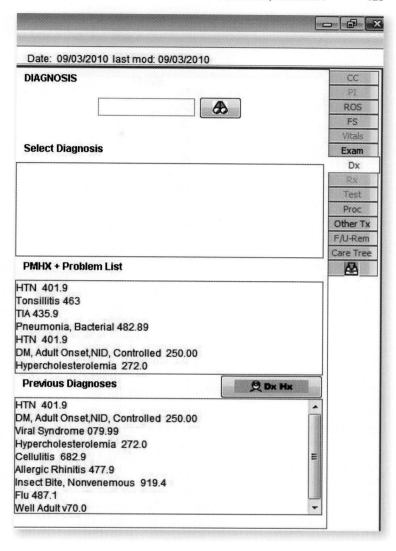

Figure 7.7

Diagnosis panel showing other resources

Activating a New Diagnosis To activate a new diagnosis, the primary care provider selects *New Diagnosis* under the *New* menu on the *Practice View* screen. The *New Diagnosis* window is displayed, as shown in Figure 7.8.

A new diagnosis can be typed directly into the appropriate text and code fields or by selecting the *Lookup* button on the bottom right side of the *New Diagnosis* screen. The *Lookup* button gives access to the ICD-9 database, allowing a search for a new diagnosis by either code or description. When the desired ICD-9 code has been selected, the *Dx Brief Name* field must be completed. Information typed into this field determines the text that the practitioner uses when searching for a medical diagnosis code in the *OV* screen. If the clinic normally uses the same text as the ICD-9 database, the user simply checks the *Use ICD name for Brief name* box.

Figure 7.8

Activating a new diagnosis code

Concept Checkup 7.1

A. What does the SOAP acronym stands for?

S. _____

O. _____

A. _____

P. _____

B. What typically appears in the right panel of the *OV* screen when a navigation tab has been selected in the *Office Visit* window? _____

C. What is the function of the [Copy Previous Note] button in the *OV* window?_____.

D. How many additional custom measurements may be added to the nine basic vitals identified by SpringCharts?_____

E. How do the diagnosis (*Dx*) and prescription (*Rx*) navigation tabs differ from other navigation tabs? _____

FOCAL POINT

American Medical Association (AMA) was founded in 1847 with the purpose of promoting the art and science of medicine.

Documentation Tip

Reassessment of the patient must be performed after administration of all types of medications in the ambulatory care setting. Documentation of the patient's response to the medication demonstrates that this standard of care has been met and protects the nurse from liability for negligence.

Legal/Ethical Considerations

Nurse practitioners may prescribe medications in all states. However, Alabama and Florida are the only two states in which NPs may not prescribe controlled substances (AANP, 2009).

Diagnosis Search button

Medication (Rx)

Nearly 3.7 billion prescriptions were filled by retail pharmacies in 2009 (Kaiser, 2010). The Institute of Medicine (IOM, 2009) estimates that 1.5 million adverse drug events (ADE) occur annually, costing billions of dollars. The primary method recommended by the IOM to reduce drug errors is increased collaboration among healthcare providers and patients where the patient assumes more responsibility for monitoring personal medications and the healthcare provider more actively listens to and educates the patient. This involves a multidisciplinary approach by primary care providers, nurses, and pharmacists. The second method to reduce drug errors recommended by the IOM is use of technology, most notably e-prescribing. Electronic prescriptions are legible and the use of technology to cross-check allergies, drug interactions, and dosages has been shown to reduce errors. In addition, e-prescribing promotes enhanced communication of patient medications among providers. SpringCharts' electronic prescriptions help to avoid costly medication errors.

The prescription (*Rx*) navigation tab allows information windows from the patient's chart related to *Allergies* and *Other Sensitivities* to be viewed in order to prevent prescribing errors, as seen in Figure 7.9. Medications can be selected from the *Routine Medications* and *Previous Prescriptions* windows. Medications prescribed during the office visit can be added to *Routine Medications* by clicking on the specific medication in the lower center window in the *Office Visit* screen and selecting *Add to Routine*, as seen in Figure 7.10. Prescribing information such as the dosage and frequency, also seen in Figure 7.10, can be edited for this specific prescription without changing the system's original medication information.

In the *Edit Rx* window, displayed when the user highlights the prescribed medication, the provider can also associate the medication with specific diagnoses, giving the indication for the prescription. The [Diagnosis Search] button in the *Edit Rx* window (see margin illustration) opens the patient's list of *Previous Diagnoses*, *PMHX*, and *Problem List*. Here, the provider can rapidly select a diagnosis or several diagnoses to accompany the medication information, thus associating an identifiable medical problem to the prescribed medication.

SpringCharts offers a prescription resource link for the prescriber in the main *Prescription* window and the *Edit Rx* window. A link to the Epocrates™ Website,

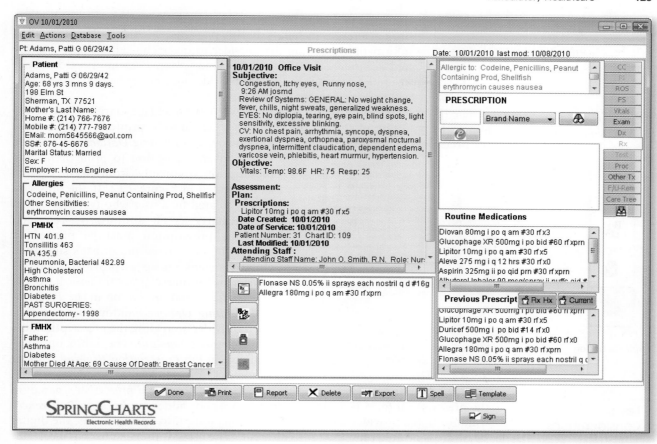

Figure 7.9

Prescription portion of the *OV* note

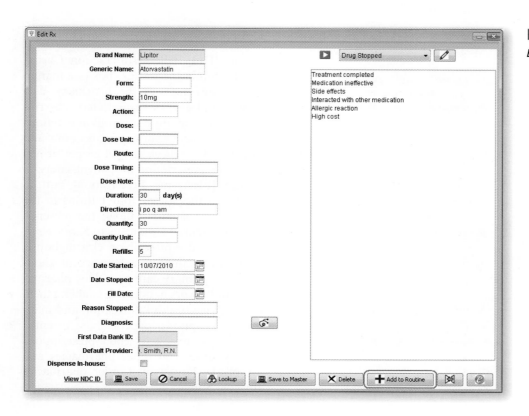

Figure 7.10

Edit Rx window

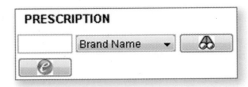

Figure 7.11

Access to the Epocrates website

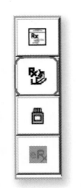

Print Rx button

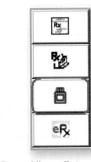

Drug Allergy/Interaction Checking button

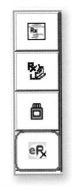

Electronic Prescription button

displayed in Figure 7.11, provides the user with a current Web-based drug reference, including health plan and Medicare **drug formulary** information, allowing the provider to make clinical decisions quickly and accurately. In addition, Epocrates™ provides information about insurance coverage so that the provider may prescribe medications that will be less costly for the patient.

The [print prescription] button in the lower left panel (see margin illustration) allows the prescription(s) from the *Office Visit* screen to be printed or faxed. Once the preferences have been selected in the *Prescription Printing Options* window the user is given the option to print or fax the prescription(s) directly from SpringCharts, as illustrated in Figure 7.12. If the prescription is created by a user who is not set up in SpringCharts as an authorized prescriber, then the prescription must be printed to receive the authorized prescriber's signature. Only clinicians set up as providers, such as physicians or nurse practitioners, have the *Use Digital Signature* option in the *Prescription Printing Options* window. If an authorized provider is creating the prescription, the *Use Electronic Signature* check-box option is available in the *Prescription Printing Options* window. If this is checked, the prescription includes the phrase: *Electronic Signature Verified* above the prescriber's name on the prescription form if a digital signature was not added to the *User Preferences* window. If the provider has added his/her signature into SpringCharts, the digital signature is printed onto the prescription(s). The prescription can be sent electronically directly to the pharmacy's fax machine from SpringCharts. The *Electronic Signature Verified* phrase informs the pharmacy that the prescription was sent by the prescriber. The program always records the provider's name on the prescription from the *Print Name As* field in the *Doctor Information* setup window on Spring-Charts server.

(See Appendix A, *Sample Documents*—Document 5: *Prescription Forms*.)

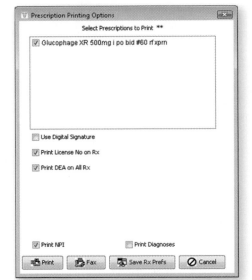

Figure 7.12

Print or fax option for prescription form

The [Drug Allergy/Interaction Checking] button in the *Rx* text box (see margin illustration) accesses the pharmacy Web service and checks the selected prescriptions for potentially dangerous interactions with the patient's current medications and allergies. This check should be performed with each prescription for patient safety.

The [Electronic Prescription] button, shown as the last of four buttons in the *Prescription* window, allows the prescription to be sent electronically to *SureScripts*, a Web-based e-prescribing clearinghouse. SureScripts connects a network of thousands of primary care providers, pharmacists, and payors nationwide enabling them to exchange health information and manage prescriptions paperlessly. Currently, prescribers are able to send e-prescriptions to any of 51,000 retail pharmacies and six of the largest mail-order pharmacies through SureScripts.

Activating a New Medication Although SpringCharts is installed with the complete AMA dictionary of drugs/medications, specific medications that are routinely prescribed by the clinic must be activated from this comprehensive database in order to appear in the active list within SpringCharts. This enables providers to prescribe medication from a limited selection rather than search through long lists of rarely prescribed drugs. To activate a new medication, the user selects *New Drug* under the *New* menu on the *Practice View* screen. The *New Drugs* window is displayed, as illustrated in Figure 7.13. The user can fill out the fields directly or search the database by clicking on the *Lookup* button. Once the drug is selected, the program automatically completes all the appropriate fields. The primary care provider can make necessary modifications within the fields. The prescriber also has access to the Epocrates™ and New-Crop™ websites from the *New Drug* window, also seen in Figure 7.13.

Discontinuing Medication To discontinue a medication that a patient is currently receiving, an *Encounter* must be created in the patient's EHR. Medications may be discontinued from within an *OV Note*, *Nurse Note*, *New TC note*, messages, or anywhere in SpringCharts where the patient's drug list can be accessed. To discontinue a patient's medication, the clinician selects the specific prescription and highlights it to open the *Edit Rx* window, seen in Figure 7.14. This graphic user interface (GUI) enables the practitioner to input a *Date Stopped* and a *Reason Stopped*. The *Reason Stopped* can be selected from preset pop-up text.

Legal/Ethical Considerations

Federal law requires that prescriptions for outpatient medications that are covered by Medicaid be written on tamper-resistant prescription forms. Prescriptions that are electronically transmitted by fax or e-prescription are exempt from this requirement (CMS, 2008).

Tests

Diagnostic tests, such as lab or imaging studies, may be ordered within the *Office Visit* by accessing the *Test* navigation tab. Once the desired tests have been selected, the user clicks the *Order Selected Tests* button, displayed in Figure 7.15, to send the tests to the lower center information window.

Note: For users to order tests in the *Office Visit* screen, they must have first selected an authorized prescriber in the *User Preferences* window—(*File* > *Preferences* > *User Preferences*). Once set up, the program allows the user to order tests.

After selecting the *Order Selected Tests* button, a window listing the primary care providers who are set up in the SpringCharts server opens. The clinician selects the provider who is ordering the tests. The tests can be printed out or faxed as an order by selecting the [printer] icon in the lower center quadrant of the screen—see Figure 7.16. The selected test(s) and the diagnoses from the *Office Visit* note are included on the printed order. Tests that are conducted in the clinic can be deleted from the order form. The user has the option

Figure 7.14
Edit Rx window

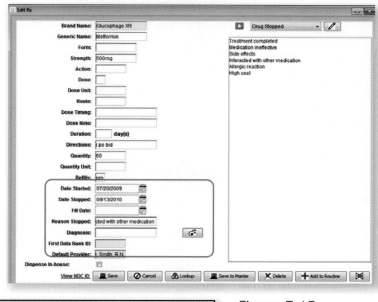

Figure 7.13
New Drug setup window

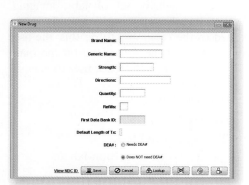

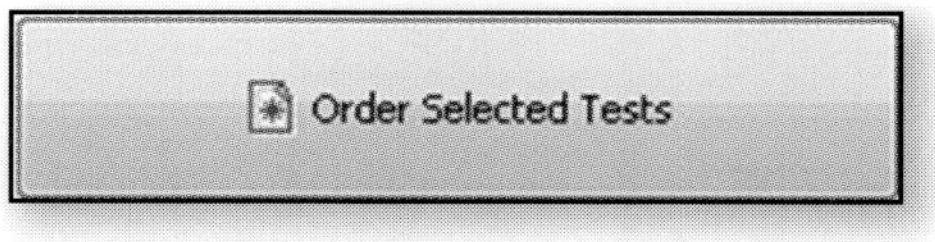

Figure 7.15
Order Selected Tests button in the *Test* panel

Figure 7.16

Printer icon for test order form

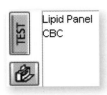

Figure 7.17

Order form showing patient's primary insurance

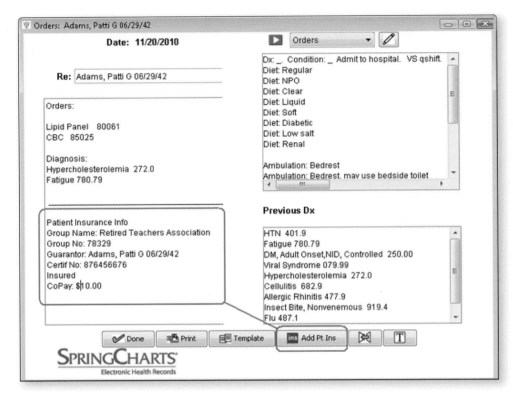

of adding selected pop-up text from the *Orders* category or adding a preset orders template by selecting the *Template* button. The patient's primary insurance information can be added to the order form by selecting the *Add Pt Ins* button, as illustrated in Figure 7.17. Often, the order form for tests to be conducted at a third-party facility are printed and given to the patient. In some cases, the orders are faxed or e-mailed.

(See Appendix A, *Sample Documents*—Document 6: *Test Order Form*.)

The order form may be used to create a referral form. The program automatically places the diagnosis codes from the *OV* note onto the form and provides the user with preset pop-up text and templates, allowing a referral form to be created quickly; printed for the patient, if necessary; and then stored in the patient's electronic chart. The form is printed with the clinic's letterhead and contains the patient's name, address, and date of birth.

Activating New Tests

Lab tests Although SpringCharts contains a very comprehensive set of labs, imaging, and other diagnostic tests, additional tests can be added to the program. To do this, the user selects *Tests* from the *Edit* menu on the main *Practice View* screen. The *Tests* window, seen in Figure 7.18, enables the user to view all installed tests and to create new ones.

The following options are displayed in the *Tests* window:

1. *New Lab Test*—creates a new laboratory test or panel.
2. *New Imaging Test*—creates a new x-ray, CT scan, or MRI test.
3. *New Medical Test*—creates any other type of diagnostic test—non-lab and non-imaging.
4. *List Lab Tests*—shows a list of all current lab tests in the program.

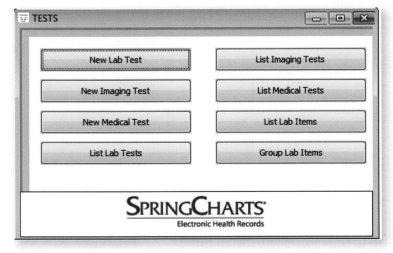

Figure 7.18

Tests window

5. *List Imaging Tests*—shows a list of all current imaging tests in the program.

6. *List Medical Tests*—shows all other diagnostic tests in the program.

7. *List Lab Items*—shows a list of all current lab items that are used to create a lab test or panel.

Whether tests are performed within the clinic or sent to an outside testing facility, all tests must be listed to be ordered from SpringCharts and create a *Pending Test* where the test results are recorded when complete.

To create a new lab test, the user clicks on the *New Lab Test* button. This displays the *Create a New Lab Test* window, as seen in Figure 7.19. Lab tests are created by adding individual components called **lab analytes** or *lab items*. Lab tests may contain one or more analytes. For example, a serum pregnancy test would consist of one lab item (a serum pregnancy lab), whereas a CBC would contain many lab items such as the WBC, RBC, Hgb, Hct. With the *Create a New Lab Test* window opened, the user enters a name in the *Test Name* field and enters the **Current Procedure Terminology (CPT) code** in the *CPT Code* field. The code is important because the test name along with the code is printed on the routing slip for billing purposes. The CPT code also prints on the order form when sent to an outside testing facility to be used by the facility for billing. The user selects the analyte from the list on the left to include in the lab testing. The order in which these lab items are selected is the order in which they appear in the pending lab test.

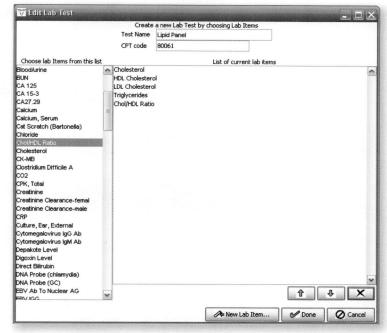

Sometimes it may be helpful for the clinic to have related labs combined together on a single order. This is useful for wellness screenings or specific male and female lab panels. To do this the user selects that *Group Lab Items* button, seen in Figure 7.18, then searches for and selects individual tests to group together. The group is given a name and can be selected in the *Test* panel of the *OV* note. Grouping labs speeds up documentation.

Creating a new analyte If an analyte (lab item) does not appear in the resource list on the left side, it can be created by choosing the *New Lab Item* button located in the bottom of the window (Figure 7.19). New lab items are set up based upon how the lab item results are presented, that is, as a positive/negative, text field, or a minimum/maximum number range, illustrated in Figure 7.20. The user selects the correct option based on the analyte result display. Once completed, the lab item appears in the list of analytes and can then be added to a *New Lab Test* panel. To edit an existing analyte listed in SpringCharts, the user chooses the *List Lab Items* button in the *Tests* window and selects the appropriate lab item. The resulting window, seen in Figure 7.21, allows the user to select and edit ranges and defaults that are displayed for each of the lab items.

Figure 7.19

Creating a new lab panel

Imaging and medical tests To create a new imaging or medical test, the user clicks on, respectively, the *New Imaging Test* or *New Medical Test* button. The *New Imaging Test* or *New Medical Test* window appears, as seen in Figure 7.22.

The test name and the CPT code (required) are typed in and the new test is saved. The user can use the *Lookup* button to access the CPT code dictionary database and have these data entered automatically. In the *Lookup* window the test can be searched by either description or code.

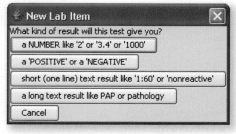

Figure 7.20

Creating a new lab analyte

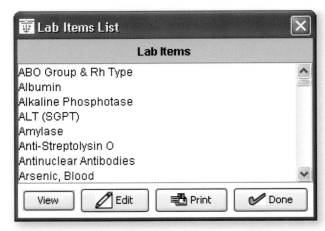

Figure 7.21

Editing an analyte

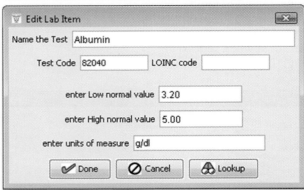

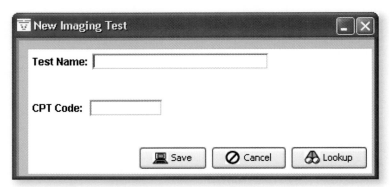

Figure 7.22

Creating a new imaging test

Procedures (Proc)

Procedures are ordered in the *OV* note by selecting first the *Proc* navigation tab in the *OV* window then the correct procedure category. Each category displays only the specific CPT codes that have been activated under these categories. Limiting the number of codes to those that the clinic typically uses facilitates selection. The user may also select procedures from the *Previous Procedure* window in the lower right corner on the *OV* screen if the procedures have been performed during previous encounters with the patient.

Often in an ambulatory setting, the primary care provider orders a treatment or medication that the office nurse performs or administers. To document these nursing actions, the ambulatory care nurse reopens the *OV* note, selects the *Proc* navigation tab, and clicks on the specific procedure. The *Edit Procedure* window displays, seen in Figure 7.23, enabling the clinician to document additional notes such as medication lot number, the **National Drug Code (NDC)** number, injection sites, medication strengths, patient response to the treatment or medication, and patient education. Pop-up text is available in the upper-right section to facilitate documentation of text. The nurse stamps the note using the date/time stamp and the initial stamp. When the *Save* button is selected, these additional notes become part of the *SOAP* note under the *Plan* segment.

Activating a New Procedure To add a new procedure, the user selects *New > New Procedure* from the *Practice View* screen. The *New Procedure* window is displayed, as seen in Figure 7.24. The *Procedure Name* and the *CPT Code* fields are completed. It is important to assign the correct type of procedure from the *Category* drop-down menu. This groups the procedures by category in a drop-down list within the *OV* screen. As mentioned earlier, choosing the procedure category first in the *OV* note speeds up the selection of the procedure by narrowing the range The *Lookup* button provides access to all the AMA procedure codes available in the SpringCharts imbedded dictionary. Although the CPT database is installed with SpringCharts, specific codes need to be manually activated by selecting them from the procedure code dictionary. This enables only the relevant codes needed for the clinic to be sorted and processed in the program during the selection process within the OV screen. The program automatically populates the code and description fields once the code has been selected in the *Lookup* window.

Procedural text can be chosen from the *PopUp Text* window on the right side of the screen as shown in Figure 7.24. It can also be manually typed into the *Procedural Text* window. However, routine text can be added to the set-up on a new procedure in order to automatically populate in the *OV* note when the procedure is selected under the *Proc* navigation tab, illustrated in Figure 7.25. This particular procedural text can be modified for a specific patient in the *OV* screen by clicking on the procedure in the lower-left quadrant, shown in Figure 7.26. Pop-up text that is modified within the *OV* screen only affects the note for the current patient; it does not change the original template text in the procedure set-up.

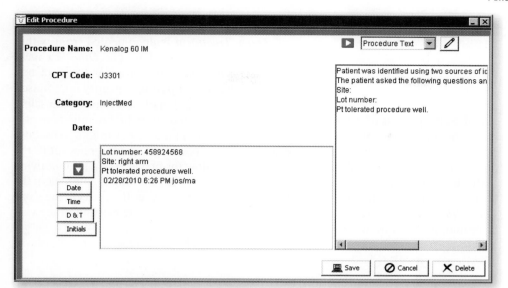

Figure 7.23
Edit Procedure window

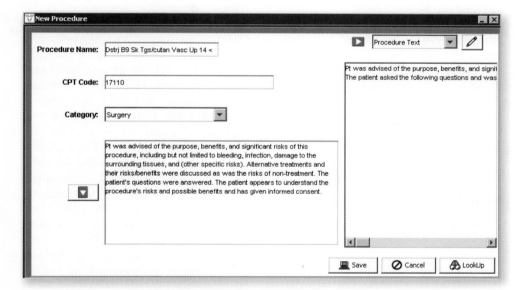

Figure 7.24
Creating a new procedure code

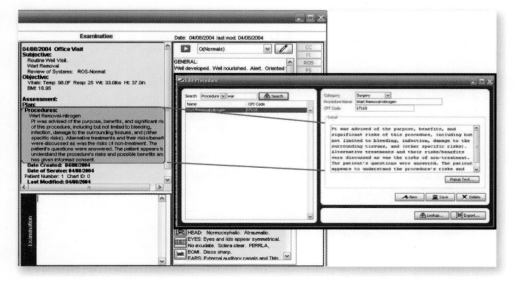

Figure 7.25
Procedure pop-up text automatically added to the *OV* note when *Procedure* selected

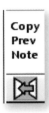

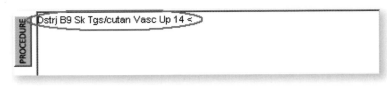

Figure 7.26

Selecting the procedure to modify the text

Copy
Prev
Note

Copy Previous Note button

Figure 7.27

New ToDo/Reminder window in *Office Visit* screen

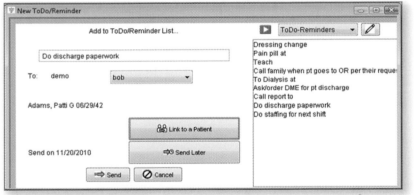

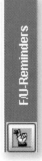

Create a Reminder icon

Other Treatment

Other Treatment is documented from within the *Office Visit* window. The *Other Tx* navigation tab allows the provider to select text from the default pop-up category for counseling or coordination of care items. Counseling involves the process of informing a patient about health matters that require cooperation and a high level of patient compliance such as weight loss or smoking cessation. Once again, text that was used in previous encounters with the patient relevant to the *Other Tx* section is available in the lower-right window for previewing and/or copying into the current visit. If the same "coordination of care" counseling is conducted, the clinician simply highlights previous text (not including the date) then selects the *Copy Prev Note* button to add this previous portion of the note to the existing office visit (see margin illustration).

Follow-up (F/U-Rem)

The *F/U-Rem* navigation tab in the *OV* window allows the selection of a follow-up time recommendation and referral notes. Text may be chosen from the default pop-up text category or selected from the previous note window containing text used in prior encounters.

In the lower left window the user finds a *Create a Reminder* icon (see margin illustration) that enables a *ToDo/Reminder* item to be sent to another person in the clinic or to be set as a personal reminder. Clicking on the icon activates the *New ToDo/Reminder* window, seen in Figure 7.27. The dialog box is automatically linked to the current patient. Pop-up text is available for rapid selection of text. The *Create a Reminder* icon may be useful for communication to the front desk personnel to schedule a follow-up appointment, call a patient, or schedule a procedure with the patient. When the recipient clicks on the item in the *ToDo List*, the patient's chart opens, giving the user the necessary information to execute the scheduled activity.

Concept Checkup 7.2

A. When editing prescription information in the *Edit Rx* window, what information is not changed? _____

B. If a provider has added a personal signature to the SpringCharts program, the digital signature can be automatically added to the _____, which is printed or electronically faxed to the pharmacy.

C. What allows individuals other than licensed independent providers to order tests within the *Office Visit* screen? _____
_____

D. What is selected first to choose a procedure? _____
_____.

LO 7.3   Modifying the OV Note

Selecting the *Sign* button in the *OV* screen provides the practitioner with the opportunity to *Initial Only* or *Permanent Sign & Lock* the office visit, as seen in Figure 7.28.

Initial Only allows the office visit note to be recalled for further edits by anyone with chart editing privileges. Portions of the *OV* note can be completed and saved into the patient's chart without the entire note being finalized, enabling various interdisciplinary team members to document their contribution to the patient's care. For example, a nurse may document the chief complaint and record the vitals in an *OV* note, then save the partial note into the patient's chart. A nurse practitioner may open the same note from another computer, complete the exam, assign medical diagnoses, prescribe medication, and create a routing slip for billing purposes. The *OV* note is placed in the patient's chart by selecting the *Done* button. A provider should not "lock" an *OV* note, even if the routing slip for billing has been completed, in case the ambulatory care nurse needs to reopen the *OV* note and document details about a medication, treatment, procedure, patient education, or the final assessment before the patient leaves the clinic.

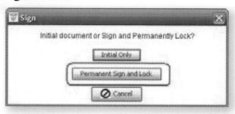

Figure 7.28
The *Sign* window in the office visit

Once the *OV* note is locked, by selecting *Permanent Sign & Lock*, it cannot be unlocked or edited, even by the individual who permanently locked it. However, an addendum can be placed at the bottom of an *OV* note, if needed. If an unlocked *OV* note is edited at a future date, the *Last Modified Date* is updated, as illustrated in Figure 7.29. The *Date Created*, *Date of Service*, and *Last Modified* date are recorded automatically at the bottom of the *OV* note.

Date Created: 11/20/2010
Date of Service: 11/18/2010
Patient Number: 31   Chart ID: 98
Last Modified: 11/20/2010

Figure 7.29
Dates automatically recorded in the office visit

The "date created" is the computer system date that is hard coded to the *OV* note when the note is first created and ***cannot be altered***. It provides the legal means of determining the date of documentation. The *Date of Service* automatically defaults to the date that the *OV* note was first created; however, it ***can be altered***. The "date of service" is important for billing and must accurately represent the actual date of the encounter, even if the note itself was created on a date subsequent to the encounter date with the patient. For this reason, the "date of service" can be modified. It is possible for the "date created" to be different from the "date of service." On the *Office Visit* menu, the provider selects *Tools > Date of Service*. The desired date of service is selected in the dialog box. This causes the office visit to be saved in the *Care Tree Encounter* category with the appropriate date of service. This date is transferred to the practice management system software for billing or printed on the routing slip used for billing.

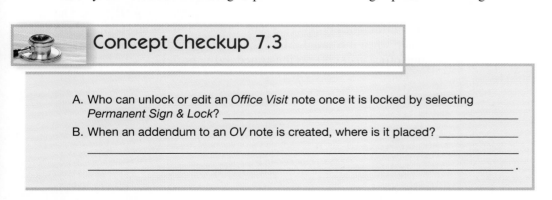

Concept Checkup 7.3

A. Who can unlock or edit an *Office Visit* note once it is locked by selecting *Permanent Sign & Lock*? _____

B. When an addendum to an *OV* note is created, where is it placed? _____
_____
_____ .

LO 7.4   Creating an Addendum

Providers have the ability to lock an *OV* note so that no additional documentation can be entered into the note. *OV* notes are locked by clicking on the *Sign* button in the *OV* screen. The user is given the option to either initial the note or *permanently sign and lock* the note, as seen in Figure 7.30. *OV* notes that have been permanently signed and locked cannot be edited but can have an addendum placed after the initial

Figure 7.30

OV notes can be permanently locked

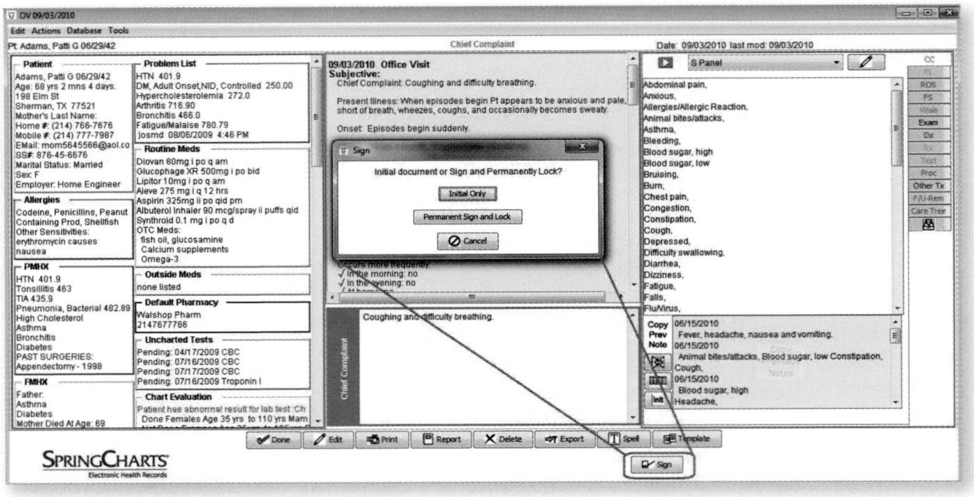

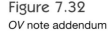

Figure 7.31

Creating an addendum to a locked *OV* note

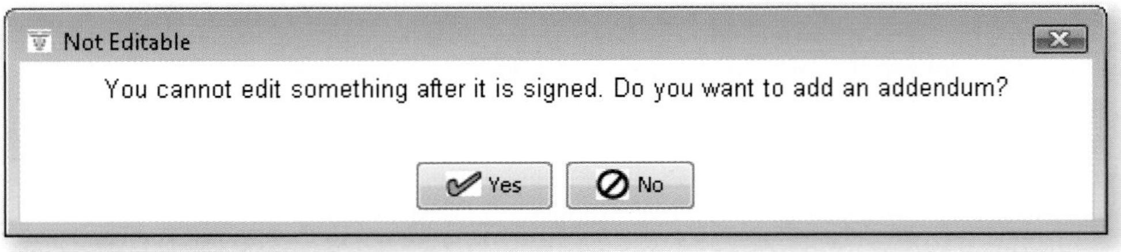

> **Not Editable** ✕
>
> You cannot edit something after it is signed. Do you want to add an addendum?
>
> ✓ Yes   ⊘ No

Figure 7.32

OV note addendum

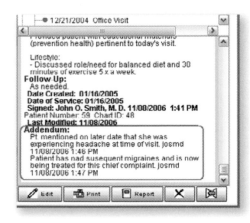

documentation for clarification or addition of facts that may have been inadvertently omitted. In an existing "Signed & Locked" office visit located in the *Care Tree*, the clinician selects the *Edit* button in the lower right panel in the patient's chart to create an **addendum** to the *OV* note, illustrated in Figure 7.31.

Note: This option does not appear if the *OV* note was not *permanently signed and locked*. In this case the *OV* note may be opened and information added or modified in the body of the existing note. The system updates the *Last Modified* date at the bottom of the note.

The addendum is placed at the bottom of the existing *OV* note. The program automatically places a date-, time-, and initial-stamp on the addendum when it is saved. More than one addendum can be placed in the same office visit note, as illustrated in Figure 7.32.

Using Terminology

Match the terms on the left with the definitions on the right.

_____ 1. SOAP

_____ 2. BMI

_____ 3. Date of Service

_____ 4. ICD-9

_____ 5. CPT

_____ 6. Pending test

_____ 7. Lab analyte

_____ 8. Date Created

_____ 9. SureScripts

_____ 10. AMA

_____ 11. Addendum

_____ 12. Office visit

A. The *International Classification of Diseases*, Vol 9.

B. This association was founded in 1847 with the purpose of promoting the art and science of medicine.

C. A note added subsequent to the original office visit encounter documentation.

D. A centralized clearinghouse that connects a network of thousands of primary care providers, pharmacists, and payors nationwide.

E. An encounter with a healthcare provider during which the patient's chief complaints are evaluated.

F. A method of documenting an OV using subjective and objective data, an assessment, and the plan for treatment.

G. Current procedure terminology.

H. The measurement of choice for studying obesity.

I. A test (lab, imaging, and diagnostic) that has been ordered but does not have results.

J. The date that the patient encounter took place.

K. A blood test item that is subject to its own specific chemical analysis.

L. The computer system date that is hard coded to the *OV* note when the note is first created.

Checking Your Understanding

Write "T" or "F" in the blank to indicate whether the statement is true or false.

_____ 13. The navigation tabs enable the provider to proceed through the office visit and includes the chief complaint (*CC*).

_____ 14. The use of Build-Your text is the most rapid way of building documentation in an office visit.

_____ 15. SpringCharts is installed with the complete AMA library of ICD-9 and CPT codes.

_____ 16. SpringCharts does not allow you to activate any of the ICD-9 or CPT codes that are listed in the AMA library.

_____ 17. SpringCharts comes with a large hardbound AMA dictionary of drugs/medications.

_____ 18. *OV* notes that have been permanently signed and locked cannot be amended.

Answer the question below in the space provided.

19. What four components make up the SOAP format?

    S. _____

    O. _____

    A. _____

    P. _____

Choose the best answer and circle the corresponding letter.

20. This panel, seen on the left side of the *Office Visit* screen, enables the clinician to view the patient's
    a) Past addendums
    b) Face sheet
    c) Various pop-up texts

21. The History & Physical report contains
    a) A combination of the patient's health history and the physical exam
    b) The history and physical location of the ambulatory clinic
    c) The details of the current SOAP note

22. The History of Present Illness is part of what component of the SOAP note?
    a) Plan
    b) Objective
    c) Subjective

23. When medication needs to be discontinued for a patient, an encounter with that patient must be created. Where can medications be recorded as discontinued? (Select all that apply)
    a) The *OV* note and *Nurse Note*
    b) *New TC Note* and messages
    c) *Routine Meds* and *Current Meds*

24. In the *F/U-Rem* section of the *Office Visit* screen, the user finds a *Create a Reminder* icon that enables the provider to send a *ToDo/Reminder* item to
    a) A patient's home e-mail
    b) Another person in the clinic
    c) An outside lab

25. The abbreviation "ROS" stands for
    a) Routine oral surgery
    b) Registered oncology school
    c) Review of systems

References

AAACN. (n.d.). About AAACN: Ambulatory Care Nursing defined. Retrieved June 24, 2010, from http://www.aaacn.org/cgi-bin/WebObjects/AAACNMain.woa/1/wa/viewSection?s_id=1073743905&ss_id=536873820&wosid=QRxZ1c45kZ5T3Kj65j01Jp7k5TY

AAACN. (2010). Frequently asked questions: Ambulatory care. Retrieved August 6, 2010, from http://www.aaacn.org/cgi-bin/WebObjects/AAACNMain.woa/1/wa/viewSection?s_id=1073744312&ss_id=536873724

AANP. (n.d.). About AANP. Retrieved August 6, 2010, from http://www.aanp.org/AANPCMS2/AboutAANP

AANP. (2009). Nurse Practitioner Prescriptive Authority. Retrieved August 6, 2010, from http://www.aanp.org/NR/rdonlyres/8A2583FC-981F-45FD-BB6D-094BDF4AEE7A/0/AuthoritytoPrescribeMap609Color.pdf

AANP. (2010a). Frequently asked questions: Why choose a nurse practitioner as your health-care provider? Retrieved August 6, 2010, from http://www.aanp.org/NR/rdonlyres/67BE3A60-6E44-42DF-9008-DF7C1F0955F7/0/2010FAQsWhatIsAnNP.pdf

AANP. (2010b). Nurse practitioner cost effectiveness. Retrieved August 6, 2010, from http://www.aanp.org/NR/rdonlyres/197C9C42-4BC1-42A5-911E-85FA759B0308/0/CostEffectiveness4pages.pdf

American Medical Association. (n.d.). Mission and history of the AMA. Retrieved August 6, 2010, from http://www.ama-assn.org/ama/pub/about-ama.shtml

Bauer, J. C. (2010). Nurse practitioners as an underutilized resource for health reform: Evidence-based demonstrations of cost effectiveness. *Journal of the American Academy of Nurse Practitioners, 22*, 228–231.

Centers for Medicaid and Medicare Services. (2008). Medicaid tamper-resistant prescription law: Pharmacist fact sheet. Retrieved August 6, 2010, from https://www.cms.gov/FraudAbuseforProfs/Downloads/pharmacisfactsheet.pdf

Haas, S. A. (2010). Priming the pipeline: Creating aspirations for new graduate nurses to enter ambulatory care nursing roles. *Nursing Economic$, 27*(1), 58–60.

Institute of Medicine. (2009). Report brief: Preventing medication errors. Retrieved August 6, 2010, from http://www.iom.edu/~/media/Files/Report%20Files/2006/Preventing-Medication-Errors-Quality-Chasm-Series/medicationerrorsnew.ashx

Kaiser Family Foundation. (2010). Total number of retail prescription drugs filled at pharmacies, 2009. Retrieved August 6, 2010, from http://www.statehealthfacts.org/comparemaptable.jsp?ind=265&cat=5

U.S. Food and Drug Administration. (2010). National drug code directory. Retrieved August 6, 2010, from http://www.fda.gov/Drugs/InformationOnDrugs/ucm142438.htm

Ambulatory

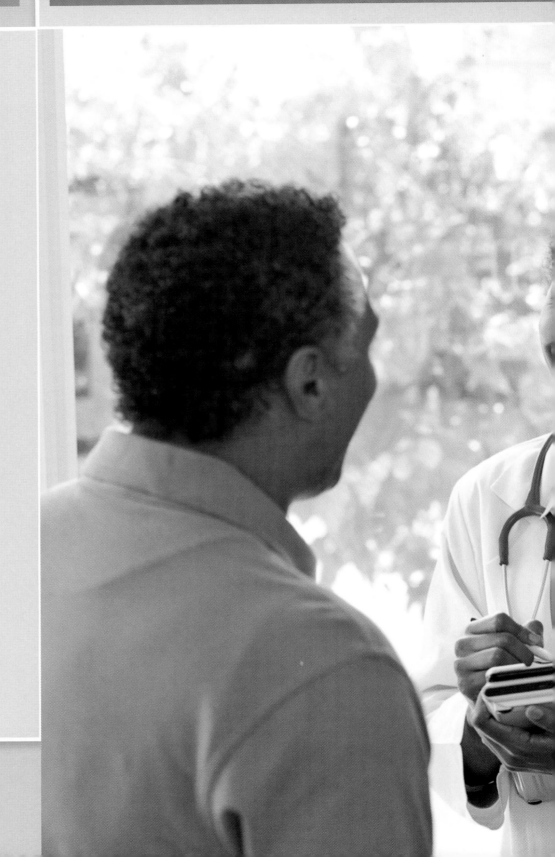

Healthcare Exercises

Learning Outcomes

When you complete Chapter 8, you will be able to:

8.1   Use SpringCharts to create an office visit note.

8.2   Use SpringCharts to modify an office visit note.

8.3   Carry out generating office visit reports.

8.4   Use SpringCharts to construct an excuse note.

8.5   Use SpringCharts to make an addendum to the office visit note.

What You Need to Know

To understand Chapter 8, you need to know:

- How to open an electronic patient chart.
- The purpose of an office visit note.
- The key elements of an office visit note.
- The function of an addendum to an office visit note.

Exercise 8.1

Building an Office Visit Note (Part 1—Ambulatory Care Nurse)

1. Open the patient's chart with your name. On the chart menu select *New > New OV*. In the *Office Visit* screen, notice the face sheet information on the left-hand side of the window.

2. Add another past health history item to the face sheet by right-clicking in the *PMHX* section and selecting *Edit*. In the *Face Sheet* window, choose another medical condition either from the list of *Preferences* in the lower left or by searching for a new medical diagnosis in the upper right. Click the *Back to Chart* button in the lower left.

Note: The *OV* screen is positioned behind the patient's chart window; you will see the top portion of the window. To bring it to the foreground, simply click on the top edge of the *OV* window.

3. A patient is visiting the nurse practitioner because of a flare-up of seasonal allergies and the ambulatory care nurse is performing an initial assessment. Click on the *CC* navigation tab on the right side of the *Office Visit* screen. In the *S Panel* of pop-up text that appears in the right-hand panel, select *Allergies/Allergic Reaction, Runny nose, Itchy eyes*. The words are added to the lower middle work area. Click on the [Time-Stamp] and [Initial] buttons in the lower right section to add the time and your initials to the note.

4. Select the *Vitals* navigation tab on the left. All previously created text is now added to the *SOAP* format. Create and enter vitals information on your patient. (Documentation of head circumference (HC) is not needed since this is not a pediatric patient.) BMI (body mass index) is grayed out because the program calculates this item from the height and weight.

5. Click on the *Done* button in the *OV* screen. Click the *Save and Skip Billing* button. The note will be finished later and a routing slip created at that time for this office visit. The *OV* note has been added to the list of *Encounters* in the *Care Tree* of your patient's chart. Close the chart.

Exercise 8.2

Building an Office Visit Note (Part 2—Primary Care Provider)

Note: Now that the ambulatory care nurse has completed the initial assessment, the office visit is handed over to the nurse practitioner. The nurse practitioner does not start a new *Office Visit* note (as the ambulatory care nurse did), but edits the existing *Office Visit* note.

1. Open your chart. Click on the + sign beside the *Encounters* heading in the *Care Tree*. Select the office visit entry started in Exercise 8.1. Click on the *Edit* button at the bottom of the window.

Note: In the *Office Visit* screen the provider can view the information already documented by the ambulatory care nurse. SpringCharts has office visit templates for some of the most common ailments, enabling the provider to quickly select the appropriate template to populate the office visit note. The provider individualizes the note to reflect this patient's condition.

2. Click on the *Template* button in the bottom right corner of the *Office Visit* screen. From the displayed list select: *Allergic Rhinitis*. Notice the entire note has been built very quickly.

3. The nurse practitioner completes the note for this patient. Click on the *PI* navigation tab on the right side. The text from the template appears in the lower middle work area. Move the scroll bar to the top of this window and complete the following sentence: *Pt c/o red, itchy eyes, congested, itchy and runny nose (clear fluid), post-nasal drip, sneezing, itchy ears, scratchy throat and occasional cough for the past_weeks*. Place your cursor in front of the word weeks, highlight the underscore mark and type: *3*. Complete the missing information in the remainder on the *PI* section by either adding or deleting information.

Note: The primary care provider continues through the entire note making changes and additions where necessary for this specific patient.

4. A diagnosis must be added. Click on the *Dx* navigation tab on the right side. This patient has had allergies in the past. The diagnosis is in the *Previous Diagnoses* window in the lower right corner. Select *Allergic Rhinitis 477.9* from this list.

5. Next the nurse practitioner prescribes a medication. Click on the *Rx* navigation tab. Once again, medications for allergies have been prescribed in the past. Select *Allegra* and *Flonase* from the *Previous Prescription* window in the lower-right corner.

6. The nurse practitioner wants the ambulatory care nurse to administer a subcutaneous allergy injection. Choose the *Proc* navigation tab on the right side. Click on the drop-down arrow beside the *All* category on the upper-right side. Select the category: *InjectMed*. From the list displayed below, choose *Kenalog 60 IM*.

7. Click on the *Done* button in the *OV* screen. Click the *Save and Skip Billing* button. The *OV* note has been added to the list of *Encounters* in the *Care Tree* of the patient's chart. Close the chart.

Exercise 8.3

Building an Office Visit Note (Part 3—Ambulatory Care Nurse)

Note: The nurse practitioner communicates with the ambulatory care nurse regarding administration of the allergy injection.

1. Open your chart. Click on the + sign beside the *Encounters* heading in the *Care Tree*. Select the *Office Visit* note you edited in Exercise 8.2. Click on the *Edit* button at the bottom of the window.

2. Click on the *Proc* navigation tab on the right side. Click on *Kenalog* injection in the lower center work area.

3. In the *Edit Procedure* window, document the injection that you just administered. Choose the pop-up text: *Lot number* and type in the lot number (*4331*).

On the next line select the pop-up text: *NDC number* and type the National Drug Code (*0003-0293-05*). On the next line choose the pop-up text: *Site* and type: *Left arm*. On a new line, document the patient's response to the injection; select the pop-up text: *Tolerated well without evidence of untoward reaction.* Click on the *D & T* button and the *Initials* button. Click the *Save* button.

4. Click on the *Done* button in the *OV* screen. Click the *Save and Skip Billing* button. It is the nurse practitioner's responsibility to complete the routing slip and bill for the encounter. The *OV* note has been added to the list of *Encounters* in the *Care Tree* of your patient's chart. Close the chart.

Exercise 8.4

Creating an Examination Report

1. Open your patient's chart. Highlight the recent *Office Visit* note. Click on the *Report* button at the bottom of the patient's chart screen. The program automatically opens the *OV* window and displays the examination report on the screen.

2. Print the report by clicking on the *Print* button in the report window. Spring-Charts automatically places the letterhead, patient's name and address, greeting, and introduction in the report letter. If you are sending an electronic document to your instructor, choose the pdf printer and e-mail the document.

3. Close the *Report* window. Submit the printed report to your instructor.

Exercise 8.5

Creating an H&P Report

1. In the *OV* window, click on the *Tools* menu and select *H&P.* The H&P contains relevant information from the current physical exam as well as documentation from the patient's face sheet.

2. Print the report and submit to your instructor or choose the pdf printer and e-mail the document to your instructor.

3. Click the *Done* button and save the H&P under the *H&Ps* category in the *Care Tree*.

(See Appendix A, *Sample Documents*—Document 7: *History & Physical Report.*)

Exercise 8.6

Creating an OV Note Report

1. With your *Office Visit* window still open, click on the *Print* button and print the entire *Office Visit* note. (To submit your coursework electronically please see section Submitting Assignments Electronically on page xxvii in the Preface of the text). The *OV* note is not pre-addressed to any entity and may be sent to a referring primary care provider or other consultant.

2. Submit the printed *OV* note to your instructor. *Office Visit* notes can be added to the body of a letter and printed, faxed, or e-mailed to the patient or others.

3. Close the *OV* window.

4. In the patient's chart, the *Report to Patient* and the *Office Visit* are saved as *Encounters* in the *Care Tree* and the *H&P* is saved under the *H&P* category in the *Care Tree*. Click on the + sign beside the *H&P* category and highlight the recently created H&P report. The report is seen in the lower-right quadrant where it can be edited and printed.

5. Close the patient's chart.

(See Appendix A, *Sample Documents*—Document 8: *Office Visit Report.*)

Exercise 8.7

Creating an Excuse Note

1. Open your patient's chart. Open the recent *Office Visit* note by clicking on the + next to *Encounters*. Click on the office visit and click *Edit* below. Click on the *Tools* menu inside the *Office Visit* screen and select *New Excuse/Note/Order > New Excuse/Note*. In the To area type: *To whom it may concern.* In the *Note* window select pop-up text to compose an excuse for the student's absence from college for the time that the student was at the doctor's office. Complete the missing information. Add your initials to the note by selecting the *Sign* button.

2. Print the excuse note and submit to your instructor or choose the pdf printer and e-mail the document to your instructor. Click on the *Done* button.

3. Click on the *Sign* button in the lower right section of the *OV* screen. Select *Permanent Sign and Lock.* Click the *Done* button and skip billing.

4. Click on the + sign to the left of the *Excuses Notes* category in the *Care Tree* and see the saved note. The note is displayed in the lower right window.

5. Click on the + sign to the left of *Encounters.* A black *Lock* icon is present to the left of the recent *Office Visit* note. No user is able to modify a locked *Office Visit* note.

Exercise 8.8

Preparing an Addendum

1. Open your patient's chart. Open the recent *Office Visit* note that you signed and locked by clicking on the *Edit* button at the bottom of the screen.

2. A warning note appears stating that you are not able to edit this note. You want to create an addendum. Click the *Yes* option.

3. In the *Office Visit Addendum* window add the following comment: *Patient complained of dull, frontal headache at time of visit. Pain level 3 on scale of 0–10.*

4. Click on the *Done* button. Close the *Office Visit* screen.

5. Scroll to the bottom of the *Office Visit* note in the lower right corner of the patient's chart. The addendum appears at the end of the *OV* note. The addendum is automatically signed and dated.

6. Using the *Print* button located at the bottom of the window, print the *OV* note and submit to your instructor. If you are transmitting an electronic document to your instructor, choose the pdf printer and send the document as an e-mail. Close the patient's chart.

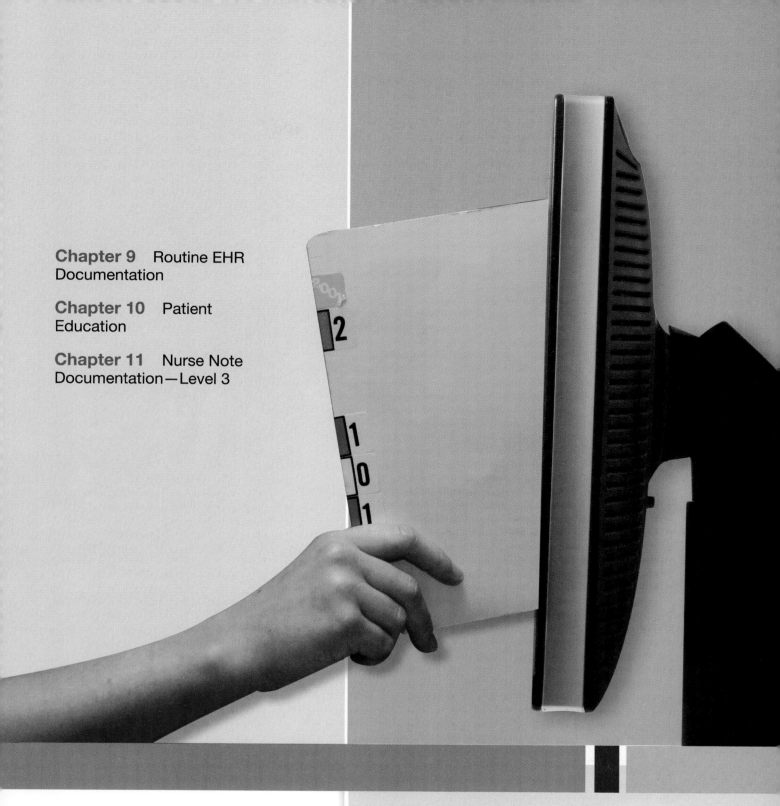

Level Three

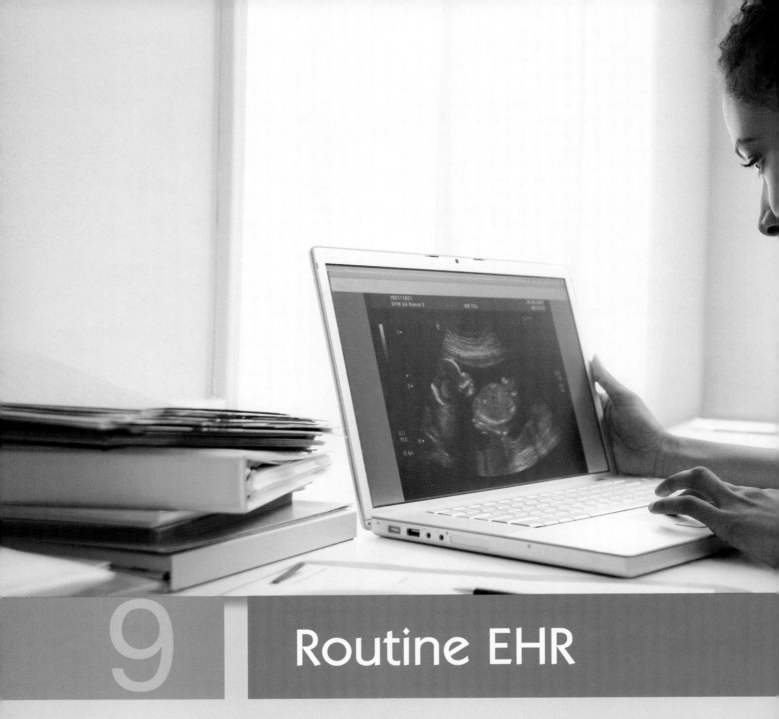

9 Routine EHR

Key Term

Term and abbreviation you will encounter in Chapter 9; they are defined in the end-of-book glossary:

Vaccination
   Information
   Statement (VIS)

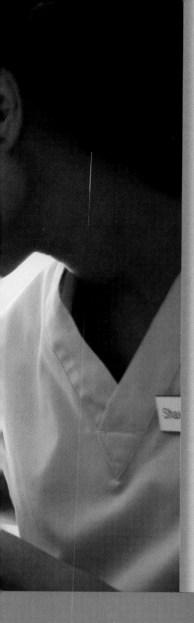

Learning Outcomes

When you complete Chapter 9, you will be able to:

9.1   Use the *ToDo List* feature.

9.2   Use internal messages.

9.3   Carry out accessing and completing the patient's immunization record.

9.4   Carry out creating and distributing a patient instruction sheet.

9.5   Use the draw program to develop illustrations to enhance documentation.

Documentation

What You Need to Know

To understand Chapter 9, you need to know how to:

- Navigate in the *Practice View* screen.
- Navigate in the *Patient Chart* screen.
- Navigate in the *Nurse Note* screen.

FOCAL POINT

The *ToDo/Reminder* feature is a user-defined item that replaces the need for hard-copy to-do lists.

Figure 9.1

New ToDo/Reminder window

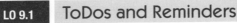

LO 9.1   ToDos and Reminders

Nurses in the clinical setting, both inpatient and outpatient, often maintain personal task reminders, or "to do" lists. For example, a nurse may make a note to check a particular lab result for a patient at the expected completion time or to follow up on medication effectiveness. With SpringCharts, this "to do" list may be maintained electronically.

The *ToDo List* is located in the lower-left quadrant of the *Practice View* screen. A *ToDo* item is set by clicking once on the *ToDo List* title bar. In the *New ToDo/ Reminder* window, illustrated in Figure 9.1, one may (1) notate the *ToDo* item, (2) send the item to another coworker, (3) link the item to a patient, and/or (4) schedule the *ToDo/Reminder* for a future date.

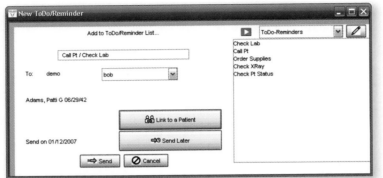

In the *New ToDo/Reminder* window, the user types the *ToDo/Reminder* message in the top text field or selects pop-up text from the list in the right window. To add to this list of pop-up text for current and future use, the user simply clicks on the [edit pencil] icon. The link opens the *Edit PopUp Text* feature enabling text to be added, deleted, or modified. When accessing the *Edit PopUp Text* window from within the *ToDo/Reminder* feature, the *ToDo/ Reminder* category of text is selected by default. Lines of text can be moved up or down using the arrows to the far left.

Figure 9.2

Items set in the *ToDo List*

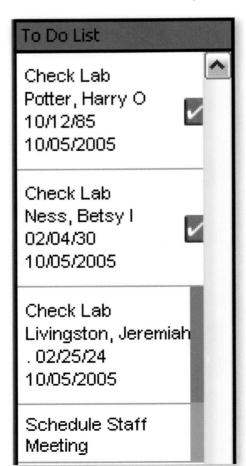

When a user sends a personal *ToDo/Reminder* item, it is stored in the user's *ToDo List*, illustrated in Figure 9.2, until the item is completed.

Patient-specific reminders may be connected to a patient's chart by selecting the *Link to a Patient* button. A search is conducted for the patient by last name. Once selected, the program adds the patient's name into the window, as seen in Figure 9.1. A *ToDo/Reminder* item linked to a patient automatically opens the patient's chart when activated, giving the nurse immediate access to the patient's demographics and health information.

A *ToDo/Reminder* item may be created for a later date. For example, the nurse may need to call a patient in three months to schedule lab work. The action date is determined by selecting the *Send Later* button, illustrated in Figure 9.1, and selecting the appropriate date. The *ToDo/ Reminder* item is added to the list on the appointed date.

ToDo/Reminder items can be sent to other coworkers in the network. As with personal *ToDo/Reminder* items, those sent to coworkers may be linked to a patient's record or programmed for a particular date. This function may be useful for items that require follow-up after change of shift. For example, if a nurse administers an analgesic just before the change of shift, a reminder can be sent to the oncoming nurse to assess and document the medication's effectiveness. Once sent, the item appears in the recipient's *ToDo List.*

When *ToDo/Reminder* items are set, they have one of four color indicators, as shown below:

1. A personal *ToDo* with a green bar on the right, as seen in Figure 9.2, is active and stays on the user's list until it is selected. Selecting the item changes it from active to completed, indicated by a red checked box, as also seen in Figure 9.2. Selecting it again reactivates the *ToDo* item and the green bar replaces the red checked box, indicating that the item is active.

2. A *ToDo* item with a blue bar on the right indicates the item is linked to a patient. When this item is selected, the patient's chart opens. When the chart is closed, the task is automatically checked as completed. The item may be clicked on with the mouse to reactivate it.

3. A *ToDo* item with an orange bar indicates a communication item between a user and an administrator regarding desired changes to the time clock feature. This kind of *ToDo* item is generated when an employee requests an adjustment to specific login to logout times that have been created when the employee used the time clock feature of SpringCharts.

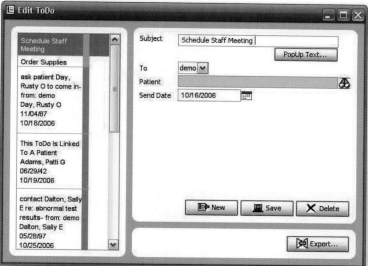

Figure 9.3
Edit ToDo window

4. A *ToDo* item with a red check is a completed item and does not appear with subsequent log-ons. Clicking on a red check box reactivates the *ToDo* item. All active items remain on the user's *ToDo List* until completed.

My ToDo List

Current and future *ToDo/Reminders* can be accessed by selecting *Edit > My ToDo List* on the main menu. From the *Edit ToDo* window, the various items can be reassigned to different users, reset to a different due date, or linked to a patient. Pop-up text can also be edited from this window. The *Save* button updates the *ToDo List*. New *ToDoReminder* items can be created from the *Edit ToDo* window as seen in Figure 9.3. Newly created items are automatically added to the user's *ToDo List* on the main screen. When a nurse plans to be away from work for an extended period of time for a vacation or other time off, arrangements should be made for future *ToDo* items that are due during the planned absence.

FOCAL POINT
The message center in SpringCharts enables the user to send and receive messages from coworkers and send and receive or e-mail messages outside of the organization.

Figure 9.4
Message list window

LO 9.2 | ## Internal Messages

The message center is located in the lower-right quadrant of the main screen. The SpringCharts message system is an intra- and interoffice mail function that enables users to send and receive messages with other SpringCharts users on the network and to e-mail messages over the Internet.

A message is viewed by clicking on it in the *Messages* list. Messages are arranged with the most recent at the top. The display shows the name of the sender, the date and time the message was sent, and the subject line, as seen in Figure 9.4.

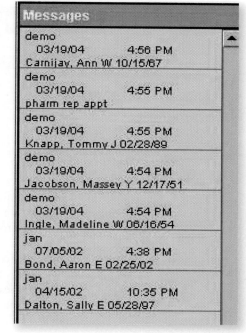

Non-Patient Messages

To create a new message, the user clicks on the *Messages* title bar or chooses *New Message* from the *New* menu on the main window. A dialog appears, asking if this message concerns a patient. If the message does not concern a patient and *No* is selected, a blank message window, shown in Figure 9.5, appears.

The user selects the recipient in the *To:* box from the pull-down list of users at the top of the message window. The subject line is completed and then the message body is typed into the text area in the middle

Figure 9.5

New non-patient message window

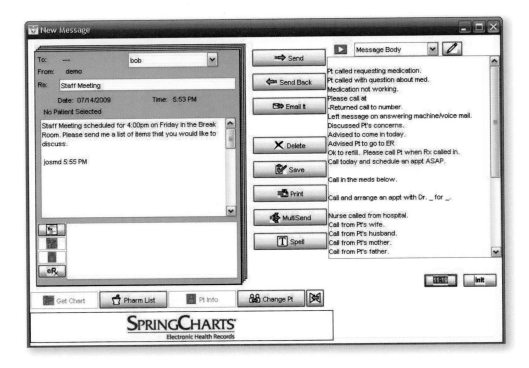

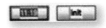

Time and *Initial* stamps

of the message. If desired, pop-up text may be selected in the window to the right. The message is electronically time- and initial-stamped by using the buttons below the pop-up text window, as seen in the margin illustration.

To add to the message pop-up text list for current and future use, the user simply clicks on the [edit pencil] icon. The link opens the *Edit PopUp Text* feature enabling the user to add, delete, or modify text in many different categories that are used in the system. The appropriate category on the left side (in this case: *Message Body*) is selected by default and necessary adjustments to the text can be made. Lines of text can be moved up or down by clicking on the arrows to the far left of the text to be moved.

The sender clicks the *Send* button to send the message to others in the office, or uses the *Email It* button to send the message as an e-mail, seen in Figure 9.5. When selecting an e-mail address, the address book entries may be used or the e-mail address may be manually entered. If the e-mail has been linked to a patient, the patient's e-mail address may be selected as illustrated in Figure 9.6.

The *Send Back* button, seen in Figure 9.5, is used to reply to the original sender as an in-office message. If the sender wishes to send the message to more than one user, the *MultiSend* button is used to allow selection of the appropriate recipients. The *Pharm List* button allows the user to see a list of all of the pharmacies entered into the SpringCharts' address book. Selecting a pharmacy from the list adds the pharmacy name and phone number to the body of the message. The *Spell* button accesses a spell checker, seen in Figure 9.7, that allows new words to be added to an in-program dictionary.

Messages that are not patient-related may be saved to private message archives. Archived messages are viewed from the *Edit* menu by selecting *Message Archive*. The message can be reactivated into the Message center from the *Message Archive* window. In addition, new messages can be created from the *Message Archive* window.

Figure 9.6

E-mail options window

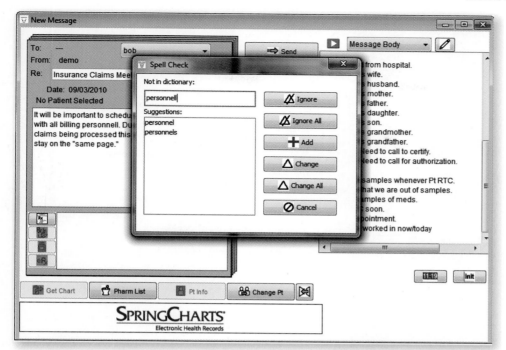

Figure 9.7

Spell Check feature in *New Message* window

Messages Concerning Patients

If a message is linked to a patient, a message window appears that provides quick access to the last patient accessed, as seen in Figure 9.8. If this is the desired patient, the user selects *Yes* and the patient's demographics are added as a left panel to the message, as seen in Figure 9.9. If this is not the desired patient, selecting the *No* option opens a search window to access the correct patient.

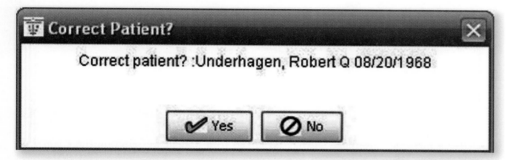

Figure 9.8

Use recent patient prompt window

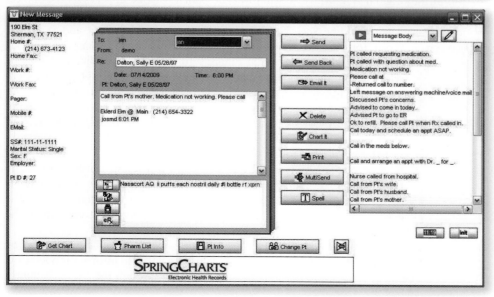

Figure 9.9

New patient-related window

Figure 9.10

Access to the patient's medications

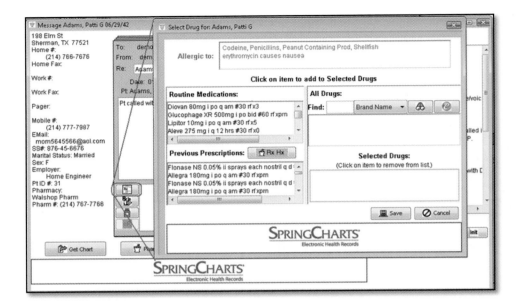

Figure 9.11

Edit Prescriptions window

FOCAL POINT

When a message concerns a patient, the patient's name and demographics are displayed with the message. The patient's chart and medications are accessible from the message screen.

FOCAL POINT

A message that does not involve a patient can be archived. A message regarding a patient can be placed in the patient's EHR.

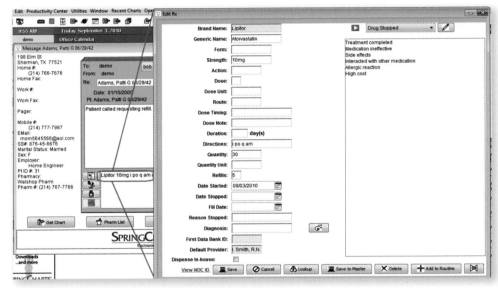

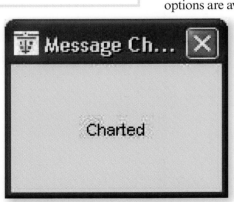

Figure 9.12

Message Charted notification

After a message is initiated, it may be linked to a patient by selecting the *Change Pt* button in the original *New Message* window. The patient's name appears as the subject and the *Get Chart* and *Pt Info* buttons are activated, as seen in Figure 9.9. All the previous options are available including *Send, Send Back, Email It, Print, MultiSend,* and *Spell*. The *Rx* button provides access to the patient's routine medications and previous prescriptions, as illustrated in Figure 9.10. Additional medications may be selected from the program's database, enabling prescriptions to be e-mailed.

As previously mentioned, the message center may be used to send prescriptions to a pharmacy. A medication may be edited by clicking on it in the *New Message* window, as illustrated in Figure 9.11. Any changes made only affect the medication information in the message, not the original medication from the patient's chart. The prescription may be printed by using the *Printer* icon in the bottom-left corner of the message. If *InterFax*™ has been activated on the SpringCharts server, the prescription can be faxed directly to the pharmacy. If the *e-Rx* button is selected, the prescription will be sent electronically to the pharmacy via the Internet clearinghouse.

Once a message is processed and no further action is needed, it is placed in the patient's record by clicking the *Chart It* button (see Figure 9.9). An information window (Figure 9.12) appears indicating that the message has been saved in the patient's chart.

The message is saved under the *Encounters* tab by default or any other custom-designed tab in the patient's *Care Tree* selected by the user. Subsequently the message may be accessed under the *Chart* tab where it was saved, as seen in Figure 9.13.

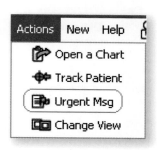

Urgent Messages

At times, a nurse may need to provide confidential patient information to a coworker quickly. The *Urgent Messages* function prevents having to locate the coworker and provides a mechanism for communicating information discreetly in order to maintain patient privacy. To send an urgent message to a coworker, the nurse clicks on the *Actions* menu and selects *Urgent Msg*, as seen in Figure 9.14. The recipient's name is selected and the message is typed or selected from available pop-up text. As with all pop-up text functions, the [edit pencil] icon enables the user to add, delete, or modify text used in this section. Once *Sent*, the urgent message instantly appears on the foreground of the receiver's screen, as illustrated in Figure 9.15. Urgent messages function like instant messaging; the information is *not* saved in the program when the *Cancel* button is selected. However, an urgent message can be printed before closing the window.

An urgent message is turned into a regular message by clicking on the *Message* button. It can then be sent or saved into the message list for follow-up at a later time.

E-mails

The message center in SpringCharts allows for communication **within** the healthcare network. However, SpringCharts also has an e-mail feature that allows patients and other entities to communicate with the facility from outside the network. E-mails in SpringCharts function like a mail sorting room. All e-mails come to a central location where they are manually forwarded to specific SpringCharts users. Because of security and electronic virus concerns, SpringCharts does not allow e-mail attachments. One e-mail account is set up for the medical facility on the SpringCharts server. Specific users are assigned the security function to receive incoming e-mails for this e-mail account. On the SpringCharts server, the user(s) responsible for **receiving** the healthcare facility's e-mails are given the security clearance as seen in Figure 9.16.

Figure 9.13
Message saved in chart's *Care Tree*

Figure 9.14
Accessing *Urgent Msg* in *Actions* menu

FOCAL POINT

Urgent messages function like instant messages and are not stored in the program.

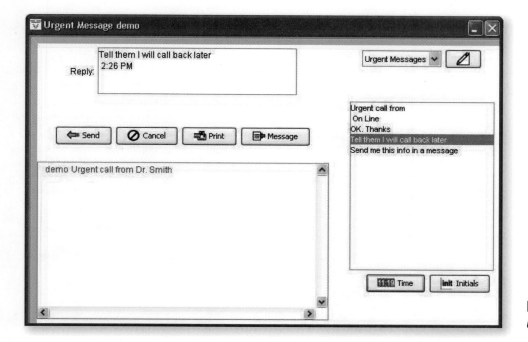

Figure 9.15
Urgent Message window

Figure 9.16

User security access window

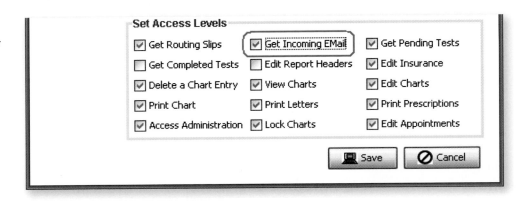

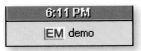

Figure 9.17

E-mail icon in *Login* window

When e-mail is received into SpringCharts, an icon appears beside the user's name who has been designated to receive company e-mail. The icon appears in the yellow login bar, as illustrated in Figure 9.17.

When the user's e-mail access authority is activated on the server, the program opens the *EMail* function located in the *Edit* menu of the main screen. The *EMail* feature is seen in Figure 9.18.

When the *EMail* feature is selected, the window that opens lists all incoming e-mails, displaying the sender's e-mail address, date and time, and subject heading. SpringCharts e-mail is integrated with the Message center and the patients' demographics. When an e-mail item is selected, the program opens a *Message* window, placing the body of the e-mail in the *Message Body* window and the subject line in the *Subject* field. If the e-mail address of the recipient is part of the patient's profile, the program recognizes the e-mail address and attaches all relevant patient demographic information to the *Message* window, as illustrated in Figure 9.19.

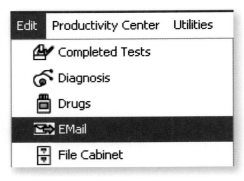

Figure 9.18

Accessing e-mail in the *Edit* menu

The e-mail administrator determines who is best suited to respond to the e-mail and forwards the e-mail message to the appropriate SpringCharts user's Message center. The e-mail message has all the functionality of a regular SpringCharts message, including accessing the patient's chart, using pop-up text, and charting the message. The user can e-mail a response to the sender from this window. Because of the central processing requirement of SpringCharts e-mail, its use in an inpatient setting is limited.

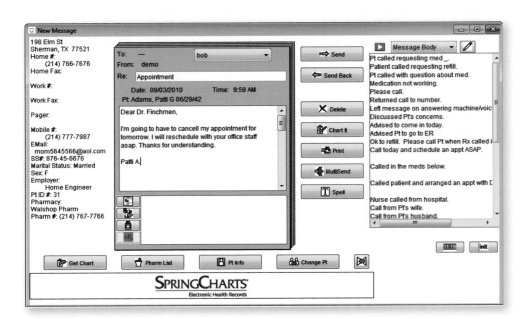

Figure 9.19

Incoming e-mail as *New Message*

Concept Checkup 9.1

A. What happens to a red-checked *ToDo* item the next time the user logs into SpringCharts? _____

B. To what two things does a user have access when a message is connected to a patient?_____

C. Where does an urgent message appear for the recipient? _____

LO 9.3   Immunization Record

Nurses in both inpatient and outpatient settings should obtain an immunization history from patients. While nurses are usually cognizant of the need to obtain pediatric immunization records, the need for obtaining an adult immunization history is often overlooked. In the inpatient setting, adult patients who meet specific criteria and have not had flu shots or pneumococcal vaccines must be offered the vaccines. According to the National Childhood Vaccine Injury Act, every healthcare provider must provide a **Vaccination Information Statement (VIS)** to the patient or legal representative before administering certain immunizations and document the edition date of the VIS that is provided as well as the date the VIS is provided to the patient or legal representative (Centers for Disease Control and Prevention, 2008). Other documentation of immunizations required by federal statutes includes the date of administration, the manufacturer and lot number of the vaccine, and the name, title, and address of the individual administering the vaccine. This documentation may be placed in the patient's health record or in a permanent office log.

In SpringCharts, a patient's immunization record may be viewed or modified by accessing the *Actions* menu within a patient's chart, as shown in Figure 9.20. Past immunizations are added to the patient's record using the submenu *Add/Edit Immunization Archives*, selecting the appropriate immunization from the list, and entering the date of inoculation in the mmddyyyy format or selecting it from the calendar icon. The immunization list is set up on the SpringCharts server under the *Category Preferences* window.

To view the patient's complete immunization list, the user selects the submenu *View Immunizations*. The list can be organized by immunization name or administration date by clicking on the appropriate heading. The immunization record can be printed or faxed as needed.

(See Appendix A, *Sample Documents—Document 9: Immunization Record*.)

Immunizations are automatically added to the immunization list when ordered in a *Nurse Note* or an *Office Visit* note. In both the *Nurse Note* and the *Office Visit* note, the nurse selects the *Proc* (procedure) navigation tab and then the procedure category heading *Immunization*, seen in Figure 9.21. The program lists all the vaccinations that have been set up as procedures in SpringCharts. The appropriate vaccine is selected and additional information such as the VIS, manufacturer, lot number, and site may be added by clicking on the vaccine name in the *Procedure* work area in the lower-left

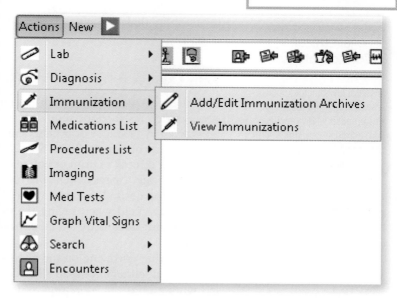

Figure 9.20

Actions menu in patient's chart

Figure 9.21

Procedure tab and *Immunization* category in *Nurse Note*

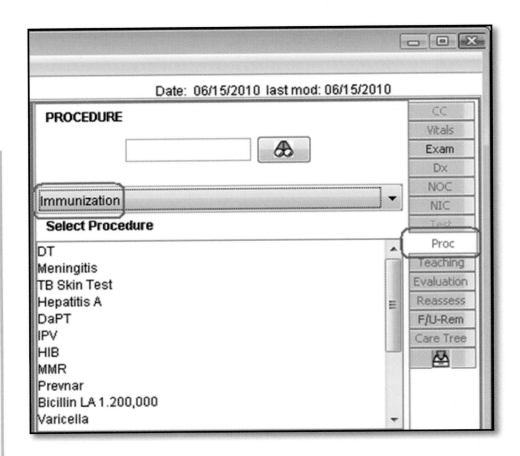

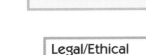
window. Because the vaccine procedures have been designated under the *Immunization* category heading, the program automatically adds the vaccines to the *View Vaccine* window, as mentioned earlier. The program also displays a complete list of prescribed immunizations in the patient's *Care Tree* under the *Immunizations* heading.

A patient's chart can be evaluated electronically to determine if the patient is up to date with immunizations. Recommendations can be customized and embedded into the program that evaluate the patient based on age, gender, and suggested procedures. (For more discussion on the chart evaluation feature, see Section 12.2.)

LO 9.4 Patient Instructions

Patient education is a key role of the nurse, as discussed in Chapter 10. Whenever possible, written instructions should be provided for patients to reinforce verbal instructions given by the nurse or primary care provider. Patient instructions can be created in SpringCharts or imported into SpringCharts, and then accessed in the *Nurse Note* and *Office Visit* screens to print or e-mail for the patient.

To generate a new patient instruction sheet in SpringCharts, users must create and save the desired document in rich text format (RTF), by selecting RTF in the *Save as type* field when saving the document, seen in Figure 9.22. In a Windows environment, documents created in Word Pad are automatically saved in the RTF format.

Under the *New* menu on the main screen, the user selects *New Patient Instruction.* The user may either import an RTF file or create a patient instruction document, as seen in Figure 9.23. If the *Write your own* option is selected, a window is displayed in which patient instructions may be typed or copied and pasted. Many routine patient instructions can be found on websites such as the Food and Drug Administration website (http://www.fda.gov/Drugs/DrugSafety/PostmarketDrugSafetyInformationfor PatientsandProviders/UCM111085) or the National Institutes of Health Medline Plus Webpage (http://www.nlm.nih.gov/medlineplus/medlineplus.html). The user saves the

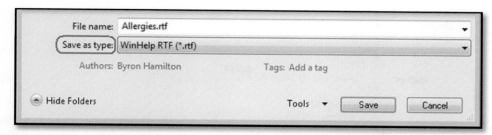

Figure 9.22
Saving as RTF document

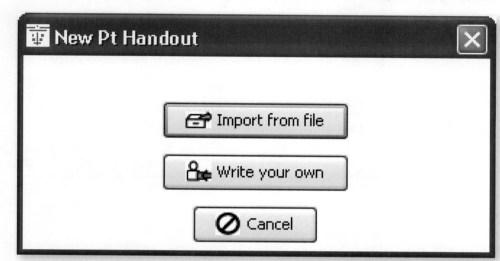

Figure 9.23
Creation options for a patient instruction

article as a "printer-friendly version" on the website, highlights the desired text, then copies and pastes it into the SpringCharts' *Patient Instruction* window. Additional information, such as the medical facility's contact information, may be added to the form. The new patient instruction sheet must be given a title before saving, as illustrated in Figure 9.24.

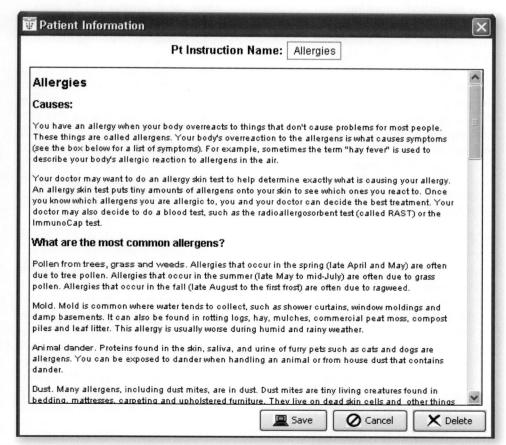

Figure 9.24
Newly imported patient instruction sheet

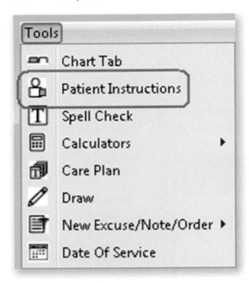

Figure 9.25

Obtaining and distributing a patient instruction sheet

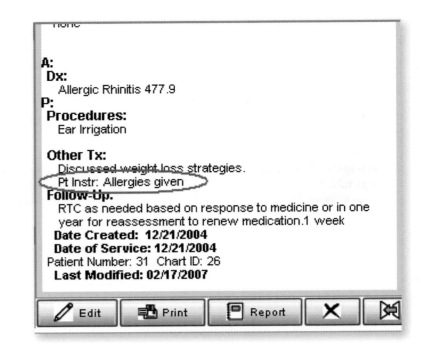

Figure 9.26

Record of patient instruction given in an *OV* note

Note: Your computer's right-click button on the mouse may not support cut/copy/paste; however, the keyboard keys can be used as follows: [Ctrl]+[X] = Cut; [Ctrl]+[C] = Copy; [Ctrl]+[V] = Paste.

Previously created patient instruction sheets may be imported by selecting the *Import from file* option, which opens a browse window where the document can be selected. Existing patient instructions can be modified and new ones created in the *Patient Instruction Manager*. The *Patient Instruction Manager* is accessed from the main window by selecting *Edit > Patient Instructions*.

To obtain and distribute a *Patient Instruction*, the provider opens either a new or existing *Office Visit* note or *Nurse Note* from a patient's chart. From within either of these two patient encounter windows, the provider selects the *Tools* menu and chooses *Patient Instructions*, as illustrated in Figure 9.25. A list of all instructions that have been created in SpringCharts is available for selection. The user is provided the option to print or e-mail the selected patient instruction sheet. Once the patient instruction sheet is selected, the program automatically notes in the *Teaching* section of the *Nurse Note* or the *Other Tx* (Treatment) section of the *Office Visit* note that the instruction/teaching document was given to the patient. Figure 9.26 displays the automatic note recorded in an *Office Visit* note.

LO 9.5   Draw Program

The old adage "a picture's worth a thousand words" may be applied to documentation in the health record. Photographs and drawings may be a useful supplement to narrative documentation for wounds or patient injuries. Photographs provide enhanced visualization of stages of healing, allowing documentation of treatment effectiveness.

The Deficit Reduction Act of 2005 mandated identification of conditions that not only increase the cost of inpatient care but may be prevented through the use of evidence-based practice (Centers for Medicare and Medicaid Services, n.d.). In October 2008, the Centers for Medicare and Medicaid Services (CMS) began withholding payment for those conditions that are acquired in the hospital setting. As a result, documentation of the presence of such conditions on admission became increasingly important to hospital reimbursement. Three conditions that may be best documented with photographs if present on admission (POA) include Stage III and IV pressure ulcers, injuries due to falls, and vascular catheter-associated infections. Coupled with accurate nurses' notes, photographs provide compelling documentation of the presence of the condition on admission and protect the hospital from accountability for the condition.

SpringCharts' *Office Visit* screen and *Nurse Note* screen provide access to a rudimentary draw program that enables the nurse to indicate the condition and location of wounds, scars, incisions, injuries, or procedures by drawing on prebuilt templates. Within either of these encounter notes, the nurse accesses the *Tools* menu and selects the *Draw* option. From the *Template* menu within the draw program, the user selects the desired body section and then uses the draw tools on the left to mark the illustration, shown in Figure 9.27. Only one draw item can be added to each encounter note. The *Edit* menu inside the draw program enables cutting, copying, pasting, and clearing of the *Simple Draw* screen.

More elaborate illustrations can be quickly imported into the draw program, as seen in Figure 9.28, by selecting *Background Image* on the menu bar, then selecting a .jpg image from within the computer or a computer on the network. A digital photo taken of the patient's body area may be imported to the draw program. Once imported, text may be added to the image by selecting the [T] icon to insert a text box which is set at a 10-point plain font, as seen in Figures 9.27 and 9.28. In addition to being useful for documenting conditions that are present on admission, sequential photographs may demonstrate response to treatment and provide pictorial evidence of healing.

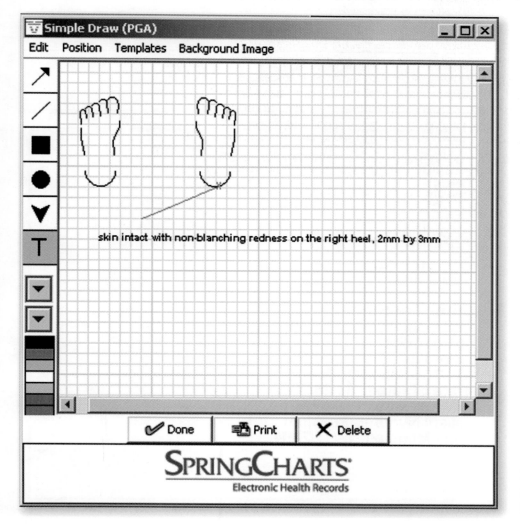

Figure 9.27

Basic templates in draw program

Figure 9.28
Images imported into
Draw program

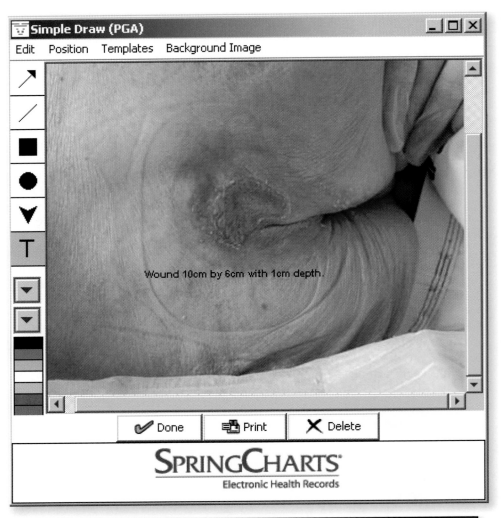

Figure 9.29
Graphic stamp in the
encounter note

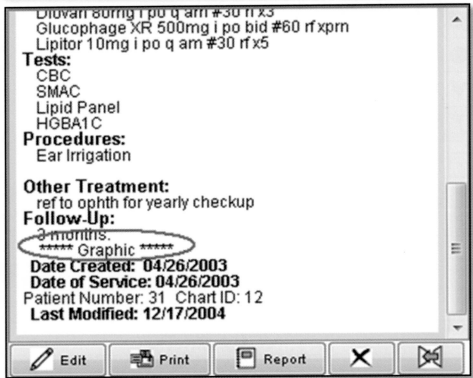

The draw image is stored with the *Office Visit* note or the *Nurse Note*. The *Follow-Up* segment on the note is stamped with the word *Graphic*, as seen in Figure 9.29. To view the attached graphic from within the patient's chart without opening the entire note screen, the user simply clicks on the specific encounter note in the *Care Tree*, then clicks the word *****Graphic***** in the lower-right detail panel of the chart. The draw item window displays along with the accompanying encounter note.

Concept Checkup 9.2

A. Immunizations are automatically added to the patient's immunization record when ordered in the _____ .

B. In what format must an existing patient instruction document be to import it into SpringCharts? _____

C. In what menu of the *Office Visit* screen is the draw feature located? _____
_____

Documentation Tip

Thorough documentation of a patient's condition on admission, particularly evidence of injuries that may be due to falls, pressure ulcers, and evidence of infection from a vascular catheter, is imperative to demonstrate that these are not hospital-acquired conditions and to ensure reimbursement. Photographs enhance this documentation.

Checking Your Understanding

Write "T" or "F" in the blank to indicate whether the statement is true or false.

_____ 1. The message center enables the user to send a message to only one other coworker at a time.

_____ 2. One may send a *ToDo/Reminder* item to another coworker.

_____ 3. Current and future *ToDo/Reminders* can be accessed by selecting *Edit > My ToDo List* on the main menu.

_____ 4. The SpringCharts message system is an intra- and interoffice mail function that enables users to send and receive messages and e-mails within and outside of the healthcare facility.

_____ 5. There are two types of messages: a message concerning a patient and a message not concerning a patient.

_____ 6. If a message concerns a patient, the user must click on the *Pt Info* button in the *New Message* window to view the patient's demographics.

_____ 7. An urgent message is similar to an instant message.

_____ 8. The draw feature does not allow a user to import a background image.

_____ 9. The draw feature allows for freehand sketching.

Answer the questions below in the space provided.

10. A patient's past immunizations are added by selecting the *Immunization* option located in the _____ menu of the patient's chart.

11. How is a current immunization added to the patient's immunization list? _____
    _____
    _____

12. List four required components of documentation for immunizations.
    _____
    _____
    _____
    _____

13. Name one website that may serve as a good resource for patient instructions.
    _____

Choose the best answer and circle the corresponding letter.

14. The *ToDo/Reminder* feature allows a user to: (Select all that apply.)
    a) Send an item to oneself or another user
    b) Send a reminder to a patient
    c) Schedule an item for the future

15. Which feature in SpringCharts facilitates discrete communication while eliminating the need to locate a coworker?
    a) *ToDo List*
    b) *Urgent Messages*
    c) Draw program

16. How many e-mail accounts may be set up within SpringCharts at one time?
    a) Only one
    b) Only one per user
    c) Only one per healthcare provider

17. Where are patient-related messages saved?
    a) *Message archive*
    b) Patient's chart
    c) *Nurse Note*

18. Where are current and future *ToDo* items found?
    a) *Edit > My ToDo List* from the main screen
    b) *Actions > My ToDo List* from the main screen
    c) *New > ToDo List* from the main screen

19. Where are non-patient-related messages saved?
    a) *Saved Messages*
    b) *Completed Messages*
    c) *Message Archive*

20. What menu is accessed from the *Nurse Note* or *Office Visit* note to select the *Draw* option?
    a) *Actions*
    b) *Tools*
    c) *Productivity Center*

21. Where are patient instructions accessed to print or e-mail for the patient? (Select all that apply.)
    a) *Office Visit*
    b) *Nurse Note*
    c) *H&P*

22. If a *ToDo* item is linked to a patient, what happens when a user selects that *ToDo* item?
    a) A patient search window appears allowing the user to find the patient's chart
    b) The patient's chart appears
    c) A check mark is placed next to the item

23. Where is a draw item stored when completed?
    a) In a chart tab that the user selects
    b) In the *Office Visit* note or *Nurse Note* in which it was created
    c) Under *My Drawings* in the patient's chart

24. Where are urgent messages saved?
    a) In the user's *Message Archive*
    b) Urgent messages cannot be saved
    c) In *My Urgent Messages* under the *Edit* menu

25. Which users may access the e-mail in SpringCharts?
    a) Only physicians may receive e-mails
    b) Only the administrator may receive e-mails
    c) A specific user or users who have been assigned to receive e-mails

References

Agency for Healthcare Research and Quality Innovations Exchange. (2009). Nurse- and pharmacist-led physician-approved inpatient Pneumococcus standing order program increases vaccination rates for at-risk patients. Retrieved August 11, 2010, from http://www.innovations.ahrq.gov/content.aspx?id=1816

Agency for Healthcare Research and Quality Innovations Exchange. (2010). Nurse-led telephone outreach more than doubles pneumococcal vaccination rates for at-risk individuals. Retrieved August 11, 2010, from http://www.innovations.ahrq.gov/content.aspx?id=1721

Centers for Disease Control and Prevention. (2008). Instructions for the use of Vaccine Information Statements. Retrieved March 21, 2010, from http://www.cdc.gov/vaccines/pubs/vis/downloads/vis-Instructions.pdf

Centers for Disease Control and Prevention. (2010). Seasonal influenza vaccination resources for health professionals. Retrieved August 11, 2010, from http://www.cdc.gov/flu/professionals/vaccination/index.htm#coverage

Centers for Medicare and Medicaid Services. (n.d.). Hospital-acquired conditions. Retrieved March 21, 2010, from http://www.cms.hhs.gov/HospitalAcqCond/06_Hospital-Acquired_Conditions.asp#TopOfPage

Grime, J. A., Blenkinsopp, D. K., Raynor, K., Pollock, P. K., & Knapp, P. (2007). The role and value of written information for patients about individual medicines: A systematic review. *Health Expectations, 10*, 286–298.

U.S. Department of Health and Human Services. (2009). Developing healthy people 2020: Immunization and infectious disease. Retrieved August 11, 2010, from http://www.healthypeople.gov/hp2020/Objectives/ViewObjective.aspx?Id=520&TopicArea=Immunization+and+Infectious+Diseases&Objective=IID+HP2020%e2%80%9324&TopicAreaId=30

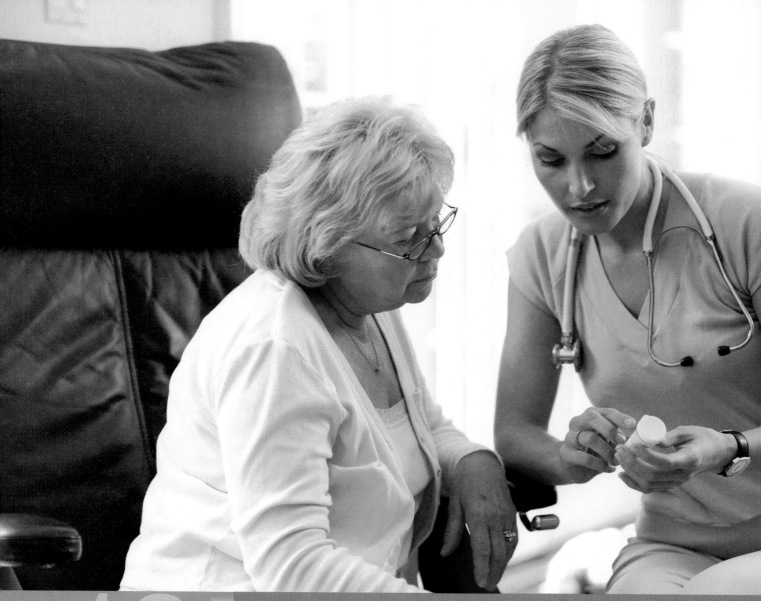

10 | Patient Education

Key Terms

Terms and abbreviations you will encounter in Chapter 10; they are defined in the end-of-book glossary:

Accreditation

National Patient
   Safety Goals
   (NPSG)

Patient Education

Patient's Bill of Rights

Standards of Practice

The Joint Commission
   (TJC)

Learning Outcomes

When you complete Chapter 10, you will be able to:

10.1 Identify patients' rights and nurses' responsibilities related to education.

10.2 Identify accreditation requirements for patient education.

10.3 Identify patients' learning needs.

10.4 Use correct nursing diagnoses, outcomes, and interventions for patient education.

10.5 Carry out implementing, evaluating, and documenting patient education.

What You Need to Know

To understand Chapter 10, you need to know how to:

- Use the nursing process to develop an individualized plan of care.

Evidence-Based Practice 10.1

Smith, Forster, and Young (2009) conducted a meta-analysis of studies of the impact of stroke education. They found that provision of patient education enhanced knowledge and satisfaction and lessened depression in patients with stroke.

FOCAL POINT

Nurses are ethically and legally obligated to provide patient education.

Evidence-Based Practice 10.2

Research funded by the Agency for Healthcare Research and Quality (2003) demonstrates that few patients have developed effective advance directives. For example, less than 50% of terminally or seriously ill patients had an advance directive in their health record. In nearly three-quarters of the cases, physicians were unaware that their patient had an advance directive. Even when advance directives existed, documentation of patient preferences in the health record was scarce.

Overview

Patient education is the very core of nursing practice. It is the patient's right to be educated and the nurse's responsibility to provide education related to health promotion, health maintenance, and adjusting to illness or disability in order to promote positive patient outcomes. The importance of patient education is highlighted by nursing's professional standards, ethical statements, and social policy statements. In addition, accrediting bodies such as **The Joint Commission (TJC)** require patient education in the provision of quality care. Federal legislation such as the Patient Self-Determination Act of 1990 and a recently introduced bill that would provide reimbursement for patient education in certain instances demonstrates the importance of educating patients (Israel, 2009). Nurses use the nursing process to assess patient education needs, formulate an education plan, and implement and evaluate the plan. Documentation is the mechanism whereby nurses demonstrate the use of the nursing process to determine that patients' educational needs are met.

LO 10.1 Patient Rights and Nurses' Responsibilities

In 1973, the American Hospital Association (AHA) embraced a **Patient's Bill of Rights** recognizing that for healthcare to be effective, healthcare professionals and patients must collaborate. In order for patients to be active participants in their care, they must be knowledgeable about their disease and its treatment. The second patient right acknowledged by the AHA states, "The patient has the right to and is encouraged to obtain from physicians and other direct caregivers relevant, current, and understandable information concerning diagnosis, treatment, and prognosis" (American Hospital Association, 1992). Recognizing patients' rights to be active decision makers in their care, the federal government passed the Patient Self-Determination Act (PSDA) of 1990 requiring that patients be given written information about their right to make decisions about their care, including end-of-life care (AHRQ, 2003). Specifically, this law gives patients the right to consent to or refuse treatment. As a result of the PSDA, most healthcare facilities provide information to patients on advance directives upon admission or initial contact.

While it is the patient's right to have the necessary information to manage his or her health and/or illness, it is the nurse's ethical and professional responsibility to provide patient education. The American Nurses Association (2004), *Nursing: Scope and Standards of Practice* identifies patient education as a **standard of practice**. Standard 5B: Health Teaching and Health Promotion states, "The registered nurse employs strategies to promote health and a safe environment" (p. 28). The following measurement criteria are used to evaluate this standard:

The registered nurse:

- Provides health teaching that addresses such topics as healthy lifestyles, risk-reducing behaviors, developmental needs, activities of daily living, and preventive self-care.
- Uses health promotion and health teaching methods appropriate to the situation and the patient's developmental level, learning needs, readiness, ability to learn, language preference, and culture.
- Seeks opportunities for feedback and evaluation of the effectiveness of the strategies used (p. 28).

The draft of the second edition of *Nursing: Scope and Standards of Practice* adds values, beliefs, health practices, spirituality, and socioeconomic status as considerations for health teaching methods (American Nurses Association, 2010). Ethically, nurses are obligated to evaluate patient understanding of the information that patients are given to "facilitate an informed judgment" (American Nurses Association, 2001, p. 8).

In addition to the nursing standards that support culturally appropriate education in a language the patient understands, the Office of Minority Health, a division of the U.S. Department of Health and Human Services, mandates the provision of language services for individuals with limited English proficiency (Office of Minority Health, 2007) The National Standards on Culturally and Linguistically Appropriate Services (CLAS) require hospitals that receive federal funds, such as Medicare, to provide interpreters for verbal communication and patient materials, including educational materials, in language easily understood by patients. Nurses are responsible to ensure that the patient's linguistic needs are met whether education is provided in written or verbal form.

Concept Checkup 10.1

A. What do patients need to be active participants in their care? _____
_____

B. According to the ANA Scope and Standards, nurses are responsible for providing patient education. List five topics for which nurses should provide patient education.

_____
_____
_____
_____
_____

C. List two mandates of the CLAS Standards.

_____
_____

LO 10.2   Accreditation Requirements

Healthcare organizations elect to become accredited or certified to demonstrate provision of quality care and to ensure eligibility for third-party reimbursement. The most widely recognized **accreditation** comes from The Joint Commission (TJC), a non-profit organization that accredits approximately 17,000 healthcare organizations (The Joint Commission, 2009a). Hospitals are evaluated based on their adherence to quality standards, including patient education. While many patient education standards are general, disease-specific requirements for patient education have also been adopted through The Joint Commission Core Measures Initiative (The Joint Commission, 2009b).

The Joint Commission requires that each patient is assessed before health education is initiated. This assessment must include readiness to learn, preferred method of learning, and barriers to learning. All hospital patients must be provided education on medications, equipment, procedures, hygiene, and nutrition in addition to being oriented to their hospital room. Effectiveness of teaching strategies must be evaluated.

The Joint Commission, the Centers for Medicare and Medicaid (CMS), and the National Quality Forum (NQF) collaborated to establish research-based, disease-specific core measures to which all hospitals are expected to adhere (The Joint Commission, 2009b). Disease-specific requirements for education include counseling for smoking cessation for all patients with a diagnosed heart attack, congestive heart failure (CHF), or pneumonia. In addition, patients with CHF have specific discharge instructions that are mandated, including medications, daily weight, and diet.

In 2002, The Joint Commission published the first **National Patient Safety Goals (NPSG)** in an effort to provide specific actions that healthcare organizations can take to reduce the likelihood of medical errors (The Joint Commission, 2010). During an accreditation survey, healthcare organizations are evaluated on their compliance with the NPSGs. The list of NPSGs has evolved and grown through the years and several

---

Legal/Ethical Considerations

The Code of Ethics for Nurses states that nurses have an ethical obligation to provide patient education to facilitate decision making.

FOCAL POINT

Accrediting agencies set standards for patient education that must be reflected in documentation.

Documentation Tip

Many facilities have disease-specific checklists to ensure that all discharge education is completed and documented.

goals emphasize patient education. The following list indicates the required elements of patient education for the 2010 NPSGs:

- NPSG.03.05.01 "Reduce the likelihood of patient harm associated with the use of anticoagulant therapy." This goal requires education for patients and families that includes content on dietary restrictions, follow-up monitoring, adverse reactions, and drug interactions.

- NPSG.07.03.01 "Implement evidence-based practices to prevent health care associated infections due to multiple drug-resistant organisms in acute care hospitals." Patients who are infected with drug-resistant organisms and their families must be educated about the facility's strategies for prevention.

- NPSG.07.04.01 "Implement best practices or evidence-based guidelines to prevent central line-associated bloodstream infections." Before insertion of central lines, patients and their families must be educated about preventing infections associated with the line.

- NPSG.07.05.01 "Implement best practices for preventing surgical site infections." Before surgery, patients and their families must receive education about preventing infections in the surgical site.

- NPSG.08.03.01 "When a patient leaves the organization's care, a complete and reconciled list of the patient's medications is provided directly to the patient, and the patient's family as needed, and the list is explained to the patient and/or family." This goal requires education about discharge medications with documentation of the education.

- NPSG.09.02.01 "The organization implements a fall reduction program that includes an evaluation of the effectiveness of the program." Patients and their families must be educated about the fall prevention program and specific strategies that are implemented for the patient.

- NPSG.13.01.01 "Identify the ways in which the patient and his or her family can report concerns about safety and encourage them to do so." In order to encourage patients' involvement in care, they must be educated about the reporting mechanisms that are available, infection control measures that should be implemented for the patient, and, if appropriate, the strategies the hospital uses to prevent adverse events during surgery.

- NPSG.16.01.01 "The organization selects a suitable method that enables health care staff members to directly request additional assistance from a specially trained individual(s) when the patient's condition appears to be worsening." The goal goes further to recommend that patients and family be taught to ask for assistance if the patient's condition is deteriorating.

 ## Concept Checkup 10.2

A. Which organization is the largest accrediting organization for hospitals?

_____

B. List two areas that The Joint Commission requires to be assessed before patient education is initiated.

_____

_____

C. List three topics of patient education required by The Joint Commission.

_____

_____

_____

Concept Checkup 10.2 *(Concluded)*

D. What is the purpose of the National Patient Safety Goals?

_____

_____

E. List five topics of patient education incorporated into the National Patient Safety Goals.

_____

_____

_____

_____

_____

LO 10.3 | ## Assessing Patients' Learning Needs

Developing a teaching strategy for a patient follows the steps of the nursing process (Potter & Perry, 2009). In the initial phase, the nurse must assess the patient's learning needs. Assessment data may be obtained from a variety of sources including the patient, family, significant others, friends, and the health record. Determining the patient's current level of knowledge and living environment is important. For example, a patient who has had diabetes for many years may have very different learning needs than a patient newly diagnosed with diabetes. A patient who receives insulin injections will require a different level of education if she lives in a nursing home where a nurse administers the insulin than if she lives at home and must be able to self-administer her insulin.

During this initial phase of the nursing process, the nurse must assess the patient's ability to learn. A nurse cannot assume that patients understand health-related information, even in the United States. Health literacy refers to an individual's ability to understand health information in order to make informed decisions (Cornett, 2009). While testing health literacy may be embarrassing to a patient, asking the patient how confident he feels completing medical forms alone has been shown to be a good indicator of health literacy (Powell, 2009). In addition, nurses should be alert to clues of low health literacy such as a patient stating he forgot his glasses or that he feels too tired. If the patient's eyes wander over the page while reading, he may not be able to read. Using a finger to point to text while reading may be another indicator of poor health literacy.

While assessing the patient, the nurse should identify barriers to learning such as language, poor vision or hearing, pain, and anxiety. Cultural norms may dictate who receives education in addition to the patient. The nurse should determine the patient's preferred method of learning. Some patients may prefer to receive pamphlets, while others prefer a video or verbal instruction.

> **FOCAL POINT**
>
> Nurses use the nursing process to assess and diagnose patient learning needs, and to plan, implement, and evaluate patient education.

> **Documentation Tip**
>
> Documentation of patient education must indicate assessment of learning preferences, barriers to learning, and readiness to learn.

LO 10.4 | ## Applying Correct Nursing Diagnoses, NOC, and NIC

Once the patient's learning needs have been assessed, the nurse assigns the appropriate NANDA-I nursing diagnoses. Typically a nursing diagnosis of knowledge, deficient is used, although nursing diagnoses of noncompliance or therapeutic regimen: ineffective management may also indicate a learning need. Specific details about the patient's learning need should be included in the nursing diagnosis. For example, a patient who needs to learn to self-administer insulin would have a nursing diagnosis of knowledge, deficient related to insulin self-administration.

In the next stage of the nursing process, the nurse identifies the priority learning needs and determines the outcome statements that are most appropriate. Nursing

Outcome Classification (NOC) outcomes related to patient education are often the "knowledge" outcomes and may include knowledge of 30 different topics including breast feeding, cardiac disease management, diabetes management, diet, disease process, medication, prescribed activity, and treatment regimen. Other NOC outcomes such as discharge readiness, fall prevention behavior, and risk control outcomes may also be appropriate outcomes for patient education (Center for Nursing Classification and Clinical Effectiveness, 2004).

The implementation phase is when the actual patient education occurs. Nursing interventions from the Nursing Interventions Classification (NIC) may include the generic health education intervention, parent education interventions, or "teaching" interventions specific to disease process, preoperative teaching, prescribed diet, and medications. In addition, other NIC interventions such as admission care, childbirth preparation, discharge planning, nutrition counseling, smoking cessation assistance, and vehicle safety promotion may also contain health education components (Center for Nursing Classification and Clinical Effectiveness, 2008).

LO 10.5   Implementing, Evaluating, and Documenting Patient Education

Nurses use a variety of educational tools and methods to teach clients and their families or significant others. For example, during medication administration, a nurse may verbally communicate the name of the medication and its mechanism of action. When the patient is discharged, the nurse may give the patient a drug information sheet for reference at home. Videos, booklets, computer programs, demonstrations, and group discussions may all be used to educate patients. Many hospitals and outpatient facilities have educational television programming that a patient may watch. Since individuals only remember about one-third to one-half of what is verbally instructed (Cornett, 2009; Powell, 2009), using a variety of teaching methods promotes learning. Accreditation standards require that nurses document who they teach as well as how.

Finally, nurses must evaluate the effectiveness of their patient education. The method of evaluation depends on the teaching content. Research indicates that one highly effective method of evaluation is the "teach-back" method (Cornett, 2009; Powell, 2009). This technique involves asking the patient to relay the instructional content back to the nurse. The teach-back method allows the nurse to evaluate the patient's understanding of the information and validate or correct as indicated. If the content of the patient education is a psychomotor skill such as insulin administration or changing an ostomy appliance, patients, or their caregivers, should be given the opportunity to demonstrate the skill to the nurse before being expected to perform the skill independently without supervision. Return demonstration gives both the patient and the nurse confidence that the skill is being performed accurately. Computerized patient education programs may use questioning at intervals to determine comprehension. Computer programs are able to give immediate feedback to the user. Nurses must document their method of evaluation of learning. In addition, mastery of content or the need for remediation should be documented. When outcomes are not met, the nurse should reevaluate the patient for barriers to learning and should consider alternate educational formats.

Concept Checkup 10.3

A. Define health literacy. _____

B. What is a simple question that may be asked to determine a client's health
   literacy? _____

C. In addition to health literacy, what other areas related to patient education
   should be assessed by the nurse?

   _____

   _____

   _____

D. List three NANDA-I diagnoses related to patient education.

   _____

   _____

   _____

E. List three NOC outcomes related to patient education.

   _____

   _____

   _____

F. List three NIC interventions related to patient education.

   _____

   _____

   _____

G. What education evaluation method has been demonstrated by research to be
   effective? _____

Using Terminology

Match the terms on the left with the definitions on the right.

_____ 1. Accreditation

_____ 2. NANDA-I

_____ 3. National Patient Safety Goals (NPSG)

_____ 4. NOC

_____ 5. Nursing diagnosis

_____ 6. Nursing standards

_____ 7. Patient education

_____ 8. Patient's rights

_____ 9. The Joint Commission (TJC)

A. A standardized list of patient outcomes that are influenced by nursing interventions

B. A process whereby a healthcare organization is evaluated for adherence to standards of care; indicates that the facility provides quality care

C. An independent, non-profit organization that sets standards of quality for healthcare organizations and evaluates compliance with these standards, providing accreditation for organizations that demonstrate excellence

D. Recommended actions to achieve overall objectives of reducing medical errors

E. Statements that describe the responsibilities of nurses

F. An organization that promotes standard usage of nursing diagnosis globally

G. Statement describing an individual's response to a health problem

H. List of basic entitlements that patients, their surrogates, or healthcare decision makers can expect from healthcare facilities and providers

I. Process in which nurses provide information to patients, families, and communities to enhance their ability to actively participate in health promotion and health maintenance or to cope with alterations in health or ability

Checking Your Understanding

Write "T" or "F" in the blank to indicate whether the statement is true or false.

_____ 10. Nurses have an ethical and professional duty to provide patients with the information they need to manage their health.

_____ 11. Standards set by accrediting agencies do not impact nurses.

_____ 12. Providing patients with a written list of discharge instructions is sufficient to meet all standards for patient education.

_____ 13. Health literacy is not a problem in the United States.

_____ 14. Nurses are continually teaching patients so there is no need to document this routine activity.

Choose the best answer and circle the corresponding letter.

15. Which of the following delineate a patient's entitlement to health information?
    a) National Patient Safety Goals
    b) Nursing Scope and Standards
    c) Nursing's Social Policy Statement
    d) Patient's Bill of Rights

16. Which of the following should nurses assess prior to patient education? (Select all that apply.)
    a) Barriers to learning
    b) Health literacy
    c) Motivation
    d) Nurse's patient load

17. A client has a new diagnosis of Diabetes Type I and will need to self-administer insulin on a routine basis. What is the best method of evaluating the patient's ability to self-administer insulin?
    a) Ask the patient questions about the procedure.
    b) Have the patient demonstrate self-administering an insulin injection.
    c) Have the patient repeat the steps in the procedure back to you.
    d) Have the patient take a computer-based learning module and complete the quiz.

18. Your client is being discharged on Coumadin 5 mg p.o. daily. Which of the following will you teach the patient before discharge? (Select all that apply.)
    a) Adverse reactions to Coumadin such as prolonged bleeding
    b) Avoid foods high in Vitamin K such as kale, swiss chard, broccoli, and spinach
    c) Avoid aspirin
    d) Monitor INR as ordered by physician

19. According to disease-specific core measures, which patients below should be taught to quit smoking? (Select all that apply.)
    a) A patient with a diagnosis of CHF
    b) A patient with an acute MI
    c) A patient with pneumonia
    d) A pregnant patient

20. Which of the following patient education methods may be used by nurses? (Select all that apply.)
    a) Demonstration
    b) Pamphlet
    c) Video
    d) Handout

References

Agency for Healthcare Research and Quality. (2003). *Research in action: Advance care planning: Preferences for care at the end-of-life*. Retrieved August 11, 2010, from http://www.ahrq.gov/research/endliferia/endria.pdf

American Hospital Association. (1992, October 21). *A patient's bill of rights*. Retrieved January 17, 2010, from http://www.aha.org/resource/pbillofrights.html

American Nurses Association. (2001). *Code of ethics for nurses with interpretive statements*. Silver Spring, MD: Author.

American Nurses Association. (2004). *Nursing: Scope and standards of practice*. Silver Spring, MD: Author.

American Nurses Association. (2010). *Draft for public comment: Nursing: Scope and standards of practice: Second edition.* Retrieved January 17, 2010, from http://www.nursingworld.org/DocumentVault/NursingPractice/Draft-Nursing-Scope-Standards-2nd-Ed.aspx

Center for Nursing Classification and Clinical Effectiveness. (2004). *Nursing outcomes classification, 4th edition.* Retrieved January 23, 2010, from http://www.nursing.uiowa.edu/excellence/nursing_knowledge/clinical_effectiveness/documents/Label%20Definitions%20NOC%204th.pdf

Center for Nursing Classification and Clinical Effectiveness. (2008). *Nursing interventions classification (NIC), 5th edition.* Retrieved January 23, 2010, from http://www.nursing.uiowa.edu/excellence/nursing_knowledge/clinical_effectiveness/documents/LabelDefinitions NIC5.pdf

Cornett, S. (2009). Assessing and addressing health literacy. *OJIN: The Online Journal of Issues in Nursing, 14*(3). Retrieved January 17, 2010, from http://www.nursingworld.org/MainMenuCategories/ANAMarketplace/ANAPeriodicals/OJIN/TableofContents/Vol142009/No3Sept09/Assessing-Health-Literacy-.aspx

Fredericks, S., Ibrahim, S., & Puri, I. (2009). Coronary artery bypass surgery patient education: A systematic review. *Progress in Cardiovascular Nursing, 24*(4), 162–168.

Israel, S. (2009, June). Legislation regarding patient education introduced in the House. *ONS Connect*, 22.

Office of Minority Health. (2007). *National standards on culturally and linguistically appropriate services (CLAS).* Retrieved August 23, 2010, from http://minorityhealth.hhs.gov/templates/browse.aspx?lvl=2&lvlID=15

Potter, P., & Perry, A.G. (2009). *Fundamentals of nursing.* St. Louis, MO: Mosby.

Powell, M. (2009). Health literacy: Implications for ambulatory care. *Nursing Economic$, 27*(5), 343–347.

Smith, J., Forster, A., & Young, J. (2009). Cochrane review: Information provision for stroke patients and their caregivers. *Clinical Rehabilitation, 23*, 195–206.

The Joint Commission. (2009a). *Facts about The Joint Commission.* Retrieved January 23, 2010, from http://www.jointcommission.org/AboutUs/Fact_Sheets/joint_commission _facts.htm

The Joint Commission. (2009b). *Improving America's hospitals: The Joint Commission's annual report on quality and safety.* Retrieved January 17, 2010, from http://www.joint commission.org/NR/rdonlyres/22D58F1F-14FF-4B72-A870-378DAF26189E/0/2009_Annual_Report.pdf

The Joint Commission. (2010). *National patient safety goals.* Retrieved January 22, 2010, from http://www.jointcommission.org/PatientSafety/NationalPatientSafetyGoals

Nurse Note

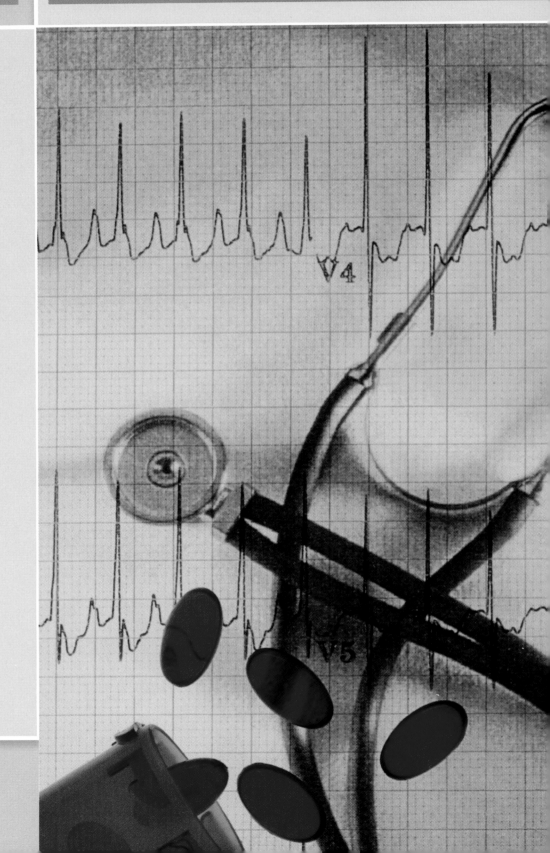

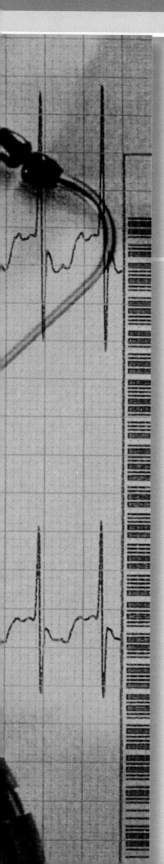

Documentation—Level 3

Learning Outcomes

When you complete Chapter 11, you will be able to:

11.1 Carry out documentation of patient education and response.

11.2 Identify patient response to interventions.

11.3 Carry out documentation of reassessment/revision of goals.

11.4 Use *ToDo/Reminders* within the *Nurse Note*.

What You Need to Know

To understand Chapter 11, you need to know how to:

- Create a new *Nurse Note* record.
- Navigate through the basic elements of a *Nurse Note*.
- Update face sheet information from the *Nurse Note*.
- Select/document applicable chief complaints.
- Document vital signs.
- Select/document an assessment.
- Select applicable NANDA-I nursing diagnoses.
- Document applicable goals using Nursing Outcomes Classification (NOC).
- Document applicable interventions using Nursing Intervention Classification (NIC).
- Document medication administration.
- Document intake and output (I&O).

Overview

Patient education was discussed in detail in Chapter 10. This chapter introduces the tools used in SpringCharts to document teaching interventions. Just as the nurse must evaluate the effectiveness of patient education, the effectiveness of all nursing interventions must be evaluated in order to determine if an outcome has been met or to adjust the goals and interventions to obtain an optimal outcome. This chapter discusses documentation of that evaluation, along with reassessment and revision of goals when necessary.

LO 11.1   Teaching (Patient Education)

SpringCharts offers the nurse the ability to document patient education by clicking on the *Teaching* tab on the right side of the screen of the *Nurse Note*, as seen in Figure 11.1. Common teaching interventions are listed under the *Other Tx* pop-up text panel, but, as always, text may be typed directly into the *Teaching* box on the bottom-left corner of the screen. Examples of pop-up text that are available in this

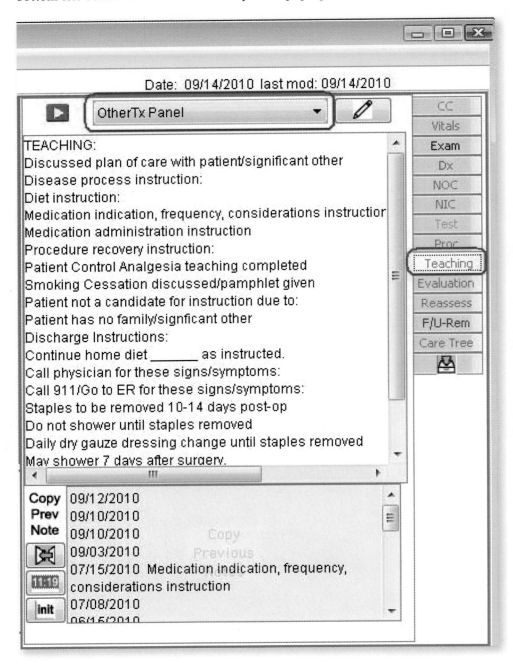

Figure 11.1

Teaching tab in *Nurse Note* screen

area are: *Discussed plan of care with patient/significant other* and *Medication indication, frequency, considerations instruction.* Sixty prebuilt entries are available for documentation of patient education. However, there are innumerable topics that nurses teach patients. Modifying this area to list education topics applicable for a particular nursing unit can be extremely useful.

Selecting the pencil icon opens the *Edit PopUp Text* window. The nurse adds the desired text into one of the open fields. The order of the list may be modified by using the up and down arrows on the left side of the screen. The user clicks *Done* when changes are complete and the newly modified text appears in the pop-up text window. When the nurse moves to the next navigation tab, text entered in the *Teaching* tab is automatically placed in the *Interventions* section of the SOAPIER note.

Concept Checkup 11.1

A. In which tab is patient education documented in SpringCharts?

_____

B. Where is the documentation of patient education placed in the SOAPIER nurse's note?

_____

LO 11.2 Evaluation

After the nurse assesses the patient and determines nursing diagnoses, the desired outcomes are identified followed by delineation of the nursing interventions to meet those outcomes. Patient progress toward meeting outcomes must be evaluated routinely to determine if the nursing interventions are effective. This evaluation process allows the nurse to determine if the outcome has been met or if the plan of care requires revision to ensure goal attainment.

Since the nurse evaluates the outcomes selected earlier under the *NOC* tab, it is necessary to copy the outcomes being evaluated into the *Evaluation* area of the nurse's note. To do this, the nurse clicks on the *NOC* tab and highlights and copies the text in the *NOC* free text area in the lower section of the screen, as seen in Figure 11.2. After returning to the *Evaluation* tab, the nurse clicks into the text field on the left and pastes the outcomes. At this point, the nurse is prepared to document the patient's progress toward a goal or resolve a goal that has been achieved.

Note: Your computer's right-click button on the mouse may not support cut/copy/paste; however, the keyboard keys can be used as follows: [Ctrl]+[X] = Cut; [Ctrl]+[C] = Copy; [Ctrl]+[V] = Paste.

Evaluation pop-up text provides common prebuilt evaluation statements such as: *Outcome met this shift*, *Outcome not met this shift*, and *Ongoing outcome*, as seen in Figure 11.3. Common variance reasons are also included in the pop-up text. The user clicks into the *Evaluation* text box on the lower left where the evaluation is placed to select preset pop-up text or type additional text to specify how the outcome was met. Sixty prebuilt entries are available for documentation of evaluation.

The pencil icon is used to individualize the evaluation pop-up text from inside the window. Selecting the pencil icon opens the *Edit PopUp Text* window. The nurse adds the desired text into one of the open fields. The nurse modifies the order of the list by using the up and down arrows on the left side of the screen. The user clicks *Done* when changes are complete. When the nurse moves to the next navigation tab, text chosen in the *Evaluation* tab area is automatically placed in the *Evaluation* section of the SOAPIER note.

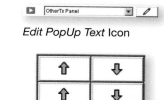

Edit PopUp Text Icon

Text order arrows in Edit PopUp Text *window*

FOCAL POINT

The *Evaluation* area provides the nurse with standardized text used to document progress toward a goal or goal attainment.

Documentation Tip

Institution policy determines the frequency of evaluation of plan-of-care goals. In the acute care setting, this is typically each shift. In addition, nursing units have standards of care that indicate how often patients are assessed. For example, in a critical care unit, a complete head-to-toe assessment may be required every two hours, whereas on a medical-surgical unit, patients may be assessed every eight hours. Nursing judgment should be used to determine if more frequent monitoring is required by the patient's condition.

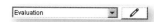

Edit PopUp Text icon

Figure 11.2
Copying *NOC* note to
Evaluation note

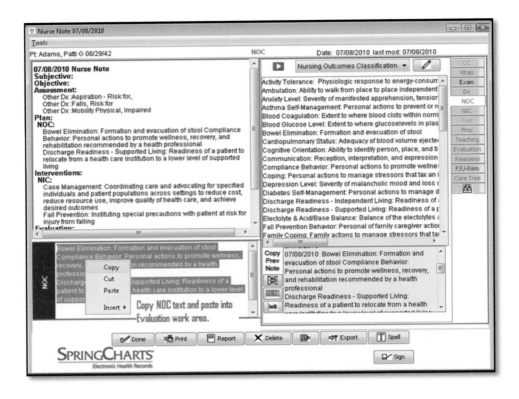

Figure 11.3
Evaluation documentation

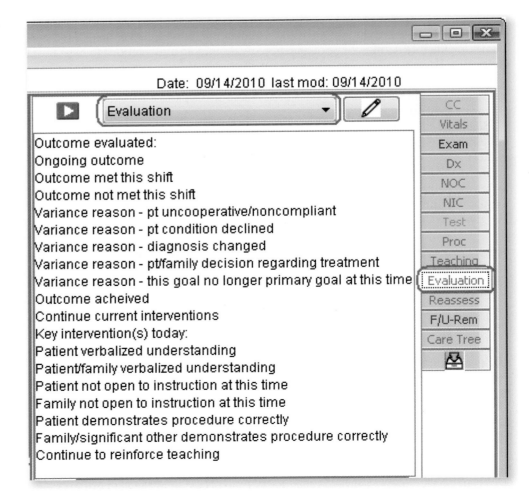

Concept Checkup 11.2

A. True or False: The *Evaluation* tab does not automatically pull the NOC information that was previously selected into the *Evaluation* field. _____
_____

B. List three common statements used to evaluate outcomes.
_____
_____
_____

LO 11.3 Reassessment

As part of the nursing process, the nurse evaluates patient responses to interventions and revises outcomes as indicated. This evaluation of outcomes is documented in the *Evaluation* section of SpringCharts, as described in the previous section. Often, the nurse needs to assess and document the patient's response to an intervention such as the administration of an analgesic or a diuretic shortly after administration. On other occasions, the patient needs frequent reassessments following a procedure such as a heart catheterization or surgery. This type of reassessment data is best documented in the *Reassessment* tab of SpringCharts.

Under the *Reassessment* navigation tab on the right side of the *Nurse Note* screen is a list of items that are typically reassessed such as vital signs and pain. In addition, prebuilt items are available to facilitate documentation.

The pencil icon in the *Reassess* pop-up text area is used to individualize text to allow for items that may not be available in the prebuilt text. Sixty entries are available in each of these areas. To individualize pop-up text, the pencil icon is selected to open the *Edit PopUp Text* window. Desired text is entered into one of the open fields. The order of the list is modified by using the up and down arrows on the left side of the screen. The user clicks the *Done* button when changes are complete and the newly modified text appears in the pop-up text window. When the nurse moves to the next navigation tab, text selected in the *Reassessment* tab is automatically placed in the *Revision* section of the SOAPIER note.

Concept Checkup 11.3

A. Name two items that are frequently reassessed by nurses: _____
_____

LO 11.4 F/U-REM (Follow-up Reminders/ToDo List)

When patients are discharged from an inpatient unit, emergency department, or ambulatory care setting, instructions are given for future healthcare follow-up. The *F/U-Rem* (follow-up/reminder) navigation tab allows the nurse to set reminders for follow-up care. Text may be chosen from the default pop-up text category, *flu Panel*, or selected from the previous note window containing text used in prior encounters. Common time frames for healthcare provider follow-up, such as *one week*, *two weeks*, and *one month*, are found under the *flu Panel*. Commonly used discharge dispositions are also available such as: *Discharged to home/self care*, *Discharged to care of family/significant other*, and *Discharged to Home Health Agency*.

Documentation Tip

The Joint Commission requires regular reassessment of pain. Typically the effectiveness of analgesics is evaluated 30 minutes after IV administration and one hour after oral administration.

Legal/Ethical Considerations

Failure to document reassessments may be a source of liability for the nurse.

Edit PopUp Text icon

FOCAL POINT

The follow-up/reminders functionality in SpringCharts allows nurses to give themselves or others reminders to perform tasks or to schedule future tasks.

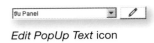

Edit PopUp Text icon

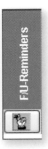

Create a Reminder icon

Referral statements are also available such as: *Pt urged to see Cardiologist promptly for . . ., Pt urged to see PCP (Primary Care Provider) promptly for . . .* As always, the nurse can click directly into the *F/U-Reminders* text box on the lower left and type directly into the field.

Next to the *flu Panel*, the pencil icon is used to individualize the text available to allow for items that may not be available in the prebuilt text. There are 60 entries available in each of these areas. Selecting the pencil icon opens the *Edit PopUp Text* window. Desired text is entered into one of the open fields. The order of the list is modified by using the up and down arrows on the left side of the screen. The user clicks *Done* when changes are complete.

In the lower-left window, the *Create a Reminder* icon is available, enabling the clinician to set a personal ToDo/Reminder or to send one to another person in the clinic. Resting the cursor over the icon causes text *Create a Reminder* to appear; clicking on the icon activates the *New ToDo/Reminder* window, seen in Figure 11.4. This feature can be used when clinicians want to send themselves a reminder to complete a task or send a task to a coworker before they exit the note.

The dialog box automatically links to the current patient. Pop-up text is available for rapid selection of *ToDo/Reminders* text. Examples of prebuilt text includes: *Teach, Dressing change,* and *Call family when pt goes to OR per their request.* The user clicks the *Send* button to send the reminder immediately, or clicks *Send Later* and designates a future date when the reminder should appear in the recipient's *ToDo List.* When the recipient clicks on the item in his or her *ToDo List,* the patient's chart opens, providing the necessary information to execute the scheduled activity.

While in the *New ToDo/Reminder* window, the pencil icon is used to individualize the *ToDo-Reminders* pop-up text to allow for items that may not be available in the prebuilt text. Sixty entries are available in each of these areas. In order to individualize pop-up text, the pencil icon is selected to open the *Edit PopUp Text* window. Desired text is added into one of the open fields. The order of the list is modified by using the up and down arrows on the left side of the screen. The user clicks *Done* when changes are complete.

Discharge instructions are created through a *New Nurse Note* by using the *Teaching* navigation tab. By using the *Teaching* and *F/U Rem* tabs, the nurse can prepare a discharge plan containing instructions and follow-up information. Preset patient instruction sheets are selected and printed by clicking on the *Tools* menu within the *Nurse Note* screen and selecting the submenu *Patient Instruction.* Upon printing a patient instruction form, a note is automatically added to the *Teaching* portion of the SOAPIER note indicating that an instruction sheet was given to the patient. The discharge *Nurse Note* containing the instructions and follow-up information can be printed out by selecting the *Print* button in the bottom section of the screen. Upon saving the *Nurse Note,* the user can add a phrase in the *Save As* field to indicate the note contains discharge instructions, as seen in Figure 11.5.

Figure 11.4

New ToDo/Reminder window

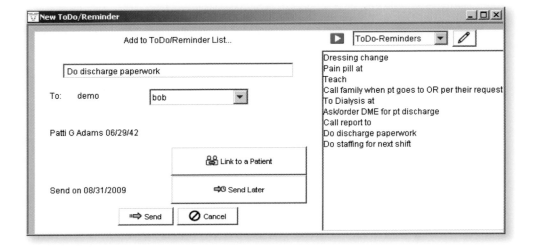

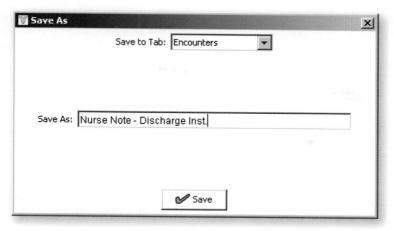

Figure 11.5
Saving a discharge note

Concept Checkup 11.4

A. Is a new ToDo/Reminder launched from within a patient's chart automatically linked to the patient?

_____

B. True or False: A ToDo/Reminder can be sent for a future date.

_____

Exercise 11.1

Stroke

Note: The MAR document is housed in the EHR Materials folder that was installed with the SpringCharts program. Your instructor or IT staff may need to inform you where this folder is kept.

1. After launching SpringCharts, from the top horizontal toolbar, click on *Actions > Open a Chart.* Type in your last name and click the *Search* button. Select your "stroke" patient and the chart opens.
2. Your patient is having difficulty communicating due to the stroke she suffered early this morning. Her significant other tells you she has a past history of Transient Ischemic Attack (TIA) and Pneumonia. Click on *PMHX* and it populates the right-lower-corner box. Click the *Edit* button below the box and a new window opens.

- In the space after *Dx* at the upper-right portion of the window, type *TIA* and click the *Search* button. TIA 435.9 appears in the box below the *Search* button. Click on *TIA* and it moves to the *Past Medical History* box on the upper left.
- In the space after *Dx* type *Pneu* and click the *Search* button. Pneumonia, bacterial 482.89 appears in the box below the *Search* button. Click on *Pneumonia, bacterial 482.89* and it moves to the *Past Medical History* box on the left.
- In the lower left corner of the window, click *Back to Chart.* Note your new entry in the *PMHX* field.

Exercises

3. You ask the patient's significant other about her social history. He states that she drinks 3 to 5 cocktails a day and has done so for the last 10 years. Click on the *Social History* field on the left and it populates the box on the lower right side of the screen

   - Click the *Edit* button and a new window opens.
   - In the right upper box below *Social History* click on *Heavy Drinker*. Heavy Drinker appears in the *Social History* box on the upper left.
   - In the *Social History* box on the upper left, click after Heavy Drinker and type: *3–5 cocktails per day for the last 10 years*.
   - In lower left corner of the window, click *Back to Chart*. The text you added appears in the *Social History* field.

4. Open your *Nurse Note*. On the top horizontal toolbar, click *New > New Nurse Note*. The *Nurse Note* opens to the *Chief Complaint* tab at the top of the vertical navigation bar on the right side of the window.

5. Your patient has no verbal complaints due to aphasia.

   - Click into the *Chief Complaint* field in the left lower box and type: *Difficulty communicating—expressive aphasia*.

6. Click on the *Vitals* tab located below the *CC* tab on the vertical navigation bar on the right side of the screen. Note that your *Chief Complaints* now appear in the *Subjective* section of the *Nurse Note*.

   - You take your patient's vital signs. Document the following in the boxes in the lower left section of the window: Temp *98.2*, Resp *16*, Pulse *76*, BP *177/96*, Ht *68 inches*, Wt *183 lbs*.
   - You measure your patient's oxygen saturation on room air and find it to be 89%. Document this in the *O2Sat%* field. You start oxygen at 2 L/minute per nasal cannula and five minutes later her oxygen saturation has increased to 94%. To document this, click into the *Notes* box on the left and document your assessment and interventions by typing in the field.
   - Under the *Vitals* text box on the right click: *BP right arm, Pt position—supine* and *Temp source—Oral, No complaints of pain*. This text is sent to the *Notes* box on the left. Separate the Temp source—Oral text from the other text by clicking in front of it and striking the [Enter] key on the keyboard.

7. Click on the *Exam* tab located below *Vitals* on the vertical navigation bar on the right. Notice the *O (Normals)* defaults in the right upper box. Select the following systems that are within normal limits when you assess your patient: *HEENT*, *Gastrointestinal*, *Heart sounds*, *Integumentary*, and *GU/GYN (female)*. Remember that you can use the [Enter] key to put these items on separate lines to streamline your documentation.

   - Click the drop-down arrow next to *O (Normals)* and select *O (Abnormals)*. Select the *General* section followed by: *generalized weakness*. Select the *Neuro* section followed by: *Aphasia*.
   - Click in the *Examination* box on the left lower side of the screen after Aphasia and type: *non-verbal at this time. Follows simple commands—squeezes hands and blinks eyes on request*.
   - You are still in the *Examination* box, click in front of generalized weakness. Delete *generalized* and type: *right sided*. Type: *Facial droop, right sided*.

8. Click into the *Dx* button below the *Exam* button in the vertical navigation bar on the right. Click on the red *NANDA* on the left bottom of the screen. The *Dx* text window populates. Remember to place nursing diagnoses in order of priority.

   - Click the following:
     - *Mobility Physical, Impaired*
     - *Communication: Impaired, Verbal*
     - *Falls, Risk for*
     - *Aspiration, Risk for*

- *Social Interaction, Impaired*
- Click the *D&T* icon to date and time the entry. Click *Done*.
- Add the etiology (related factor) and symptoms (as evidenced by) by typing into the field after each nursing diagnosis.

9. Click the *NOC* button in the vertical navigation bar on the right located below the *Dx* button. Notice that your nursing diagnosis documentation populates the *Nurse Note*.

   - Click into the *Nursing Outcomes Classification* text field on the lower left and type: *Aspiration Prevention: Personal actions to prevent the passage of fluid and solid particles into the lung*.
   - Below the *Nursing Outcomes Classification* on the right upper side, select the following:
     - *Communication: Reception, interpretation, and expression of spoken, written, and non-verbal messages*.
     - *Fall Prevention Behavior: Personal or family caregiver actions to minimize risk factors that might precipitate falls in the personal environment*.
     - *Knowledge—Disease Process: Extent of understanding conveyed about a specific disease process and prevention of complications*.
     - *Mobility: Ability to move purposefully in own environment independently with or without assistive device*.
   - Remember that you can use the [Enter] key to put these items on separate lines to streamline your documentation.

10. Click the *NIC* button on the right below the *NOC* button. Notice that your outcomes populate the *Nurse Note*.

    - Select the following interventions:
      - *Respiratory Monitoring: Collection and analysis of patient data to ensure airway patency and adequate gas exchange*.
      - *Embolus Precautions: Reduction of the risk of an embolus in a patient with thrombi or at risk for thrombus formation*.
      - *Emotional Support: Provision of reassurance, acceptance, and encouragement during times of stress*.
      - *Fall Prevention: Instituting special precautions with patient at risk for injury from falling*.
      - *Medication Administration: Preparing, giving, and evaluating the effectiveness of prescription and nonprescription drugs*.
      - *Teaching: Disease Process: Assisting the patient to understand information related to a specific disease process*.
      - *Vital Signs Monitoring: Collection and analysis of cardiovascular, respiratory, and body temperature data to determine and prevent complications*.
    - In the *Nursing Interventions Classifications* box on the lower left, click after the Embolus Precautions entry and type: *Sequential compression devices (SCDs) placed on bilateral lower extremities*
    - Click after the Fall Prevention line and type: *Fall prevention teaching with family, verbalized understanding. They will inform the nurse when they leave the room or if the patient needs to get out of bed*.
    - Strike the [Enter] key to put the cursor on a new line. Type: *Aspiration Precautions: Prevention or minimization of risk factors in the patient at risk for aspiration*

11. You receive an order for Lovenox 250 (3 mg/kg) subcutaneous every 12 hours.

    - Move the *Nurse Note* by clicking the minimize icon in the upper right corner. This will bring you back to the patient's chart. Click the *New* menu and *Import Items* at the bottom of the list. Select *Import File Cabinet Document* and the *File Cabinet* window appears.

Evidence-Based Practice 11.1

In a review of 36 studies, Muller-Staub et al. (2009) found that the use of nursing diagnoses without signs and symptoms and etiology statements was ineffective. However, when patient needs are more accurately reflected by including signs and symptoms (AEB) and etiology (R/T), more effective nursing interventions were implemented, resulting in enhanced patient outcomes.

- Type: *MAR* into the *Document name*.
- In the *Chart* tab select the drop-down box on the right and choose *Nursing Documentation*. In the *Description* field type: *MAR*.
- Click *Attach*. Select *Existing*. Use the search mechanism to select the blank MAR document.
- Click *Done*. The document appears in the *Care Tree* on the right in the *Nursing Documentation* tab.
- Click on the + in front of *Nursing Documentation*. Highlight the *MAR* and click *Edit* at the lower right side of the screen. The *File Cabinet* window appears.
- Click on the blue hyperlink next to the word *File*. The *MAR* document opens.
- Enter the Patient, Date of Birth, Date, Admit date, Doctor, and Room #.
- On the left enter the *Lovenox* on the blank field above Strength and Dose. In the *Dose* field type: *250 mg*.
- Under *Directions* type: *Subq every 12 hrs*. Indicate the scheduled administration times of 0900 and 2100.
- Type your name and initials in the *Initial & Name* area at the bottom of the document.
- Type your initials in the 9am top time box and type: *RLQ* (right lower quadrant of abdomen) in the bottom box to indicate the injection location.
- Click the *Save* diskette icon to save your work.
- Click the *X* on the far right upper corner to close the *MAR*. A pop-up will ask you if you want to save the changes you have made, select *Yes*. The *File Cabinet* window is still present.
- Click *Done*. A pop-up appears: "The Attached file may have changed. Do you want to send a new version to the server?" Click *Yes*. The window closes.

12. Your patient is NPO until a swallowing assessment is completed.
- Click the *New* menu and then *Import Items* at the bottom of the list.
- Select *Import File Cabinet Document* and the *File Cabinet* window appears.
- Type: *Intake and Output* into the *Document name*.
- In the *Chart* tab select the drop-down box on the right and choose *Nursing Documentation*.
- In the *Description* field type: *Intake and Output*.
- Click *Attach*. Select *Existing*. Use the search mechanism to select the blank Intake and Output document. The I&O document is found in the *EHR Materials* folder.
- Click *OK*. Click *Done*. The document appears in the *Care Tree* on the right in the *Nursing Documentation* tab.
- Click on the + in front of *Nursing Documentation*.
- Highlight the *Intake and Output* and click *Edit* at the lower right side of the screen. The *File Cabinet* window appears.
- Click on the blue hyperlink next to the word *File*. The *Intake and Output* document opens.
- Type in the Patient Name and Date.
- Your patient urinated 200 mL in the bedpan at 0930. Document this.
- Click the *Save* diskette icon to save your work.
- Click the *X* on the far right upper corner to close the I&O sheet. A pop-up will ask you if you want to save the changes you have made, select *Yes*. The *File Cabinet* window is still present.
- Click *Done*. A pop-up appears: "The Attached file may have changed. Do you want to send a new version to the server?" Click *Yes*. The window closes.

Legal/Ethical Considerations

Nurses may delegate measuring and documenting I&O to unlicensed assistive personnel who have demonstrated competence in monitoring I&O.

13. The *Nurse Note* may be located at the bottom of the screen due to minimizing it earlier. Return to the *Nurse Note* by clicking the maximize icon on the upper right side of the *Nurse Note*. Click the *Teaching* button on the vertical navigation bar on the right.

    • Under the *Other Tx Panel* at the upper right select the following: *Discussed plan of care with patient/significant other.*

    • Click into the *Teaching* text box on the lower left of the screen and type: *Patient unable to participate verbally in discussion but nods understanding.*

14. Click into *Evaluation* on the vertical navigation bar on the right. Using the *Evaluation* text on the right side, add the text below manually. (The NOC item for the patient is referenced by the first word.)

    • *Communication: Outcome met this shift for reception and interpretation as evidenced by nodding and following instructions to move left side. Outcome not met this shift for expression of spoken messages due to aphasia.*

    • *Fall Prevention Behavior: Outcome met this shift, no falls. Ongoing outcome.*

    • *Knowledge—Disease Process: Outcome met this shift—teaching completed with family and patient. Continue to reinforce. Ongoing outcome.*

    • *Mobility: Right-sided weakness limits mobility. Bed rest maintained this shift. Ongoing outcome.*

    • *Continue current interventions.*

    • Use the [Enter] key on the keyboard to place text on separate lines to streamline your documentation.

15. Click into *Reassess*. Under the *Reassessment* text box on the right click: *New/Added Intervention*. The text moves to the *Reassessment* text box on the lower left side of the screen.

    • Click after *New/Added Intervention*: and type: *Add Thicket to all liquids for dysphagia.*

16. Click into *F/U-Rem*. Notice your documentation from the *Reassess* area populates the *Nurse Note*. On the lower left side of the screen below the *F/U-Reminders* text, click on the icon of a finger with a piece of string tied around it.

    • The *Add to ToDo/Reminder List . . .* window populates. Click into the free text field at the upper left and type: *Move patient close to nursing station when room available.*

    • Notice that your patient's name displays in the middle left side of the window. *F/U-Rem* is linked to a patient when accessed within the *Nurse Note*. Click *Send*.

    • Look to the far left of the screen to the SpringCharts fields that are open outside of the *Nurse Note*. Your new entry is visible in the *ToDo List* in dark pink below the calendar.

17. Click *Done*. The *Save As* screen populates. Click *Save*.

18. A pop-up appears asking if you want to create a routing slip. Click *No*.

19. In the *Care Tree*, click the + next to *Encounters*. Click on the date of your *Nurse Note* and it appears in the bottom right corner box.

    • Click *Edit*. Click *Sign*. Select *Permanent Sign and Lock* when finished with your *Nurse Note*.

Exercise 11.2

Cellulitis

1. After launching SpringCharts, click on *Actions > Open a Chart*. Type in your last name and click the *Search* button. Select your "cellulitis" patient and the chart opens.

2. Your patient tells you she scraped her arm getting groceries out of her car a week ago and now her entire right arm is infected. She tells you she has taken Synthroid 0.1 mg by mouth daily for the past year. The Synthroid is not in her *Routine Meds* list. You check her chart and find that her physician has ordered this medication to be continued during her hospital stay. Click on *Routine Meds* and it populates in the bottom right corner of the screen. Click *Edit* below this box.

   - The *Routine Med* screen populates. In the space after *Brand Name* in the upper right portion of the window type: *Synthroid* and click the *Search* icon. Options appear in the box below. Click on the *Synthroid 0.1 mg po daily*, which sends the medication information to the *Routine Meds* list at the upper left side of the window.

   - Click on the *Synthroid* in the *Routine Meds* field on the left side of the screen. The *Edit Rx* window opens. Put a date of one year ago in the *Date Started* and click *Save*.

   - In the left lower portion of the window, click *Back to Chart*. Your entry appears in the *Routine Meds* field.

3. Open your *Nurse Note*. On the top horizontal toolbar, click *New > New Nurse Note*. The *Nurse Note* opens to the *Chief Complaint* tab at the top of the vertical navigation bar on the right side of the window.

4. Your patient complains of pain and swelling in her right arm. Select *Pain* and select *Swelling in legs* in the *S Panel* text and it populates the *Chief Complaint* box on the bottom left of the screen. Click in to the *Chief Complaint* box after Swelling in legs and delete *legs* and type: *right arm*.

5. Click on the *Vitals* button located below the *CC* button in the vertical navigation bar on the right side of the screen. Note that your *Chief Complaints* now appear in the *Subjective* section of the *Nurse Note*.

   - You take your patient's vital signs. Document the following: Temp *102.4*, Resp *18*, Pulse *102*, BP *148/74*, Ht *55 inches*, Wt *180 lbs.*, O2Sa% *92*.

   - Also select: *BP left arm, Pt position—supine* and *Temp source—tympanic*.

   - Under the *Vitals* text box on the lower right click: *Pt Complains of pain, Pain location, Pain rating 0–10 scale, Pain Description, Factors affecting pain*, and *Factors relieving pain*. The text is sent to the *Notes* box on the left. Use the [Enter] key to place each entry on a separate line.

   - Fill in the following information in the *Notes* box that your patient conveys to you: Pain location: *Right arm pain*, Pain rating 0–10 scale: *3*, Description: *aching*, Factors affecting pain: *movement*, Factors relieving pain: *aspirin*.

6. Click on the *Exam* tab located below the *Vitals*. Notice the *O (Normals)* defaults in the right upper box. In this area select the following systems that are within normal limits when you assess your patient: *HENT, Heart sounds, Lungs/Respiratory, GU/GYN (female)*, and *Neurological*.

   - Click the drop-down arrow next to *O (Normals)* in the right upper box and select *O (Abnormals)*. Select the *Skin* section followed by: *abrasions*. Select the *Extremities* section followed by: *edema*.

   - Click into the *Examination* box on the lower left after abrasions and type: *4 cm by 6 cm abraded area to right forearm. Inflammation present*. After edema type: *to right arm, 14 cm circumference measured and marked*.

7. Click into the *Dx* tab below the *Exam* tab in the vertical navigation bar on the right. Click on the red *NANDA* on the left bottom of the screen. The *Dx* text window populates.

   - Click *Infection, Risk for*; *Pain, Acute*; *Skin Integrity, Impaired*. Remove the *Risk for* after Infection as this is an actual problem. Click the *D&T* icon to date and time the entry. Click *Done*. Use the [Enter] key to place each nursing diagnosis on a separate line. Consider your assessment data and add one additional nursing diagnosis.

   - Add the etiology (related factor) and symptoms (as evidenced by) by typing them into the field after each nursing diagnosis to individualize the diagnosis for your patient.

   - Place the nursing diagnoses in order of priority.

8. Click the *NOC* tab on the right located below the *Dx* tab. Notice that your *NANDA* documentation populates the *Nurse Note*.

   - Below the *Nursing Outcomes Classification* at the upper right select the following:

     - *Infection Severity: Severity of infection and associated symptoms.*

     - *Tissue Integrity: Skin and Mucous Membranes: Structural intactness and normal physiological function of skin and mucous membranes.*

     - *Knowledge—Disease Process: Extent of understanding conveyed about a specific disease process and prevention of complications.*

     - *Pain Control: Personal actions to control pain.*

     - *Vital Signs: Extent to which temperature, pulse, respiration, and blood pressure are within normal range.*

   - Consider the nursing diagnoses above and add other NOCs as indicated.

   - Use the [Enter] key on the keyboard to place text on separate lines to streamline your documentation.

9. Click the *NIC* button on the right below the *NOC* button. Notice that your outcomes populate the *Nurse Note*.

   - Select the following interventions:

     - *Intravenous (IV) Insertion: Administration and monitoring of intravenous fluids and medications.*

     - *Medication Administration: Preparing, giving, and evaluating the effectiveness of prescription and nonprescription drugs.*

     - *Pain Management: Alleviation of pain or a reduction in pain to a level of comfort that is acceptable to the patient.*

     - *Skin Survellance: Collection and analysis of patient data to maintain skin and mucous membrane integrity.*

     - *Vital Signs Monitoring: Collection and analysis of cardiovascular, respiratory, and body temperature data to determine and prevent complications.*

     - *Wound Care: Prevention of wound complications and promotion of wound healing.*

   - Click after the Intravenous (IV) Insertion line and type: *IV started with 20-G catheter in left forearm, first attempt.*

   - Click after the Wound Care line and type: *Neosporin applied to abrasions on right arm per physician order.*

   - Consider the nursing diagnoses and outcomes above and add other interventions as indicated.

10. Move the *Nurse Note* by clicking on the minimize icon in the upper right corner. This will bring you back to the patient's chart.
    Your patient is NPO so you do not administer her oral medication.

    - To document this, click the *New* menu, and then *Import Items* at the bottom of the list.

- Select *Import File Cabinet Document* and the *File Cabinet* window appears.
- Type: *MAR* into the *Document name*.
- In the *Chart* tab select the drop-down box on the right and choose *Nursing Documentation*. In the *Description* field, type: *MAR*.
- Click *Attach*. Select *Existing*. Use the search mechanism to select the blank MAR document as before.
- Click *OK*. Click *Done*. The document appears in the *Care Tree* on the right in the *Nursing Documentation* tab.
- Click on the + in front of *Nursing Documentation*. Highlight the *MAR* and click *Edit* at the bottom right-hand side of the screen. The *File Cabinet* window appears.
- Click on the blue hyperlink next to the word *File*. The *MAR* document opens.
- Enter the Patient, Date of Birth, Date, Admit date, Doctor, and Room #.
- On the left enter the *Synthroid* on the blank field above Strength and Dose.
- In the *Strength* field type: *0.1 mg* and in the *Dose* field type: *1*. Under *Directions* type: *po daily*. Add *0900* as scheduled administration time.
- Type your name and initials in the *Initial & Name* area at the bottom of the document.
- Type: *NPO* in the 0900 top time box and your initials in the bottom box.
- Click the *Save* diskette icon to save your work. Your shift coordinator receives an order for Lactated Ringers at 100 mL/hr IV and Clindamycin 600 mg IVPB every 8 hours from the physician.
- On the left enter the *Clindamycin* on a blank field above Strength and Dose. In the *Strength* field type: *600 mg* and in the *Dose* field type: *1*.
- Under *Directions* type: *IVPB every 8 hours*. Add *0800*, *1600*, and *2400* as scheduled administration times.
- Type your initials in the 8am top field to indicate the time you initiated the Clindamycin.
- Click the *Save* diskette icon to save your work.
- On the left enter the *Lactated Ringers* on a blank field above Strength and Dose. In the *Dose* field type: *100 mL/hr*. Under *Directions* type: *continuous IV infusion*.
- Type your initials in the 8am top field to indicate the time you initiated the Lactated Ringers.
- Click the *Save* diskette icon to save your work.
- Click the *X* on the far right upper corner to close the *MAR*. A pop-up will ask you if you want to save the changes you have made, select *Yes*. The *File Cabinet* window is still present.
- Click *Done*. A pop-up appears stating, "The Attached file may have changed. Do you want to send a new version to the server?" Click *Yes*. The window closes.

11. Your patient remains NPO, so she has no oral intake during your shift. In order to document intake and output, import the I&O form.
    - Click the *New* menu and then *Import Items* at the bottom of the list.
    - Select *Import File Cabinet Document* and the *File Cabinet* window appears.
    - Type: *Intake and Output* into the *Document name*. In the *Chart* tab select the drop-down box on the right and choose *Nursing Documentation*. In the *Description* field type: *Intake and Output*.
    - Click *Attach*. Select *Existing*. Use the search mechanism to select the blank *Intake and Output* document as before.

- Click *OK*. Click *Done*. The document appears in the *Care Tree* on the right in the *Nursing Documentation* tab.
- Click on the + in front of *Nursing Documentation*. Highlight the *Intake and Output* and click *Edit* at the bottom right-hand side of the screen. The *File Cabinet* window appears.
- Click on the blue hyperlink next to the word *File*. The *Intake and Output* document opens.
- Type the Patient Name and Date.
- She has received 600 mL of Lactated Ringers since 0800, and it is currently 1400, so document the intake including the shift total.
- Your patient has voided 350 mL over the course of the shift, 150 mL at 1000 hours and 200 mL at 1330 hours. Document her output, including the shift total.
- Click the *X* on the far right upper corner to close the I&O sheet. A pop-up will ask you if you want to save the changes you've made, select *Yes*. The *File Cabinet* window is still present.
- Click *Done*. A pop-up appears stating, "The Attached file may have changed. Do you want to send a new version to the server?" Click *Yes*. The window closes.

12. The *Nurse Note* may be located at the bottom of the screen due to minimizing it earlier. Return to the *Nurse Note* by clicking the maximize icon on the upper right side of the *Nurse Note*. Click into the *Nurse Note*. Click the *Teaching* button on the right. Under the *Other Tx Panel* at the upper right, select the following:
    - *Discussed plan of care with patient/significant other*.
    - *Medication indication, frequency, considerations instruction*.

13. Click into *Evaluation* on the right. Using the *Evaluation* text on the right, add the text below by clicking on it. (The NOC item for the patient is referenced by the first word.) Add text manually where directed to type.
    - *Infection Severity: Ongoing outcome*.
    - *Knowledge—Disease Process: Outcome met this shift*. Type: *continue to reinforce*.
    - *Pain Control: Outcome met this shift*.
    - *Vital Signs: Ongoing outcome*.
    - Add an outcome for the nursing diagnosis that you added earlier.
    - Continue current interventions.

14. Click into *Reassess*. Click into the *Reassessment* text box on the left and click: *Temperature* and *Temp source: Oral*. Click into the *Reassessment* box on the left and separate the two entries by using the [Enter] key. After temperature type: *100.4 after Tylenol administration in ED*.

15. The family has gone to the cafeteria to get something to eat but they want to accompany your patient to surgery and wait in the surgical waiting room.
    - Click into *F/U-Rem*. Notice your documentation from the *Reassess* area populates the *Nurse Note*. On the lower left side of the screen below the *F/U-Reminders* text, click on the icon of a finger with a piece of string tied around it.
    - The *Add to ToDo/Reminder List* window populates. Under the *ToDo-Reminders* text field on the right click on: *Call family when pt. goes to OR per their request*. This populates into the text field on the left. Notice your patient's name displays in the middle left section of this window. *F/U-Rem* is linked to a patient when accessed within the *Nurse Note*. Click *Send*.

Documentation Tip

The response to medications is documented to indicate effectiveness.

- Look to the far left of the software, to the SpringCharts fields that are open outside of the *Nurse Note*. You will see the dark pink *ToDo List* below the calendar with your new entry visible below it.

16. Click *Done* at the bottom left of the screen. The *Save As* screen populates. Click *Save*.

17. A pop-up appears asking if you want to create a routing slip. Click *No*.

18. In the *Care Tree*, click the + next to *Encounters*. Click on the date of your *Nurse Note* and it appears in the bottom right corner box.
    - Click *Edit*. Click *Sign*. Select *Permanent Sign and Lock* when finished with your *Nurse Note*.

Exercise 11.3

Chest Pain

1. After launching SpringCharts, click on *Actions > Open a Chart*. Type in your last name and click the *Search* button. Select your "chest pain" patient and the chart opens.

2. Your patient informs you he has heart disease, diabetes, and high cholesterol. Click on the *PMHX* box and it populates in the bottom right corner. Click *Edit*.
    - In the *Preferences* box on the far right bottom of the screen, click the three conditions your patient related. They appear under other *PMHX* on the left.
    - Click *Back to Chart*. The items are now listed in the *PMHX*.

3. Your patient has been married for 47 years. He is a nonsmoker and drinks 24 ounces of beer a day.
    - Click in the *Social History* box. The box appears on the far bottom right-hand side of the screen. Click *Edit*.
    - Under *Social History* click *Nonsmoker*, *Ounces per day*, and *Married*. The items appear on the left side of the screen under *Social History*. Click into the area and type the information into the field as your patient related it to you. Use the [Enter] key to move each item to a separate line.
    - Click *Back to Chart*.

4. Your patient has been taking Nitrolingual 0.4 mg sublingual every 3–5 minutes x 3 doses prn chest pain for the last month. Click on the *Routine Meds* box and it populates in the bottom right corner. Click *Edit*.
    - Click in the space after *Brand Name* and type: *Nitro*. Click the *Search* icon.
    - Click on the *Nitrolingual 0.4 mg* to send the medication to the *Routine Medications* list.
    - Click on the *Nitrolingual 0.4 mg* in the *Routine Medications* list. The *Edit Rx* window opens. Click into *Directions* and type: *sublingual every 3–5 minutes x 3 as needed for chest pain*. Click in the calendar to the right of *Date Started* and choose a date one month ago. Click *Save*.
    - Click *Back to Chart*. The Nitrolingual 0.4 mg is now listed in the *Routine Meds*.

5. Open your *Nurse Note*. Click *New > New Nurse Note*.

6. Your patient complains of chest pain. Select *Chest pain* from the *S Panel* text and it populates the *Chief Complaint* box on the bottom left of the screen.

7. Sensing the urgency of responding to your patient's chest pain, you assess his vital signs and pain level. Click on the *Vitals* button located below the *CC* button on the vertical navigation bar on the right side of the screen. Note that your *Chief Complaints* now appear in the *Subjective* section of the *Nurse Note*.

- You take your patient's vital signs. Document the following: Temp *99.2*, Resp *18*, Pulse *114*, BP *110/72*, O2SAT% *97*. You defer measuring height and weight due to the patient's chest pain.
- Under the *Vitals* text box on the right click: *BP left arm, Pt position—supine* and *Temp source—Oral*. These items populate the *Notes* textbox on the left.
- Under the *Vitals* text box on the right click: *Pt Complains of pain*, *Pain Location*, *Pain rating 0–10 scale*, *Pain Radiation*, *Pain Description*, *Factors affecting pain*, and *Factors relieving pain*.
- Click into the *Notes* section on the left and add the following information: pain location substernal, 10 on 0–10 scale, radiating to the jaw, description "feels like an elephant is on my chest," Factors affecting pain— "everything," Factors relieving pain—"nothing so far."

8. You quickly assess your patient while another nurse obtains his Nitrolingual. Click on the *Exam* button located below the *Vitals*. Notice the *O (Normals)* defaults. In this area select the following systems that are within normal limits when you assess your patient: *HEENT, Musculoskeletal, GU (male), Lungs/ Respiratory*, and *Neurological*.
   - Click the drop-down arrow next to *O (Normals)* and select *O (Abnormals)*. Select the *General* section followed by: *diaphoretic*. Select the *Chest/ABD* section followed by: *irregular*.
   - Click into the *Examination* field in front of irregular and type: *heart rhythm*.

9. Move the *Nurse Note* by clicking the minimize icon in the upper right corner. This will bring you back to the patient's chart.
   You administer the Nitrolingual to your patient for his chest pain.
   - In order to document, click the *New* menu and then *Import Items* at the bottom of the list.
   - Select *Import File Cabinet Document* and the *File Cabinet* window appears.
   - Type: *MAR* into the *Document name*. In the *Chart* tab, select the drop-down box on the right and choose *Nursing Documentation*.
   - In the *Description* field, type: *MAR*. Click *Attach*. Select *Existing*. Use the search mechanism to select the blank MAR document as before.
   - Click *Done*. The document appears in the *Care Tree* on the right in the *Nursing Documentation* tab.
   - Click on the + in front of *Nursing Documentation*. Highlight the *MAR* and click *Edit* at the bottom right of the screen. The *File Cabinet* window appears.
   - Click on the blue hyperlink next to the word *File*. The *MAR* document opens.
   - Enter the Patient, Date of Birth, Date, Admit date, Doctor, and Room #.
   - On the left enter the *Nitrolingual* on the blank field above Strength and Dose. In the *Strength* field type: *0.4 mg* and in the *Dose* field type: *1*.
   - Under *Directions* type: *sublingual every 3–5 minutes x3 doses prn chest pain*.
   - Type your name and initials in the *Initial & Name* area at the bottom of the document.
   - Type your initials in the 1000 top time box. Click the *Save* diskette icon to save your work.
   - Click the *X* on the far right upper corner to close the *MAR*. A pop-up will ask you if you want to save the changes you have made, select *Yes*. The *File Cabinet* window is still present.
   - Click *Done*. A pop-up appears: "The Attached file may have changed. Do you want to send a new version to the server?" Click *Yes*. The window closes.

10. The *Nurse Note* may be located at the bottom of the screen due to minimizing it earlier. Return to the *Nurse Note* by clicking the maximize icon on the upper right side of the *Nurse Note*. Your patient's chest pain is relieved after the initial dose of Nitrolingual so you develop his plan of care. Click into the *Dx* tab below the *Exam* tab on the right. Click on the red *NANDA* lettering on the left bottom of the screen. The *Dx* text window populates.

   • Click *Pain, Acute*. Click into the text field after acute and type: *chest*. Click the *D&T* icon to date and time the entry. Click *Done*.

   • Add the etiology (related factor) and symptoms (as evidenced by) by typing them into the field after the nursing diagnosis to individualize the nursing diagnosis.

11. Click the *NOC* tab on the right located below the *Dx* tab in the vertical navigation bar on the right. Notice that your *NANDA* documentation populates the *Nurse Note*.

   • Below the *Nursing Outcomes Classification* select the following:

      • *Cardiopulmonary Status: Adequacy of blood volume ejected from the ventricles and exchange of carbon dioxide and oxygen at the alveolar level.*

      • *Pain Control: Personal actions to control pain.*

      • *Knowledge—Cardiac Disease Management: Extent of understanding conveyed about heart disease, its treatment, and the prevention of complications.*

      • *Vital Signs: Extent to which temperature, pulse, respiration, and blood pressure are within normal range.*

   • Use the [Enter] key to place text on separate lines to streamline your documentation.

12. Click the *NIC* button on the right below the *NOC* button. Notice that your outcomes populate the *Nurse Note*.

   • Select the following interventions:

      • *Intravenous (IV) Insertion: Administration and monitoring of intravenous fluids and medications*

      • *Medication Administration: Preparing, giving, and evaluating the effectiveness of prescription and nonprescription drugs*

      • *Pain Management: Alleviation of pain or a reduction in pain to a level of comfort that is acceptable to the patient*

      • *Teaching: Disease Process: Assisting the patient to understand information related to a specific disease process*

      • *Vital Signs Monitoring: Collection and analysis of cardiovascular, respiratory, and body temperature data to determine and prevent complications*

13. In order to document intake and output, import the I&O form.

   • Move the *Nurse Note* by clicking the minimize icon in the upper right corner. This will bring you back to the patient's chart. Click the *New* menu and then *Import Items* at the bottom of the list. Select *Import File Cabinet Document* and the *File Cabinet* window appears.

   • Type: *Intake and Output* into the *Document name*. In the *Chart* tab select the drop-down box on the right and choose *Nursing Documentation*.

   • In the *Description* field type: *Intake and Output*. Click *Attach*. Select *Existing*. Use the search mechanism to select the blank Intake and Output document.

   • Click *Done*. The document appears in the *Care Tree* on the right in the *Nursing Documentation* tab.

   • Click on the + in front of *Nursing Documentation*. Highlight the *Intake and Output* and click *Edit* at the bottom right-hand side of the screen. The *File Cabinet* window appears.

- Click on the blue hyperlink next to the word *File*. The *Intake and Output* document opens.
- Type in the Patient Name and Date.
- Your patient consumed 240 mL orally today at 1130. He voided 200 mL at 1000 when he first arrived. Document these items. Your shift is not over, so don't fill in shift totals at this time.
- Click the *X* on the far right upper corner to close the I&O sheet. A pop-up will ask you if you want to save the changes you have made, select *Yes*. The *File Cabinet* window is still present.
- Click *Done*. A pop-up appears: "The Attached file may have changed. Do you want to send a new version to the server?" Click *Yes*. The window closes.

14. The *Nurse Note* may be located at the bottom of the screen due to minimizing it earlier. Return to the *Nurse Note* by clicking the maximize icon on the right upper side of the *Nurse Note*. Click in the *Teaching* button on the right.
    - Under the *Other Tx Panel* select the following: *Patient not a candidate for instruction due to:* and it populates into the *Teaching* area on the left of the screen.
    - Click into the *Teaching* area after the selected text and type: *acute chest pain*.

15. Click into *Evaluation* on the right. Using the *Evaluation* text on the right side, add the text below by clicking on it. (The NOC item for the patient is referenced by the first word.) Add text manually where directed to type.
    - *Cardiopulmonary Status:* Type: *Chest pain controlled by Nitrolingual. Ongoing outcome*.
    - *Knowledge—Cardiac Disease Management: Outcome not met this shift. Variance reason—pt condition*.
    - *Pain Control: Outcome met this shift*. Type: *Chest pain resolved with Nitrolingual*.
    - *Vital Signs: Ongoing outcome*.
    - *Continue current interventions*.

16. Click into *Reassess*. Click into the *Reassessment* text box on the left and type: *patient reports his pain has decreased to a 0 on a scale of 0–10 four minutes after taking the Nitrolingual*.

17. Click into *F/U-Rem*. Notice your documentation from the *Reassess* area populates the *Nurse Note*. On the left side of the screen below the *F/U-Reminders* text, click on the icon of a finger with a piece of string tied around it.
    - The *Add to ToDo/Reminder List . . .* window populates. Under the *ToDo-Reminders* text field on the right, click on *Teach*. It populates into the text field on the left.
    - Click after the word Teach and type: *cardiac disease management when patient receptive*.
    - Notice that your patient's name displays in the middle left portion of the screen. Click *Send*.
    - Look to the far left of the software, to the SpringCharts fields that are open outside of the *Nurse Note*. Your entry appears in the dark pink *ToDo List* below the calendar.

18. Click *Done*. The *Save As* screen populates. Click *Save*.

19. A pop-up appears asking if you want to create a routing slip. Click *No*.

20. In the *Care Tree*, click the + next to *Encounters*. Click on the date of your *Nurse Note* and it appears in the bottom right corner box.
    - Click *Edit*. Click *Sign*. Select *Permanent Sign and Lock* when finished with your *Nurse Note*.

Reference

Muller-Staub, M., Lunney, M., Odenbreit, M., Needham, I., Lavin, M. A., van Achterberg, T. (2009). Evaluation of the implementation of nursing diagnoses, interventions, and outcomes. *International Journal of Nursing Terminologies and Classifications, 20*(1), 9–15.

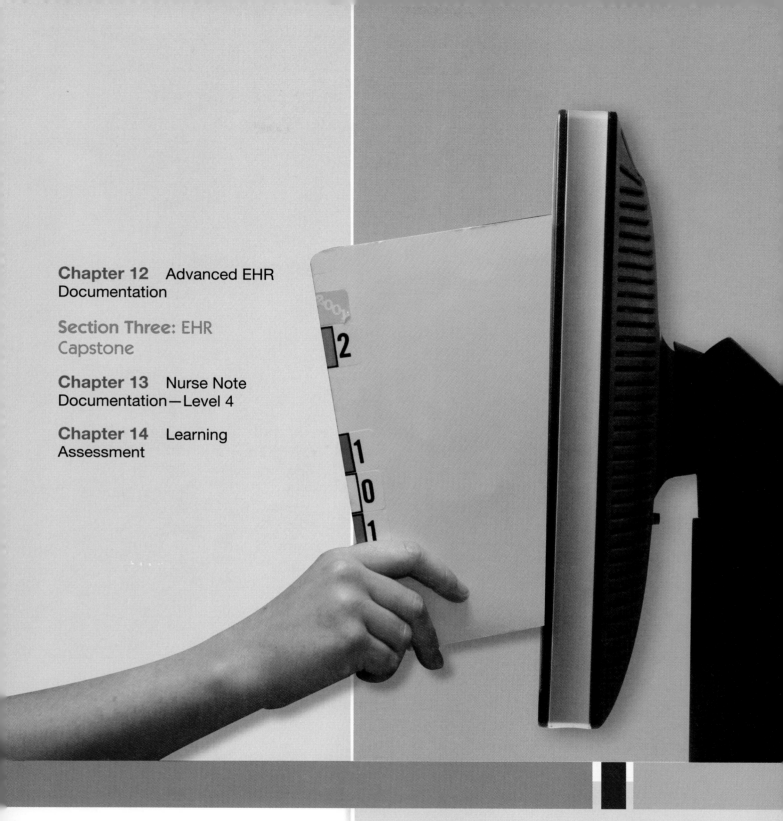

Level Four

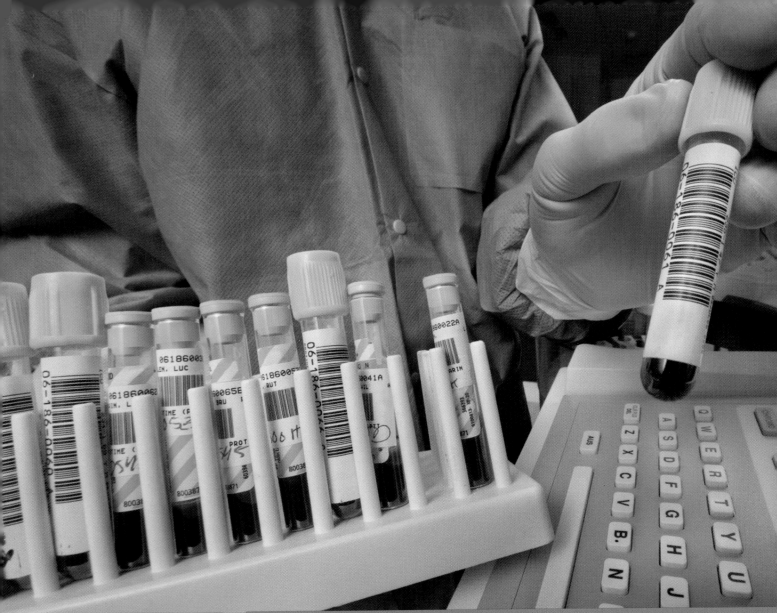

12 Advanced EHR

Key Terms

Terms and abbreviations you will encounter in Chapter 12; they are defined in the end-of-book glossary:

Critical Results

Critical Test

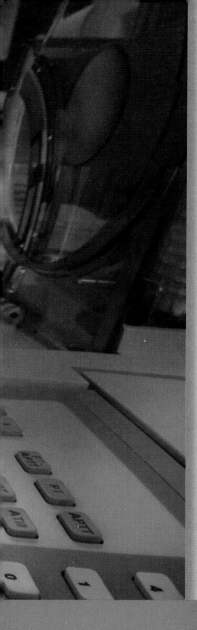

Learning Outcomes

When you complete Chapter 12, you will be able to:

12.1   Use EHR to order diagnostic tests.

12.2   Carry out a chart evaluation.

12.3   Use a *New Note* to create an *Addendum* to a *Nurse Note*.

12.4   Carry out printing a *Nurse Note*.

12.5   Carry out exporting and printing elements of a patient's chart.

Documentation

What You Need to Know

To understand Chapter 12, you need to know how to:

- Navigate in the *Practice View* screen.
- Navigate in the *Patient Chart* screen.
- Navigate in the *Nurse Note*.

Documentation Tip

Healthcare facilities and practices have Release of Records forms that patients may sign to release their healthcare records to other providers.

FOCAL POINT

The *Test* area allows the nurse to order diagnostic tests for a patient using the EHR.

Overview

Diagnostic testing and screening are key components of healthcare that enable the provider to determine necessary treatment. Once the primary care provider orders diagnostic or screening tests, the appropriate department must be notified to conduct the test. These tests may be requested by a primary care provider, a unit clerk, office administrative personnel, or the nurse using the EHR. Following completion of the testing, results are placed in the EHR, allowing immediate access by other healthcare professionals and promoting timely response to abnormalities. Diagnostic and screening evaluations are requested in SpringCharts using the *Test* area.

On occasions, hard copies of portions of a patient's health record or the entire record may be necessary. In the outpatient setting, a copy of a consultation record or procedural report may be needed to send to a primary care provider. Often, a history and physical examination are conducted in the outpatient setting or the primary care provider may write admission orders before a patient is admitted to the hospital and send hard copies to the facility. In the inpatient setting, copies of the health record may be sent to other facilities in the event a patient is transferred or discharged to a long-term care or sub-acute setting. Discharge instructions are routinely printed and given to the patient. In addition, patients may request copies of portions of their records for personal use or to take to other healthcare providers. In these situations, one must be able to print the health record. However, as use of technology expands, electronic transfer of portions of the EHR will become the norm. Before an individual's health record may be released, electronically or in hard copy, to an insurance company or another healthcare provider, the individual must give written consent. SpringCharts enables the nurse to export an electronic file or print elements of the patient's chart.

LO 12.1   Diagnostic Tests

Diagnostic and screening procedures may consist of lab tests, imaging studies, and other tests ordered by the primary care provider. To order these tests from the appropriate department, the user clicks on the *Test* tab on the right side of the *Nurse Note* screen—see Figure 12.1. Next, the user clicks into the search field and types the name of the study to be completed, such as CBC (complete blood count). By typing the

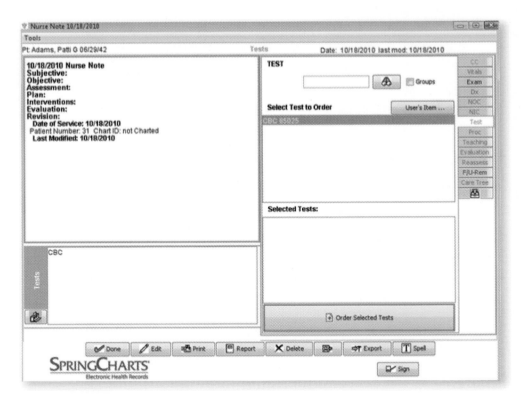

Figure 12.1

Selecting *Test* in *Nurse Note*

first few letters of the test name and clicking on the *Search* icon, choices appear in the *Select Tests to Order* field. The user then selects the appropriate test from the list to send the item into the *Selected Tests* field below. This can be done as many times as necessary to create a list of desired tests. When the user clicks the *Order Selected Tests* button at the bottom of the *Selected Tests* field, the test(s) populates the *Test* field on the left of the *Nurse Note* screen, also seen in Figure 12.1. If the incorrect test is inadvertently selected, the user clicks on the test in the left *Tests* field and answers *Yes* to the "Do you want to delete this reference to this test?" query to delete the test. Diagnostic tests may also be ordered from the *Office Visit Note* or from the *Actions* menu in the patient's chart.

Once ordered, diagnostic procedures are sent to the *Pending Tests* area of Spring-Charts, where they remain until the results are entered either manually or electronically through an interface with the testing facility. After results are entered, the test moves into the *Completed Tests* list. Here, the test results are viewed by the care provider; comments may be added and stored in the patient's chart.

In the inpatient setting, results are posted in the EHR by the department that conducts the test or procedure. In an outpatient setting, however, results may be called, mailed, or electronically transmitted to the facility. In this case, the results may need to be manually entered into the EHR. To manually enter results, the user selects *Pending Tests* from the main *Edit* menu, illustrated in Figure 12.2. The *Pending Tests* window, Figure 12.3, appears, showing all outstanding tests for all patients in SpringCharts. The user selects the specific test for which results are to be entered. Some results require simply clicking the radio button to enter a *Positive* or *Negative* result. Others require clicking the *Normal Test* button and yet others may require more elaborate text to define the results. Results that have been received by e-mail or fax can be copied and pasted into the *Pending Tests* window. Test results received in hard copy must be scanned into an electronic file. When the electronic file is opened, the clinician highlights the result, copies it, and then pastes it into the text field of the *Pending Test*, as seen in Figure 12.4.

Once the results are entered, the user clicks the *Tech Sign* button to indicate the source of the data entry and then clicks the *Testing Facility* button to choose the appropriate originating facility, as illustrated in Figures 12.4 and 12.5. If the facility is not listed, it must be set up in the address book under the *New* menu or the *Productivity Center* menu. The data entry technician may use the *ToDo* or *Message* button to notify the appropriate healthcare professional that results are

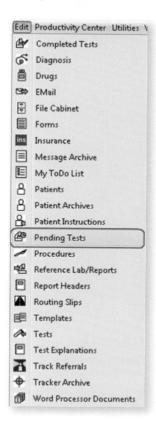

Figure 12.2

Accessing *Pending Tests* through *Edit* menu

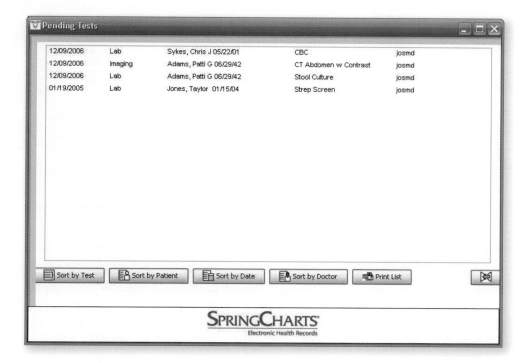

Figure 12.3

Pending Tests window

Figure 12.4

Test results copied and pasted into *Pending Test*

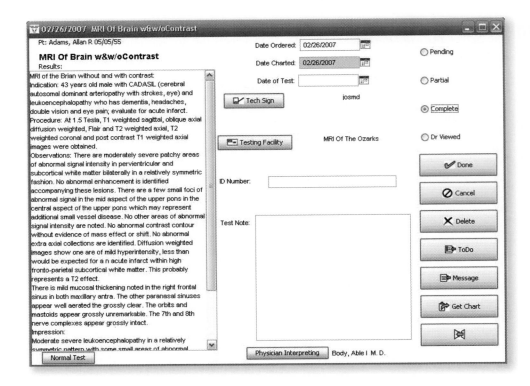

Figure 12.5

Results entry into *Pending Test*

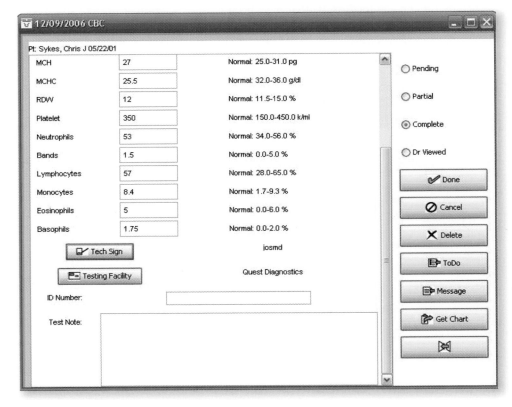

available. To complete this process, the user clicks the *Complete* radio button on the right side of the screen and then the *Done* button to move the *Pending Tests* to the *Completed Tests* list.

When ready to evaluate a completed test, the clinician opens the *Completed Tests* window from the *Practice View* screen by selecting *Edit > Completed Tests*. The *Completed Tests* window displays all results that were entered. The list of tests can

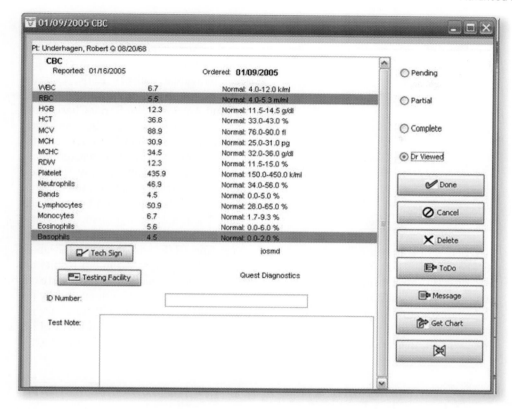

Figure 12.6
Completed test results

be organized by the test name, the patient name, the test order date, or the ordering primary care provider to facilitate finding the desired results.

When a completed test is selected by clicking on the item, test results display. Abnormal results are highlighted in a color bar, as seen in Figure 12.6. From this screen, the healthcare provider can perform all the administrative functions necessary to process the test. The patient's chart can be opened to look for other health information, a *ToDo/Reminder* for follow-up may be created, or a *Message* may be sent to another user. Free text can be typed in the *Test Note* window to record an observation or a plan of care. The nurse may document that the primary care provider was notified of the results and the provider's response.

Certain test results require immediate communication of results to the primary care provider. These tests are considered **critical tests** and their results must be reported urgently, even if they are normal. For example, some facilities identify all tests that are ordered STAT (immediately) as critical tests. Other test findings must be communicated quickly if they have a **critical result**, one that is grossly abnormal and may be life-threatening to the patient. National Patient Safety Goal 2.03.01 requires that healthcare facilities define critical tests and critical results (The Joint Commission, 2010). Upon receipt of the results of a critical test or critical result, the nurse is responsible to notify the appropriate licensed healthcare provider immediately. While each facility has policies that dictate what must be documented, a minimal requirement is who was notified, the time of notification, the critical test/result that was reported, and the provider's response.

A nurse may review test results and leave them in the *Completed Test* section of the EHR until the primary care provider reviews them. The tests are not stored in the patient's EHR until the *Dr Viewed* button is selected. If the clinician clicks the *Done* button without first selecting *Dr Viewed*, the completed test remains in the *Completed Test* window awaiting further analysis, as shown in Figure 12.7. When the results have been evaluated by the primary care provider, the practitioner selects the *Dr Viewed* radio

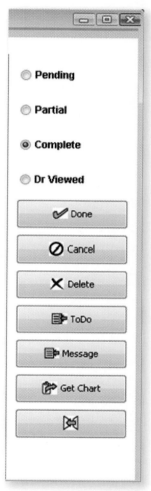

Figure 12.7
Navigation buttons in *Completed Tests* window

Legal/Ethical Considerations

Failure to notify a primary care provider of abnormal results may be considered nursing negligence. If unable to reach the primary care provider, the nurse must follow the facility's chain-of-command policy.

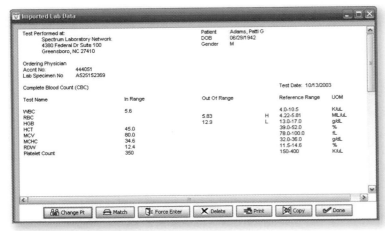

Figure 12.8

Reference lab results

button on the right side of the screen, and then clicks the *Done* button to remove the results from the *Completed Tests* list and save them to the patient's EHR.

In the individual patient's EHR, tests are stored in three categories in the *Care Tree*: *Lab*, *Imaging*, and *Medical Tests*. SpringCharts automatically stores the tests under the appropriate category. The test results may be viewed from the *Nurse Note* or *Office Visit Note* where initially ordered. To view test results from one of these encounter notes, the user clicks on the name of the test under the *Test* navigation tab to display the results. The results are automatically printed when a *History & Physical Report* is generated.

When a hospital interface is in place between the EHR and the hospital lab or between the ambulatory care EHR and an outside lab company, the lab results are sent directly into SpringCharts over a secure Internet connection using Electronic Data Interchange (EDI) standards and protocols. The results may be reviewed by the physician (or any other healthcare provider who has been set up with test viewing security) in the *Reference Lab* submenu of the main *Edit* menu, as seen in Figure 12.8. Once viewed, the results are stored in the *Care Tree* of the patient's electronic chart.

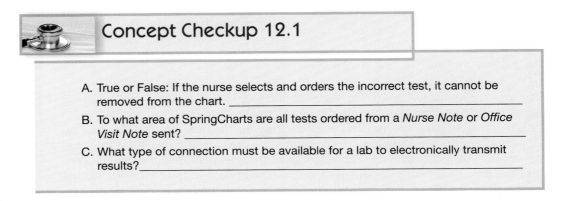

Concept Checkup 12.1

A. True or False: If the nurse selects and orders the incorrect test, it cannot be removed from the chart. _____

B. To what area of SpringCharts are all tests ordered from a *Nurse Note* or *Office Visit Note* sent? _____

C. What type of connection must be available for a lab to electronically transmit results?_____

FOCAL POINT

Chart Evaluation criteria vary by clinic based on specialty.

LO 12.2   Chart Evaluations

EHRs promote quality patient care through the use of reminders and alerts. These reminders are particularly useful to ensure that recommended preventive health guidelines, such as immunizations and screenings, are followed. SpringCharts' *Chart Evaluation* feature allows the nurse to define preventive health guidelines and then evaluate patients' charts to ensure guideline adherence.

In order to set up chart evaluations, *Chart Evaluation* is selected from the *Administration* menu as seen in Figure 12.9. From the *Chart Evaluation Items* window, the user can access the National Guideline Clearinghouse (NGC) through the Internet to determine the latest evidence-based practice guidelines for preventive healthcare. The information from NGC can be used within SpringCharts to set the evaluation criteria such as age, gender, family history, and frequency for each health maintenance intervention.

Selecting the *New* button presents the *Edit Chart Evaluation Item* window for setting up evaluation criteria, illustrated in Figure 12.10. In the setup window, administrators define specifications for each preventive health measure by:

1. *Gender*—Select whether an intervention or procedure is specific to male, female, or both.
2. *Age*—Select the age range for which the criteria should be met.

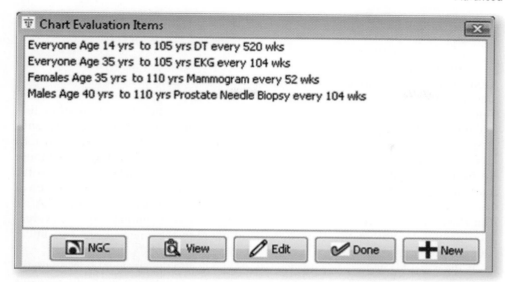

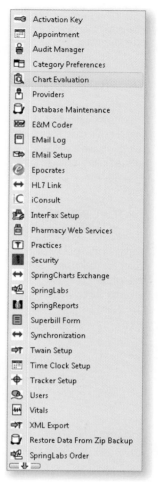

Figure 12.9

Accessing the *Chart Evaluation* from the *Administration* menu

3. **Actions**—Indicate the *Test*, *Procedure*, or *Encounter* for which the guideline is recommended.

4. **Recurring**—Specify if this is a recurring procedure or one-time event. If recurring, enter the time span in number of weeks or the number of screenings/procedures needed in the patient's lifetime.

5. **Diagnosis(es)**—Specify if this criterion is required only if a patient has a specific diagnosis(es) or it is linked to a family history of a particular diagnosis(es).

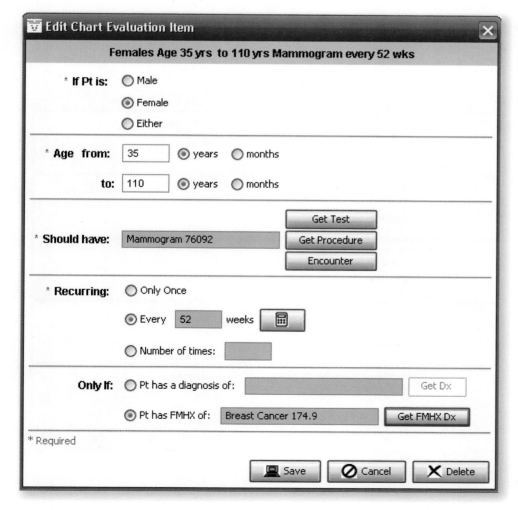

Figure 12.10

Edit Chart Evaluation Item window

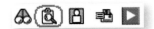

Perform Chart Evaluation
speed button

Documentation Tip

Patients have the right to
refuse healthcare. Such
refusal should be docu-
mented in the health record.

FOCAL POINT

SpringCharts can conduct a
chart evaluation on specific
patients or run an evalu-
ation on the entire patient
database.

Having the wellness screening item linked to a diagnosis from the patient's chart is optional. These preventive guidelines can be accessed on the SpringCharts server in the future and modified if guidelines change.

Individual patient charts can be screened by accessing *File > Evaluate Chart* from within the patient's chart. A speed icon on the patient chart's tool bar also activates this feature (see margin illustration). A chart evaluation should be conducted with each patient encounter. Once activated, the chart evaluation lists recommendations, as seen in Figure 12.11, with a field to document the patient's response. While a recommendation may be made to the patient, the patient may decline to have the test, injection, or procedure. The clinician may also choose to override automated prompts and not make a specific recommendation to the patient, based on individual clinical assessment. If a verbal recommendation is made to the patient, the clinician checks the *Mark this Done* radio button. After the *Done* button is selected, the patient's response and a summary of the evaluation item(s) are automatically recorded and dated in the chart's *Care Tree* under the *Encounter* category.

If the patient is up to date with evaluations and health management screenings, the clinician receives a message: *Pt up to date with recommendations* when the *Evaluate Chart* feature is activated in the chart. The message: *No criterion set* indicates that no chart evaluations have been set up on the SpringCharts server.

SpringCharts EHR also has the ability to scan the entire patient database and apply the chart evaluation criteria to all patient charts. When this activity is necessary, the administrator clicks on the *Utilities* menu on the main *Practice View* screen and selects *Evaluate All Charts*. SpringCharts lists all patients in the database and indicates the outstanding preventive health interventions or screenings. *UTD* indicates that a patient is "up to date" with the health maintenance activities, as displayed in Figure 12.12.

Note: Because all charts are evaluated, this process is time-consuming and should be conducted after hours.

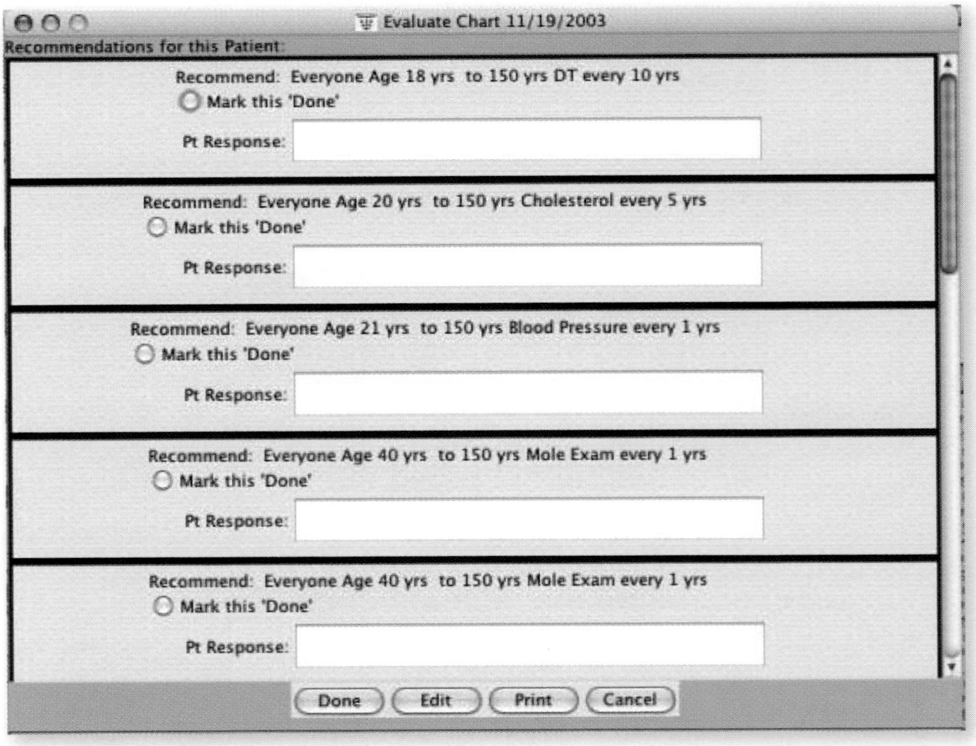

Figure 12.11
Chart Evaluation window

Evaluate Chart 11/19/2003

Recommendations for this Patient:

Recommend: Everyone Age 18 yrs to 150 yrs DT every 10 yrs
○ Mark this 'Done'
Pt Response:

Recommend: Everyone Age 20 yrs to 150 yrs Cholesterol every 5 yrs
○ Mark this 'Done'
Pt Response:

Recommend: Everyone Age 21 yrs to 150 yrs Blood Pressure every 1 yrs
○ Mark this 'Done'
Pt Response:

Recommend: Everyone Age 40 yrs to 150 yrs Mole Exam every 1 yrs
○ Mark this 'Done'
Pt Response:

Recommend: Everyone Age 40 yrs to 150 yrs Mole Exam every 1 yrs
○ Mark this 'Done'
Pt Response:

(Done) (Edit) (Print) (Cancel)

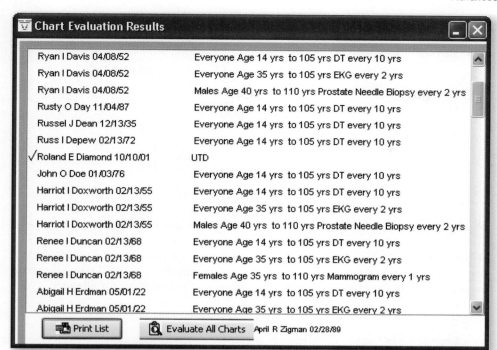

Figure 12.12

Chart evaluation results from database

Concept Checkup 12.2

A. List the four required fields that are necessary to create a new *Chart Evaluation* item.

1. _____
2. _____
3. _____
4. _____

B. What is the purpose of the *Chart Evaluation* feature in SpringCharts?

_____
_____

C. What does the message *No criterion set* indicate?

_____
_____

> **Documentation Tip**
>
> When creating an addendum to a nurse's note, document the addendum as a "late entry" and note specific details about the actual date and time of the occurrence in the narrative note.

LO 12.3 Addenda to a Nurse Note

Upon completion, a *Nurse Note* is locked for security so that no additional material can be entered into the note. *Nurse Notes* are locked by clicking on the *Sign* button in the *Nurse Note* screen. The user is given the option to either initial the note or permanently sign or lock the note, as seen in Figure 12.13. *Nurse Notes* that have been *permanently signed and locked* cannot be amended.

On occasion, after completing and locking a *Nurse Note* entry, a nurse may realize that all appropriate information was not documented. The *New Note* under the *New* menu in the patient chart allows the nurse to do additional charting, or what is commonly referred to as a late entry or addendum. An addendum should always begin with the words "Late entry" to indicate that documentation occurred after the initial record

> **FOCAL POINT**
>
> The *Addendum* functionality can be used by the nurse to document after a *Nurse Note* has been permanently signed and locked.

Figure 12.13
Nurse Note completion options

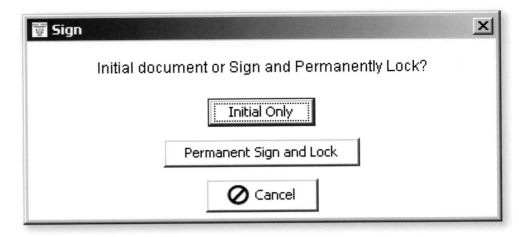

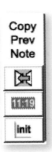

Figure 12.14
Copy Prev Note

of the event. In the *New Note* window, the nurse may use pop-up text or copy a previous entry. A time- and initial-stamp must be included in the additional note, as seen in Figure 12.14. These notes are saved as *Encounters* and are viewable for all users.

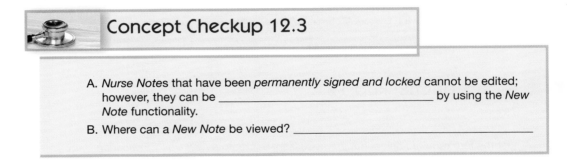

Concept Checkup 12.3

A. *Nurse Notes* that have been *permanently signed and locked* cannot be edited; however, they can be _____ by using the *New Note* functionality.

B. Where can a *New Note* be viewed? _____

LO 12.4   Printing a Nurse Note

Both the *Print* button within the *Nurse Note* screen and the *Print* button located in the patient's chart allow printing/faxing of the *Nurse Note* itself. The *Nurse Note* prints in the SOAPIER format with the patient identifiers in the footer of each page. Test results can be included in the *Nurse Note* as well. Upon completion, tests ordered within the *Nurse Note* will be included in the printed *Nurse Note*. If the test results are not complete, the *Nurse Note* will simply state *pending* beside the name of the test. This concept is also true when printing an *Office Visit Note*. If test results have been processed and completed, the results become part of the *OV Note* and a *History & Physical Report*. If the results have not been entered, the *OV Note* and the *H&P Report* have the phrase *pending* printed beside the name of the ordered test.

The *Nurse Note* does not include any letter formatting like letterhead or salutation; it simply prints/faxes the note in the *SOAPIER* format.

(See Appendix A, *Sample Documents*—Document 10: *Nurse Note Report*.)

FOCAL POINT

Some or all of the elements of a patient's chart can be exported to other software programs and text-capturing devices.

Concept Checkup 12.4

A. What two functions does the *Print* button have for a *Nurse Note*?

_____

_____

B. If test results have not been entered into SpringCharts, what word appears after the name of the test in the printed *Nurse Note*? _____

LO 12.5 Exporting and Printing the Chart

The *Export Chart* feature enables any portion of the chart to be exported as a text file. To access the *Export Chart* feature, a user selects *File > Export Chart* from the patient chart screen. The *Export Chart* window seen in Figure 12.15 opens, detailing all the items from the patient's chart. Each item is checked by default. The list can be unchecked by selecting the *Clear List* button. The user is presented with several export options, including (1) saving the selected material as a text file that can be emailed, (2) copying the material to a clipboard to be pasted into another program, (3) opening the selected material in the computer's default word processing program, or (4) exporting the material to a personal digital assistant (PDA).

Like the *Export Chart* feature, the *Print Chart* feature enables the user to print either the entire chart or selected portions. If a fax server program has been set up on the network, then the selected portions of the patient's chart can be faxed from within the program.

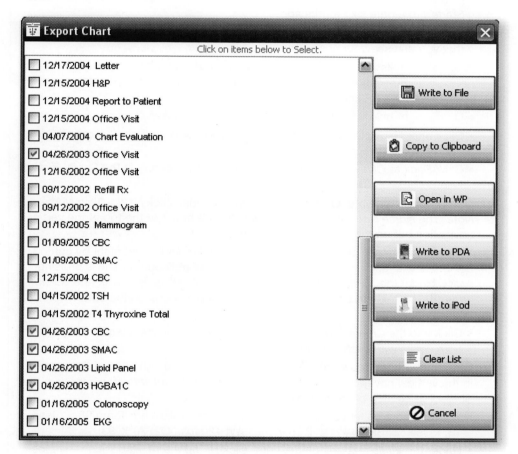

Figure 12.15
Export Chart selection list window

Exercise 12.1

Bipolar Affective Disorder

1. After launching SpringCharts, click on *Actions > Open a Chart*. Type in your last name and click the *Search* button. Select your "bipolar" patient and the chart opens.
2. Your patient tells you she has a past history of bipolar disorder and liver disease. Click on *PMHX* and it populates the right corner box. Click the *Edit* button.

- In the space after *Dx,* type: *Bipolar* and click the *Search* button. A list appears in the box below the *Search* button. Click on *Bipolar Affective Disorder 296.63* and it moves to the *Past Medical History* box on the left.

- In the *Preferences* text box at the lower right, click on *Liver Disease* and it moves to the *Other PMHX* box on the left.

- Click *Back to Chart* in the lower left section of the screen. Note that you can see your new entry under *PMHX.*

3. You ask your patient about her daily medications. She tells you she has taken Lithobid 600 mg by mouth twice daily for the past six months. Click on the *Routine Meds* field and it populates the right lower corner. Click *Edit.*

   - In the space after *Brand Name* at the upper right, type: *Lithobid* and click the *Search* icon. A list of options populates. Click on *300 mg po bid* to send it to the *Routine Medications* list on the left.

   - Click on *Lithobid* in the *Routine Medications* area on the left. The *Edit Rx* window appears. Click in the *Strength* and change it to *600 mg.* Change the *Date Started* to a date six months ago.

   - Click *Save.* Click *Back to Chart* in the lower left portion of the window. Note that you can see your new entry.

4. Your patient tells you she harmed her liver through a combination of drinking and her bipolar medications. Click on the *Social History* field and it populates in the right lower corner. Click *Edit.*

   - On the right below *Social History* click on *Heavy Drinker.*

   - Click after Heavy Drinker and type: *Quit drinking 4 years ago. 3–5 mixed drinks per day for 20 years.*

   - Click *Back to Chart.* Note that you can see your new entry in the *Social History* field.

5. Open your *Nurse Note.* On the top horizontal toolbar, click *New > New Nurse Note.* The *Nurse Note* opens to the *Chief Complaint* tab at the top of the vertical navigation bar on the right side of the window.

6. Your patient states she is anxious and tried to take her life last night by cutting her wrists with a kitchen knife. She states she has noticed that she is bruising easily. Under the *S Panel* in the text box click on *Anxious, Bruising,* and *Suicide attempt.* The text will populate in the *Chief Complaint* box on the bottom left of the screen.

   - Click into the *Chief Complaint* field and type after Suicide attempt: *Lacerated both wrists with kitchen knife.*

7. Click on the *Vitals* tab located below the *CC* tab on the right side of the screen in the vertical navigation bar. Note that your *Chief Complaints* now appear in the *Subjective* section of the *Nurse Note.*

   - You take your patient's vital signs. Document the following: Temp 98.6, Resp *16,* Pulse *88,* BP *144/80,* Ht *59 inches,* Wt *120 lbs.,* O2SAT% *93.*

   - Under the *Vitals* text box on the right, click *BP right arm, Pt position—supine* and *Temp source—Oral, Pt Complains of pain, Pain Location, Pain rating 0–10 scale, Pain Radiation, Pain Description, Factors affecting pain,* and *Factors relieving pain.* This sends this text to the *Notes* box on the lower left. Place each of these items on a separate line by clicking in front of it and striking the [Enter] key on the keyboard.

   - Click into the *Notes* box and enter the following information regarding your patient's description of her pain: location—bilateral wrists, 7 on 1–10 scale, does not radiate, stinging type of pain, clenching fists makes it worse, medication makes it better.

8. Click on the *Exam* button located below the *Vitals.* Notice the *O (Normals)* defaults in the right upper portion of the screen. Select the following systems that are within normal limits when you assess your patient: *HEENT, Heart sounds,*

Lung/Respiratory, and *GU/GYN (female)*. Use the [Enter] key to place these items on separate lines to streamline the documentation.

- Click the drop-down arrow next to *O (Normals)* and select *O (Abnormals)*. Select the *General* section followed by: *restless*. Select the *Skin* section followed by: *wound: location*, *stage*, *width/length/depth*, *color*, *drainage*.

- Click in the *Examination* box on the lower left and enter information regarding the wounds after the appropriate heading: *Bilateral wrists, 10 cm each, lacerations, closed with sutures, small amount sanguineous drainage, dry gauze dressings applied*.

- Your patient tells you she has been having black, tarry stools for the last week. Click back into the *CC* (Chief Complaint) button on the top right and then click into the *Chief Complaint* box on the left side of the screen. Type: *Reports black, tarry stools for the last week*.

9. Click into the *Dx* tab below the *Exam* tab in the vertical navigation bar on the right. Click on the red *NANDA* on the left bottom of the screen. The *Dx* text window populates.

- Click on the following nursing diagnoses and click [Enter] after each to place on a separate line:
  - *Anxiety*.
  - *Coping, Ineffective*.
  - *Hopelessness*.
  - *Infection, Risk for*.
  - *Pain, Acute*.
  - *Skin Integrity, Impaired*.
- Click the *D&T* icon to date and time the entry. Click *Done*.
- Click into the *NANDA* text box on the left. Place your cursor in the text field and type: *Suicide, risk for*. Strike your [Enter] key to put the cursor on a new line. Type: *Tissue perfusion, altered: gastrointestinal*.
- Place the nursing diagnoses in order of priority. Complete the nursing diagnoses with the etiology (R/T) and signs and symptoms (AEB).

10. Click the *NOC* tab in the vertical navigation bar on the right located below the *Dx* tab. Notice that your *NANDA* documentation populates the *Nurse Note*.

- Below the *Nursing Outcomes Classification* select the following:
  - **Anxiety Level:** *Severity of manifested apprehension, tension, or uneasiness from an unidentifiable source*.
  - *Coping: Personal actions to manage stressors that tax an individual's resources*.
  - **Depression Level:** *Severity of melancholic mood and loss of interest in life events*.
  - *Knowledge—Depression Management: Extent of understanding conveyed about depression and interrelationships among causes, effects, and treatments*.
  - *Pain Control: Personal actions to control pain*.
  - *Wound Healing: Primary Intention: Extent of regeneration of cells and tissue following intentional closure*.
- Click into the *Nursing Outcomes Classification* text field on the left and type: *Blood Loss Severity of internal or external bleeding/hemorrhage* as the second nursing outcome.
- *Mood Equilibrium: Appropriate adjustment of prevailing emotional tone in response to circumstances*.
- Place in order of priority.

11. Click the *NIC* tab on the right below the *NOC* tab. Notice that your outcomes populate the *Nurse Note*.

- Select the following interventions:
  - *Anxiety Reduction: Minimizing apprehension, dread, foreboding, or uneasiness related to an unidentified source of anticipated danger.*
  - *Crisis Intervention: Use of short-term counseling to help the patient cope with a crisis and resume a state of functioning comparable to or better than the pre-crisis state.*
  - *Incision Site Care: Cleansing, monitoring, and promotion of healing in a wound that is closed with sutures, clips, or staples.*
  - *Medication Administration: Preparing, giving, and evaluating the effectiveness of prescription and nonprescription drugs.*
  - *Pain Management: Alleviation of pain or a reduction in pain to a level of comfort that is acceptable to the patient.*
  - *Suicide Prevention: Reducing risk of self-inflicted harm with intent to end life.*
  - *Teaching: Disease Process: Assisting the patient to understand information related to a specific disease process.*
  - *Vital Signs Monitoring: Collection and analysis of cardiovascular, respiratory, and body temperature data to determine and prevent complications.*
  - *Wound Care: Prevention of wound complications and promotion of wound healing.*
- Click into the *Nursing Interventions Classification* text field on the left and type: *Bleeding reduction, gastrointestinal: Limitation of the amount of blood loss from the upper and lower gastrointestinal tract and related complications. Monitor amount, character, and frequency of stools.*
- Click after the Incision Site Care and type: *Bilateral wrist incisions closed with suture, to remove in 7–10 days. Daily dry gauze dressing change.*
- Click after the Suicide Prevention line and type: *Every 15 minute nursing checks/observation.*
- Place interventions in order of priority.

12. Click into *Test* in the vertical navigation bar on the right. The nurse practitioner ordered a CBC, PT, and Liver Panel on your patient.

- Click into the space after *Test* at the right upper side of the screen.
  - Type: *CBC*. Click the *Search* icon. CBC 85025 appears in the *Select Test to Order* field. Click on *CBC*. It appears in the *Selected Tests* field at the bottom right. Click the *Order Selected Tests* button at the bottom right side of the screen and the test populates into the *Tests* field on the left.
  - Type: *Liver Panel* in the space after *Test* at the right upper side of the screen. Click the *Search* icon. Liver Panel 80058 appears in the *Select Test to Order* field. Click on *Liver Panel*. It appears in the *Selected Tests* field below. Click the *Order Selected Tests* button at the bottom right side of the screen and the test populates into the *Tests* field on the left.
  - Type: *PT*. Click the *Search* icon. PT 85610 appears in the *Select Test to Order* field. Click on *PT*. It appears in the *Selected Tests* field. Click the *Order Selected Tests* button at the bottom right side of the screen and the test populates into the *Tests* field on the left.

Note: To complete segments 13 and 14 of this exercise, you must access certain files contained in the *EHR Materials Folder*. Your instructor or IT staff may need to inform you of the location of this folder.

13. The admission orders indicate that the patient is to continue Lithobid 600 mg by mouth twice daily.

- Move the *Nurse Note* by clicking the minimize icon in the upper right corner. This will bring you back to the patient's chart. In order to document, click the *New* menu and then *Import Items* at the bottom of the list.
- Select *Import File Cabinet Document* and the *File Cabinet* window appears. Type: *MAR* into the *Document name*.
- In the *Chart* tab select the drop-down box on the right and choose *Nursing Documentation*. In the *Description* field type: *MAR*. Click *Attach*.
- Select *Existing*. Use the search mechanism to go out and select the blank MAR document.
- Click *Done*. The document appears in the *Care Tree* on the right in the *Nursing Documentation* tab.
- Click on the + in front of *Nursing Documentation*. Highlight the *MAR* and click *Edit* at the bottom right-hand side of the screen. The *File Cabinet* window appears.
- Click on the blue hyperlink next to the word *File*. The *MAR* document opens.
- Enter the Patient, Date of Birth, Date, Admit date, Doctor (Nurse Practitioner), and Room #.
- On the left enter the *Lithobid* on the blank field above Strength and Dose. In the *Strength* field type: *600 mg* and in the *Dose* field type: *1*.
- Under *Directions*, type: *po BID* and schedule administration times for 0900 and 2100. Type your name and initials in the *Initial & Name* area at the bottom of the document.
- Type your initials in the 0900 top time box. Click the *Save* diskette icon to save your work.
- Your patient has Tylenol 650 mg po ordered every four hours prn pain. On the left enter the *Tylenol* on the blank field above Strength and Dose.
- In the *Strength* field type: *650 mg* and in the *Dose* field type: *1*. Under *Directions* type: *every 4 hours prn pain*.
- Recognizing that Tylenol is often contraindicated with liver disease, the previous nurse verified the order with the nurse practitioner. The nurse practitioner gave the order to administer the Tylenol because the patient is not a candidate for aspirin or nonsteroidal anti-inflammatory drugs due to her black tarry stool that indicates gastrointestinal bleeding. This was documented in detail by the previous nurse.
- Document administration by typing your initials in the 1300 time box.
- Click the *X* on the far right upper corner to close the *MAR*. A pop-up will ask you if you want to save the changes you have made, select *Yes*. The *File Cabinet* window is still present. Click *Done*.
- A pop-up appears: "The Attached file may have changed. Do you want to send a new version to the server?" Click *Yes*. The window closes.

14. In order to document intake and output, import the I&O form.

- Click the *New* menu and then *Import Items* at the bottom of the list. Select *Import File Cabinet Document* and the *File Cabinet* window appears.
- Type: *Intake and Output* into the *Document name*. In the *Chart* tab select the drop-down box on the right and choose *Nursing Documentation*.
- In the *Description* field type: *Intake and Output*. Click *Attach*.
- Select *Existing*. Use the search mechanism to select the blank Intake and Output document. Your instructor or IT staff may need to inform you where these documents are kept.
- Click *Done*. The document appears in the *Care Tree* on the right in the *Nursing Documentation* tab.

- Click on the + in front of *Nursing Documentation*. Highlight the *Intake and Output* and click *Edit* at the bottom right-hand side of the screen.
- The *File Cabinet* window appears. Click on the blue hyperlink next to the word *File*. The *Intake and Output* document opens.
- Type in the Patient Name and Date. Your patient drank 480 mL of fluid with her breakfast at 0800 this morning. She urinated 150 mL at 0800 and 200 mL at 1100.
- Document her intake/output. Complete the eight-hour totals for the shift.
- Click the *X* on the far right upper corner to close the *I & O* document. A pop-up will ask you if you want to save the changes you have made, select *Yes*. The *File Cabinet* window is still present. Click *Done*.
- A pop-up appears: "The Attached file may have changed. Do you want to send a new version to the server?" Click *Yes*. The window closes.

15. The *Nurse Note* may be located at the bottom of the screen due to minimizing it earlier. Return to the *Nurse Note* by clicking the maximize icon on the upper right side of the *Nurse Note*. Click the *Teaching* button on the right.
    - Under the *Other Tx Panel* at the upper right portion of the screen, select the following:
        - *Discussed plan of care with patient/significant other.*
        - *Disease process instruction completed. Continue to reinforce.*
        - *Medication indication, frequency, considerations instruction.*
    - Click into the *Teaching* field on the left bottom of the screen after Disease process instruction and type: *Suicide watch explained. No-harm contract signed with patient.*

16. Click into *Evaluation* on the right. Using the *Evaluation* text on the right side, add the text below by clicking on it. (The NOC item for the patient is referenced by the first word.) Add text manually where directed to type.
    - *Anxiety Level:* Type: *Pt reports anxiety has decreased since she's been in the hospital. Ongoing outcome.*
    - *Blood Loss: Severity of internal or external bleeding/hemorrhage.* Type: *Two small black, tarry stools. Awaiting CBC results. Ongoing outcome.*
    - *Coping:* Type: *Reports primary stressors are family relationships and job stress. Ongoing outcome.*
    - *Depression Level:* Type: *Pt reports feeling like she just cannot go on. Ongoing outcome.*
    - *Knowledge—Depression Management: Outcome not met this shift. Variance reason—pt uncooperative/noncompliant.* Type: *Pt states she is not willing to discuss at this time. Will attempt to discuss tomorrow.*
    - *Pain Control:* Type: *Reports pain level decreased to 3 after administration of Tylenol.*
    - *Wound Healing: Primary Intention:* Type: **Incisions dry, intact, approximated, secured with sutures. No swelling or redness. Dry gauze dressing applied. Ongoing outcome.**
    - *Continue current interventions.*
    - Use the [Enter] key on the keyboard to place text on separate lines to streamline your documentation.

17. Click into *Reassess*. Click in the *Reassessment* text box on the left side of the screen and type: *Every 15 minute observation suicide watch*. Enter times *1045, 1100, 1115, 1130*.
    - *1045—pt watching TV.*
    - *1100—pt watching TV.*
    - *1115—Instructed patient that sutures will be removed in approximately one week.*
    - *1130—pt watching TV.*

18. Click into *F/U-Rem*. Notice your documentation from the *Reassess* area populates the *Nurse Note*. On the left side of the screen below the *F/U-Reminders* text click on the icon of a finger with a piece of string tied around it.

   • The *Add to ToDo/Reminder List* window populates. Under the *ToDo-Reminders* text field click *Teach* to populate the free text field to the left. Click after Teach and type: *regarding bipolar disease process*.

      • Notice that your patient's name displays in the left middle section of this window. Select your name in the *To* dropdown. *F/U-Rem* is linked to a patient when accessed within the *Nurse Note*. Click *Send Later*. Select tomorrow's date on the calendar. Click *Send*.

      • Look to the far left of the software, to the SpringCharts fields that are open outside of the *Nurse Note*. The *ToDo List* appears in dark pink color below the calendar with your new *ToDo-Reminder* below it.

19. With your *Nurse Note* window still open, click on the *Print* button at the bottom of the screen and click *Print* in the *Document Print Options* screen to print the entire *Nurse Note*.

20. Click *Done*. The *Save As* screen populates. Click *Save*.

21. A pop-up appears asking if you want to create a routing slip. Click *No*.

22. In the *Care Tree*, click the + next to *Encounters*. Click on the date of your *Nurse Note* and it appears in the bottom right corner box.

   • Click *Edit*. Click *Sign*. Select *Permanent Sign and Lock* when finished with your *Nurse Note*.

23. You realize that you forgot to document suicide watch on the patient at 1145 and 1200. Click *New > New Note* (not *New > New Nurse Note*).

   • Click into the free text field at the lower left, enter *late entry*, and add the times above. After 1145 type: *Pt resting in bed with eyes closed*. After 1200 type: *Pt watching TV*.

   • Click *Done*. The *Save As* window opens. Click *Save* and skip billing.

Final Text Review

Using Terminology

Match the terms on the left with the definitions on the right.

_____ 1. SOAP(IER)

_____ 2. e-MAR

_____ 3. Care Plan

_____ 4. Electronic Chart

_____ 5. NANDA-I

_____ 6. Face Sheet

_____ 7. Nursing standards

_____ 8. EHR

_____ 9. AANP

_____ 10. The Joint Commission

_____ 11. CCHIT

_____ 12. VIS

_____ 13. Lab analyte

_____ 14. History & Physical Report

_____ 15. Tablet PC

A. The repository for patient health data created through computer automation in the healthcare office/hospital/clinic. It holds such static information as the patient's health history and health problems as well as the dynamic information including encounter notes, tests, letters, and reports concerning the patient.

B. Contains more constant patient information such as allergies, problem list, past health history (PMHX), etc.

C. An organization that promotes standard usage of nursing diagnoses globally.

D. An electronic method for documentation of drug administration to patients.

E. An expanded method of documentation that allows for extended discussion of nursing interventions, evaluation comments, and revisions to the plan based on progress toward outcome attainment.

F. Specific documents that provide a "road map" to guide all who are involved with a patient's care, outlining the appropriate treatment to ensure the optimal outcome.

G. Defined by the American Nurses Association (2004) as "authoritative statements by which the nursing profession describes the responsibilities for which its practitioners are accountable."

H. Vaccination Information Statement sheets developed by the Centers for Disease Control and Prevention that delineate the risks and benefits of a vaccine.

I. A blood test compound that is subject to its own specific chemical analysis. Used in combination to form a lab panel.

J. Certification Commission for Health Information Technology, an independent initiative that seeks to accelerate the adoption of EHRs with a credible certification program.

K. Documentation of the patient's health history combined with the physical exam; contains the initial clinical evaluation and examination of the patient.

L. The most commonly accepted term for software with a full range of functionalities to store, access, and use patient health information.

M. Founded in 1985 to promote excellence in advanced nursing practice, research, and education.

N. An independent, non-profit organization that sets standards of quality for healthcare organizations and evaluates compliance with these standards, providing accreditation for organizations that demonstrate excellence.

O. A portable, handheld computer that allows documentation on the screen with a stylus pen.

Checking Your Understanding

Write "T" or "F" in the blank to indicate whether the statement is true or false.

_____ 16. Using e-MARs allows the nurse to administer medications to a patient without the necessity of checking the five rights of medication administration.

_____ 17. Voice recognition systems cannot be used with electronic health records.

_____ 18. Providing patients with a written list of discharge instructions is sufficient to meet all standards for patient education.

_____ 19. *OV Notes* that have been permanently signed and locked can be amended.

_____ 20. A high-speed Internet connection is not necessary for an ASP.

_____ 21. The SpringCharts message system does not support e-mail.

_____ 22. Nurses have an ethical obligation to provide patient education to facilitate decision making.

_____ 23. The use of *Templates* is the most rapid way of building documentation in an office visit.

_____ 24. Sixty lines of preset type can be added to each pop-up text category in SpringCharts.

_____ 25. One may not send an item to another coworker in the *New ToDo/Reminder* window.

_____ 26. A patient's chart notes can be added to a letter created in SpringCharts.

_____ 27. Nurses are continually teaching patients so there is no need to document this routine activity.

_____ 28. Order forms in SpringCharts are used to record the ordering of specific medications.

_____ 29. The nursing process fits with the PART(IER) charting method.

_____ 30. Information to complete the electronic face sheet is taken from intake forms that patients complete regarding their PMHX, routine meds, and current health problems.

Choose the best answer and circle the corresponding letter.

31. Which of the following features is most appropriate to use when documenting only a blood pressure check with a patient?
    a) *New TC* note
    b) *New Nurse Note*
    c) *New Vitals Only*
    d) *New OV*

32. A client has a new diagnosis of Diabetes Type I and needs to self-administer insulin on a routine basis. What is the best method of evaluating the patient's ability to self-inject insulin?
    a) Ask the patient questions about the procedure.
    b) Have the patient demonstrate self-administration of an insulin injection.
    c) Have the patient repeat the steps in the procedure back to you.
    d) Have the patient take a computer-based learning module and complete the quiz.

33. What did CCHIT specifically address?
    a) EHR costs
    b) Security issues
    c) Lack of industry standards
    d) The appropriation of government money

34. The Exam is part of what component of the SOAP note?
    a) Subjective
    b) Objective
    c) Assessment
    d) Plan

35. Which feature in SpringCharts eliminates the need to locate a staff member and allows discrete communication?
    a) *ToDo List*
    b) *Urgent Message*
    c) *Patient Tracker*
    d) *Care Tree*

36. The panel seen on the left side of the *Office Visit* screen in SpringCharts enables the clinician to view the patient's
    a) Past OV addenda
    b) Face sheet
    c) Various pop-up texts
    d) Available templates

37. When a nurse creates practice guidelines in SpringCharts, which website is accessible to import recommended guidelines?
    a) Family Doctor
    b) American Medical Association
    c) National Guideline Clearinghouse
    d) CCHIT

38. What does MIPPA mean?
    a) Medical Improvements per Patient Annually
    b) Medicaid Improvement for Patients Act
    c) Medicare Improvement for Patients and Providers Act
    d) Medicare Installments for Patients Pay Plan Act

39. When a user modifies personal pop-up text: (Select all that apply.)
    a) It only changes it for the same type of users (i.e., nurses, providers, etc.).
    b) SpringCharts must be shut down and restarted to see the modifications.
    c) It is also modified for all users at the same time.
    d) It only modifies that user's pop-up text.

40. SpringCharts EHR was chosen as the training tool for this text because of its
    a) Customization, cost, and bright colors.
    b) Scheduling and patient-tracking features.
    c) Nurse note, office note, and MAR form.
    d) Ease of use, full features, and customization.

41. Which of the following should nurses assess prior to patient education? (Select all that apply.)
    a) Barriers to learning
    b) High blood pressure
    c) Preferred method of instruction
    d) Social history

42. A student nurse sits down to review a patient's chart. Which of the following purposes of documentation is being fulfilled?
    a) Legal and ethical
    b) Communication
    c) Reimbursement
    d) Education

43. How may a user convert a *Vitals Only Note* to an *OV Note*?
    a) A user cannot convert a *Vitals Only Note* to an *OV Note*. A new *OV Note* must be created.
    b) By selecting the *Convert to OV Note* icon at the bottom of the *Vitals Only* screen.
    c) By selecting the *New* menu in the *Patient's Chart* screen then selecting *Convert to OV Note*.
    d) By creating an *OV Note*, selecting the *Vitals* tab, then highlighting the previous vitals and using the *Copy Prev Note* button.

44. Which of the following is a way to edit a patient's face sheet? (Select all that apply.)
    a) Select an item from the *Edit* menu in the *Patient's Chart* screen.
    b) Use the *Open Face Sheet* button on the toolbar of the *Patient's Chart* screen.
    d) Right-click on an item in the *Face Sheet* and select *Edit*.
    c) Type the face sheet subheading in the *Find Text* feature and conduct a search.

45. What is the acronym for the Certification Commission for Health Information Technology?
    a) CHIT
    b) HIT
    c) CCHIT
    d) CHCIT

46. Where can patient instructions be accessed in SpringCharts? (Select all that apply.)
    a) *Message Center*
    b) *Nurse Note*
    c) *New Note*
    d) *Office Visit*

47. When medication is discontinued for a patient, an encounter with that patient needs to be created. Where are medications recorded as discontinued? (Select all that apply.)
    a) *New Vitals Only*
    b) *New TC* note and messages
    c) The *OV Note* and *Nurse Note*
    d) *New Rx Refill*

48. Where are previous *Patient Tracker* records stored in SpringCharts?
    a) On the SpringCharts Server application
    b) In the *Tracker Archive* found in the main *Edit* menu
    c) In *Tracker History* found in the *Patient's Chart Actions* menu
    d) In the *Tracker Archive* found in the main *Utilities* menu

49. For security, data are encrypted on what kind of a network?

   a) ASP network

   b) Wireless network

   c) 3G network

   d) Mobile network

50. Nursing outcomes criteria (NOC) best fit into which part of the SOAP(IER) charting method?

   a) Interventions

   b) Subjective data

   c) Plan

   d) Assessment

References

American Nurses Association. (2004). *Nursing: Scope and standards of practice*. Silver Spring, MD: Author.

The Joint Commission. (2010). National Patient Safety Goals. Retrieved November 28, 2010 from http://www.jointcommission.org/NR/rdonlyres/868C9E07-037F-433D-8858-0D5FAA4322F2/0/July2010NPSGs_Scoring_HAP2.pdf

Jamal, A., McKenzie, K., & Clark, M. (2009). The impact of health information technology on the quality of medical and health care: A systematic review. *Health Information Management Journal 38*(3), 26–37.

The Medical Records Confidentiality Act of 1995. (n.d.) Retrieved July 1, 2010, from http://optout.cdt.org/privacy/medical/950000mrca_summary.shtml

U.S. Department of Health and Human Services. (n.d.). *Understanding health information privacy*. Retrieved April 2, 2010, from http://www.hhs.gov/ocr/privacy/hipaa/understanding/index.html

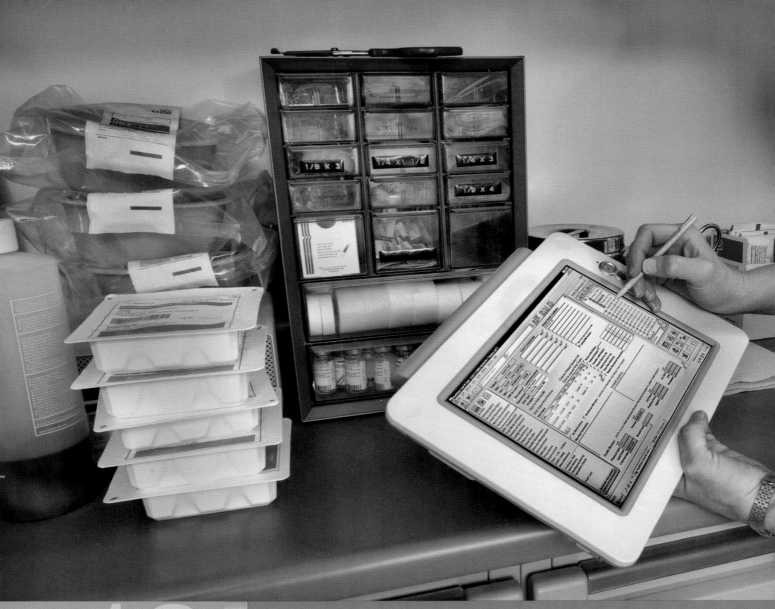

13 | Nurse Note

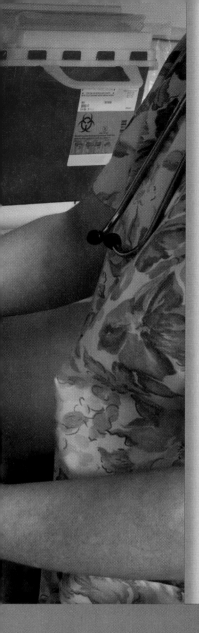

Learning Outcomes

When you complete Chapter 13, you will be able to:

13.1 Use all aspects of the SpringCharts program successfully.

Documentation—Level 4

What You Need to Know

To understand Chapter 13, you need to know how to:

- Navigate in the *Patient Chart* screen.
- Navigate in the *Nurse Note* screen.
- Navigate in the *Office Visit* screen.

A.   Patient Chart Screen

Exercise 13.1

1. Set up a new female patient: Use the first name of Jade. Make up a middle initial and last name for your new patient.

   Address: 6021 Hodges Place

   Mansfield, TX 76063

   DOB: 10/5/73

   SS#: 456-78-2371

   Home Phone: (817) 473-0328

   Work Phone: (817) 966-2484

   Cell Phone: (817) 504-0903

   E-mail: jade@nofencedland.net

   Employer: No Fenced Land Company

   Jade is married and has two children.

   She carries insurance on the family through her employer. Her assigned physician is Dr. Stephen C. Finchman, the family's primary care physician.

2. Set up Jade's allergies.

   Jade is allergic to Amoxicillin, Sulfa, and Phenergan.

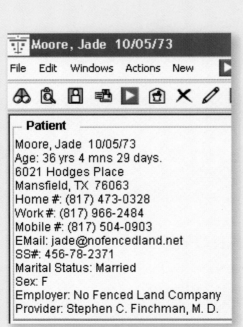

Figure 13.1a

Patient demographics

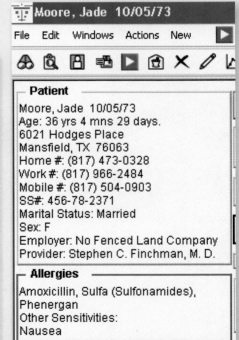

Figure 13.1b

Patient demographics and allergies

Exercise 13.2

1. Document Jade's PMHX: Past Medical History: asthma, bronchitis, fracture of rib. She has given birth to two children with normal, vaginal deliveries.

2. Family Medical History: Using the *Preferences* list, build the following family health history data:

   Brother: Heart Disease

   Mother: Hypercholesterolemia

   Father Died At Age: 59

   Cause of Death: Heart Disease

3. Social History: Tobacco Use: Nonsmoker.

   Alcohol Use: 1–2 mixed drinks/month

   Caffeine Use: Yes. Cups Per Day: 4.

   Marital Status: Married.

   Occupation: Sales.

   Education: College.

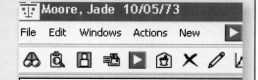

Moore, Jade 10/05/73

File   Edit   Windows   Actions   New

Patient

Moore, Jade 10/05/73
Age: 36 yrs 4 mns 29 days.
6021 Hodges Place
Mansfield, TX 76063
Home #: (817) 473-0328
Work #: (817) 966-2484
Mobile #: (817) 504-0903
SS#: 456-78-2371
Marital Status: Married
Sex: F
Employer: No Fenced Land Company
Provider: Stephen C. Finchman, M. D.

Allergies

Amoxicillin, Sulfa (Sulfonamides),
Phenergan
Other Sensitivities:
Nausea

PMHX

Asthma 493
Bronchitis 490
Fracture Of Rib 807.00
Vaginal birth x2

FMHX

Brother: Heart Disease
Mother: Hypercholesterolemia
Father Died At Age: 59 Cause Of
Death: Heart Disease

Social History

Tobacco Use: Nonsmoker.
Alcohol Use: Social Drinker.
Caffeine Use: Cups Per Day: 4
Marital Status: Married.
Occupation: Sales
Education: College.

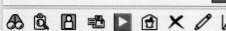

Moore, Jade 10/05/73

File   Edit   Windows   Actions   New

Patient

Moore, Jade 10/05/73
Age: 36 yrs 4 mns 29 days.
6021 Hodges Place
Mansfield, TX 76063
Home #: (817) 473-0328
Work #: (817) 966-2484
Mobile #: (817) 504-0903
SS#: 456-78-2371
Marital Status: Married
Sex: F
Employer: No Fenced Land Company
Provider: Stephen C. Finchman, M. D.

Allergies

Amoxicillin, Sulfa (Sulfonamides),
Phenergan
Other Sensitivities:
Nausea

PMHX

Asthma 493
Bronchitis 490
Fracture Of Rib 807.00
Vaginal birth x2

FMHX

Brother: Heart Disease
Mother: Hypercholesterolemia
Father Died At Age: 59 Cause Of
Death: Heart Disease

Figure 13.2a

Patient face sheet data

Figure 13.2b

Patient face sheet data

Exercise 13.3

1. Add Routine Meds for Jade:

   Azmacort Inhaler 100 micrograms 4 puffs twice daily

   Singulair 10 mg by mouth every evening

   Allegra 180 mg by mouth every morning

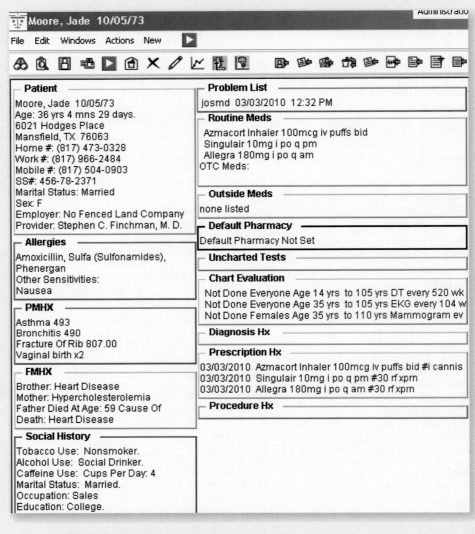

Figure 13.3 Patient face sheet

B.   Nurse Note

Exercise 13.4

1. Import the MAR and I&O forms into the *Nursing Documentation* portion of the *Care Tree* in the patient's chart.
2. Jade tells you that she's here because "I can't breathe." Document this as the *Chief Complaint*.

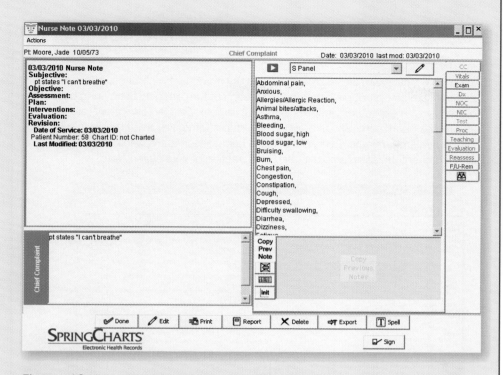

Figure 13.4a *Nurse Note Chief Complaint* window

3. You take Jade's vital signs: Temp 101.6 oral, Resp 22, Pulse 108, BP 144/80, pulse oximetry 94% on oxygen at 2 Liters/minute by nasal cannula, Ht 59 inches, Wt 120 lbs. Jade complains of pain in her chest due to the constant cough she has had for the last two days. She describes it as an "ache" and rates it a "7" on a 0–10 scale. She tells you coughing makes it worse and nothing has really made it better. Document this in the *Vital Signs* section of your *Nurse Note*.

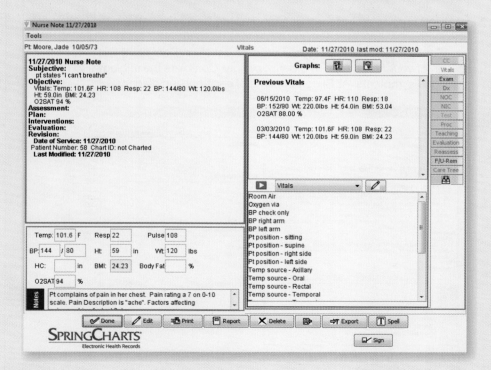

Figure 13.4b *Nurse Note Vitals* window

1. Jade's physical exam (assessment) reveals dry mucous membranes, sclera reddened bilaterally, productive cough with green sputum, rhonchi in her lung bases bilaterally with expiratory wheezes in the left upper lobe. Her respiratory rate is 22 breaths per minute. She is voiding dark amber urine. Her heart rate is regular at 108 beats per minute. Everything else in her assessment is within normal limits. Document the assessment in the *Exam* section of your *Nurse Note*.

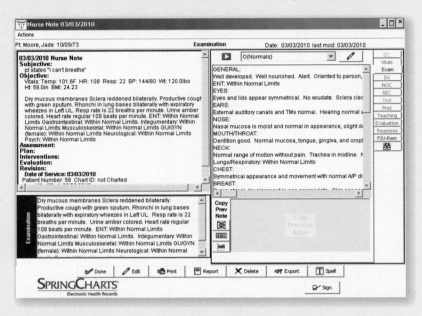

Figure 13.5a *Nurse Note Examination* window

2. NANDA-I nursing diagnoses that apply include Breathing Pattern, Ineffective, Gas Exchange, Impaired, Fatigue, Fluid volume, Deficient, Risk for, Pain, acute, Infection, and Knowledge, disease process deficient. Document this in the *Dx* section of your *Nurse Note* in order of priority. Complete the etiology (R/T) and signs and symptoms (AEB) components of each nursing diagnosis.

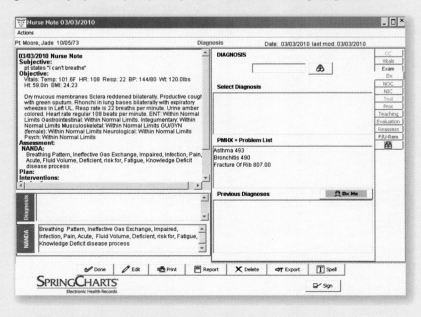

Figure 13.5b *Nurse Note Diagnosis* window

3. Nursing outcomes that pertain to Jade are: Fluid Balance, Infection severity, Knowledge—disease process, Pain Control, Respiratory status, and Discharge readiness, independent living. Enter these in the *NOC* section of your *Nurse Note*.

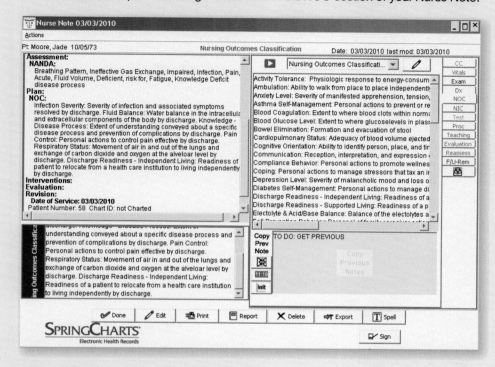

Figure 13.5c *Nurse Note NOC* window

4. Nursing interventions that pertain to Jade are: Discharge planning, Fluid/ Electrolyte management, IV insertion and therapy, Medication Administration, Pain Management, Teaching—disease process, Respiratory monitoring, and Vital Signs Monitoring. Enter these in the *NIC* section of your *Nurse Note*.

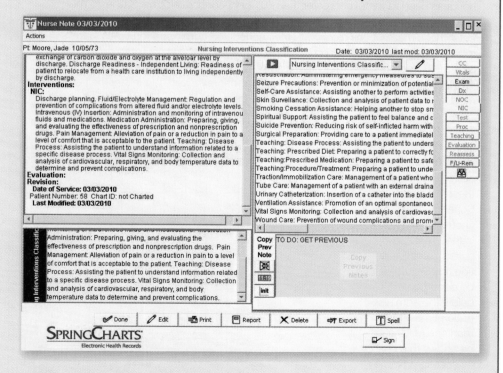

Figure 13.5d *Nurse Note NIC* window

Exercise 13.6

1. You call the physician and she gives you a verbal order for an electrolyte panel and urine culture. (A sputum culture was obtained in the emergency room.) Enter these two orders in the *Test* area of the *Nurse Note*.

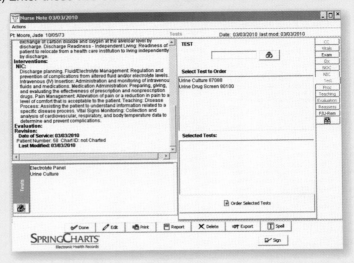

Figure 13.6 *Nurse Note Test* window

Exercise 13.7

1. You receive the following physician orders: Tylenol 650 mg by mouth every 4–6 hours as needed for fever greater than 101 or headache. Normal Saline 75 mL/ hr IV. Levofloxacin 750 mg/150 mL D5W IV every 24 hours. Open the *MAR* and enter these medications along with their scheduled administration times. Jade's routine medications have been continued; make sure these are listed on the *MAR* as well. (Remember you may have to import the document on your patient.) You give Jade 650 mg of Tylenol orally at 0900 for her fever and administer the Levofloxacin at 1000. You started the Normal Saline at 0800. The Singulair and Allegra were given at 0800.

The Azmacort inhaler was given at 0900. Document administration of these medications. Scheduled times should be placed in the *MAR* and actual administration times should be documented below the administration times. More than one *MAR* can be added to a chart if necessary. Name additional *MARs* MAR2, MAR3, etc.

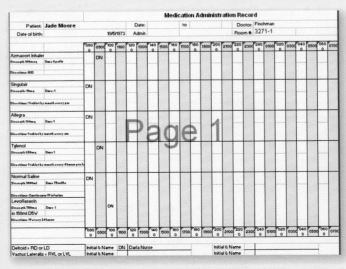

Figure 13.7a *Nursing Documentation File Cabinet MAR* form

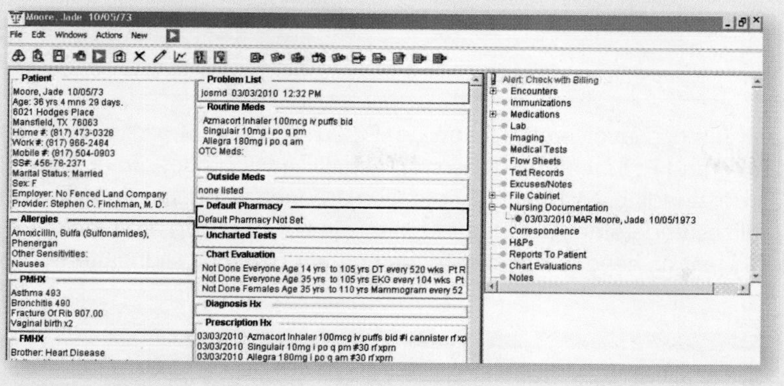

Figure 13.7b Patient's *MAR* saved in *Care Tree*

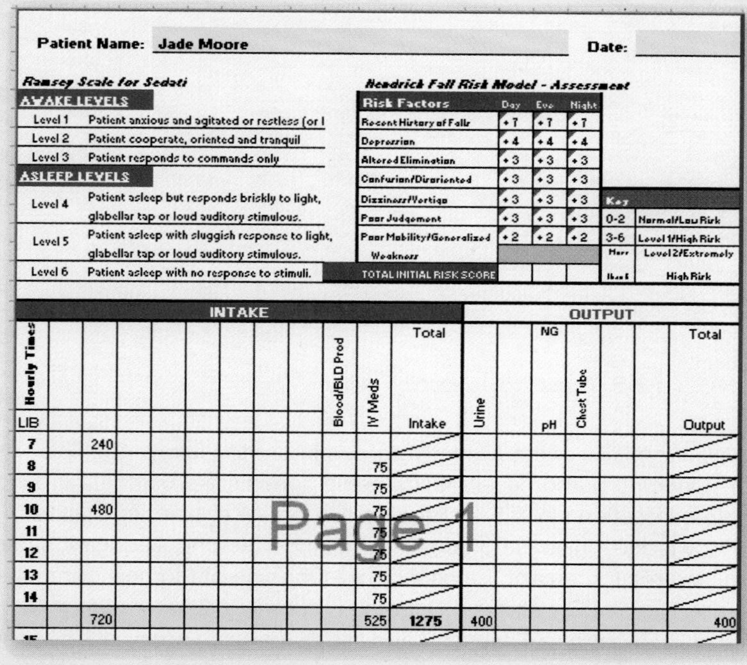

Figure 13.7c *Nursing Documentation File Cabinet Input and Output* form

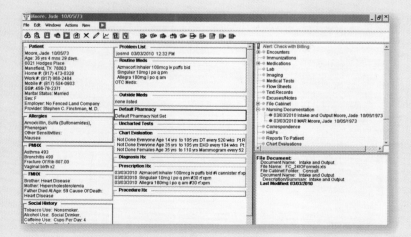

Figure 13.7d Patient's *Input and Output* form saved in *Care Tree*

Teaching this shift has involved the following: Discussed plan of care with patient/ significant other and Pt verbalizes understanding. Disease process instruction: Pt verbalizes understanding. Medication indication, frequency, considerations instruction. Pt verbalizes understanding. Document this in the *Teaching* area of your *Nurse Note*. Add free text as needed to indicate the content of patient education.

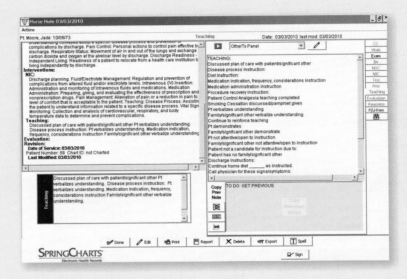

Figure 13.8a *Nurse Note Teaching* window

1. In the *Evaluation* area of the *Nurse Note* document the following: Fluid balance—Ongoing outcome—IV fluids being administered, urinating dark amber urine; Infection severity—Ongoing outcome—antibiotics initiated, febrile; Knowledge—disease process—Ongoing outcome—education initiated, requires reinforcement; Pain Control—Ongoing outcome—controlled with Tylenol; Respiratory status—Ongoing outcome, O2 saturation > 92% on O2 at 2 L/min per nasal cannula; and Discharge readiness, independent living—will address tomorrow.

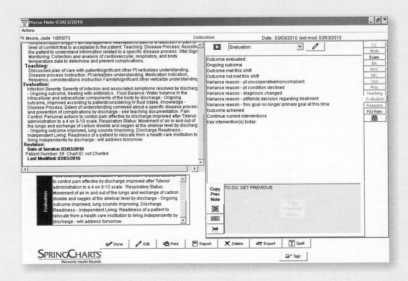

Figure 13.8b *Nurse Note Evaluation* window

2. You have reassessed the following at 10am: Temp 99.4, Pulse 94 beats per minute, Respirations 18 per minute, Pain level in her chest Pain location) 4 on a 0–10 scale, O2 saturation 94% on O2 at 2 L/min. At 2pm the patient stated, "I'm feeling a little bit better." Document this in the *Reassess* area of the *Nurse Note*.

3. It is near the end of your shift, 0630–1500. Document intake and output including IV normal saline, 720 mL of oral intake, and 400 mL of urine output. Complete your shift totals. (Remember you may have to import the document on your patient.)

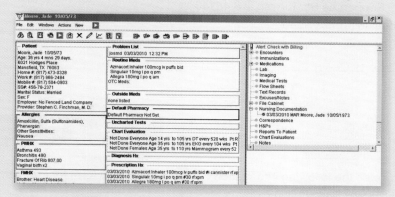

Figure 13.8c *Nursing Note Reassessment* window

Exercise 13.9

1. You have completed the documentation for this shift. Click *Sign* and *Permanent Sign and Lock*. Answer *No* to the routing slip question. The *Nurse Note* is in the *Care Tree* under the *Encounters* heading. Click the + sign to view your *Nurse Note*.

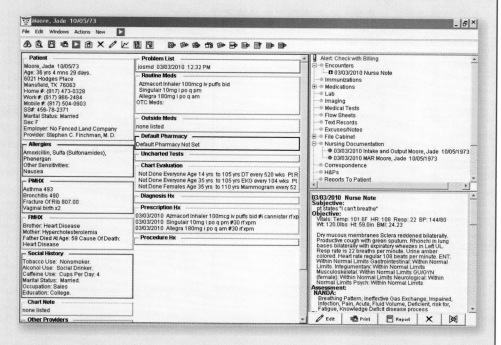

Figure 13.9 *Nurse Note* saved in patient's *Care Tree*

Exercises

C.   Office Visit Screen

Exercise 13.10

Tarra has arrived at the nurse practitioner's office with her toddler, Emmasyn Grace. Enter Emmasyn as a new patient.

Address: 5 Peppertree St., Kirwan, KS 48140

Home Phone: (614) 773-4586

D.O.B.: 3/11/2008

Exercise 13.11

Tarra completes the following information on the health intake form for Emmasyn.

ALLERGIES: Penicillins, Pollen Extracts

PMHX: Chicken Pox

FMHX: Father—Hypercholesterolemia

Father, Mother, Sister have consistent problems with allergies.

REFERRALS: Harry Hart, MD

MEDS: Allegra 30mg i po q am and Nasacort AQ 55mcg ii puffs each nostril q am

From your analysis of the patient you make the following notation:

PROBLEM LIST: Allergic Rhinitis

Chart Note: Allergies should be watched as child grows. Consider referral to allergist at next physical.

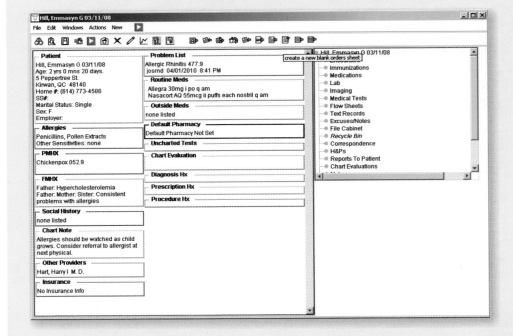

Figure 13.11   Patient Chart screen

Exercise 13.12

Emmasyn and her mother are taken from the waiting room to the nurse station, where you note the chief complaint and vitals. After a brief interview with the mother, you determine that Emmasyn needs to be seen by the nurse practitioner.

Open a new *OV Note* and record the following:

CHIEF COMPLAINTS: Nasal and chest congestion, cough, itchy eyes

Time-Stamp and initial the *CC* section

HX PRESENT ILLNESS: Patient's mother reports symptoms began gradually 1 week ago and have been constant since onset.

Alleviated by: Benadryl

VITALS: 98.0 F, Resp—25, HR—88, Ht—36.2 ins, Wt—27 lbs

Close the *OV Note* and skip billing.

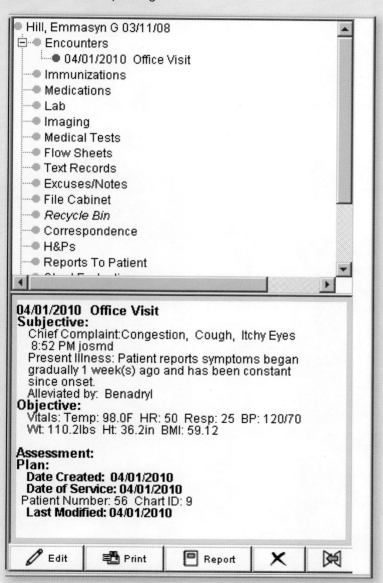

Figure 13.12 Saved and completed *Chief Complaint* and *Vitals*

Exercises

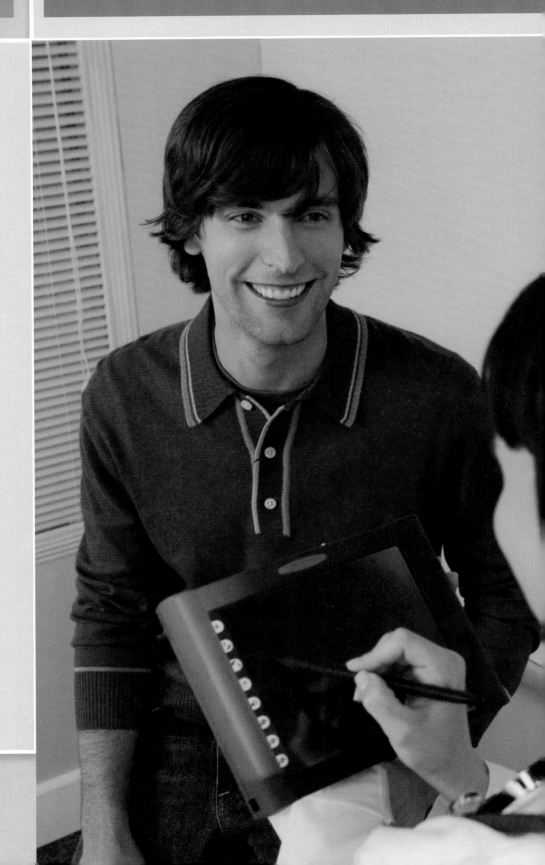

Assessment

Learning Outcomes

When you complete Chapter 14, you will be able to:

14.1   Use all aspects of the SpringCharts program successfully.

What You Need to Know

To understand Chapter 14, you need to know how to:

- Navigate in the *Patient Chart* screen.
- Navigate in the *Nurse Note* screen.

The purpose of Chapter 14 is to test your ability to enter the information from a hard-copy patient health record into SpringCharts. In the exercises below, source documents refer to sample hard-copy health records found in Appendix B. Remember, to record information onto the Medication Administration Record and Intake & Output documents for a new patient, the forms must be imported into SpringCharts first. If you have been requested to submit your work to your instructor via e-mail, create a pdf document of your exercises by choosing the PDF printer and e-mailing the pdf file. Do this rather than printing the document as instructed in the following exercises. Please add the patient's name and date of birth to the source documents in Appendix B where appropriate. The documents in Appendix B do not have a patient name or biographical data. Please use your own name and data.

Exercise 14.1

1. *Using Source Document 1: Admission Data Base (see Appendix B, pages 259–262)*, complete *Allergies* and *PMHX*.
2. Print the face sheet. Record your name on the document and submit to your instructor.

Exercise 14.2

1. *Using Source Document 2: Admission Medication Reconciliation Form (see Appendix B, page 263)*, enter the *Routine Meds* in SpringCharts.
2. Print the face sheet. Record your name on the document and submit to your instructor.

Exercise 14.3

1. *Using Source Document 1: Admission Data Base (see Appendix B, pages 259–262)*, add the *Social History* to SpringCharts.
2. Print the face sheet. Record your name on the document and submit to your instructor.

Exercise 14.4

1. *Using Source Document 1: Admission Data Base (see Appendix B, page 259)*, add the *Chief Complaint* to SpringCharts.
2. Using the *Print* button, print the *Nurse Note*. Record your name on the document and submit to your instructor.

Exercise 14.5

1. *Using Source Document 3: Critical Care Flow Sheet (see Appendix B, pages 264–265)*, complete the *Vital Signs* documented at 0700 in the *Nurse Note*.

2. Using the *Print* button, print the *Nurse Note*. Record your name on the document and submit to your instructor.

Exercise 14.6

1. *Using Source Document 4: Initial Shift Assessment (see Appendix B, pages 266–267)*, add a new *Exam* in SpringCharts.

2. Using the *Print* button, print the *Nurse Note*. Record your name on the document and submit to your instructor.

Exercise 14.7

1. *Using Source Document 5: Plan of Care (see Appendix B, pages 268–271)*, document the *NANDA-I/Dx* in the *Nurse Note*.

2. Using the *Print* button, print the *Nurse Note*. Record your name on the document and submit to your instructor.

Exercise 14.8

1. *Using Source Document 5: Plan of Care (see Appendix B, pages 268–271)*, document the *Nursing Outcomes* (NOC) in the *Nurse Note*.

2. Using the *Print* button, print the *Nurse Note*. Record your name on the document and submit to your instructor.

Exercise 14.9

1. *Using Source Document 5: Plan of Care (see Appendix B, pages 268–271)*, update the *Nursing Interventions* (NIC) in the patient's chart.

2. Using the *Print* button, print the *Nurse Note*. Record your name on the document and submit to your instructor.

Exercise 14.10

1. *Using Source Document 6: Physician Orders (see Appendix B, page 272)*, update the *Test* in the patient's chart.
2. Using the *Print* button, print the *Nurse Note*. Record your name on the document and submit to your instructor.

Exercise 14.11

1. *Using Source Document 7: Medication Administration Record (see Appendix B, pages 273–274)*, record the notation into a *MAR* in a patient's *Care Tree*.
2. Using the *Print* button, print the *eMAR*. Record your name on the document and submit to your instructor.

Exercise 14.12

1. Write the name and date of birth of your patient on Source Document 8.
2. *Using Source Document 8: Intake and Output Record (see Appendix B, page 275)*, record the notation into an *I&O* form in a patient's *Care Tree*.
3. Using the *Print* button, print the *Intake and Output* document. Record your name on the document and submit to your instructor.

Exercise 14.13

1. Write the name and date of birth of your patient on Source Document 9. Create an ID number for your patient and record it under the DOB in the Addressograph area.
2. *Using Source Document 9: Interdisciplinary Education (see Appendix B, page 276)*, record the notation into the *Teaching* area of the *Nurse Note*.
3. Using the *Print* button, print the *Nurse Note*. Record your name on the document and submit to your instructor.

Exercise 14.14

1. Write the name and date of birth of your patient on Source Document 10.
2. *Using Source Document 10: Discharge Paperwork (see Appendix B, pages 277–278)*, create a *F/U-Rem* for the patient within the patient's chart.
3. Print the reminder. Record your name on the document and submit to your instructor.

Exercise 14.15

1. *Using Source Document 11: Nurses Supplement Record (see Appendix B, page 279)*, create an addendum to a *Nurse Note*.

2. Using the *Print* button, print the addendum. Record your name on the document and submit to your instructor.

Appendix A

Sample Documents

1. Patient's Face Sheet (Referenced in LO 3.7—The Face Sheet/Chart Alert)

Suburban Medical Group
101 Elm Street Sherman, TX 77521
(214) 674-2000

Name: Patti G Adams 06/29/42
Address: 198 Elm St Sherman, TX 77521
Home Phone: (214) 766-7676
Home Fax:
Work Phone:
Work Fax:
Pager:
Mobile Phone: (214) 777-7987
EMail: mom5645566@aol.com
SS#: 876-45-6676
Marital Status: Married
Sex: F
Pt ID #: 31
Employer: Home Engineer
  Date Entered: 04/02/2002
  Last Modified: 04/02/2002
Allergies:
Codeine   entered 04/26/2003 1507:39 PM by demo note:
Patient Number: 31 Chart ID: 3
  Last Modified: 11/18/2006
Other Sensitivities
  erythromycin causes nausea
Patient Number: 31 Chart ID: 4
  Last Modified: 04/26/2003
Social History
  Tobacco Use: Moderate Smoker
  Alcohol Use: Social Drinker
Patient Number: 31 Chart ID: 11
  Last Modified: 11/27/2006
PMHX
  HTN 401.9
  DM, Adult Onset,NID, Controlled 250.00
  HTN 401.9
    cholecystectomy 1998, TAH BSO 1999
Patient Number: 31 Chart ID: 5
  Last Modified: 12/15/2004
FMHX
  HTN 401.9
    F died of MI age 48. PGF died of MI age 53.
Patient Number: 31 Chart ID: 6
  Last Modified: 04/26/2003
Problem List
 Dx:

Patient: Adams, Patti G 06/29/42   **Page 1 of 2**

1. Patient's Face Sheet *cont.*

HTN 401.9
DM, Adult Onset,NID, Controlled 250.00
Hypercholesterolemia 272.0

Patient Number: 31 Chart ID: 7
Last Modified: 04/26/2003

Routine Meds
Diovan 80mg i po q am
Glucophage XR 500mg i po bid
Lipitor 10mg i po q am
Aleve 275 mg i q 12 hrs
Aspirin 325mg ii po qid prn

OTC Meds:
fish oil, glucosamine
Patient Number: 31 Chart ID: 8
Last Modified: 01/16/2005

Referring Dr:
Physician Body, Able
Patient Number: 31 Chart ID: 9
Last Modified: 04/26/2003

Chart Notes
Friend of Mrs Bibi.
Received informational letter on Naproxen.
Patient Number: 31 Chart ID: 10
Last Modified: 01/16/2005

Patient Insurance Info
Group Name: Retired Teachers Association
Group/Policy No: 78329
Certif No: 876456676
Insured's relation to patient: Insured
CoPay: 10.0

2. Letter to a Patient (Referenced in LO 5.3—Creating a Letter to a Patient or About a Patient)

Suburban Medical Group

101 Elm Street
Sherman, TX 77521
(214) 674-2000   Fax (214) 674-2100

September 7, 2010

Patti G Adams
198 Elm St
Sherman, TX 77521

Re:

Dear Ms. Adams;

An appointment has been scheduled for you on March 3rd, 2011. Please contact our office as soon as possible if you need to change the appointment.

Please arrive for your appointment 15 minutes early in order to complete your new patient forms. You will need to bring all medications that you are currently taking with you.

If you have any questions regarding this appointment, please call our office at (214) 674-2000.

Sincerely,

John O. Smith

3. Letter About a Patient (Referenced in LO 5.3—Creating a Letter to a Patient or About a Patient)

Suburban Medical Group
101 Elm Street
Sherman, TX 77521
(214) 674-2000   Fax (214) 674-2100

November 27, 2006

Harry I Hart M. D.
220 Elm St
Sherman, TX 77521

Re: Chris J Sykes 05/22/01

Dear Dr. Hart;

Thank you for allowing me to participate in this patient's care. If you have any questions or observations for me, please do not hesitate to call.

I will update you on this patient's progress after our next appointment.

Below please find a copy of the patient's recent lab results.

01/09/2005 Strep Screen

Strep Screen   negative   Normal: negative

  ID:
  Note:
  Tech: josmd
  Test Facility: Quest Diagnostics
  Reported: 01/09/2005 Last Modified: 01/09/2005
  ID#:
  Note:

Sincerely,

---

4. Test Report to Patient (Referenced in LO 5.5—Sending a Test Report to a Patient)

Suburban Medical Group
101 Elm Street
Sherman, TX 77521
(214) 674-2000   Fax (214) 674-2100

November 27, 2006

Patti G Adams
198 Elm St
Sherman, TX 77521

Dear Ms. Adams

This is a report of your recent examination results.

04/26/2003 Lipid Panel
Cholesterol: 170.0   Normal:0.0-180.0 mg/dl
HDL Cholesterol: 40.0   Normal:40.0-100.0 mg/dl
LDL Cholesterol: 100.0   Normal:0.0-130.0 mg/dl
Triglycerides: 100.0   Normal:0.0-180.0 mg/dl
Chol/HDL Ratio: 4.2   Normal:0.0-4.0
Test Description: These four tests measure different fats in the bloodstream. Their main importance is in determining the risk of blood vessel disease. Elevated Cholesterol, LDL cholesterol and Triglycerides are all associated with increased risk of heart disease and strokes. A high HDL cholesterol is currently thought to be protective against heart disease and strokes. The ratio of total cholesterol to HDL cholesterol (also called the coronary risk factor) is a calculation which yields a number useful in prediction overall risk from abnormal tests.
Problems:
Elevated Cholesterol.
Recommendations:
Low cholesterol diet.
Regular exercise program.
Please make an appointment to see the doctor as soon as possible.

Report for Pt: Adams, Patti G 06/29/42   Page 1 of 1
Suburban Medical Group

Prepared by
SpringChartsEMR

5. Prescription Forms (Referenced in LO 7.2—Building an Office Visit Note/Medication-Rx)

Suburban Medical Group
101 Elm Street
Sherman, TX 77521
Office:(214) 674-2000 Fax:(214) 674-2100
EMail:doc@sfischermd.com

John O. Smith, M.D.
Lic: J87877 DEA: AJ3434343
NPI: 07V000XYZ
July 01, 2010

Pt: Patti G Adams
198 Elm St
Sherman, TX 77521
DOB: 06/29/1942

℞ Allegra 180mg
disp: 30 thirty
sig: i po q am
Refill: prn

John O. Smith, M.D.
**** Electronic Signature Verified ****

John O. Smith, M.D.

A generically equivalent drug product may be dispensed unless
the practitioner hand writes the words 'BRAND NECESSARY'
or 'BRAND MEDICALLY NECESSARY' on the prescription face

Suburban Medical Group
101 Elm Street
Sherman, TX 77521
Office:(214) 674-2000 Fax:(214) 674-2100
EMail:doc@sfischermd.com

John O. Smith, M.D.
Lic: J87877 DEA: AJ3434343
NPI: 07V000XYZ
July 01, 2010

Pt: Patti G Adams
198 Elm St
Sherman, TX 77521
DOB: 06/29/1942

℞ Flonase NS 0.05%
disp: 16g
sig: ii sprays each nostril q d
Refill: prn

John O. Smith, M.D.
**** Electronic Signature Verified ****

John O. Smith, M.D.

A generically equivalent drug product may be dispensed unless
the practitioner hand writes the words 'BRAND NECESSARY'
or 'BRAND MEDICALLY NECESSARY' on the prescription face

Suburban Medical Group
101 Elm Street
Sherman, TX 77521
Office:(214) 674-2000 Fax:(214) 674-2100
EMail:doc@sfischermd.com

John O. Smith, M.D.
Lic: J87877 DEA: AJ3434343
NPI: 07V000XYZ
July 01, 2010

Pt: Patti G Adams
198 Elm St
Sherman, TX 77521
DOB: 06/29/1942

℞ Tamiflu 60mg/5cc
disp: 50cc
sig: i tsp po bid
Refill: 0 zero

John O. Smith, M.D.
**** Electronic Signature Verified ****

John O. Smith, M.D.

A generically equivalent drug product may be dispensed unless
the practitioner hand writes the words 'BRAND NECESSARY'
or 'BRAND MEDICALLY NECESSARY' on the prescription face

6. Test Order Form (Referenced in LO 7.5—Building an Office Visit Note/Tests)

Suburban Medical Group
101 Elm Street
Sherman, TX 77521
(214) 674-2000   Fax (214) 674-2100

Date: 11/27/06
Pt: Adams, Patti G 06/29/42
Address: 198 Elm St   Sherman, TX 77521

Physician Order

Orders:
CBC 85025
SMAC 80054

Diagnosis:
HTN 401.9

Patient Insurance Info
Group Name: Retired Teachers Association
Group/Policy No: 78329
Guarantor: Adams, Patti G 06/29/42
Certif No: 876456676
Insured
CoPay: 10.0

Insurance Company: United Healthcare
Mail Claim To: Claims
Attention:
Address: 19900 Molson Dr.
City: San Antonio
State: TX
Zip: 77890
Phone: 8008880404
Details:
EMail:
URL:

Prepared by
SpringChartsEMR

Suburban Medical Group

7. History & Physical Report (Referenced in Exercise 8.5—Creating an H&P Report)

History and Physical
Patient: Sykes, Chris J 05/22/01
Date of Service: 11/27/2006
Chief Complaint:
 Acute Diarrhea.
Present Illness:
 Pt c/o watery diarrhea which began 2 days ago. Notes the diarrhea is moderate.
 Comes on suddenly. - Pt denies nausea, vomiting, pain. - Pt has not noted stools
 floating or food particles within stool. - History of sick contacts, antibiotic use,
 foreign travel, bad food exposure. Past Hx of similar episodes: Negative. Family Hx
 of similar episodes: Negative.
Allergies:
 Penicillin
 pollen
Current Medications:
 Allegra 30mg i po q am
 Nasacort AQ 55mcg ii puffs each nostril q am
 Children's aspirin, benedryl
Past Medical History:
 Chickenpox
Family Medical History:
 HTN, Mother, father and sister have had consistent problems with allergies.
Social History:
Review Of Systems:
 GENERAL: + - no weight change, fever, chills, night sweats, generalized
 weakness Gastrointestinal: + -Appetite is normal. No dysphagia, dyspepsia, abd.
 pain, heartburn, nausea, vomiting, vomiting blood or coffee ground material,
 jaundice, constipation, melena, blood in or on stools, hemorrhoids.
Examination:
 Vitals: Temp: 98.6 Wt: 42.0 Ht: 41.0
 GENERAL: + - Well developed. Well nourished. In no distress / evident discomfort /
 Appears ill. ABDOMEN: + - Bowel sounds present and normal. - No evidence of
 scarring or past surgical procedures. - Flat, soft, nontender, without rebound or
 guarding. No fluid wave elicited. - No evidence of masses, organomegaly or
 abdominal aneurysm. - Normal to percussion. RECTAL: + - No abnormality. No
 masses, hemorrhoids, no fissures. - Hemoccult: Negative.
Impression:
 Diarrhea, Acute 787.91
Plan:
 Flagyl 500mg i po bid #10 rf x0
 Discussed keeping up hydration and eating crackers until diarrhea remits. Once
 better add complex carbohydrates to diet (cereals, rice, potatoes, bread). Avoid
 fatty foods until well. Watch for lactose intolerance. Pt Instr: Diarrhea given

Suburban Medical Group
H&P for Pt: Sykes, Chris J 05/22/01   Page 1 of 2

8. Office Visit Report (Referenced in Exercise 8.6—Creating an OV Note Report)

Suburban Medical Group
101 Elm Street Sherman, TX 77521
(214) 674-2000

04/28/2003 Office Visit

S:

Needs medications refilled. Follow-Up.

O:

Vitals: 97.5 F   80   14   130/74   Wt: 180.0 lbs   Ht: 64.0 in
BMI: 30.89

EAC/TM's nl. Pharynx nl. Neck supple s adenopathy. Thyroid normal to palpation. Chest clear to auscultation. Heart rrr s m or g. Abdomen: BS nl. nontender no organomegaly or masses. Extremities: pulses symmetrical UE and LE's. motor strength normal extrem x 4. cap refill < 2 sec extrem x 4. Neurological: CN II - XII nl. DTR's symm no sens defects. Gait nl.

A:

  Dx:

HTN 401.9
DM, Adult Onset,NID, Controlled 250.00
Hypercholesterolemia 272.0

P:

  Rx:

Diovan 80mg i po q am #30 rf x3
Glucophage XR 500mg i po bid #60 rf xprn
Lipitor 10mg i po q am #30 rf x5

  Tests:

CBC
SMAC
Lipid Panel
HGBA1C

  Procedures:

Ear Irrigation

Other Tx:

ref to ophth for yearly checkup

Follow-Up:

3 months.
***** Graphic *****
Date Created: 04/26/2003
Date of Service: 04/28/2003
Patient Number: 31 Chart ID: 12
Last Modified: 11/22/2006

9. Printed Immunization Record (Referenced in LO 9.3—Immunization Record)

Suburban Medical Group
101 Elm Street
Sherman, TX 77521
(214) 674-2000   Fax (214) 674-2100

Immunizations for Sykes, Chris J 05/22/01
DPT 04/08/2002
MMR 04/08/2002
HepatitisB 02/15/2002
HepatitisB 04/17/2002
DaPT 03/15/2002
HFlu 03/15/2002
IPV 03/15/2002
Pneumococcus 05/18/2002
HFlu 05/18/2002
IPV 05/18/2002
DaPT 07/16/2002
HFlu 07/16/2002
Pneumococcus 07/16/2002
Varicella 01/08/2003
MMR 01/08/2003
Flu Shot 12/21/2004
date printed: 11/27/06

Prepared by
SpringChartsEMR

Suburban Medical Group

10. Nurse Note Report (Referenced in LO 12.4—Printing a Nurse Note)

Suburban Medical Group
101 Elm Street Sherman, TX 77521
(214) 674-2000

11/06/2010 Nurse Note
  Subjective:
     Swelling in right arm.

  Objective:
     Vitals: Temp: 102.4F HR: 102 Resp: 18 BP: 148/74 Wt: 180.0lbs Ht: 55.0in BMI: 41.83 O2SAT 92.00 %

     BP left arm. Pt position-supine. Temp source-Tympanic.

     Pt complains of pain. Pain Location right arm. Pain rating 3 0-10 scale.

     Pain Description aching. Factors affecting pain movement. Factors relieving pain "took aspirin earlier today".

     ENT: Within Normal Limits.

        Heart sounds: Within Normal Limits.

        Lungs/Respiratory: Within Normal Limits.

        GU/GYN (female): Within Normal Limits.

        Neurological: Within Normal Limits.

     SKIN: abrasions 4cm by 6cm abraded area right forearm.

     EXTREM ITIES: edema right arm 14cm circumference measured and marked.

  Assessment:
     Other Dx :Infection of right arm r/t_ AEB fever, swelling.
     Other Dx :Pain related to edema/infection right arm. AEB pt. report of pain rating of 3 on 0-10 scale.
     Other Dx :Acute Skin Integrity, Impaired as evidenced by abrasion to right arm.
     11/06/2010 10:26 AM

  Plan: NOC:
     Infection Severity: Severity of infection and associated symptoms.

     Tissue Integrity: Skin and Mucous Membranes: Structural intactness and normal physiological function of skin and mucous membranes.

Patient: Adams, Patti G 06/29/42   Page 1 of 2
  Prepared by

SpringChartsEMR   Suburban Medical Group

10. Nurse Note Report *cont.*

Knowledge -Disease Process: Extent of understanding conveyed about a specific disease process and prevention of complications.

Pain Control: Personal actions to control pain.

Vital Signs: Extent to which temperature, pulse, respiration, and blood pressure are within normal range.

Interventions: NIC:

Intravenous (IV) Insertion: Administration and monitoring of intravenous fluids and medications. IV started #20 catheter left forearm first attempt.

Medication Administration: Preparing, giving, and evaluating the effectiveness of prescription and nonprescription drugs.

Pain Management: Alleviation of pain or a reduction in pain to a level of comfort that is acceptable to the patient.

Skin Surveillance: Collection and analysis of patient data to maintain skin and mucous membrane integrity.

Vital Signs Monitoring: Collection and analysis of cardiovascular, respiratory, and body temperature data to determine and prevent complications.

Wound Care: Prevention of wound complications and promotion of wound healing. Neosporin applied to abrasions on right arm per physician order.

Teaching:

Discussed plan of care with patient/significant other. Medication indication, frequency, considerations instruction.

Evaluation:

Patient/family verbalized understanding.

Infection Severity: Ongoing outcome

Knowledge -Disease Process: Outcome met this shift, continue to reinforce.

Pain Control: Outcome met this shift. Continue to monitor.

Vital Signs: Ongoing outcome.

Continue current interventions.

Revision: Reassessment:

Temperature 100.4 after Tyelonol administration in ED. Temp source -Tympanic.

Patient: Adams, Patti G 06/29/42   Page 2 of 2
    Prepared by   SpringChartsEMR   Suburban Medical Group

Appendix B

Source Documents

Source Document 1   Admission Data Base—Page 1

ADMISSION DATA BASE

Page 1

PATIENT IDENTIFICATION

For In & Out Surgery Patients, complete shaded areas

INITIAL NURSING ASSESSMENT

Arrived From: ☐ Home   ☐ ER-see ER Triage Record   ☑ Physician's Office   ☐ Other: _____
☐ Nursing Home   ☐ ER-see ER Fax Report   ☐ Surgical Services

Date of Arrival: _____   Time of Arrival: 0700   (Military Time)

Chief Complaint / History Present Illness: Chest Pain

Information Given by: Patient

Past Med History: ☑ Heart Disease   ☑ Hypertension   Past Surgical History: None
☐ Angina   ☐ Hypotension   ☐ Chest Pain
☐ Circulation   ☐ Kidney/Bladder   ☐ Cancer   ☑ Diabetes   ☐ Thyroid
☐ Anemia   ☐ Seizures   ☐ Stroke   ☐ TB   ☐ Lung Disease   ☐ Glaucoma
Other (specify): _____

Inoculations: PPD ☐Y ☑N Date _____   Tetanus ☑Y ☐N Date 2009   Flu ☑Y ☐N Date Oct 2010   Pneumonia ☐Y ☑N Date _____

Previous Anesthesia: ☐ Yes   ☑ No   Difficulties with Anesthesia: ☐ Yes   ☑ No
If yes, specify   Clinical Pathways Initiated: ☐ Yes   ☑ No

Adm VS: T 98.2   HR: 114   RR: 22   BP (R) 172 / 104   (L) __/__   SaO2 (ASU) 86 %   Ht 5'10"   Wt 260 lbs

NPO Status: _____   Valuables: Belongings Log Completed: ☐ Yes   ☑ No

CURRENT MEDICATIONS

Name of Med ☐ No Medications	Dose / Schedule	Last Dose	Name of Med ☐ No Medications	Dose / Schedule	Last Dose
Lopressor	100 mg BID	yesterday	Coumadin ERROR RN	2 mg Daily	yesterday
HCTZ	50 mg Daily	yesterday	Nitroglycerin	0.4 mg SL PRN	3 months ago
K-Dur	10 mEq BID	yesterday			
Glucophage	500 mg BID	yesterday			

Disposition of Medication: ☐ N/A   ☑ Home   ☐ Given to Family   ☐ Bedside   ☐ Valuables Envelope

ALLERGIES

Drugs, Food, Environment: ☐ None Known   ☐ Latex Allergy   **Specify Reaction:**
Amoxicillin   Hives

PERSONAL & SOCIAL

Marital Status: Married   Occupation: Retired   Role in Family: _____
Decision Maker: _____   Tel #: _____   Relationship: _____
Contact Person in event of emergency:
Name: Mary   Relationship: Spouse   Phone (Day): 569-9767   (Eve): _____

LIFE STYLE

☐ SMOKING - How many packs / day? _____   For how many years? _____   Smoking Cessation Information given? ☐ Yes ☐ No ☑ N/A
☑ ALCOHOL - Amount 2 beers a day   Date Last Used: yest   ☐ Denies alcohol use
☐ DRUGS - Type (Cocaine, Heroin, etc.) _____   Date Last Used: _____   ☑ Denies substance abuse

COPING / STRESS

Stress in your life (health, relationships, finances) fixed income
Recent changes / losses (job, move, new baby, divorce, death): retirement
What do you do under stress? eat
Due to the increase in domestic violence, we ask all adult patients. "Are you being hurt, hit or frightened by anyone in your life?" ☐ Yes ☑ No
If yes, explain: _____
Would you like assistance in dealing with this problem?   ☐ Yes ☐ No   **If patient states "Yes", contact Social Services:** _____
☐ Patient denies   ☐ Patient is unable to communicate   ☐ Pamphlet given

BEHAVIOR ASSESSMENT

Previous Psychiatric Therapy / Counseling / Admissions: ☑ None _____

☐ Depression   ☐ Self-Destructive Thoughts / Attempts   ☐ HALLUCINATIONS: ☐ Auditory ☐ Visual ☐ Other   ☐ Anxiety

SPIRITUAL / CULTURAL

Do you have any spiritual or cultural practices than may affect your medical care or hospitalization?   ☐ Yes ☑ No
If yes, explain: _____

ADVANCED DIRECTIVES

Do you have **Advanced Directives?** ☑ Yes ☐ No   Copy placed on chart? ☑ Yes   Date today   ☐ Not Available
Do you have a **Durable Power of Attorney** for Health Care decision making?   ☑ Yes ☐ No
Requested from Patient / Family ☐ Yes ☐ No ☑ N/A
Written information on advanced directives given to patient? ☐ Yes ☑ No

PART OF THE MEDICAL RECORD

Source Document 1 Admission Data Base—Page 2

ADMISSION DATA BASE
Page 2

For In & Out Surgery Patients, complete shaded areas

SENSORY / COGNITION

HISTORY

SENSORY / COGNITION ☐ No Impairment

Hearing: ☐ Impaired ☐ R ☑ L
☐ Deaf ☐ R ☐ L ☐ Aid
Vision: ☐ Impaired ☐ R ☐ L ☐ R ☐ L
☐ Blind ☐ R ☐ L
☑ Glasses ☐ Contacts ☐ Eye Prosthesis

Comment: _____ Glasses on _____

Are you having any difficulty reading? ☐ Yes ☑ No
Explain:
☐ Seizures ☐ Syncope ☐ Memory Loss ☐ Other _____

Sleep / Rest Problems: ☑ Yes ☐ No
If "Yes", what do you do at home to sleep? _Sleep in recliner_

ASSESSMENT

EYES:
☑ PERLA If unequal, specify: _____
☐ Redness ☐ Drainage ☐ Other: _____
☐ Speech ☑ Clear ☐ Slurred ☐ Non Verbal
☐ Foreign Language: _____

What is patient's response to Questions 1 - 4?
1) Today's date? _today_
2) Your birthday and age? _correct_
3) Name of hospital? _correct_
4) Where is the hospital located? _correct_

Level of consciousness: ☑ Alert ☐ Lethargic ☐ Unresponsive
Oriented: ☑ To Time ☑ To Place ☑ To Person
☐ Confused ☑ Easily Distracted ☐ Unable to Focus

BEHAVIOR: ☑ Cooperative ☑ Restless ☐ Agitated ☐ Depressed
☐ Angry ☐ Anxious ☐ Fearful ☐ Tearful ☐ Tremulous
☐ Inappropriate Behavior or Responses ☐ Guarded ☐ Combative
☐ Assaultive ☐ Threatening ☐ Resistant

PAIN

ACUTE PAIN: ☐ No Acute pain
Location: _Chest_
Intensity (0-10): _9_ Scale _0-10/NuM_
Comfort Goal: _4_
Quality (Patient's own words): _PRESSURE_
Onset: _hour ago_ Pattern _getting worse_
Aggravating Factors: _movement, walking_
Alleviating Factors: _NONE_
Impact on Functional Ability: _yrs_
Impact on Quality of Life: _yrs_
PAIN MANAGEMENT HISTORY: _N/A_
Helpful:
NOT Helpful:

CHRONIC PAIN: ☑ No Chronic pain
Location:
Intensity (0-10): _____ Scale _____
Comfort Goal:
Quality (Patient's own words):
Onset: _____ Pattern _____
Aggravating Factors:
Alleviating Factors:
Impact on Functional Ability:
Impact on Quality of Life:
PAIN MANAGEMENT HISTORY:
Helpful:
NOT Helpful:

PAIN SCALES:

WONG-BAKER: (Faces) 0   1   2   3   4   5
0-10 VISUAL: (Numerical) 0 1 2 3 4 5 6 7 8 (9) 10
VERBAL: No Hurt   Hurts Little Bit   Hurts Little More   Hurts Even More   Hurts Whole Lot   Worst Pain
NON-COGNITIVE: (FLACC Scale)

FLACC PAIN SCALE:
1. Sum of FACE, LEGS, ACTIVITY, CRY & CONSOLABILITY Scores = FLACC
2. Record FLACC Score using the 0-10 VISUAL (NUMERIC) Scale above

___ = FACE Score
0 = No particular expression or smile
1 = Occasional grimace or frown, withdrawn, disinterested
2 = Frequent to constant frown, clenched jaw, quivering chin
___ = LEGS Score
0 = Normal position, or relaxed
1 = Uneasy, restless, tense
2 = Kicking, or legs drawn up
___ = ACTIVITY Score
0 = Lying quietly, normal position, moves easily
1 = Squirming, shifting back & forth, tense
2 = Arched, rigid, or jerking
___ = CRY Score
0 = No crying (asleep or awake)
1 = Moans or whimpers, occasional complaint
2 = Crying steadily, screams or sobs, frequent complaints
___ = CONSOLABILITY Score
0 = Content, relaxed
1 = Reassured by touching/hugging/talking to, distractable
2 = Difficult to console or comfort

SEDATION SCALE:
S = NORMAL SLEEP, EASY TO AROUSE, ORIENTED WHEN AWAKENED, APPROPRIATE COGNITIVE BEHAVIOR
1 = WIDE AWAKE - ALERT (OR AT BASELINE), ORIENTED, INITIATES CONVERSATION
2 = DROWSY, EASY TO AROUSE, BUT ORIENTED AND DEMONSTRATES APPROPRIATE COGNITIVE BEHAVIOR WHEN AWAKE
3 = DROWSY, SOMEWHAT DIFFICULT TO AROUSE, BUT ORIENTED WHEN AWAKE
4 = DIFFICULT TO AROUSE, CONFUSED, NOT ORIENTED
5 = UNAROUSABLE

INTERVENTION:
1 = DISCUSS PAIN MANAGEMENT PLAN WITH PHYSICIAN
2 = PHARMACOLOGICAL (See MED KARDEX)
3 = NON-PHARMACOLOGICAL   A. Position Changed
B. Relaxation Technique   C. Splinting   D. Imagery
E. Music   F. Education   G. Other: _____

REPRODUCTIVE / SEXUALITY

LMP _N/A_ ☐ Regular ☐ Irregular ☐ Postmenopausal ☐ Penile Discharge ☐ Vaginal Discharge ☐ Abnormal Bleeding
Pregnancy Hx: _N/A_ Gr _____ P _____ A _____ Specify: _____
Type of Delivery: ☐ Full-Term ☐ Pre-term ☐ Vaginal ☐ C/S Lesions (Specify): _____
STD's: _Denies_ Do you practice breast self-exam? ☐ Yes ☑ No
Sexual Function Issues: _Denies_ Do you practice testicular self-exam? ☑ Yes ☐ No ☐ N/A
Contraception: _____ ☑ No reproductive / sexual issues identified

PART OF THE MEDICAL RECORD

8850016 Rev. 05/05   Admission Data Base_NURSING   PAGE 2 of 4

Source Document 1   Admission Data Base—Page 3

ADMISSION DATA BASE

Hospital's Logo Here

Page 3

For In & Out Surgery Patients, complete shaded areas

PATIENT IDENTIFICATION

CARDIOVASCULAR

HISTORY

- ☐ No Impairment
- ☑ Hypertension   ☐ CHF
- ☐ Pacemaker   Insert Date:
- ☑ Angina / Chest Pain   ☐ Previous M.I.
- ☐ Palpitations / Dysrhythmias
- ☐ Very Cold / Numb Extremities
- ☐ DVT / PE
- ☑ CABG
- ☐ Other (Specify)

ASSESSMENT

Skin Condition   ☑ Dry   ☐ Diaphoretic
Color: ☐ Normal ☑ Pale ☐ Cyanotic ☐ Other (specify)
Apical Pulse: 114   / min
Radial Pulse: ☐ Regular   ☐ Irregular
Pedal Pulse: ☐ Present   ☐ R Absent   ☐ L Absent
Edema ☐ None ☐ R Arm ☐ L Arm ☑ R Leg ☑ L Leg
Comments:
Vascular Access (specify kind & location): R FA #18

RESPIRATORY

- ☑ No Respiratory Problems
- ☐ Asthma
- ☐ Bronchitis
- ☐ Chronic Obstructive Pulmonary Disease
- ☐ Sleep Apnea
- ☐ Pneumonia
- ☐ Home O2
- ☐ Other (specify)

☐ Orthopnea   ☐ Dyspnea   ☐ Tachypnea   ☐ SOB
☐ Cough
☐ Sputum Production   Specify Color: Amt:
CHEST APPEARANC Symmetrical   Retraction   Deformities
Left Lung ☑   CLEAR   ☑ Right Lung
Left Lung ☐   DIMINISHED   ☐ Right Lung
Left Lung ☐   RALES   ☐ Right Lung
Left Lung ☐   RHONCHI   ☐ Right Lung
Left Lung ☐   WHEEZES   ☐ Right Lung
☐ Oxygen ☐ Chest Tube   ☐ Trach   ☐ ET Tube   ☐ Other

NUTRITION

Unplanned weight loss (10-15 lbs) in the last 6 months)   ☐ Yes   ☑ No
Difficulty chewing or swallowing   ☐ Yes   ☑ No
If yes, Liquids?   ☐ Yes   ☐ No   Solids?   ☐ Yes   ☐ No
☐ sore mouth   ☐ dentures   ☐ inability to feed self
Nausea, vomiting or diarrhea daily for 3 days pre-admission? ☐ Yes   ☐ No
A "YES" answer to any item results in a dietary consult

Dentures   ☐ None   ☐ Upper   ☐ Lower   ☐ Partial

☐ N/G Tube   ☐ Small-bone Feeding Tube
☐ PEG Tube   ☐ Jejunostomy Tube   ☐ Gastrostomy Tube

ELIMINATION

Bowel: ☐ Diarrhea ☐ Constipation ☐ Rectal Bleeding ☐ Incontinence
Last BM   YESTERDAY   Usual Pattern
Bladder: ☐ Urgency ☐ Nocturia ☐ Incontinence ☐ Burning
☐ Retention ☐ Frequency ☐ Anuria ☐ Dialysis
☐ No elimination problems noted

☑ Abdomen Soft ☐ Abdomen Tender ☐ Abdomen Distended
Bowel Sounds: ☑ Present   ☐ Absent

☐ Foley Catheter   ☐ Urostomy *   ☐ Colostomy / Ileostomy *
☐ External Catheter   * If YES, Request ET Consult

EDUCATION

☐ Needs full knowledge about:
☑ Needs refresher about: DISEASE PROCESS
Patient's preference for learning information: ☐ TV / Video   ☐ Reading   ☑ Teaching 1:1   ☐ Groups   ☐ Tapes
Interdisciplinary Patient Educational Assessment Form Initiated: ☐ Yes   ☐ No

DISCHARGE

DISCHARGE ASSESSMENT (ANTICIPATED ASSISTANCE NEEDED)   ☐ None Anticipated at Present
Place of Residence: ☑ Home   ☐ Nursing Home ☐ Res. Facility   ☐ Senior Housing   ☐ Shelter   ☐ Homeless
Source of Medical Care: ☐ None   ☐ Private MD   ☐ Clinic   ☐ Other:
Health Services at Home (Specify) ☑ None   ☐ Nurse   ☐ Homemaker   ☐ Social Worker ☐ PT   ☐ OT   ☐ Speech   ☐ Hospice
☐ Other: / ☐ Home Health Aide
Do you feel you will need additional help with care at home? ☑ No   ☐ Yes (describe):

REFERRALS

BASED ON ADMISSION ASSESSMENT, PLEASE CHECK NEEDED SERVICES: ☐ None anticipated at present
☐ Case Management Dept   ☐ Food & Nutrition Services   ☐ Wound, Ostomy & Continence Nurse (ET)
☑ Diabetes Nurse Educator   ☐ Rehabilitative Services   ☑ Other: Social Worker

Reason for Referrals: High blood sugar, financial issues

PART OF THE MEDICAL RECORD

Source Document 1   Admission Data Base—Page 4

ADMISSION DATA BASE   Page 4

For In & Out Surgery Patients, complete shaded areas

ACTIVITY

MUSCULOSKELETAL   GAIT: ☐ Normal ☐ Abnormal
- ☑ No muscoulskeletel problems
- ☐ Limited ROM: ☐ Rt. Arm ☐ Lt. Arm ☐ Rt. Leg ☐ Lt. Leg
- ☐ Amputation ☐ Rt. Arm ☐ Lt. Arm ☐ Rt. Leg ☐ Lt. Leg

DEVICES: ☐ Cane ☐ Quad Cane ☐ Crutches ☐ Walker
☐ W/C ☐ Braces ☐ Prosthesis ☐ Other

FALL RISK ASSESSMENT CRITERIA
INSTRUCTIONS: For any "YES" response, initiate the Fall Risk Assessment Protocol and include safety problem on Patient Care Portfolio.

	Yes	No
A. History of falls, use of restraints.	☐	☑
B. Ambulation / gait problems, use of adaptive devices (i.e., canes, walkers, prosthesis)	☐	☑
C. Weakness / paresis	☐	☑
D. Confusion, disorientation, impulsiveness, agitation, combativeness, seizures	☐	☑
E. Incontinence / urgency, diarrhea, frequent toileting	☐	☑
F. Post-op within 48 hours, sedatives, narcotic analgesics	☑	☐

ADL'S

PRE ADMISSION:

	Self	Assist	Complete
AMBULATION:	☑	☐	☐
DRESSING:	☑	☐	☐
MEAL PREPERATION:	☑	☐	☐
FEEDING:	☑	☐	☐
BATHING:	☑	☐	☐
TOILETING:	☑	☐	☐

REHAB TRIGGERS: A "YES" answer to above items triggers request to physician for consult for appropriate rehab discipline
PT - Recent and significant decline in functional mobility (ambulation, transfers, bed mobility): ☐ Yes ☑ No
OT - Recent and significant change in ADL's: ☐ Yes ☑ No
Speech - Consistently coughs when eating and/or drinking: ☐ Yes ☑ No

SKIN INTEGRITY

PHYSICAL MARKINGS: Any Pressure Ulcer should be staged, measured & described in Admitting Nurse's Notes.
- ☑ NONE
- ☐ ABRASIONS
- ☐ SCARS
- ☐ CONTUSIONS
- ☐ RASH
- ☐ PRESSURE ULCERS *
- ☐ HEALED PRESSURE ULCER * - or - FLAP *
- ☐ OTHER

* OBTAIN Dietary Consult + Stamp ORDER SHEET w/ Serum Albumin Request

Braden Score for Pressure Ulcer Risk

BRADEN SCORE FOR PREDICTING PRESSURE ULCER RISK
INSTRUCTIONS: Circle the number in each column that best describes the criteria.

SENSORY PERCEPTION	MOISTURE	ACTIVITY	MOBILITY	NUTRITION	FRICTION & SHEAR
1 COMPLETELY LIMITED	1 CONSTANTLY MOIST	1 BEDREST	1 COMPLETELY IMMOBILE	1 VERY POOR	1 PROBLEM
2 VERY LIMITED	2 VERY MOIST	2 CHAIRFAST	2 VERY LIMITED	2 PROBABLY INADEQUATE	2 POTENTIAL PROBLEM
3 SLIGHTLY LIMITED	3 OCCASIONALLY MOIST	3 WALKS OCCASIONALLY	3 SLIGHTLY LIMITED	3 ADEQUATE	3 NO APPARENT PROBLEM
4 NO IMPAIRMENT	4 RARELY MOIST	4 WALKS	4 NO LIMITATIONS	4 EXCELLENT	
SCORE 4	SCORE 4	SCORE 3	SCORE 4	SCORE 3	SCORE 2

A total score of < 17 = high risk pressure ulcer patient. Implement Pressure Ulcer Prevention Protocol.   **TOTAL SCORE:** 20

NURSING NOTES

PRINT NAME / TITLE	SIGN NAME	DATE	Military TIME
Student Nurse	Student Nurse	today	0745
PRINT NAME / TITLE	SIGN NAME	DATE	Military TIME

PART OF THE MEDICAL RECORD

Source Document 2 Admission Medication Reconciliation Form

COMPLETE THE YELLOW SHADED COLUMNS FIRST!
THEN REMOVE THE TOP COPY OF THE FORM TO COMPLETE THE REMAINING INFORMATION.

ALLERGIES: Amoxicillin

Home Medications Dose / Route/ Frequency (Include Herbal/OTC/Vitamins) Patient takes no medications ( )	Indication	Continue Medication On Admission?	
Lopressor 100mg ↑ po BID	HTN	✓ Yes	☐ No
HCTZ 50mg ↑ po daily	HTN	✓ Yes	☐ No
K-Dur 10meq ↑ po BID	Electrolytes	✓ Yes	☐ No
Glucophage 500mg ↑ po BID	DM	✓ Yes	☐ No
Nitrolingual 0.4mg SL prn chest pain	Chest pain	✓ Yes	☐ No
Coumadin 2mg ↑ po daily	Anticoagulation	☐ Yes	✓ No
		☐ Yes	☐ No
		☐ Yes	☐ No
		☐ Yes	☐ No
		☐ Yes	☐ No
		☐ Yes	☐ No
		☐ Yes	☐ No
		☐ Yes	☐ No

IMMUNIZATION RECORD (Record the month/year of last dose taken, if known)

Pneumonia Vaccine: Never   Flu Vaccine(s): last month   Other:

Information obtained:
✓ Patient/Family   ☐ Bottles/List   ☐ Old Records   ☐ Retail Pharmacy   ☐ MD Office Records   ☐ Unable to Obtain

Comments: None

PHYSICIAN SIGNATURE: _[signature]_   DATE: today   TIME: 0730

Page 1 of 3
Chart Copy File with History and Physical

ADMISSION MEDICATION
RECONCILIATION FORM

Patient Label

Source Document 3   Critical Care Flow Sheet—Page 1

ADMISSION DATA BASE

CRITICAL CARE FLOW SHEET

PATIENT IDENTIFICATION

START DATE: _today_   STOP DATE: _today_

SIGNATURE / TITLE / INITIALS	SIGNATURE / TITLE / INITIALS
Student Nurse, SN	

Registered/IV

2/7 Today _2400_	KG	HT: _5' 6"_	TYPE:	PA Catheter	Arterial Line	Central Line	Cordial Line	Sheath	Other
OUT Yesterday (LBS)			Insertion Date	N/A	N/A	N/A	N/A	N/A	_today_
PAST 24° Intake _N/A_		BALANCE 24°	Insertion Site						_RBFA_
_N/A_ Output			Removal Date						

LAB DATA

LABWORK		RESULTS				LABWORK		RESULTS			
TIME						Time					
BS						Albumin					
BUN						WBC					
Cr						Hgb					
Na						Hct					
K						PT					
Cl						INR					
CO2						PTT					
Ca						Platelets					
Phos						CPK					
Magnesium						CK-MB					
Cholesterol						CPK Index					
Total Bili						Troponin					
Alk. Phos						Lactic Acid					
SGOT						NH3					
SGPT						Pre-Albumin					
Total Protein						Digoxin					

TIME	STAT MEDS	INITIALS	TIME	STAT MEDS	INITIALS

ISOLATION	☐ YES ☒ NO	ISOLATION TYPE:	NEGATIVE FLOW MAINTAINED:	☐ YES ☐ NO	☐ N/A ☐ HEPAFILTER
PATHWAY	☒ NO	☐ YES, IF 'YES', SPECIFY:			
CODE STATUS	☒ FULL CODE	☐ DNR	☐ OTHER:		

Source Document 3   Critical Care Flow Sheet—Page 2

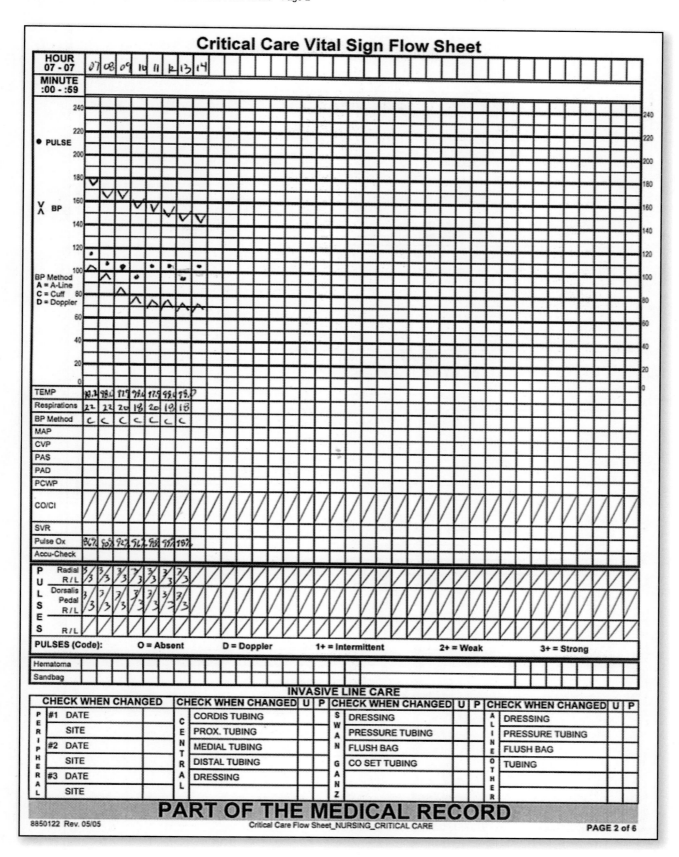

Critical Care Vital Sign Flow Sheet

HOUR 07 - 07	07	08	09	10	11	12	13	14					

MINUTE :00 - :59

PULSE / BP graph (240 down to 0)

BP Method
A = A-Line
C = Cuff
D = Doppler

TEMP	98.1	98.6	97.9	97.6	97.9	98.0	98.0							
Respirations	22	22	20	18	20	18	18							
BP Method	C	C	C	C	C	C	C							
MAP														
CVP														
PAS														
PAD														
PCWP														
CO/CI														
SVR														
Pulse Ox	86%	90%	92%	96%	98%	99%	99%							
Accu-Check														

P U L S E S	Radial R/L	3/3	3/3	3/3	3/3	3/3	3/3	3/3							
	Dorsalis Pedal R/L	3/3	3/3	3/3	3/3	3/3	3/3	3/3							
	R/L														

PULSES (Code):   O = Absent   D = Doppler   1+ = Intermittent   2+ = Weak   3+ = Strong

Hematoma														
Sandbag														

INVASIVE LINE CARE

CHECK WHEN CHANGED			CHECK WHEN CHANGED	U	P	CHECK WHEN CHANGED	U	P	CHECK WHEN CHANGED	U	P
P E R I P H E R A L	#1 DATE		C E N T R A L	CORDIS TUBING			S W A N	DRESSING			A L I N E	DRESSING		
	SITE			PROX. TUBING				PRESSURE TUBING				PRESSURE TUBING		
	#2 DATE			MEDIAL TUBING			G	FLUSH BAG			O T H E R	FLUSH BAG		
	SITE			DISTAL TUBING			A N Z	CO SET TUBING				TUBING		
	#3 DATE			DRESSING										
	SITE													

PART OF THE MEDICAL RECORD

Source Document 4   Initial Shift Assessment—Page 1

Date _today_

INITIAL SHIFT ASSESSMENT   SHIFT: 7-3

☑ Patient ID Bracelet On   ☐ Special Care Bed   ☐ Isolation

NEUROLOGICAL / SAFETY

LOC/ORIENTATION	Oriented x 3
GAG/SWALLOW/COUGH	WDL
EMOTION	Anxious
PUPILS/MOTOR	WDL

RESPIRATORY

OXYGEN DELIVERY	3L per NC
	☐ Pulse Oximeter On / Low Alarm Limit Set At ( )
CHARACTER OF RESP.	Unlabored
BREATH SOUNDS	Clear Bil
CHEST TUBES N/A	Amount: Site:
	Suction: Drainage:
SECRETIONS N/A	
TRACH INSERTION DATE	N/A Shiley #:

CARDIOVASCULAR

IV LINES – TYPE	L (2) FA #18 + Fluids?
LOCATION/DRESSING	Dry / Intact
REDNESS/SWELLING?	No
WAVEFORM	N/A

IV LINES – TYPE	TLC N/A	PIV N/A	PIV N/A	PIV N/A	SHILEY N/A
LOCATION					
REDNESS/SWELLING?					
DRESSING					

CARDIAC MONITOR	Sinus tach
?	☐ Alarms On / Limits Set At (/)
BLOOD PRESSURE	☑ Alarms On / Limits Set At (160 / 90)
HEART SOUNDS	Regular
CARDIAC INFUSIONS N/A	
PACEMAKER N/A	Wires: Epicardial or TVP Type: Rate:
	AV Interval: MA: Threshold:

GI/NUTRITION

BOWEL SOUNDS	Active all quadrants
CHARACTER OF ABD	Round soft
LAST BM	yesterday
NG TUBE OFF/FRM N/A	
JT/GT N/A	
TUBES N/A	
DIET	Diabetic 1800 calories/Day

GU

URINATION	voiding
COLOR/CLARITY	yellow/clear
AMOUNT	225 mls

SKIN

TEMP/TURGOR	Warm/pink
COLOR/EDEMA	+2 non-pitting Edema bil LE
SKIN INTEGRITY	intact
LEG/ARM INCISION	Intact/Non Reddened ☐ Stage____ Refer to pressure ulcer doc. record
INCISION CARE	

Signature: _Student Nurse_   Shift: _today_

INTERMEDIATE CARE FLOW SHEET   MEDICAL RECORD   PAGE 5   REV 6/29/04

Source Document 4 Initial Shift Assessment—Page 2

Date _today_

INITIAL SHIFT ASSESSMENT SHIFT: 7-3	INITIAL SHIFT ASSESSMENT SHIFT:
☑ Patient ID Bracelet On ☐ Special Care Bed ☐ Isolation	☐ Patient ID Bracelet On ☐ Special Care Bed ☐ Isolation

☑ Pulse Oximeter On / Low Alarm Limit Set At (90 %)   ☐ Pulse Oximeter On / Low Alarm Limit Set At (   )

| Airleak: N/A | Site: | Airleak: | Site: |
| Suction: N/A | Drainage: | Suction: | Drainage: |

A-Line N/A   A-Line

TLC	PIV	PIV	PIV	SHILEY	TLC	PIV	PIV	PIV	SHILEY

N/A NO ART LINE

☐ Alarms On / Limits Set At (/   )   ☐ Alarms On / Limits Set At (/   )
☐ Alarms On / Limits Set At (/   )   ☐ Alarms On / Limits Set At (/   )

Wires Epicardial or TVP Type: N/A   Rate: Wires Epicardial or TVP Type: Rate:
AV Interval N/A   mA: Threshold   AV Interval   mA: Threshold

Intact/Non Reddened ☐ Stage_____ Refer to pressure ulcer doc. record   Intact/Non Reddened ☐ Stage_____ Refer to pressure ulcer doc. record

Signature _Student Nurse_   Shift 7-3   Signature   Shift

INTERMEDIATE CARE FLOW SHEET   MEDICAL RECORD PAGE 6   REV 6/29/04

Source Document 5 Plan of Care—Page 1

Plan reviewed with patient ☑ Yes ☐ No
Plan reviewed with family ☐ Yes ☐ No
Plan reviewed with significant other ☑ Yes ☐ No
If NO, Explain: _____

PLAN OF CARE

PATIENT IDENTIFICATION

DATE / INITIAL	PROB. NO.	PROBLEMS RELATED TO (NURSING DIAGNOSIS)	EXPECTED OUTCOME (SHORT TERM GOAL)	NURSING INTERVENTION (NURSING ORDERS)	FREQUENCY	DATE RESOLVED	INITIAL
Today sn	1	☑ Physiologic Problems Risk for Altered tissue perfusion: Cardiac	Cardiac pump effective on discharge as evidenced by: Normal vital signs, orientation, tolerance for ADLs	Vital Signs Monitoring As Indicated, Neurologic Assessment, Assist with ADLs as needed			
Today sn		☑ Lack of Knowledge Regarding Health / Illness State ☐ Not Applicable	☑ Pt will demonstrate an increase in knowledge related to health / illness state ☑ Pt will verbalize knowledge about selfcare activities ☑ Pt will demonstrate application of health teaching into daily activities	☑ Patient teaching plan initiated	q 24 hr or as indicated		
Today sn		☑ Discharge Planning	☑ Pt will have appropriate supportive care at time of discharge ☑ Self care ☐ Family Care ☐ Home Care Agency ☐ Placement in long term care facility	☐ Resources Required / Date contracted: ☑ Social Services ☐ Home Care Agency: ☐ Equipment ☐ Continuity of Care Coordinator ☐ Assess home support system	As indicated		
				☐ Discuss patient needs at discharge planning rounds	Weekly		

PART OF THE MEDICAL RECORD

Plan of Care_NURSING

8850026 Rev. 05/05

PAGE 1 of 5

Source Document 5 Plan of Care—Page 2

DATE / INITIAL	PROB. NO.	PROBLEMS RELATED TO (NURSING DIAGNOSIS)	EXPECTED OUTCOME (SHORT TERM GOAL)	NURSING INTERVENTION (NURSING ORDERS)	FREQUENCY	DATE RESOLVED	INITIAL
		☐ Alteration in Bowel Elimination related to:	☐ Bowel sounds are present by:	☐ Assess for presence of bowel sounds & abd. distention	q shift or as indicated		
				☐ Record number of BM's			
		☑ Not Applicable	☐ Normal elimination pattern is re-established	☐ Monitor diet for proper roughage			
				☐ Obtain order for ☐ laxative			
				☐ Antidiarrheal as needed			
				☐ Give ___ cc fluid per 24 hours			
				☐ Obtain dietary consult			
				☐ Encourage mobility by ___ q ___ i.e., ambulation, turning, OOB / chair			
		☐ Alteration in Urinary Elimination related to:	☐ Pt will have a normal pattern of urinary elimination by:	☐ Monitor and maintain accurate intake & output	q shift		
				☐ Palpitate bladder for distention	q shift		
			☐ Voiding spontaneously 6 - 8 hours after surgery	☐ Monitor for symptoms and signs of distention: (sm. freq. Amt of urine, abd discomfort, character of urine	q shift		
		☑ Not Applicable	☐ Removal of catheter	☐ Offer bedpan ☐ Offer urinal			
				☐ BSC ☐ Bathroom q ___			
			☐ Absence of bladder distention	☐ Provide means to induce voiding			
		☐ Potential for: ___ or Alteration in: Skin Integrity	☐ Patient's skin will remain intact	☐ Skin Care Protocol Started	q shift or as indicated		
				☐ Pressure Ulcer Progress Chart Initiated	indicated		
		☐ Not Applicable	☐ Patient will exhibit evidence of wound healing				
SW		☑ Potential for Injury	☑ Patient will be free of physical injury	☑ Fall Prevention Protocol Initiated	q shift or as indicated		

PART OF THE MEDICAL RECORD

Source Document 5 Plan of Care—Page 3

DATE / INITIAL	PROB. NO.	PROBLEMS RELATED TO (NURSING DIAGNOSIS)	EXPECTED OUTCOME (SHORT TERM GOAL)	NURSING INTERVENTION (NURSING ORDERS)	FREQUENCY	DATE RESOLVED	INITIAL
SV		☑ Alteration in Comfort / pain related to: *Chest Pain*	☑ Patient will verbalize decreased discomfort and / or pain	☑ Assess onset of pain (location, duration, intensity)	q shift or as indicated		
			☑ Patient will perform ADL with minimal difficulty	☑ Change position of patient to facilitate comfort	As indicated		
				☑ Allow patient to verbalize feelings about pain	As indicated		
		☐ Not Applicable		☑ Administer analgesics as per physician's order & evaluate / record effectiveness	As indicated		
		☐ Alteration in Mobility	☐ Pt will demonstrate maximum mobility for their physical condition as evidence by	☐ Maintain proper positioning	As indicated		
				☐ Perform passive ROM [ ]			
				☐ Encourage patient to perform active ROM [ ]			
			☐ Transfers with assistance	☐ Encourage use of assistive device			
			☐ Turning independently	☐ Turn q2 hours			
		☑ Not Applicable	☐ Ambulating with assistance	☐ Maintain g safe environment			
			☐ Ambulating independently	☐ Collaborate with PT / OT for rehab			
				☐ Place call light and bedside table within reach			

PART OF THE MEDICAL RECORD

Plan of Care_NURSING

Source Document 5 Plan of Care—Page 4

DATE / INITIAL	PROB. NO.	PROBLEMS RELATED TO (NURSING DIAGNOSIS)	EXPECTED OUTCOME (SHORT TERM GOAL)	NURSING INTERVENTION (NURSING ORDERS)	FREQUENCY	DATE RESOLVED	INITIAL

REVIEW DATES / SIGNATURES

DATE	SIGNATURE / TITLE	DATE	SIGNATURE / TITLE
	Student Nurse /sn		

PART OF THE MEDICAL RECORD

Plan of Care_NURSING

Source Document 6 Physician Orders

| Physician Orders | System Downtime Tool

1) CBC
2) Liver Panel
3) Serum Protein

Stephen Finchberg M.D. today 0730

	PATIENT ID STICKER

Last Revised: March 2008

Source Document 7   Medication Administration Record—Page 1

Medication Administration Record

Patient:

Date of birth:

Date:

Admit:

Doctor: Steven Finchman)

to

Room #:

	0800	0900	1000	1100	1200	1300	1400	1500	1600	1700	1800	1900	2000	2100	2200	2300	2400	0100	0200	0300	0400	0500	0600	0700
Normal Saline Strength 0.9% Dose Directions 75 mL/hr IV																								SN 0715
Strength Dose Directions																								
Strength Dose Directions																								
Strength Dose Directions																								
Strength Dose Directions																								
	0800	0900	1000	1100	1200	1300	1400	1500	1600	1700	1800	1900	2000	2100	2200	2300	2400	0100	0200	0300	0400	0500	0600	0700

Initial & Name   SN   Student Nurse

Initial & Name

Initial & Name

Initial & Name

Initial & Name   SN   Student Nurse

Initial & Name

Initial & Name

Initial & Name

Deltoid = RD or LD
Vastus Lateralis = RVL or LVL
Lower Abdominal = RLA or LLA
Anterior Gluteal = RAG or LAG
Posterior Gluteal = RPG or LPG

Source Document 7 Medication Administration Record—Page 2

Medication Administration Record

Patient:
Date of birth:

Date:
Admit:

Doctor: Steven Finchman
Room #: 3205

Medication	0800	0900	1000	1100	1200	1300	1400	1500	1600	1700	1800	1900	2000	2100	2200	2300	2400	0100	0200	0300	0400	0500	0600	0700
Lopressor Strength 100 mg Dose 1 Directions PO BID		900 SN												2100										
HCTZ Strength 25mg Dose 1 Directions PO Daily	800 SN																							
K-Dur Strength 10 MEQ Dose 1 Directions PO BID		900 SN												2100										
Glucophage Strength 500mg Dose 1 Directions PO BID		900 SN												2100										
Nitrolingual Strength 0.4mg Dose 1 Directions Sublingual PRN chest pain																								

Initial & Name
Initial & Name
Initial & Name
Initial & Name

SN   Student Nurse

Initial & Name
Initial & Name
Initial & Name
Initial & Name

Deltoid = RD or LD
Vastus Lateralis = RVL or LVL
Lower Abdominal = RLA or LLA
Anterior Gluteal = RAG or LAG
Posterior Gluteal = RPG or LPG

Source Document 8 Intake and Output Record

Patient Name: _____   **Date:** __today__

Ramsey Scale for Sedation

AWAKE LEVELS	
Level 1	Patient anxious and agitated or restless (or both)
Level 2	Patient cooperate, oriented and tranquil
Level 3	Patient responds to commands only

ASLEEP LEVELS	
Level 4	Patient asleep but responds briskly to light, glabellar tap or loud auditory stimulous.
Level 5	Patient asleep with sluggish response to light, glabellar tap or loud auditory stimulous.
Level 6	Patient asleep with no response to stimuli.

Hendrich Fall Risk Model - Assessment Tool

Risk Factors	Day	Eve	Night		
Recent History of Falls	+7	+7	+7		
Depression	+4	+4	+4		
Altered Elimination	+3	+3	+3		
Confusion/Disoriented	+3	+3	+3	Key	
Dizziness/Vertigo	+3	+3	+3	0-2	Normal/Low Risk
Poor Judgement	+3	+3	+3	3-6	Level 1/High Risk
Poor Mobility/Generalized	+2	+2	+2	More than 6	Level 2/Extremely High Risk
Weakness					
TOTAL INITIAL RISK SCORE					

Hourly Time	INTAKE										OUTPUT					
	Oral						Blood/BLD Prod	IV Meds	Total Intake		Urine	NG pH	Chest Tube			Total Output
LIB																
7	240							75								
8								75								
9								75								
10	480							75								
11								75								
12								75								
13								75								
14								75								
TOTALS	720							525	1245		400					400
15																
16																
17																
18																
19																
20																
21																
22																
8 Hour Total																
23																
24																
1																
2																
3																
4																
5																
6																
8 Hr total																
24 Hr total																

Source Document 9   Interdisciplinary Education

County HOSPITAL

Interdisciplinary Education

Patient/Family Learning Needs: _Disease process_

ADDRESSOGRAPH STAMP HERE

Factors that may influence patient's ability and readiness to learn:

☑ None   ☐ Culture   ☐ Religion   ☐ Emotional Barriers   ☐ Language Barriers   ☐ Motivation

☐ Hearing/Vision/Speaking Impairment   ☐ Cognitive Limitation   ☐ Psychological Factors   ☐ Physical Limitations

☐ Financial Implications of Care Choices   Explanation: _____

Preferred methods of learning   ☑ Verbal   ☐ Written   ☐ Audio Visual   ☐ Demonstration

Is patient a minor?   ☐ Yes   ☑ No   If yes, do the patient's academic needs require addressing?

Signature: _Student Nurse_

KEY:

Taught to whom:
P - Patient
F - Family
O - Other
(if family member or other identify person)

Methods:
W - Written
P - Pamphlet
D - Demonstrated
F - Film/Video
V - Verbal Discussion

Department Codes:
D - Dietary
F - Financial Services
L - Laboratory
MD - Physician
N - Nursing

P - Pharmacy
PT - Physical Therapy
R - Radiology
RC - Respiratory Care
S - Social Services
ST - Speech Therapy

Evaluation:
RT - Reteach
NP - Needs Practice
RC - Reinforce Content
NT - No further teaching required

Response: V - Verbalizes Understanding   VP - Verbalizes Partial Understanding   RI - Returns Demo. Independently
RA - Returns Demo. with Assistance   NC - Noncompliant   U - Unable to Learn

DEPT. CODE	TAUGHT TO	METHOD	RESPONSE	EVALUATION	SUBJECT	Date/Time	INTERDISCIPLINARY NOTES
N	P	V	✓	RC	CAD		Importance of med administration
N	P	V	✓	RC	DM		Diet, surveillance of blood sugar, exercise

Rev 4/00

continued on back

Source Document 10   Discharge Paperwork—Page 1

UNIVERSITY MEDICAL CENTER

PATIENT DISCHARGE SUMMARY

Discharge Date: _today_   Time: _1430_

DISCHARGED VIA: **DISCHARGED TO:**

- ☑ Wheelchair   ☑ Home   ☐ Rehab Facility   Patient Name _____   MR# _____
- ☐ Ambulatory   ☐ Subacute ☐ Long Term Care
- ☐ Ambulance   ☐ Hospice   ☐ Other _____

ACCOMPANIED BY: _spouse_

DISCHARGE VITAL SIGNS: BP: _115_ / _70_   Pulse: _80_   Resp: _16_   Temp: _98.0_   Weight: _258_   Blood Sugar: _107_

Barrier(s) to communication/learning: _None_

Steps taken to overcome barrier(s): _N/A_

Follow-up education needed: _Diabetes management_

DIET: **ACTIVITY AS TOLERATED:** ✓
- ☐ No Restrictions   ☐ Restrictions: _____
- ☐ Diet Consult Completed
- ☑ Diet Instructions Given for _Diabetic Diet_
- ☐ Increase Intake of Clear Liquids   ☐ Return to School/Work on: _____

WEIGHT MONITORING:

You should weigh yourself: ☑ Daily   ☐ Weekly   ☑ Other _Call physician if weight gain of 5 or more pounds in 2 days_

SPECIALIZED DISCHARGE INSTRUCTIONS GIVEN FOR:

- ☐ Asthma   ☐ CVA   ☐ Myocardial Infarction   ☐ Wound/Incision Care
- ☐ Atrial Fibrillation ☑ Diabetes   ☐ Pneumonia   ☐ Other _____
- ☑ CHF   ☐ Influenza & Pneumococcal Vaccine   ☐ Post Operative Care   ☐ Other _____
- ☐ COPD   ☑ Medications   ☑ Weight Monitoring

If patient is on Coumadin, Education Booklet Given ☐

Smoking Cessation: If patient has smoked within the last year or lives with a smoker, Smoking Cessation Information Given ☐

☐ Follow-up Bloodwork (PT / INR) on: _____

FOLLOW UP WITH:

- ☑ Dr. _Stephen Finchman_   Phone: _542-6906_   to arrange office visit within _2_ days / (weeks)
- ☐ Dr. _____   Phone: _____   to arrange office visit within _____ days / weeks

LAB WORK TO FOLLOW UP WITH: _N/A_ _____ Date _____

REFERRALS: ☐ Home Care   ☐ Physical Therapy   ☐ Occupational Therapy
                  ☐ Speech Therapy   ☑ Social Services   ☐ Other: _____

EMERGENCY INSTRUCTIONS: Call 911 for persistent chest pain and shortness of breath or recurrence of symptoms that brought you to the hospital _Chest pain_

PATIENT EDUCATION MATERIALS GIVEN TO PATIENT/FAMILY (ex. Care Notes):
CHF, Diabetes, Medication handouts

INSTRUCTIONS GIVEN TO: _patient, spouse_

COMMENTS / RESPONSE TO INSTRUCTIONS: _Verbalized understanding_

I have received and understand the above instructions given to me by the nurse / physician.

_____   _____   _today_
PATIENT / REPRESENTATIVE SIGNATURE   RELATIONSHIP TO PATIENT   DATE

Student Nurse   _Student Nurse_
NURSE'S NAME (PLEASE PRINT)   NURSE'S SIGNATURE

PATIENT DISCHARGE SUMMARY   PART OF MEDICAL RECORD   REV. 9/29/05
                                 PAGE 1   CHART COPY

Source Document 10 Discharge Paperwork—Page 2

UNIVERSITY MEDICAL CENTER

NURSING MEDICATION
DISCHARGE INSTRUCTIONS

❑ Flu Vaccine N/A   Date: _____

❑ Pneumococcal Vaccine Date: N/A

Patient Name _____ MR# _____

* Review Current Medication Profile, MAR, Admission Reconciliation Form for Reconciling ALL medications at discharge.

🛑 STOP	Stop Taking These Medications at Home (Drug Name)	Allergies
	NONE	Amoxicillin

New Medications to Start Taking at Home

Drug Name	Dose	Route	How Often	How Long	Next Dose	Script Given	Reason for Taking/ Education
Lipitor	1 10mg	by mouth	Daily			☑ Yes ❑ No	High cholesterol
						❑ Yes ❑ No	
						❑ Yes ❑ No	
						❑ Yes ❑ No	
						❑ Yes ❑ No	

Continue Home Medications (continue until instructed to stop by your physician)

Drug Name	Dose	Route	How Often	Next Dose	Reason for Taking/ Education
Lopressor	1 50mg	by mouth	twice/day		blood pressure
HCTZ	1 50mg	by mouth	daily		blood pressure
K-Dur	1 10meq	by mouth	twice/day		electrolyte
Glucophage	1 500mg	by mouth	twice/day		diabetes
Nitrolingual	1 0.4mg	under tongue	as needed	for chest pain

Fax to the following physician(s): _____ Stephen Fischman _____

Patient / Parent Signature: _____   Nurse's Signature: _____ Student Nurse _____

Date/Time: _today_ 1400

* **PLEASE TAKE THIS FORM TO YOUR NEXT PHYSICIAN APPOINTMENT**
* **NOTIFY YOUR PHYSICIAN IF YOU STOP TAKING ANY OF YOUR MEDICATIONS**

PATIENT DISCHARGE SUMMARY   PART OF MEDICAL RECORD
                                   PAGE 2   REV 6/29/06
                                        CHART COPY

Source Document 11   Nurses Supplement Record

NURSES SUPPLEMENT RECORD

Date	
Today	Pain Reassessment after first Nitrolingual was 5 on scale 0-10 scale. Patient stated "It's easing up a bit." —————— Student Nurse

Concept Checkup Answer Key

Chapter 1: An Introduction to Electronic Health Records

Concept Checkup 1.1

A. Improvement of patient healthcare

B. 1. Keyboard typing
   2. Voice recognition
   3. Electronic handwriting
   4. Templates

C. 1. Internet
   2. Intranet

D. EHR—Electronic Health Record

Rationales:

A. Having comprehensive health information available when needed spurred the innovation of storing patient information electronically. Improvement of patient healthcare has been the catalyst for implementation of the electronic health record.

B. Traditionally, a keyboard was the only source for data entry. However, the need for convenience, efficiency, and speed has mandated other methods of input. Voice recognition systems adapt to a person's voice and speech patterns so that the computer inputs data as the operator speaks. Electronic handwriting recognition is now available. Also, large bodies of preset text known as "templates" can be used to easily input data into the patient's record.

C. Internet and intranet technologies have increased the availability of healthcare databases that can be shared and accessed across large distances. This remote access gives healthcare providers accessibility to EHR from remote locations such as nursing homes, a patient's home, a home office, or hospitals.

D. EHR—Electronic Health Record: Currently, this term is the most commonly accepted term for storing and accessing patient health information electronically. The EHR meets interoperability standards and therefore is able to be used across many healthcare organizations.

Concept Checkup 1.2

A. Standardizing how information is coded or termed for use in exchanging data to or from an EHR.

B. 1. Health Level Seven (HL7)
   2. National Council on Prescription Drug Programs (NCPDP)
   3. Institute of Electrical and Electronics Engineers 1073 (IEEE)
   4. Digital Imaging Communications in Medicine (DICOM)
   5. The Laboratory Logical Observation Identifier Name Codes (LOINC)
   Other acceptable answers may include:
   Systematized Nomenclature of Medicine Clinical Terms (SNOMED-CT)
   The Health Information Portability and Accountability Act's Transaction and Code Sets
   The United States Food and Drug Administration (FDA)
   The Human Gene Nomenclature (HUGN)
   The Environmental Protection Agency (EPA)

C. Standardization and interoperability promote safety, quality, cost savings, research, and identification of nursing's contribution to patient outcomes.

Rationales:

A. The CHI standards required common clinical vocabularies and standard methods for transmitting health information. By May of 2004, a set of 20 standards were announced and became the point of reference to standardize how information is coded or termed for use in exchanging data to or from an EHR.

B. CHI standards are not required by law. However, vendors doing business with the federal government voluntarily adopt these standards. The federal government, as the largest purchaser of healthcare services, uses these standards to promote interoperability between EHR systems. The many different standards and organizations and their descriptions can be found on page 7.

C. The nursing profession has recognized the importance of standardization in promoting the exchange of information since the days of Florence Nightingale (Ozbolt & Saba, 2008) and has taken steps to ensure nursing input into the standardization of the EHR. Standardization and interoperability promote saftety, quality, cost savings, research, and identification of nursing's contribution to patient outcomes (Halley, Brokel, & Sensmeier, 2009). Safety and quality are enhanced by the communication of information such as patient allergies, past health history, and current medications across organizations and from one level of care to another. Cost savings are achieved by reduction in duplicate tests and procedures. Finally, standardization promotes data collection for research purposes and allows nursing to identify the relationships among nursing interventions and patient outcomes.

Concept Checkup 1.3

A. "Accelerate the adoption of health information technology by creating an efficient, credible, and sustainable product certification program."

B. 1. Functionality
   2. Interoperability
   3. Security

C. Its purpose was to serve as a resource to the entire health system, to support the adoption of health information technology, and to promote a nationwide health information exchange in order to improve healthcare in the United States.

Rationales:

A. The Certification Commission states its mission is "to accelerate the adoption of health information technology by creating an efficient, credible and sustainable product certification program."

B. CCHIT certification demonstrated that an EHR product met basic requirements for:
   - Functionality—ability to carry out specific tasks.
   - Interoperability—compatibility and communication with other products.
   - Security—ability to keep patients' information safe.

C. In 2004, the Office of the National Coordinator for Health Information Technology (ONC) was established within the Office of the Secretary for the U.S. Department of Health and Human Services (HHS). Its purpose was to serve as a resource to the entire health system, to support the adoption of health information technology, and to promote a nationwide health information exchange in order to improve healthcare in the United States.

Concept Checkup 1.4

A. Enhanced accessibility to clinical information
B. Patient safety
C. Quality of patient care
D. Efficiency and savings

Rationales:

A. EHRs provide enhanced accessibility of clinical information for the healthcare provider. Access to the patient's healthcare information is not limited to the location of the paper chart, but is available at the point of care. The healthcare provider can easily retrieve information such as past health history, family health history, and immunization records. Up-to-date data, including test results, routine and current medications, and allergy information are crucial for informed decision making.

B. The EHR contributes to patient safety in several ways. For example, illegible handwriting is recognized as the source of many medical errors. The challenge of reading handwritten notes, orders, and prescriptions has been eliminated with the EHR. Patient information is clear and legible. Reports and letters to other specialists and patients are comprehensive, professional, and easy to create, promoting safe patient handoffs and continuity of care. Information is readily accessible in the EHR.

C. As healthcare becomes more complex, healthcare providers rely increasingly on evidence-based practice guidelines to support their practice. Through incorporation into the EHR as decision support systems, these guidelines are readily available to healthcare professionals, and promote adherence, ensuring quality care for patients.

D. An obvious financial savings is in the elimination of the paper-based chart, storage costs, and retrieval costs. Electronic messaging enables speedy communication between staff members. Job processes can be streamlined and reporting expedited. Often the need for a transcriptionist can also be eliminated.

Concept Checkup 1.5

A. 2014
B. 1. Automatic drug and allergy interaction checking
   2. Elimination of medication errors due to poor handwriting
   3. Greater efficiency to prescribing process
C. Its purpose is to aid in the development of a healthcare infrastructure and to assist individual providers and other entities such as hospitals in adopting and using health information technology, including EHRs.
D. (Any of the following are suitable answers.) Nursing informatics specialists are involved in streamlining documentation; integrating safety measures online; and participating in new medication distribution systems, telemedicine, privacy protection programs, and wireless applications.

Rationales:

A. President George W. Bush, in his 2004 State of the Union address, stated, "By computerizing health records, we can avoid dangerous medical mistakes, reduce costs, and improve care." President Bush subsequently created a sub-Cabinet-level position for a national health information coordinator at the Department of Health and Human Services (HHS). Then in April of 2004, he outlined a plan "to ensure that most Americans have electronic health records within the next 10 years."

B. Electronic prescribing is intended to bring greater safety to patients by providing for automatic drug and allergy interaction checking and the elimination of medication errors due to poor handwriting. E-prescribing is also designed to bring greater efficiency to the prescribing process for providers. It will dramatically decrease communication from pharmacies requesting clarification of prescriptions, resulting in enhanced efficiency and faster medication delivery to the recipient.

C. The Health Information Technology for Economic and Clinical Health (HITECH) Act was passed as part of ARRA and included over $20 billion to aid in the development of a healthcare infrastructure and to assist individual providers and other entities such as hospitals in adopting and using health information technology, including EHRs. These incentives through the Medicare and Medicaid reimbursement systems have assisted providers in adopting EHRs.

D. Nursing informatics is far more than simply understanding how to operate a computer. This growing field promotes access to current evidence-based nursing practice for integration into patient care. Nursing informatics specialists are involved in streamlining documentation; integrating safety measures online; and participating in new medication distribution systems, telemedicine, privacy protection programs, and wireless applications.

Chapter 2: Nursing Documentation Overview

Concept Checkup 2.1

A. 1. Confidentiality of patient records
    2. Power outages
    3. Computer "crashes"
    4. Computer viruses
B. 1. Readily accessible information
    2. Elimination of illegible handwriting
    3. Automatic alert systems
    4. Decision support
    5. Reduction in duplicate diagnostic testing
C. They enhance the quality of documentation and ultimately promote safe, effective patient care.
D. The primary purpose of HIPAA is to protect the privacy of patient health information.

Rationales:

A. In addition to privacy concerns, opponents fear that EHRs may be subject to power outages, computer "crashes," and computer viruses that may alter patient data without the knowledge of the healthcare team or the patient.

B. Some benefits of the EHR include readily accessible information, elimination of illegible handwriting, automatic alert systems, decision support, and reduction in duplicate diagnostic testing.

C. Healthcare providers and organizations are increasingly implementing EHRs in order to enhance the quality of documentation and ultimately promote safe, effective patient care.

D. In April 2003, healthcare organizations became responsible for adherence to the Health Insurance Portability and Accountability Act (HIPAA) that was passed in 1996 to protect the privacy of patient health information. All healthcare members, teams, and systems are held accountable to this legislation, which gives greater control to patients for their care, provides patient education on privacy protection, ensures patient access to personal records, ensures patient consent prior to release of medical information, and provides recourse if privacy violations occur.

Concept Checkup 2.2

A. 1. Comprehensive
   2. Concise
   3. Clear
B. 1. Prevent medical errors
   2. Communicate with other healthcare providers
   3. Demonstrate the delivery of care to ensure appropriate reimbursement
   4. Demonstrate adherence to accreditation standards
   5. Provide a source of evidence in the event of legal proceedings
      Another acceptable answer would be to promote knowledge development through research.
C. 1. Failure to record pertinent health or drug information
   2. Failure to record nursing actions
   3. Failure to record medication administration
      Other acceptable answers may include: failure to record drug reactions, changes in a patient's condition, and discontinued medications.
D. DRGs are used to establish the quantity of services for which a hospital, ambulatory care center, or home health agency will receive payment.

Rationales:

A. Documentation should be comprehensive, concise, and clear.
B. All patient care must be documented in the patient's record in order to:
   1. prevent medical errors,
   2. communicate with other healthcare providers,
   3. demonstrate the delivery of care to ensure appropriate reimbursement,
   4. adhere to accreditation standards,
   5. provide a source of evidence in the event of legal proceedings, and
   6. promote knowledge development through research. Documentation is critical for patient safety.
C. To ensure patient safety, healthcare providers must avoid documentation errors, such as the failure to record pertinent health or drug information, nursing actions, medication administration, drug reactions, changes in a patient's condition, and discontinued medications.
D. Appropriate documentation is critical for reimbursement purposes. Diagnostic-related groups (DRGs) are used to establish the quantity of services for which a hospital, ambulatory care center, or home health agency will receive payment. Healthcare organizations receive a standard payment for Medicare and Medicaid claims regardless of the time the patient received services or the type of services rendered. DRG determination is dependent on documentation. Documentation omissions may result in the assignment of a DRG that results in lower reimbursement.

Concept Checkup 2.3

A. The key to thorough, legal, and ethical documentation is to follow the nursing process to ensure the accuracy and comprehensiveness of the patient health record.
B. The problem-oriented medical record allows for documentation based on the patient's problems. Data are organized by problem or category and a plan of care emerges from this newly created problem database.
C.
   S: Subjective data
   O: Objective data
   A: Assessment

P: Plan

 I: Intervention

E: Evaluation

R: Revision

Rationales:

A. The key to thorough, legal, and ethical documentation is to follow the nursing process to ensure the accuracy and comprehensiveness of the patient health record. Approaching documentation of nursing care in a systematic manner minimizes the risk of missed or inaccurate information.

B. The problem-oriented medical record (POMR) allows for documentation based on the patient's problems. In the POMR, data are organized by problem or category and a plan of care emerges from this newly created problem database. Data are recorded using the PIE, SOAP, SOAP(IE), or SOAP(IER) format.

C. SOAP, SOAP(IE), and SOAP(IER) are widely used among healthcare professionals, including nursing, because of the ability to chart assessment findings. However, the SOAP model is primarily a medical model and does not allow for nursing diagnosis and evaluation of interventions. Consequently, nurses often use the SOAP(IER) note format since this style allows for the entire nursing process to be addressed. SOAP(IER) represents:

- S—subjective data (verbalizations of the patient)
- O—objective data (measurable and observable data)
- A—assessment (diagnosis based upon data)
- P—plan (what the nurse plans to do)
- I—interventions (actions taken)
- E—evaluation (patient response to the intervention)
- R—revision (modifications to the plan based on the evaluation)

Concept Checkup 2.4

A. Documentation of medication name, dosage, route of administration, date and time of administration, and the signature of the nurse who administers the medication.

B. 1. Reduces the number of medication errors
   2. Allows efficient tracking of medications within the healthcare system
   3. Reduces time spent searching for missing medications

Rationales:

A. While healthcare organizations use a variety of methods to record administration of medications, the critical aspects of recording medication administration remain the same. These critical aspects include documentation of the medication name, dosage, route of administration, date and time of administration, and the signature of the nurse who administers the medication. Patient allergies are routinely recorded on the medication administration record for ease of reference and to prevent administration of a drug to which a patient is allergic.

B. Electronic MARs (e-MARs) reduce the number of medication errors, protecting the patient from harm and the nurse from liability. In addition, e-MARs allow for more efficient tracking of medications within the healthcare system. e-MARs are usually user-friendly and reduce the time spent searching for missing medications.

Concept Checkup 2.5

A. Nursing diagnoses, NOC, and NIC are relevant because of the need to communicate quality, effective standard terminology for nursing data.

B. Traditionally used in schools of nursing and inpatient care, nursing diagnoses, NOC, and NIC may be used in any healthcare system.

C. 1. Selection of diagnostic criteria enables the nurse to develop a plan of care in a variety of settings including hospitals, home healthcare, hospice, ambulatory care, schools, and nursing homes.

   2. Standardized classification of outcomes and interventions.

   3. Permitting comparison of nursing care across settings.

Rationales:

A. The need to communicate quality, effectiveness, and the value of nursing services led to the creation of databases accessible to all nurses to assist with accurate, legal, and reimbursable documentation criteria. In 1991 the National Center for Nursing Research of the National Institutes of Health recommended the development of standard terminology for nursing data. This led to the formation of standardized nursing diagnoses, nursing outcomes, and nursing interventions.

B. The use of nursing diagnoses, NOC, and NIC has traditionally been limited to schools of nursing and hospitals where the focus is on inpatient care. However, accurate and appropriate patient care documentation is critical in any healthcare setting.

C. NANDA-I nursing diagnosis classifications are used to guide nursing decisions and plans of care for individual patients. Selection of diagnostic criteria enables the nurse to develop a plan of care in a variety of settings including hospitals, home healthcare, hospice, ambulatory care centers, schools, and nursing homes. NOC and NIC reflect nursing practice and permit comparison of nursing care across settings.

Chapter 3: Essential Documentation

Concept Checkup 3.1

A. 1. Ease of use
   2. Richness in features
   3. Customizable for multiple healthcare specialties

B. 1. Functionality
   2. Interoperability
   3. Security

Rationales:

A. The SpringCharts EHR™ software has been chosen as the training tool for this textbook because of its ease of use, richness in features, and ability to be customized to suit a wide range of healthcare specialties. SpringCharts is an international program and is used by over 1,500 physicians and many thousands of nurses, MAs, and other healthcare support staff.

B. The Falcon version of SpringCharts EHR was certified with ARRA in 2010 to qualify for financial rebates to physicians under the HITECH ACT for Ambulatory EHRs. That means that SpringCharts EHR has met a comprehensive set of criteria for:

- Functionality—setting features and functions to meet a basic set of requirements.

- Interoperability—establishing basic functionality enabling standards-based data exchange with other sources of healthcare information in future versions of the product.

- Security—ensuring data privacy and robustness to prevent data loss.

Concept Checkup 3.2

A. Primary provider, practice name
B. Multiple locations
C. When nurse practioners or other providers at the healthcare facility prescribe medication.

Rationales:

A. In the *Set User Preferences* window, each user sets:
   1. The primary provider's name that appears as the default for the user on reports and letters. The list of providers is based upon those set up in the administration panel of the SpringCharts server.
   2. The practice name or healthcare facility that defaults for letterheads. Although the provider's and the practice's name are chosen here as "default," they can be changed within the program at the time of creating various letters and reports. A clinic may have several practices set up in various locations but use the same database for SpringCharts across the Internet. This enables the complete patient health record to be viewed by any of the practices.
B. The *Tracker Group* displays the list of patients in the *Patient Tracker* window of the *Practice View* screen. Clinics that have several locations and work from the same patient database over the Internet are able to track patients separately for each location. The various tracker groups are set up in the administrative panel of the SpringCharts server. *Show All* displays all patients in the *Patient Tracker* window from all locations. If the healthcare facility has only one location, the *Tracker Group* field will be left blank.
C. The selection of a practitioner in the *Rx Print Attending* field prints this name as the attending provider on the pharmacy prescription forms. Based on state laws, nurse practitioners and other support providers may be required to indicate the attending physician when creating prescriptions.

Concept Checkup 3.3

A. To access the *Edit PopUp Text* window so that a user can add or modify pop-up text.
B. It means that each user has a personal set of pop-up texts that can be modified without affecting any other user's pop-up text.

Rationales:

A. SpringCharts pop-up text can be edited from multiple locations. In any dialogue box within SpringCharts that displays pop-up text, the edit icon gives access to the *Edit PopUp Text* window where text can be added, deleted, or modified.
B. Pop-up text is stored in the SpringCharts database by the user login name; therefore, each user has a personal set of pop-up texts that can be modified without affecting any other user's pop-up text.

Concept Checkup 3.4

A. Patient medical data
B. Charts opened during the current logon session
C. Multiple users,
D. Multiple users, editing

Rationales:

A. The electronic chart is the repository for patient medical data created through computer automation in the healthcare setting. Similar to the traditional paper chart, it holds such static information as the patient's demographics, allergies, medical history, and medical problems as well as the dynamic information including encounter notes, nurse notes, tests, letters, and reports concerning the patient.

B. The *Recent Charts* menu provides a drop-down window that allows the user to access charts that have been opened during the current logon session.

C. A patient's chart can be opened by multiple users in SpringCharts at the same time. In fact, all users can be editing the same chart at the same time. However, because of data protection, the same specific area of the chart cannot be edited simultaneously by different users. Many different patient electronic charts can be opened simultaneously by the same user.

D. All users can be editing the same chart at the same time. However, because of data protection, the same specific area of the chart cannot be edited simultaneously by different users. Many different patient electronic charts can be opened simultaneously by the same user.

Concept Checkup 3.5

A. From the paper intake forms that the patient completes or from interviewing the patient

B. The *Chart Alert* section

C. Category preferences table on the SpringCharts server

Rationales:

A. Information to complete the electronic face sheet is taken from the paper intake forms that the patient completes containing information such as past health history, routine medications, and current health problems. These intake forms are typically completed by patients in the waiting room while they wait to be seen or admitted. The paper intake forms may be designed to cover the same categories and data flow that appear in the SpringCharts face sheet. In the inpatient setting, this information is often obtained through patient interview.

B. A newly completed face sheet can be printed for new patients. This allows patients another opportunity to confirm the accuracy of their health information. The face sheet is printed by selecting the *Print Face Sheet* button. All information in the *Edit Face Sheet* window is printed except the *Chart Alert*, preventing the *Chart Alert* information from being seen by the patient.

C. The social history, past medical history, and family medical history sections contain health history items that are set up in the category preferences table on the SpringCharts server. The category preferences table enables the administrator to create predetermined customized lists of healthcare data. The lists are displayed in SpringCharts on each computer and enable rapid selection of items from these checklists to build the face sheet.

Concept Checkup 3.6

A. They can be altered or edited

B. 30 categories

Rationales:

A. There are preset categories in the *Care Tree* that cannot be altered or edited. When certain documents and tests are saved, they are automatically positioned in these appropriate *Care Tree* categories. The preset list includes all categories from *Encounters* through *Recycle Bin*.

B. An additional 30 categories can be added to the *Care Tree* list. This provides all users the opportunity to store created documents and imported files under these added categories.

Chapter 4: Nurse Note Documentation—Level 1

Concept Checkup 4.1

A.

     S. Subjective

     O. Objective

     A. Assessment

     P. Plan

     I. Intervention

     E. Evaluation

     R. Revision

B. *Show Chart Summary*

Rationales:

A. The SOAPIER format:

The Subjective component consists of the patient's description of his/her current health condition. It generally includes the symptoms, the history of the present illness, and a review of the patient's body systems as stated by the patient.

The Objective component contains the nurse's observations and generally includes the vital signs and findings from the physical exam.

The Assessment component details the nursing diagnosis(es) (NANDA-I) based on the examination. Nursing diagnoses should be listed in order of priority.

The Plan component includes the nursing goals applicable to the patient stated in Nursing Outcomes Classification (NOC) format. In the planning phase, the nurse sets the anticipated time frame for goal attainment. Outcomes are reviewed periodically, typically every shift to determine patient progress.

The Intervention component is made up of the list of patient-specific actions that the nurse takes stated in Nursing Intervention Classification (NIC) format. These interventions, including patient education, are designed to positively impact the patient and move the patient toward achieving the planned goals.

The Evaluation component involves reviewing the outcomes that have been set and the patient's progress toward achieving these goals.

The Revision component, based on the evaluation, involves streamlining, adding, and reassessing goals to continually make them appropriate and achievable for the patient.

B. Upon opening a new *Nurse Note* form, the *Show Chart Summary* icon at the bottom right side shows the patient's *Face Sheet Overview* panel. This panel allows the nurse to access the patient's chart without having to exit the *Nurse Note* window.

Concept Checkup 4.2

A. False

B. *Copy Prev Note*

Rationales:

A. The navigation tabs along the right side of the screen enable the nurse to proceed through the *Nurse Note* in a logical flow; however, the various panels may be selected in any order.

B. The *Chief Complaint, Exam, NOC, NIC, Teaching, Evaluation, Reassessment,* and *Follow-up* areas allow the addition of notes from previous encounters in the bottom right window. A clinician can highlight previous note text and copy it to the present note by clicking on the *Copy Prev Note* icon.

Concept Checkup 4.3

A. By selecting any other navigation tab

B. True

Rationales:

A. The selected text is moved into the body of the SOAPIER format by clicking on any other navigational tab. *CC* (Chief Complaint), *Vitals*, *Exam* (Examination), *Dx* (NANDA/Diagnosis), *NOC* (Nursing Outcomes Classification), *NIC* (Nursing Interventions Classification), *Test* (Tests), *Proc* (Procedures), *Teaching*, *Evaluation*, *Reassess* (Reassessment), and *F/U-Rem* (F/U-Reminders) all operate in a similar manner with the appropriate pop-up text appearing on the right side once a different tab in the note is selected.

B. The *Chief Complaint* area can also be individualized to allow for symptoms that are specific to a certain area, for example, orthopedics or neurology. In order to individualize pop-up text, the user selects the pencil icon to open the *Edit PopUp Text* window.

Concept Checkup 4.4

A. Height and Weight

B. Height, Weight, Blood Pressure, and BMI

Rationales:

A. The BMI is automatically calculated for the user based upon the patient's height and weight.

B. SpringCharts displays four vital charts (Height, Weight, Blood Pressure, and BMI) by accessing the *Height/Weight Graph* or *BP/BMI Graph* icons at the top right in the *Vitals* panel.

Concept Checkup 4.5

A. True

B. *Permanent Sign and Lock* prevents further changes to an entry, even by the user who locked it. It should be used when an entry is completed.

Rationales:

A. Using the defaulted text, *O (Normals)*, the nurse clicks on systems that are within normal limits upon examination to send that text to the *Examination* text field in the lower left section of the window. Using the *O (Abnormals)* drop-down selection box, the nurse can easily choose the applicable text and modify it as necessary. The user also has the ability to type text if the desired text is not available by clicking directly into the *Examination* text field.

B. Once the *Nurse Note* is locked, which is accomplished by clicking the *Sign* button, then *Permanent Sign and Lock*, it cannot be unlocked or edited, even by the user who permanently locked it. Nurses should sign and lock each entry as completed to prevent editing of entries by other users.

Chapter 5: Fundamental EHR Functionality

Concept Checkup 5.1

A. When patients need frequent vital sign monitoring

B. False

Rationales:

A. SpringCharts EHR has a feature that allows vital signs to be recorded outside of a regular note. This feature in SpringCharts is only used when patients need frequent vital sign monitoring in either the inpatient or outpatient setting. For example, hypertensive patients may come to an outpatient healthcare clinic for the sole purpose of having their blood pressure monitored. In the inpatient setting, patients may have vital signs monitored frequently following procedures or if their condition is unstable.

B. The body mass index is grayed out; the program calculates this item from the patient's height and weight.

Concept Checkup 5.2

A. Telephone call encounter

B. *Add Chart Notes* button

C. *Edit > Tests Explanations*

Rationales:

A. *New TC note* creates a new telephone call encounter form. A user may create a *New TC note* by selecting *New > New TC note* from the patient's chart screen.

B. All entries in the patient's *Care Tree* are available to add into the body of a letter by selecting the *Add Chart Notes* button. This is useful when sending office visit notes, such as test results, encounter notes, or information from the face sheet, to a referring physician.

C. Test descriptions for test reports are created and edited by selecting *Edit > Tests Explanations* from the main screen.

Concept Checkup 5.3

A. 1. Labs
   2. Imaging
   3. Medical tests

B. The nurse selects the *Tools* menu from within the *Nurse Note* screen and chooses *Care Plan*.

C. 1. Conversion Calculator
   2. Pregnancy Expected Date of Delivery
   3. Simple Calculator

Rationales:

A. Order forms are used to record orders for lab, imaging, and medical tests that are conducted at a third-party facility.

B. To access a practice guideline, the nurse selects the *Tools* menu from within the *Nurse Note* screen and chooses *Care Plan*.

C. SpringCharts contains three types of calculators: a Conversion Calculator, a Pregnancy Expected Date of Delivery (EDD) Calculator, and a Simple Calculator. The three types of calculators may be selected either from the *Utilities* menu from the main screen or from the *Tools* menu in the *Nurse Note* screen.

Chapter 6: Nurse Note Documentation—Level 2

Concept Checkup 6.1

A. 1. Comparison of nursing activities and outcomes
   2. Positive patient outcomes
   3. Enhanced quality of patient care

B. False

Rationales:

A. In nursing, standard language reflects the nursing process: nursing diagnoses, nursing outcomes, and nursing interventions. In addition to facilitating the use of technology, standard language allows for comparison of nursing activities and outcomes in diverse settings and locations, thereby enabling nursing research to demonstrate the value of nursing in promoting positive patient outcomes. Another benefit of standardized terminology is enhanced quality of patient care through promotion of compliance to standards of care.

B. NANDA-I defines nursing diagnosis as "a clinical judgment about individual, family, or community experiences and responses to actual or potential health problems and life processes."

Concept Checkup 6.2

A. Short, long, time frame for achievement

B. False

Rationales:

A. Once an outcome is selected, the nurse designates a specific time frame for achievement of the goal. Nursing outcomes may be either short-term or long-term goals.

B. The *NOC* area can be individualized from inside the *NOC* window to allow for Nursing Outcomes Classifications that may not be available in the prebuilt text.

Concept Checkup 6.3

A. To facilitate wellness or movement toward wellness

B. True

Rationales:

A. Interventions are the activities the nurse provides in order to facilitate wellness or movement toward wellness.

B. In order to individualize pop-up text, the user selects the pencil icon. This opens the *Edit PopUp Text* window where the nurse can add useful text into the open fields. The order of the intervention list may be modified by using the up and down arrows on the left-hand side of the screen.

Concept Checkup 6.4

A. 1. Drug name
    2. Route
    3. Dosage
    4. Frequency
    5. Time

B. Under the *Nursing Documentation* tab in the *Care Tree* within a patient's chart.

Rationales:

A. New medications are typed into the MAR, including the drug name, route, dosage, frequency, and time.

B. The MAR is located within the *Nursing Documentation* tab within the *Care Tree* of a patient's chart.

Concept Checkup 6.5

A. The *Care Tree* tab

B. Each shift

Rationales:

A. Like the *MAR*, in SpringCharts, *I&O* documentation is in the *Nursing Documentation* area, which is accessed via the *Care Tree* tab in the *Nurse Note.*

B. *I&O* may be documented hourly and shift totals are calculated by the user each shift on the *I&O* form.

Chapter 7: Ambulatory Healthcare

Concept Checkup 7.1

A.

    S. Subjective

    O. Objective

    A. Assessment

    P. Plan

B. Pop-up text relevant to that topic appears.

C. Copy previous note text into the present note

D. Three

E. By offering a search feature of the database rather than using pop-up text.

Rationales:

A. The middle panel of the *OV Note* is the portion where the notes are stored in the SOAP format, containing subjective, objective, assessment, and plan categories.

B. Once a tab has been selected from the navigation panel, a list of pop-up text relevant to that topic appears in the third panel of the screen.

C. Past encounter notes enable clinicians to refresh their memory of past visits and copy similar notes quickly into the current office visit if necessary. A clinician can highlight previous note text and copy it to the present note by clicking on the *Copy Prev Note* icon.

D. Along with the nine vital signs defined by SpringCharts, three additional custom measurements can be added to the program, such as peak flow rate or oxygen saturation.

E. The diagnosis (*Dx*) and prescription (*Rx*) navigation tabs differ from other navigation tabs by offering a search feature of the database rather than using pop-up text.

Concept Checkup 7.2

A. Changing the system's original medication information

B. Prescription(s)

C. By selecting an authorized prescriber in the User Preferences window

D. Procedures are chosen by first selecting the *Proc* navigation tab then the correct procedure category.

Rationales:

A. Prescribing information, such as the dosage and frequency, can be edited for a specific prescription without changing the system's original medication information.

B. If the provider has added her signature into SpringCharts, the digital signature is printed onto the prescription(s). The prescription can be sent electronically directly to the pharmacy's fax machine from SpringCharts.

C. For a non-authorized prescriber to order tests in the *Office Visit* screen, the user must have first selected an authorized prescriber in the *User Preferences* window—(*File > Preferences > User Preferences*). Once set up, the program allows the user to order tests.

D. Procedures are chosen by first selecting the *Proc* navigation tab then the correct procedure category.

Concept Checkup 7.3

A. No one
B. At the bottom of the existing *OV Note*

Rationales:

A. Once the office visit is locked, by selecting *Permanent Sign and Lock*, it cannot be unlocked or edited, even by the individual who permanently locked it. However, an addendum can be added to the bottom of an *Office Visit Note*, if needed.

B. The addendum is placed at the bottom of the existing *Office Visit Note*. The program automatically places a date-, time-, and initial-stamp on the addendum when it is saved. More than one addendum can be placed in the same *Office Visit Note*.

Chapter 9: Routine EHR Documentation

Concept Checkup 9.1

A. It is removed.
B. Patient's chart, patient's routine medications, and previous prescriptions.
C. It appears on the foreground of the recipient's SpringCharts' screen.

Rationales:

A. A *ToDo* item with a red check is a completed item and does not appear with subsequent log-ons. Clicking on a red check box reactivates the *ToDo* item. All active items remain on the user's *ToDo List* until completed.

B. After a message is initiated, it may be linked to a patient by selecting the *Change Pt* button in the original *New Message* window. The patient's name appears as the subject and the *Get Chart* and *Pt Info* buttons are activated. If needed, the *Rx* button provides access to the patient's routine medications and previous prescriptions.

C. Once *Sent*, the urgent message instantly appears on the foreground of the receiver's screen.

Concept Checkup 9.2

A. *Nurse Note* or an *Office Visit Note*
B. RTF (rich text format)
C. The *Tools* menu

Rationale:

A. Immunizations are automatically added to the immunization list when ordered in a *Nurse Note* or an *Office Visit Note*.

B. Under the *New* menu on the main screen, the user selects *New Patient Instruction*. The user has the option to either import an RTF (rich text format) file or create a patient instruction document.

C. SpringCharts' *Office Visit* screen and the *Nurse Note* screen provide access to a rudimentary draw program that enables the nurse to indicate the condition and location of wounds, scars, incisions, injuries, or procedures by drawing on prebuilt templates. Within either of these encounter notes, the nurse accesses the *Tools* menu and selects the *Draw* option.

Chapter 10: Patient Education

Concept Checkup 10.1

A. Patients need to be knowledgeable about their disease and its treatment.
B. 1. Healthy lifestyle
   2. Risk-reducing behaviors
   3. Developmental needs
   4. Activities of daily living
   5. Preventive self-care
C. 1. Interpreters for verbal communication
   2. Patient materials in language easily understood by patients

Rationale:

A. In order for patients to be active participants in their care, they must be knowledgeable about their disease and its treatment.
B. Standard 5B: Health Teaching and Health Promotion states, "The registered nurse employs strategies to promote health and a safe environment" The following is one measurement criterion that is used to evaluate this standard: Provides health teaching that addresses such topics as healthy lifestyles, risk-reducing behaviors, developmental needs, activities of daily living, and preventive self-care.
C. The National Standards on Culturally and Linguistically Appropriate Services (CLAS) require hospitals that receive federal funds, such as Medicare, to provide interpreters for verbal communication and patient materials, including educational materials, in language easily understood by patients. Nurses are responsible to ensure that the patient's linguistic needs are met whether education is provided in written or verbal form.

Concept Checkup 10.2

A. The Joint Commission
B. 1. Readiness to learn
   2. Preferred method of learning.
      Also an acceptable answer is: Barriers to learning
C. 1. Medications
   2. Equipment
   3. Procedures
      Other acceptable answers include: Hygiene, nutrition, hospital room orientation.
D. To provide specific actions that healthcare organizations can take to reduce the likelihood of medical errors.
E. 1. Reduce the likelihood of patient harm associated with the use of anticoagulant therapy.
   2. Implement evidence-based practices to prevent healthcare-associated infections due to multiple drug-resistant organisms in acute care hospitals.
   3. Implement best practices or evidence-based guidelines to prevent central line–associated bloodstream infections.
   4. When a patient leaves the organization's care, a complete and reconciled list of the patient's medications is provided directly to the patient, and the patient's family as needed, and the list is explained to the patient and/or family.
   5. The organization implements a fall reduction program that includes an evaluation of the effectiveness of the program.
      Other acceptable answers include: Identify the ways in which the patient and his or her family can report concerns about safety and encourage them to do so, and The organization selects a suitable method that enables healthcare

staff members to directly request additional assistance from a specially trained individual(s) when the patient's condition appears to be worsening.

Rationales:

A. The most widely recognized accreditation comes from The Joint Commission, a non-profit organization that accredits approximately 17,000 healthcare organizations (The Joint Commission, 2009a).

B. The Joint Commission requires that each patient be assessed before health education is initiated. This assessment must include readiness to learn, preferred method of learning, and barriers to learning.

C. All hospital patients are required to be provided education on medications, equipment, procedures, hygiene, and nutrition in addition to being oriented to their hospital room. Effectiveness of teaching strategies must be evaluated.

D. In 2002, The Joint Commission published the first National Patient Safety Goals (NPSG) in an effort to provide specific actions that healthcare organizations can take to reduce the likelihood of medical errors (The Joint Commission, 2010).

E. The list of NPSGs has evolved and grown through the years and several goals emphasize patient education. The following list indicates the required elements of patient education for the 2010 NPSGs:

- NPSG.03.05.01 "Reduce the likelihood of patient harm associated with the use of anticoagulant therapy." This goal requires education for patients and families that includes content on dietary restrictions, follow-up monitoring, adverse reactions, and drug interactions.

- NPSG.07.03.01 "Implement evidence-based practices to prevent health care associated infections due to multiple drug-resistant organisms in acute care hospitals." Patients who are infected with drug-resistant organisms and their families must be educated about the facility's strategies.

- NPSG.07.04.01 "Implement best practices or evidence-based guidelines to prevent central line-associated bloodstream infections." Before insertion of central lines, patients and their families must be educated about preventing infections associated with the line.

- NPSG.07.05.01 "Implement best practices for preventing surgical site infections." Before surgery, patients and their families must receive education about preventing infections in the surgical site.

- NPSG.08.03.01 "When a patient leaves the organization's care, a complete and reconciled list of the patient's medications is provided directly to the patient, and the patient's family as needed, and the list is explained to the patient and/or family." This goal requires education about discharge medications with documentation of the education.

- NPSG.09.02.01 "The organization implements a fall reduction program that includes an evaluation of the effectiveness of the program." Patients and their families must be educated about the program and specific strategies that are implemented for the patient.

- NPSG.13.01.01 "Identify the ways in which the patient and his or her family can report concerns about safety and encourage them to do so." In order to encourage patients' involvement in care, they must be educated about the reporting mechanisms that are available, infection control measures that should be implemented for the patient, and, if appropriate, the strategies the hospital uses to prevent adverse events during surgery.

- NPSG.16.01.01 "The organization selects a suitable method that enables health care staff members to directly request additional assistance from a specially trained individual(s) when the patient's condition appears to be worsening." The goal goes further to recommend that patients and family be taught to ask for assistance if the patient is worsening.

Concept Checkup 10.3

A. Health literacy refers to an individual's ability to understand health information in order to make informed decisions.

B. How confident do you feel completing medical forms?

C. 1. Language barriers
   2. Poor vision
   3. Poor hearing
   Other acceptable answers include pain, anxiety.

D. 1. Knowledge deficit
   2. Noncompliance
   3. Therapeutic regimen
   Another acceptable answer is ineffective management.

E. 1. Diet
   2. Diabetes management
   3. Disease process
   Other acceptable answers include breastfeeding, cardiac disease management, medication, prescribed activity, treatment regimen, discharge readiness, fall prevention behavior, risk control.

F. 1. Generic health intervention
   2. Parent education interventions
   3. Teaching interventions specific to disease process
   Other acceptable answers include admission care, childbirth preparation, discharge planning, nutrition counseling, smoking cessation assistance, vehicle safety promotion.

G. Teach-back

Rationales:

A. Health literacy refers to an individual's ability to understand health information in order to make informed decisions (Cornett, 2009).

B. While testing health literacy may be embarrassing to a patient, asking the patient how confident he feels completing medical forms alone has been shown to be a good indicator of health literacy (Powell, 2009).

C. While assessing the patient, the nurse should identify barriers to learning such as language, poor vision or hearing, pain, and anxiety.

D. Once the patient's learning needs have been assessed, the nurse assigns the appropriate NANDA-I nursing diagnoses. Typically, a nursing diagnosis of knowledge, deficient is used although nursing diagnoses of noncompliance or therapeutic regimen: ineffective management may also indicate a learning need.

E. Nursing Outcomes Classification (NOC) outcomes related to patient education are often the "knowledge" outcomes and may include knowledge of 30 different topics including breastfeeding, cardiac disease management, diabetes management, diet, disease process, medication, prescribed activity, and treatment regimen. Other NOC outcomes such as discharge readiness, fall prevention behavior, and risk control outcomes may also be appropriate outcomes for patient education (Center for Nursing Classification and Clinical Effectiveness, 2004).

F. Nursing interventions from the Nursing Interventions Classification (NIC) may include the generic health education intervention, parent education interventions, or "teaching" interventions specific to disease process, preoperative teaching, prescribed diet, and medications. In addition, other NIC interventions such as admission care, childbirth preparation, discharge planning, nutrition counseling, smoking cessation assistance, and vehicle safety promotion may also contain health education components.

G. This technique involves asking the patient to relay the instructional content back to the nurse. It allows the nurse to evaluate the patient's understanding of the information and validate or correct as indicated.

Chapter 11: Nurse Note Documentation—Level 3

Concept Checkup 11.1

A. The *Teaching* tab

B. *Interventions*

Rationales:

A. SpringCharts offers the nurse the ability to document patient education by clicking on the *Teaching* tab on the right side of the screen of the *Nurse Note*.

B. When the nurse moves to the next navigation tab, text entered in the *Teaching* tab is automatically placed in the *Interventions* section of the SOAPIER note.

Concept Checkup 11.2

A. True

B. 1. Outcome met this shift

2. Outcome not met this shift

3. Ongoing outcome

Rationales:

A. Since the nurse evaluates the outcomes selected earlier under the *NOC* tab, it is necessary to copy the outcomes being evaluated into the evaluation area of the nurse's note. To do this, the nurse clicks on the *NOC* tab and highlights and copies the text in the *NOC* free text area in the lower section of the screen. After returning to the *Evaluation* tab, the nurse clicks into the text field on the left and pastes the outcomes. At this point, the nurse is prepared to document the patient's progress toward a goal or resolve a goal that has been achieved.

B. Evaluation pop-up text provides common prebuilt evaluation statements such as *Outcome met this shift*, *Outcome not met this shift*, and *Ongoing outcome*.

Concept Checkup 11.3

A. 1. Vital signs

2. Pain

Rationale:

A. The patient needs frequent reassessments following a procedure such as a heart catheterization or surgery. This type of reassessment data is best documented in the *Reassessment* tab of SpringCharts. Under the *Reassessment* navigation tab on the right side of the *Nurse Note* screen is a list of items that are typically reassessed such as vital signs and pain.

Concept Checkup 11.4

A. Yes

B. True

Rationales:

A. In the lower left window of *flu Panel* within an *Office Visit* or *Nurse Note* screen, the *Create a Reminder* icon is available, enabling the clinician to set a personal ToDo/Reminder or to send one to another person in the clinic. The ToDo/Reminder is automatically linked to the patient's chart.

B. In the *New ToDo/Reminder* window a user clicks the *Send* button to send the reminder immediately, or clicks *Send Later* and designates a future date when the reminder should appear in the recipient's *ToDo List*.

Chapter 12: Advanced EHR Functionality

Concept Checkup 12.1

A. False
B. *Pending Tests*
C. Interface

Rationales:

A. When the user clicks the *Order Selected Tests* button at the bottom of the *Selected Tests* field, the test populates the *Tests field on the left of the Nurse Note* screen. If the incorrect test is inadvertently selected, the user clicks on the test in the left *Tests* field and answers *Yes* to the "Do you want to delete this reference to this test?" query to delete the test from the field.

B. Once ordered, diagnostic procedures are sent to the *Pending Tests* area of SpringCharts.

C. Diagnostic procedures remain in the *Pending Tests* area until the results are entered either manually or electronically through an interface with the testing facility.

Concept Checkup 12.2

A. 1. Gender
   2. Age
   3. Actions
   4. Recurring
B. To define preventive health guidelines and to evaluate guideline adherence
C. No chart evaluations have been set up on the SpringCharts server

Rationales:

A. In the setup window for *Chart Evaluations*, administrators define specifications for each preventive health measure by:
   1. Gender—Select whether an intervention or procedure is specific to male, female, or both.
   2. Age—Select the age range for which the criteria should be met.
   3. Actions—Indicate the *Test, Procedure*, or *Encounter* for which the guideline is recommended.
   4. Recurring—Specify if this is a recurring procedure or one-time event. If recurring, enter the time span in number of weeks or the number of screenings/procedures needed in the patient's lifetime.

B. SpringCharts' *Chart Evaluation* feature allows the nurse to define preventive health guidelines and then evaluate patients' charts to recommend guideline adherence.

C. The message *No criterion set* indicates that no chart evaluations have been set up on the SpringCharts server.

Concept Checkup 12.3

A. Amended
B. *Encounters*

Rationales:

A. *Nurse Note*s that have been permanently signed and locked cannot be amended. On occasion, after completing and locking a *Nurse Note* entry, a nurse may realize that all appropriate information was not documented. The *New Note* under the *New* menu in the patient chart allows the nurse to do additional charting, or what is commonly referred to as a late entry or addendum. An addendum should always begin with the words "Late entry" to indicate that documentation occurred after the initial record of the event.

B. Notes are saved as *Encounters* and are viewable for all users under the *Encounters* tab in the *Care Tree*.

Concept Checkup 12.4

A. Printing, faxing

B. Pending

Rationales:

A. Both the *Print* button within the *Nurse Note* screen and the *Print* button located in the patient's chart allow printing/faxing of the *Nurse Note* itself. The *Nurse Note* prints in the SOAPIER format with the patient identifiers in the footer of each page.

B. Test results can be included in the *Nurse Note*. If test results are complete and have been entered into a test that was ordered within the *Nurse Note*, the printed *Nurse Note* will contain the name and results of the test. If test results have not been entered into the pending test area, the *Nurse Note* will simply state *pending* beside the name of the test.

A

AAACN American Academy of Ambulatory Care Nursing. Founded in 1978, the mission of the AAACN is to advance the specialty of ambulatory nursing. Ambulatory nursing occurs in a variety of settings such as primary care clinics, physician practices, nurse practitioner practices, ambulatory surgery centers, and urgent care centers. It is characterized by brief patient encounters that include intense education to allow the patient and family to manage the patient's health (AAACN, n.d.).

AANP American Academy of Nurse Practitioners. Founded in 1985, the AANP is the professional organization for nurse practitioners with a mission to promote excellence in practice, education, and research. In addition, the AANP influences healthcare policy and promotes the image of nurse practitioners (AANP, n.d.).

Accreditation A process whereby a healthcare organization is evaluated for adherence to standards of care; indicates that the facility provides quality care.

Addendum An addendum is a note added subsequent to the original documentation to provide supplemental clinical information.

AMA American Medical Association. Founded in 1847, the AMA's purpose is to promote the art and science of medicine in order to improve professional and public health concerns in America's healthcare system (AMA, n.d.).

Ambulatory The ability to walk or move from one place to another.

Ambulatory Healthcare Provision of healthcare services in brief episodes to patients who are not admitted overnight to a hospital; may include, but is not limited to, outpatient clinics, urgent care centers, emergency rooms, ambulatory or same-day surgery centers, diagnostic and imaging centers, primary care centers, community health centers, occupational health centers, mental health clinics, and group practices.

ARRA American Recovery and Reinvestment Act. Legislation passed by Congress in 2009 to stimulate the economy through investments in infrastructure, unemployment benefits, transportation, education, and healthcare.

ASP Application Server Provider. Enables access to an EHR via the Internet; the EHR software and database are housed and maintained by a separate company in a remote location.

B

BMI Body Mass Index. Measurement of choice for studying obesity. Calculated by a mathematical formula that divides weight by height in meters squared ($BMI = kg/m^2$).

C

Care Tree List of categories in the EHR that includes encounters (progress notes), tests, excuse notes, letters, reports, and other current records.

Category Preferences Table on the SpringCharts server that enables the clinic administrator to create customized predetermined lists of healthcare data that are displayed in SpringCharts on each computer to enable rapid selection of items to build the face sheet.

CBE Charting by Exception. Method of documentation in which normal parameters are delineated; only documentation of deviations to the preestablished parameters is required.

CCD Continuity of Care Document. A core set of provider-oriented health data reflecting the most relevant and timely facts about a patient's health care. It is vendor and technology neutral, enabling the electronic access of patient information between healthcare providers and other entities.

CCHIT Certification Commission for Health Information Technology. An independent initiative to accelerate the adoption of EHRs with a credible certification program.

Chart Alert Text that appears in red above the *Encounters* category on the EHR's *Care Tree* to notify the user of important patient information.

CHI Consolidated Health Informatics. A federal government initiative that seeks to provide adoption of health information interoperability standards for health vocabulary and messaging.

Clinical Practice Guidelines Statements used to direct care that indicate evidence-based diagnosis and treatment for clinical conditions.

CMS Centers for Medicare and Medicaid Services, formerly known as the Health Care Financing Administration (HCFA). Federal agency responsible for administering Medicare, Medicaid, the Health Insurance Portability and Accountability Act (HIPAA), and other health-related programs.

Computerized Charting Use of electronic sources and databases to record data relating to patient care.

Connectivity The ability to make and maintain a connection between two or more points in a telecommunications system allowing for viewing and/or transfer of data from one computer system to another.

COW/WOW Computers on Wheels, known also as WOW—workstation on wheels. A computer placed on a mobile device to allow movement around an office, unit, and patient rooms.

CPT Codes Current Procedure Terminology Codes. Five-digit codes developed by the American Medical Association (AMA); adopted by insurance carriers and managed care companies as the means to identify common procedures, e.g., "82270—Fecal occult blood test."

Critical Pathway/Care Map A comprehensive, preestablished, interdisciplinary, standardized plan of care for stable patients experiencing a particular disease process or procedure; outcomes are usually predictable.

Critical Results Grossly abnormal test results that may be life-threatening to the patient.

Critical Test A diagnostic test that requires rapid communication of results whether normal or abnormal.

D

Database A computer-based, comprehensive collection of related information organized for convenient access.

Diagnostic Related Group (DRG) System to classify patients into one of approximately 500 groups which are expected to have similar hospital resource use; developed for Medicare as part of the prospective payment system. DRGs are grouped by medical diagnoses, procedures, age, gender, and the presence of complications or co-morbidities; healthcare agencies are reimbursed a predetermined amount per DRG or procedure regardless of the patient's length of stay or cost of treatment.

DICOM The Digital Imaging and Communications in Medicine Standard. Created to aid distribution and viewing of medical images, such as CT scans, MRIs, ultrasound, and x-rays.

Documentation Act of recording patient information and patient care activities in written or electronic format; serves as legal evidence of care provided and poses ethical concerns regarding a patient's right to privacy.

Drug Formulary A database of approved medications in drug therapy categories and includes information on preparation, safety, effectiveness, and cost.

E

EDD Estimated Date of Delivery. Pregnancy due date calculated from the date of a pregnant woman's last menstrual period.

EHR Electronic Health Record. A computerized systematic collection of health information in digital format about individual patients. An EHR is interoperable, having the capable of sharing information across different health care settings.

Electronic Chart Repository for patient health data created through computer automation in the healthcare office/hospital/clinic. Similar to the traditional paper chart, it holds such static information as the patient's health history and health problems as well as the dynamic information including encounter notes, tests, letters, and reports concerning the patient.

e-MAR Electronic Medication Administration Record. Computerized method for documentation of drug administration.

E&M Code Evaluation and Management Code. Five-digit number used by healthcare providers to report evaluation and management services with a patient such as obtaining a health history, a physical examination, and healthcare decision making. E&M encounters may be inpatient, outpatient, or a consultation and occur in a variety of healthcare settings.

Encounters A tab in the SpringCharts *Care Tree* that stores many documents created from encounters with the patient.

Encrypted Change of electronic data from its original format so that it is secure and unintelligible to unauthorized parties and then "decrypted" back into its original form for use.

E-prescribing Electronic prescribing. Use of computerized tools, usually embedded in an EHR program, to create and sign prescriptions for medicines; replaces handwritten prescriptions. Electronic prescriptions are sent to pharmacies over the Internet via a clearinghouse.

F

Face Sheet Portion of the EHR that contains more constant patient information such as allergies, problem list, past health history (PMHX), and so on.

FMHX Family Medical History. SpringCharts category for recording family health history in the patient's face sheet.

Focus Charting/DAR Documentation format in which all entries are related to a patient problem, or focus, which may be expressed as a nursing diagnosis. D (data), A (actions), R (response) are recorded for each focus using a three-column format to chart patient assessment data, actions taken based on the assessment, and the response of the patient to the actions.

G

Graphic User Interface Software program screen that can display icons, sub-windows, text fields, and menus designed to standardize and simplify the use of the computer program by typing in fields and by using a mouse to manipulate text and images.

H

HL7 Health Level Seven. International computer language by which various healthcare systems communicate; currently the selected standard for the interfacing of clinical data between software programs in most institutions.

H&P Report History & Physical Report. Documentation of the patient's health history and physical examination; typically the initial clinical evaluation and examination of the patient that is updated with subsequent visits.

I

ICD-9 Codes International Classification of Diseases, Volume 9. The international standard diagnostic classification for all data dealing with the incidence and prevalence of disease in large populations and for other health management purposes, e.g., 474.00—Tonsillitis (chronic).

Imperial Units Having to do with weights and measures that conform to standards legally established in Great Britain and widely used in the United States.

Inpatient Care Care provided to patients in a hospital or long-term setting that involves staying overnight after admission is ordered by a primary care provider.

Interoperability Ability of a software program to accept, send, or communicate data from its database to other software programs from multiple vendors allowing programs to exchange and use information (Sensmeier, 2007).

Intranet Technologies Privately maintained computer network that provides secure accessibility to authorized people enabling sharing of software, databases, and files.

IOM Institute of Medicine. Federal agency that gives advice and information about government policies affecting human health.

L

Lab Analyte Blood test compound subject to specific chemical analysis. A lab panel is composed of multiple analytes that undergo analysis. For example, an electrolyte panel is composed of sodium, potassium, chloride, and carbon dioxide analytes.

LAN Local Area Network. A wired or wireless connection of computers on a single campus or facility.

Licensed Independent Practitioner Individual licensed to provide healthcare without supervision.

M

MAR Medication Administration Record. Form used to document drug administration.

Medical Diagnosis Identification of an illness or disease.

Medicare Part A Part of the federally funded Medicare insurance program that covers hospitals, skilled nursing facilities, home health agencies, and other non-ambulatory services.

Medicare Part B Part of the federally funded Medicare insurance program that covers medical providers' supervision, outpatient hospital care, diagnostic tests, ambulance services, and other ambulatory services.

Metric Units Having to do with weights and measures relating to the metric system, also known as the International System of Units. Commonly used in healthcare measurement.

MIPPA Medicare Improvements for Patients and Providers Act of 2008. Establishes Medicare reimbursement for providers, reduces racial and ethnic disparities among Medicare recipients, and places limits on certain rapidly growing Medicare supplemental insurance policies.

N

NANDA-I North American Nursing Diagnosis Association–International. Organization responsible for developing standardized diagnostic terminology to reflect nursing practice (nursing diagnoses).

Narrative Charting Chronologic recounting of relevant patient information throughout the course of the nurse's time with the patient; documentation is recorded in paragraph form.

NDC National Drug Code. Ten-digit, three-segment number that serves as a unique identifier for each prescription drug and insulin product and indicates the medication labeler, strength, dosage form, formulation, package size, and type (U.S. Food & Drug Administration, 2010).

NIC Nursing Interventions Classification. Standardized classification of actions performed by nurses, both independent and collaborative.

NOC Nursing Outcomes Classification. Standardized classification of statements for evaluating the effectiveness of nursing interventions.

NPSG National Patient Safety Goals. A set of objectives developed by The Joint Commission (2010) with specific actions to reduce medical errors.

Nurse Note In SpringCharts, documentation of nursing care of a patient within an acute care facility including the patient's chief complaints, vital signs, physical assessment, goals, interventions, and so on.

Nursing Diagnosis "Statement that describes the client's actual or potential response to a health problem that the nurse is licensed and competent to treat" (Potter & Perry, 2009, p. 248). The client may be a person, family, or community.

Nursing Informatics Nursing specialty that integrates nursing, computer, and information sciences to manage and communicate data, information, and knowledge in nursing practice; supports patients and nurses in decision making in a variety of healthcare settings.

Nursing Standards of Care Statements that describe a nurse's responsibilities and accountabilities; indicate the minimum acceptable level of nursing care.

O

Objective Data Information collected by the nurse through observation, auscultation, palpation, or smell. May include information obtained from the health record such as diagnostic results and medical diagnoses.

ONC The Office of the National Coordinator for Health Information Technology. The ONC is organizationally located within the Office of the Secretary for the U.S. Department of Health and Human Services (HHS). It is charged with coordination of nationwide efforts to implement and use the most advanced health information technology and the electronic exchange of health information.

OV Office Visit. Used in SpringCharts to designate the graphic user interface window in which the encounter note is created.

P

Patient Education Process in which healthcare professionals provide information to patients, families, and communities that ideally results in enhanced ability of the patient, family, or community to actively participate in health promotion and health maintenance or to cope with alterations in health or ability.

Patient's Bill of Rights List of basic entitlements that patients, their surrogates, or healthcare decision makers can expect from healthcare facilities and providers.

PHR Personal Health Records. Electronic access to personal health information via the Internet that allows individuals to update and send inquires to their healthcare provider about prescriptions, appointments, or concerns.

PIE P—problem, I—interventions, E—evaluation. Method of documentation that focuses on patient problems or nursing diagnoses, interventions to address/resolve the problems, and evaluation of the effectiveness of the intervention; PIE notes are in narrative format and are labeled according to the patient's problems.

PMHX Past Medical History. SpringCharts category for recording past health history in the patient's face sheet.

PMS Practice Management Software. A software program that manages financial transactions, billing of insurance claims, patient statements, and so on.

Point of Care Time and location of care being given to a patient from a healthcare provider.

POMR Problem-Oriented Medical Record. Method of documentation that emphasizes the patient's problems; data are gathered and organized, then a problem list is generated followed by a nursing plan of action to alleviate the problems; PIE, SOAP, and SOAP(IER) are traditional POMR formats.

Q

Quality Improvement (QI) The continuous efforts of healthcare professionals, patients and caregivers, to make the necessary changes that will lead to better patient care outcomes and better system performances

R

Record All information pertaining to the patient; includes electronic and handwritten data.

S

Server A main computer designed to provide services to client, workstation, or desktop computers over a local network or the Internet. Many network software programs have a server component and workstation component.

SOAP S—subjective, O—objective, A—assessment, P—plan. Method of charting that focuses on gathering both patient-reported and nurse-observed data, drawing conclusions about the problems the patient is experiencing, and creating a plan to address the problems; commonly used in both inpatient and outpatient settings.

SOAP(IE) S—subjective, O—objective, A—assessment, P—plan, I—intervention, and E—evaluation. Method of charting that adds documentation for interventions and evaluation to the SOAP note and enables nurses in an inpatient setting to detail the nursing process more thoroughly.

SOAP(IER) S—subjective, O—objective, A—assessment, P—plan, I—intervention, E—evaluation, I—interventions, E—evaluation, and R—revisions. Expanded method of documentation that allows for documentation of nursing actions, evaluation of patient response to those actions, and changes to the plan of care based on progress toward outcome attainment; used in many areas of nursing since it reflects the nursing process.

Source-Oriented Charting/Source Records Form of narrative charting in which each discipline documents in a separate section of the chart.

Standardized Language. Common terminology that supports interoperability, security, and privacy; an approved format agreed upon by experts.

Standards An approved format agreed upon by experts that established common terminology that supports interoperability, security, and privacy (Sensmeier, 2007).

Standards of Practice Defined by the American Nurses Association (2004) as "authoritative statements by which the nursing profession describes the responsibilities for which its practitioners are accountable" (p. 1).

Subjective Data Descriptions given by the patient or family about the patient's condition.

T

Tablet PC Tablet Personal Computer. A portable, handheld computer that may allow the user to document directly on the screen with a stylus pen.

Telehealth The use of electronic and communication technology to deliver health information and services from distances through a standard telephone line.

TJC The Joint Commission. An independent, non-profit organization that sets standards of quality for healthcare organizations and evaluates compliance with these standards, providing accreditation for organizations that demonstrate excellence (TJC, 2010).

U

User Preferences Setup window in SpringCharts that enables each user to preset the default practice name, provider name, schedule, and various other features that are displayed when the user logs into the program.

V

VIS Vaccination Information Statement. Forms developed by the Centers for Disease Control and Prevention (CDC) to explain the risks and benefits of vaccines; must be given to a patient or guardian before administration of certain immunizations.

Photo Credits

Chapter 1 opener: © Van D. Bucher/Photo Researchers, Inc.

Chapter 2 opener: © Jose Inc/Blend Images RF/ Photolibrary RF

Chapter 3 opener: © Tetra Images/Agefotostock RF

Chapter 4 opener: © FURGOLLE/BSIP/Corbis

Chapter 5 opener: © Helen King/Corbis RF

Chapter 6 opener: © Purestock/Getty Images RF

Chapter 7 opener: © Michael N. Paras/Corbis RF

Chapter 8 opener: © Tripod/Getty Images

Chapter 9 opener: © Rachel Frank/Corbis RF

Chapter 10 opener: © Corbis Super/Alamy RF

Chapter 11 opener: © Ocean/Corbis RF

Chapter 12 opener: © Lester Lefkowitz/Getty Images

Chapter 13 opener: © Lester Lefkowitz/Getty Images

Chapter 14 opener: © Jupiterimages/Getty Images

Index

List of Exercises by Diagnosis

SRA Reading Mastery

Signature Edition

Language Arts
Presentation Book A
Grade 2

Siegfried Engelmann
Karen Lou Seitz Davis
Jerry Silbert

 SRA

Columbus, Ohio

Table of Contents

Curriculum Map *following final lesson*

Before presenting the program, see the Placement section of the guide. If students have completed the Grade 1 Language Arts program, start the students on Lesson 5.

Note: Each student will need a set of crayons that includes pink, purple and gray.

Objectives

- **Follow directions involving left and right.** (Exercise 2)
  Note: To demonstrate **left** and **right,** do not face the students. Face the same direction they are facing.
- **Answer questions involving all, some, and none.** (Exercise 3)
- **Fix up pictures to show a true some statement.** (Exercise 4)
- **Apply an if-then rule.** (Exercise 5)
- **Compose and write a parallel sentence based on a single picture.** (Exercise 6)
- **Listen to a story and answer comprehension questions.** (Exercise 7)
- **Make a picture consistent with the details of a story.** (Exercise 8)

WORKBOOK

EXERCISE 1 Introduction

1. (Hand out student workbooks.)
   These are workbooks for your language program. This program is very tough, and you have to work very hard. You'll also get to do some things like color, make up pictures and tell stories. But for most of the things you'll work on, I'll try to fool you. And I will fool you unless you listen very carefully.

2. We'll start with left and right.
   Remember, if you don't listen carefully, I'll fool you.

EXERCISE 2 Actions

Left/Right

1. I'm going to show you about **left** and **right.** (Face the same direction the students are facing.)
- (Hold out your right hand.)

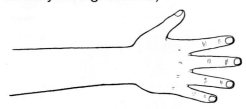

- This is my **right** hand. Everybody, hold out your **right** hand. ✔
  Hands down.
- (Hold out your left hand.)
- This is my **left** hand. Everybody, hold out your **left** hand. ✔

2. I'll hold out my hands. You tell me if I hold out my left hand or my right hand.
- (Hold out your left hand.)
  Everybody, which hand? (Signal.) *Left.*
- (Hold out your right hand.)
  Everybody, which hand? (Signal.) *Right.*
- (Repeat step 2 until firm.)

3. Your turn: Hold out your **right** hand. ✔
  Hands down.
- Hold out your **left** hand. ✔
  Hands down.
- Everybody, stand up.
  (Face the same direction the students are facing.)

4. I'll show you how to turn a corner to the **right.** Watch. (Turn a 90° corner to the right.)
- Here's another corner to the **right.** Watch. (Turn another 90° corner to the right.)

5. Your turn: Turn a corner to the **right.** ✔
- Turn another corner to the **right.** ✔
- Turn a corner to the **left.** ✔
- Turn another corner to the **left.** ✔
- Everybody, sit down.
  Good following directions.

EXERCISE 3 All, Some, None

Introduction

1. You're going to do a lot of work with statements that tell about **all, some** or **none.**
- Watch. (Hold up **all** 5 fingers on a hand.)
  I'm holding up **all** the fingers on this hand.

- (Hold up 2 fingers.)
  Now I'm holding up **some** of the fingers.
- What am I holding up now? (Signal.) *Some of the fingers.*
- (Hold up all 5 fingers.)
  What am I holding up now? (Signal.) *All of the fingers.*
- (Hold up closed fist.)
  Now I'm holding up **none** of the fingers.
- What am I holding up now? (Signal.) *None of the fingers.*
2. Watch. (Hold up 4 fingers.)
   What am I holding up now? (Signal.) *Some of the fingers.*
- (Hold up 3 fingers.)
  What am I holding up now? (Signal.) *Some of the fingers.*
- (Hold up fist.)
  What am I holding up now? (Signal.) *None of the fingers.*
- (Hold up all 5 fingers.)
  What am I holding up now? (Signal.) *All of the fingers.*
- (Repeat step 2 until firm.)

EXERCISE 4   All, Some, None

Application

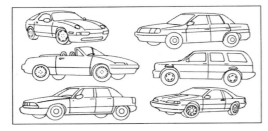

1. Everybody, take out your crayons.
- (Write on the board:)

> **Lesson 1**

- This says **lesson 1.** Open your workbook and find the page that has **lesson 1** written at the top of the page. It's right near the beginning of the workbook. ✔
2. For some things you'll be doing in your workbook, you'll have to find the right numbers or letters.
- Everybody, touch the big **A.** That's part A. ✔
- Everybody, touch part **B.** ✔
- Everybody, touch part **C.** ✔
3. Everybody, touch part **A** again. ✔
   Look at the cars.
- I'll say statements about the cars. Some of these statements are wrong. You'll say **yes** or **no** for each statement.

4. Listen: **Some** of those cars are blue. Is that right? (Signal.) *No.*
- Listen: **All** of those cars are blue. Is that right? (Signal.) *No.*
- Listen: **None** of those cars are blue. Is that right? (Signal.) *Yes.*
- (Repeat step 4 until firm.)
5. This time, I'll say statements. You'll say **true** or **false.** You'll say **true** if what I say is right. You'll say **false** if it's wrong.

6. Listen: **All** of those cars are blue. True or false? (Signal.) *False.*
- Listen: **None** of those cars are blue. True or false? (Signal.) *True.*
- Listen: **Some** of those cars are blue. True or false? (Signal.) *False.*
- (Repeat step 6 until firm.)
7. I'm going to say a statement about those cars that is **false.** You'll fix up the picture to make the statement **true.**
- Here's the statement: **Some** of those cars are blue. Is that true or false? (Signal.) *False.*
- You can make it true by coloring **some** of the cars so they are blue.
- Quickly color **some** of the cars, not **all** of them. Raise your hand when you're finished.
  (Observe students and give feedback.)
8. Everybody, hold up your workbook if you fixed up the picture so that **some** of the cars are blue. ✔
- You did it the right way.

EXERCISE 5   If-Then Application

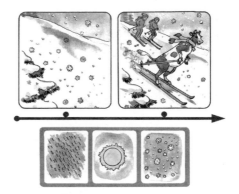

1. Everybody, find part B. ✔
   The pictures on the arrow show what the weather will do and what a cow named Clarabelle will do.
2. Everybody, touch the arrow. ✔
   The first picture shows what the weather will do.

- Everybody, what's coming out of the sky in that picture? (Signal.) *Snow.*
- Touch the second picture. ✔
  That picture shows what Clarabelle will do. Everybody, what will Clarabelle do? (Signal.) *Go skiing.*
3. We have to make up a rule for these pictures. The rule starts with **if.** The **if** part tells about the **first** picture. Listen to the **if** part: If it snows . . .
- Your turn: If it snows, what will Clarabelle do? (Signal.) *Go skiing.*
- Yes, **if it snows, Clarabelle will go skiing.**
4. Everybody, say the whole **if** rule. Get ready. (Signal.) *If it snows, Clarabelle will go skiing.*
- (Repeat step 4 until firm.)
5. That's the rule for these pictures. Look at the pictures below the arrow. They show things that **might** happen. You have to figure out what Clarabelle will do.
- Touch the first picture **below** the arrow. ✔
  Everybody, what's happening in that picture? (Signal.) *It's raining.*
- My turn: What will Clarabelle do if it rains? We don't know. We only know what she'll do if it **snows.**
- Your turn: What will Clarabelle do if it rains? (Signal.) *We don't know.*
- Right, we don't know.
6. Touch the second picture below the arrow. ✔
  What's happening in that picture? (Call on a student. Idea: *The sun's shining.*)
- Think big. Everybody, what will Clarabelle do if the sun shines? (Signal.) *We don't know.*
- Right, we don't know.
7. Touch the last picture below the arrow. ✔
  Everybody, what's happening in that picture? (Signal.) *It's snowing.*
- Everybody, what will Clarabelle do if it snows? (Signal.) *Go skiing.*
- Right, that's the rule: **If it snows, Clarabelle will go skiing.**
8. Two of the pictures below the arrow show things that our rule does **not** tell us about. So we don't know what Clarabelle will do if these things happen. Listen: Cross out the two pictures that show things our rule does **not** tell us about. Raise your hand when you're finished.
  (Observe students and give feedback.)

9. (Call on a student.) Which two pictures did you cross out? (Idea: *The picture that shows it's raining and the picture that shows the sun's shining.*)
- Why did you cross them out? (Call on a student. Idea: *Our rule does not tell us about them.*)
10. Raise your hand if you crossed out the pictures of it raining and the sun shining. ✔ I couldn't fool you.

EXERCISE 6 Writing Parallel Sentences

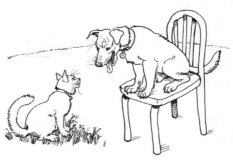

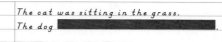

The cat was sitting in the grass.
The dog ██████████████████████.

1. Find part C. ✔
  You're going to write about this picture on lined paper. (Hand out a piece of lined paper to each student.) Write your name on the top line of the paper. ✔
2. The picture shows what the cat and the dog were doing. The cat and the dog were sitting. One of them was sitting in the grass. Which animal was that? (Signal.) *The cat.*
- Where was the dog sitting? (Call on a student. Idea: *On the chair.*)
3. (Point to the first sentence below the picture.)
  The first sentence is written and part of the next sentence is written.
- The first sentence says: **The cat was sitting in the grass.** Everybody, say that sentence. (Signal.) *The cat was sitting in the grass.*
- The second sentence should say: **The dog was sitting on the chair.** Say that sentence. (Signal.) *The dog was sitting on the chair.*

4. I'll say the first sentence. You tell me what the second sentence should say.
   - **The cat was sitting in the grass.** Tell me about the dog. (Signal.) *The dog was sitting on the chair.*

5. Look at your lined paper. ✔
   - The line that goes up and down is the margin. What is the up-and-down line? (Signal.) *The margin.*
   - Here's the rule about the margin: You start writing words just after the margin. Where do you start writing words? (Signal.) *Just after the margin.*

6. Now copy the first sentence just as it's written below the picture. Remember, start the sentence just after the margin. Begin the sentence with a capital **T.** Don't write capital letters anywhere except at the beginning of the sentence. Put a period at the end of the sentence. Raise your hand when you're finished with the first sentence. (Observe students and give feedback.)

7. (Write on the board:)

chair	on

   - Here are words you'll need: **chair . . . on.** Spell them correctly in your second sentence. Copy and complete the second sentence. Remember to start with a capital letter and put a period at the end of the sentence. Begin your sentence just after the margin.
     (Observe students and give feedback. Praise students with specific comments such as:) Good starting with a capital; good starting just after the margin; good spelling; good putting a period at the end of the sentence.

8. **(Optional:)** Skip a line on your paper and write both sentences again. Write: The cat was sitting in the grass. The dog was sitting on the chair.
   (Observe students and give feedback.)

9. (Collect and correct papers. Students who do not complete writing both pairs of sentences may complete their work after the lesson or for homework.)

EXERCISE 7   Paul Paints Plums

Storytelling

- Everybody, I'm going to read you a silly story. Listen to the things that happen in the story because you're going to fix up a picture that shows part of the story.
- This is a story about Paul. Listen:

Everybody has favorite colors. Some people love red. Some people love yellow. Others love blue or green. Some like brown or black. Well, Paul had his favorite colors, too. But his favorite colors were not red or blue, or brown or black, or even white or yellow. His two favorite colors were pink and purple. It's hard to say which color Paul liked the most. Sometimes, he would prefer pink. At other times, he preferred purple.

Well, Paul also loved to paint. And whenever he painted, he'd use one of his favorite colors. One day, he was on his porch painting a picture of purple plums.

- Everybody, what was Paul's favorite color on that day? (Signal.) *Purple.*

Paul said, "Painting pictures of purple plums on the porch is perfect."

- That's hard to say. Listen again: Painting pictures of purple plums on the porch is perfect.
- Who can say that? (Call on a student.) *Painting pictures of purple plums on the porch is perfect.*

As Paul was painting, he dripped some purple paint on the floor of the porch. "Oh, pooh," he said. "Puddles of purple paint are on the porch, but I can fix it." So he got a great big brush and started to paint the whole floor of the porch purple.

- Everybody, is that the way **you** would fix up the purple puddles? (Signal.) *No.*
- How would you fix up the purple puddles? (Call on a student. Praise reasonable response.)

But here's what Paul did: He got a great big brush and started to paint the whole porch purple. But just when he was almost finished, he backed into his painting and the painting fell against the window. It didn't break the window, but it got purple paint on the window pane.

Listen: Why did purple paint get on the window pane? (Call on a student. Idea: *The painting fell against the window.*)
- So now the floor of the porch is purple and there is purple paint on the window pane.

"Whoa," Paul said. "Now there are patches of purple paint on the pane. But I can fix it."

He tried wiping the purple paint from the pane, but that didn't work. At last Paul said, "I fixed the floor of the porch and I can fix that pane the same way."

- What do you think he'll do? (Call on a student. Idea: *Paint the whole window pane purple.*)

Paul said, "A purple pane may look perfectly pleasing." And he painted the whole window pane purple. But just as he was painting the last corner of the pane, some purple paint dripped on the wall.

- What do you think he'll do? (Call on a student. Idea: *Paint the whole wall purple.*)
- Let's see.

The purple paint dripped on the wall. "Wow," Paul said, "perhaps purple paint would look perfect on the wall." So you know what he did next. He painted the whole wall purple. And just as he was finishing up the last corner

of the wall, his brother came out of the house. As his brother walked onto the porch, he rubbed against the wall and got a great smear of purple paint on his pants. Paul's brother tried to wipe the purple paint from the pants, but he just smeared the paint.

"I'm a mess," his brother said.

"So you are," Paul agreed. Then Paul smiled at his brother and said, "But brother, don't worry. I can fix it." And he did just that.

- What do you think he did? (Call on a student. Ideas: *Paul painted his brother purple* or *Paul painted his brother's pants purple.*)

EXERCISE 8 **Details**

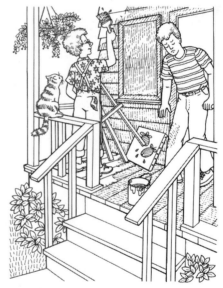

1. Everybody, find the picture of Paul. That's part D. It's on the next page of your workbook. ✔

   This picture takes place after Paul had already painted some things.
   - What did he start out painting? (Call on a student. Idea: *A picture of purple plums.*)
   - What did he paint purple next? (Call on a student. Idea: *The floor of the porch.*)
   - Why did he paint the floor of the porch purple? (Call on a student. Idea: *Because he dripped purple paint on the porch.*)

- What did he paint after the floor of the porch? (Call on a student. Idea: *The whole window pane.*)
- Why did he paint the window pane purple? (Call on a student. Idea: *Because he got purple paint on the window pane.*)
- What did he paint after he painted the window pane? (Call on a student. Idea: *The wall.*)
- Why did he paint the wall purple? (Call on a student. Idea: *Because paint dripped on the wall.*)
- What's he doing in the picture? (Call on a student. Idea: *Painting the wall.*)
- Who is that coming out the door? (Signal.) *His brother.*
  I can see that smear of paint on his brother's pants.
- What's Paul going to do after this picture? (Signal.) *Paint his brother's pants.*

2. Listen: Get a purple crayon and put a little purple mark on everything that is **already** purple. Don't put a purple mark on anything that Paul hasn't painted purple yet. Raise your hand when you're finished. (Observe students and give feedback.)
- Name the things you marked with purple. (Call on several students. Praise students who name the plums, the floor of the porch, the window, the wall and the smear on the pants.)
3. Your turn: Fix up the picture so that all these things are purple—the plums, the floor of the porch, the window, the smear on Paul's brother's pants and most of the wall. Later, you can color the other parts of the picture any color you wish.

Objectives

- Compose and write a parallel sentence based on a single picture. (Exercise 1)
- Follow directions involving **left** and **right**. (Exercise 2)
- **Fix up pictures to show a true all statement. (Exercise 3)**
- Apply an if-then rule. (Exercise 4)
- **Determine which clue eliminates specific members of a class. (Exercise 5)**
- Listen to a story and answer comprehension questions. (Exercise 6)
- **Circle the word true or false for statements about a story. (Exercise 7)**
- Make a picture consistent with details of a story. (Exercise 8)

EXERCISE 1 Writing Parallel Sentences

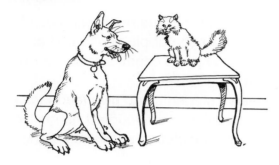

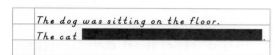

1. Open your workbook to lesson 2 and find part A. ✔
   You're going to write about this picture on lined paper. **(Hand out a piece of lined paper to each student.)** Write your name on the top line of the paper. ✔

2. The picture shows what the dog and the cat were doing. The dog and the cat were sitting. One of them was sitting on the table. Which animal was that? (Signal.) *The cat.*

   - Where was the dog sitting? (Signal.) *On the floor.*

3. (Point to the first sentence below the picture.)
   The first sentence is written and part of the next sentence is written.

- The first sentence says: **The dog was sitting on the floor.** Say that sentence. (Signal.) *The dog was sitting on the floor.*

- The second sentence should say: **The cat was sitting on the table.** Say that sentence. (Signal.) *The cat was sitting on the table.*

4. I'll say the first sentence. You tell me what the second sentence should say.

- **The dog was sitting on the floor.** Tell me about the cat. (Signal.) *The cat was sitting on the table.*

5. (Write on the board:)

table

- Here's a word you'll need: **table.** Spell it correctly in your sentence.

6. Write both sentences on your lined paper. Start writing just after the margin. Copy the sentence that is written and complete the second sentence. Remember to start both sentences with a capital letter and put a period at the end of each sentence. (Observe students and give feedback.)

7. **(Optional:)** Skip a line on your paper and write both sentences again. Write: The dog was sitting on the floor. The cat was sitting on the table.
   (Observe students and give feedback.)

8. (Collect and correct papers. Students who do not complete writing both pairs of sentences may complete their work after the lesson or for homework.)

EXERCISE 2   Actions

Left/Right

1. Get ready to follow some directions that involve **left** and **right**.
   (Face the same direction the students are facing.)
   - Watch me. I'm going to take two tiny steps to my **right**.
     (Move **sideways** two tiny steps to your right.)
   - Watch again. I'm going to take two tiny steps to my **left**.
     (Move **sideways** two tiny steps to your left.)
2. Now it's your turn: Everybody, stand up.
   - Take two tiny steps to your **right**. ✔
   - Take two tiny steps to your **left**. ✔
   - Turn a corner to your **left**. ✔
   - Turn another corner to your **left**. ✔
   - Turn **two** corners to your **right**. ✔
   - Sit down.
3. Here come some tough directions.
   - Everybody, listen: You're going to put your **right** hand on your desk and your **left** hand on your head. Listen again: Put your **right** hand on your desk and your **left** hand on your head. Do it.
     (Praise students who respond correctly.)
   - Hands down.
4. Everybody, listen: You're going to put your **left** hand on your desk and your **right** hand on your left hand.
   - Listen again: Put your **left** hand on your desk and your **right** hand on your left hand. Do it. (Praise students who respond correctly.)
5. Raise your right hand if you followed all those tough, tough directions. ✔
   Good for you.

WORKBOOK

EXERCISE 3   All, Some, None

Application

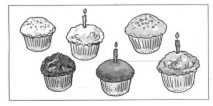

1. Everybody, find part B. ✔
   - Look at the cupcakes.

- I'll say statements about the cupcakes. You'll say **true** or **false**. Remember, say **true** if the statement is right; say **false** if the statement is wrong.
2. Listen: **All** of the cupcakes have a candle. True or false? (Signal.) *False.*
   - Listen: **Some** of the cupcakes have a candle. True or false? (Signal.) *True.*
   - Listen: **None** of the cupcakes have a candle. True or false? (Signal.) *False.*
   - (Repeat step 2 until firm.)
3. I'm going to say a statement about the cupcakes that is **false**. You'll fix up the picture to make the statement **true**.
   - Here's the statement. **All** of the cupcakes have a candle. Is that true or false? (Signal.) *False.*
   - You can make it true by drawing candles. Quickly fix up your picture so that **all** of the cupcakes have a candle. Raise your hand when you're finished.
     (Observe students and give feedback.)
4. Everybody, hold up your **left** hand if you fixed up your picture so that **all** of the cupcakes have a candle.
   - You did it the right way.

EXERCISE 4   If-Then Application

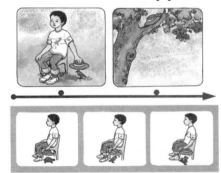

1. Everybody, find part C. ✔
   - You're going to say a rule about the pictures on the arrow. That rule starts with **if** and it tells what happened in the first picture and what happened in the second picture.
   - Touch the first picture on the arrow. ✔
     The boy in the picture is named Roger. Roger is putting his hat on top of something in that picture. What's he putting his hat on top of? (Signal.) *A bird.*
   - Touch the second picture on the arrow. ✔
     Where's his hat in that picture? (Signal.) *In a tree.*

- Touch the first picture again. ✔
Everybody, what's Roger doing in that picture? (Signal.) *Putting his hat on top of a bird.*
2. Here's the first part of the **if** rule: If Roger puts his hat on top of a bird . . .
- Everybody, say that part. (Signal.) *If Roger puts his hat on top of a bird . . .*
- Listen: If Roger puts his hat on top of a bird, his hat will end up some place. Where will it end up? (Signal.) *In a tree.*
- I'll say the whole rule. Touch the first picture and the second picture as I tell about each picture. Listen: **If Roger puts his hat on top of a bird . . . ✔ . . . his hat will end up in a tree.** ✔
3. Your turn to touch the pictures and say both parts of the rule. Remember, start with **if** and tell about **Roger** for the first picture. Tell about **his hat** for the second picture.
4. Tell about the first picture. (Signal.) *If Roger puts his hat on top of a bird . . .*
- Tell about the second picture.
  . . . his hat will end up in a tree.
- (Repeat step 4 until firm.)
5. Everybody, say the whole **if** rule. Get ready. (Signal.) *If Roger puts his hat on top of a bird, his hat will end up in a tree.*
- (Repeat step 5 until firm.)
6. That rule tells what will happen if Roger puts his hat on top of a bird. It doesn't tell what will happen if Roger puts his hat on top of an elephant, a skunk, a gopher or anything but a bird.
7. Touch the pictures below the arrow. ✔
Some of the pictures below the arrow show things our rule does not tell us about.
- Listen: Cross out the two pictures that our rule doesn't tell about. Raise your hand when you're finished.
(Observe students and give feedback.)
8. (Call on a student.) Which two pictures did you cross out? (Idea: *The picture with a turtle and the picture with a frog.*)
- Raise your hand if you crossed out the picture with a turtle and the picture with a frog.
9. Everybody, what will happen if Roger puts his hat on top of a turtle? (Signal.) *We don't know.*
- What will happen if Roger puts his hat on top of a frog? (Signal.) *We don't know.*

- Our rule **does** tell us about one of those pictures.
- Everybody, if Roger puts his hat on top of that bluebird, what will happen to the hat? (Signal.) *It will end up in a tree.*
- I'll bet Roger will have trouble figuring out how his hat ended up in a tree.

EXERCISE 5   Classification

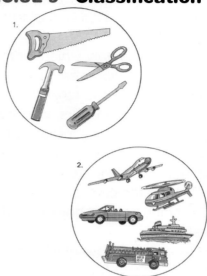

1. Everybody, find part D. ✔
- Touch circle 1. ✔
The objects in circle 1 are **tools.** Listen: A tool is made to help you do work.
- Touch circle 2. ✔
The objects in circle 2 are **vehicles.** Listen: A vehicle is made to take things places.
2. Everybody, what is a vehicle made to do? (Signal.) *Take things places.*
- What is a tool made to do? (Signal.) *Help you do work.*
- (Repeat step 2 until firm.)
3. Get ready to play a game. Listen carefully: I'm thinking of an object in one of the circles. I'm going to give you clues.
4. Here's the first clue: The object I'm thinking of is a **tool.** So you know which **circle** it must be in.
- Touch that circle. ✔
5. Here's the next clue: You use this tool to **cut.**
- Everybody, do you know which tool I'm thinking of yet? (Signal.) *No.*
- But you should know some tools I could not be thinking of.
I could **not** be thinking of a hammer. Why not? (Call on a student. Idea: *You don't cut with a hammer.*)

- I could **not** be thinking of a screwdriver. Why not? (Call on a student. Idea: *You don't cut with a screwdriver.*)
- I **could** be thinking of the saw because it's a tool and you use a saw to cut. Or I **could** be thinking of scissors.
- How do you know I could be thinking of scissors? (Call on a student. Idea: *It's a tool and you use scissors to cut.*)

6. Here's the next clue: This kind of tool cuts wood.
- Everybody, do you know which tool I'm thinking of yet? (Signal.) *Yes.*
- Which tool? (Signal.) *The saw.*
- Listen: You cut with scissors. How do you know I wasn't thinking of scissors? (Call on a student. Idea: *They don't cut wood.*)

7. New game: I'm thinking of a different object in one of the circles.
- Here's the first clue: The object I'm thinking of is a **vehicle.**
- Everybody, do you know which object I'm thinking of? (Signal.) *No.*
- Who can name some of the vehicles I **might** be thinking of? (Call on a student. Accept any vehicle in circle 2.)
- Everybody, how do you know I'm **not** thinking of a hammer? (Signal.) *A hammer is not a vehicle.*

8. Here's the next clue: This vehicle has wheels. Everybody, do you know which vehicle I'm thinking of yet? (Signal.) *No.*
- But you should know some vehicles I could **not** be thinking of. Who can name all the vehicles in the circle I'm not thinking of? (Call on a student. Ideas: *The helicopter and ship.*)
- I couldn't be thinking of a helicopter. Why not? (Call on a student. Idea: *It doesn't have wheels.*)
- I couldn't be thinking of a ship. Why not? (Call on a student. Idea: *It doesn't have wheels.*)

9. Here's the next clue: This vehicle goes on roads.
- Everybody, do you know which vehicle I'm thinking of? (Signal.) *No.*
- There's one vehicle with wheels I could not be thinking of.
- Touch that vehicle. ✔
  Everybody, which vehicle are you touching? (Signal.) *The airplane.*

- An airplane has wheels. Why couldn't I be thinking of an airplane? (Call on a student. Idea: *It doesn't go on roads.*)
10. Here's the next clue: This vehicle takes people to put out fires.
- Everybody, do you know which vehicle I'm thinking of? (Signal.) *Yes.*
- Which vehicle? (Signal.) *The fire truck.*
- A sports car goes on roads. How do you know I wasn't thinking of a sports car? (Call on a student. Idea: *It doesn't take people to put out fires.*)
- Let's see how well you remember the clues I gave you for the last game.
11. I gave you a clue that lets you know the object is in circle 2. Raise your hand if you remember that clue.
- What clue? (Call on a student. Idea: *The object is a vehicle.*)
- I gave you a clue that lets you know the vehicle is not a ship or a helicopter. What clue? (Call on a student.) *The vehicle has wheels.*
- I gave you a clue that lets you know the vehicle is not an airplane. What clue? (Call on a student.) *The vehicle goes on roads.*
- I gave you a clue that lets you know the vehicle is not a sports car. What clue? (Call on a student.) *The vehicle takes people to put out fires.*
- (Repeat step 11 until firm.)
12. You're pretty good at working with clues.

EXERCISE 6   The Bragging Rats Race

Storytelling

- Everybody, I'm going to read you a story. Listen to the things that happen in the story because you're going to answer some questions.
- This is a story about the bragging rats. Listen:

A bunch of rats lived near a pond that was on a farm. The rats got along well, except for two of them. The other rats called these two the bragging rats because they were always bragging, quarreling and arguing about something.

One day they'd argue about who could eat the most. Another day they'd squabble and quarrel over who was the best looking. Neither one of them was very good looking. One was a big gray rat with the longest tail you've ever seen on a rat. The other one wasn't big, but he had the biggest, yellowest teeth you ever saw.

The other rats in the bunch didn't pay much attention to the bragging and quarreling until the two rats started bragging about who was the fastest rat in the whole bunch. This quarrel went on for days, and the other rats got pretty sick of listening to the rats shout and yell and brag about how fast they were.

On the third day of their quarrel, the two rats almost got into a fight. The rat with the yellow teeth was saying, "I'm so fast that I could run circles around you while you ran as fast as you could."

The big gray rat said, "Oh, yeah? Well I could run circles around your circles. That's how fast I am."

The two rats continued yelling at each other until a wise old rat said, "Stop! We are tired of listening to all this shouting and yelling and bragging. There is a way to find out who is the fastest rat on this farm."

- How could they find out who was the fastest? (Call on a student. Idea: *Have a race.*)

The wise old rat continued, "We will have a race for any rat that wants to race. Everybody will line up, run down the path to the pond, then run back to the starting line. The first rat to get back is the winner. And then we'll have no more arguing about which rat is the fastest."

- Get a picture in your mind of how they're going to run. They'll start at the starting line, run down the path to the pond, turn around at the pond and run all the way back to the starting line. The wise old rat said there would be no more arguing about who could run the fastest.

- Why wouldn't there be any more arguing about which rat was the fastest? (Call on a student. Idea: *Because the race would prove who was the fastest.*)

The rats agreed, and early the next morning they were lined up, ready for the big race. Six rats entered the race. The bragging rats were lined up right next to each other, making mean faces and mumbling about how fast they were going to run.

The rats put their noses close to the ground, ready to take off like a flash.

"Everybody, steady," the wise old rat said, "Everybody, ready. Go!"

The rats took off toward the pond. The big gray rat got ahead of the others, with the yellow-toothed rat right behind him. But just before they got to the pond, the yellow-toothed rat stepped on the long tail of the gray rat, and both rats tumbled over and over in a cloud of dust.

They tumbled down the dusty path and right into the pond.

The other rats finished the race. The winner was a little black rat. It was hard for her to finish the race because she was laughing so hard over the bragging rats who were still splashing and sputtering around in the pond.

After the race, all the other rats went back to the pond. The bragging rats were still splashing and sputtering. The wise old rat said to them, "So now we know who the fastest runner on this farm is. It's neither one of you, so we will have no more arguments from either of you about who can run the fastest!"

The bragging rats looked at each other. Then the rat with yellow teeth suddenly smiled and said, "I may not be the fastest **runner** in this bunch, but there is no rat in the world that can **swim** as fast as I can."

"Oh, yeah?" said the gray rat. "I can swim so fast that I could go all the way across this pond without even getting my fur wet."

The wise old rat and the other rats just walked away from the pond, slowly shaking their heads.

- Why do you think they were shaking their heads? (Call on a student. Idea: *The race didn't settle anything.*)
- I don't think these bragging rats will ever stop bragging and arguing.

EXERCISE 7 True/False

Story Comprehension

1. Everybody, find part E. ✔
- Get ready to circle **true** or **false** to answer questions about the story.
- Touch number 1. ✔
  Listen: There were three bragging rats that argued and bragged all the time. Circle **true** or **false.**
- Number 2: One of the rats had yellow teeth and a very long tail. Circle **true** or **false.**
- Number 3: The two bragging rats got into a terrible argument about who could run the fastest. Circle **true** or **false.**
- Number 4: The rats argued for days until a little black rat said, "There's a way to find out who is the fastest rat." Circle **true** or **false.**
- Number 5: The rats had a race down the path to the pond and then back to the starting line. Circle **true** or **false.**
- Number 6: The rat with yellow teeth stepped on the tail of the gray rat and both of them went into the pond. Circle **true** or **false.**
- Number 7: At the end of the story, the bragging rats started a new argument about who could swim the fastest. Circle **true** or **false.**

2. Check your answers.
- Number 1: There were three bragging rats that argued and bragged all the time. Is that true or false? (Signal.) *False.*
- How many bragging rats were there? (Signal.) *2.*
- Number 2: One of the rats had yellow teeth and a very long tail. Is that true or false? (Signal.) *False.*
- Yes, that's false. One rat had yellow teeth. The other rat was gray with a big long tail.
- Number 3: The two bragging rats got into a terrible argument about who could run the fastest. Is that true or false? (Signal.) *True.*
- Number 4: The rats argued for days until a little black rat said, "There's a way to find out who is the fastest rat." Is that true or false (Signal.) *False.*
- Who said, "There's a way to find out who is the fastest rat"? (Signal.) *The wise old rat.*
- Number 5: The rats had a race down the path to the pond and then back to the starting line. Is that true or false? (Signal.) *True.*
- Number 6: The rat with yellow teeth stepped on the tail of the gray rat and both of them went into the pond. Is that true or false? (Signal.) *True.*
- Number 7: At the end of the story, the bragging rats started a new argument about who could swim the fastest. Is that true or false? (Signal.) *True.*

EXERCISE 8 Details

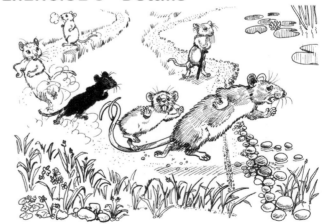

1. Find part F. ✔
   This picture shows part of the story.
- Everybody, what are all the rats doing in this picture? (Signal.) *Racing.*
2. Touch the rat with the big teeth. ✔
   He's the one stepping on the tail of the other bragging rat.

- In the story, what color are those big teeth? (Signal.) *Yellow.*
3. Touch the rat with the long tail. ✔
- In the story, what color is that rat? (Signal.) *Gray.*
4. Touch that little rat running behind the bragging rats. ✔

   That's the rat that ended up winning the race.
- Everybody, what color is that rat? (Signal.) *Black.*

5. Who remembers what happened just after this picture? (Call on a student. Idea: *The bragging rats tumbled into the pond.*)
6. Later you'll color the picture. Remember the color of that one rat's big teeth, the color of the rat with the long tail and the color of the rat that ended up winning the race.

> ***Note:*** If gray crayons are not available, direct students to use their pencil to color the gray rat.

Objectives

- **Identify letters that are 1st, 2nd or 3rd to the left or right.** (Exercise 1)
- Fix up pictures to show a true **all** statement. (Exercise 2)
- **Use clues to eliminate specific members of a class.** (Exercise 3)
- **Construct sentences for different illustrations.** (Exercise 4)
- Listen to a story and answer comprehension questions. (Exercise 5)
- Make a picture consistent with the details of a story. (Exercise 6)

EXERCISE 1   Left/Right

1. Let's see how well you remember **left** and **right.**
   - Everybody, hold your **right** hand out to your right side. ✔
     Hands down.
   - Everybody, hold your **left** hand out to your left side. ✔
     Hands down.
   - (Repeat step 1 until firm.)
2. (Write on the board:)

$$\boxed{\text{B T A} \;\bigcirc\; \text{C M K}}$$

   - You're going to tell me the letters that are to the **left** or to the **right** of the circle.
3. You start at the circle. If you go to the **left,** you'll come to the **A** first.
   - Watch. (Touch the circle.)
     Here I go to the **left.** (Move to the **A.**)
   - Everybody, what's the **first** letter I come to? (Signal.) *A.*
   - So the **A** is the **first** letter to the **left** of the circle.
   - Everybody, what's the **second** letter to the **left** of the circle? (Signal.) *T.*
   - What's the **third** letter to the **left** of the circle? (Signal.) *B.*
4. Listen: If you go to the **right** of the circle, you start at the circle and go **right.** Here I go to the **right.**
   - Watch. (Touch the circle and move to the **C.**)
   - What's the **first** letter I come to when I go **right?** (Signal.) *C.*
   - So the **C** is the **first** letter to the **right** of the circle.

- Everybody, what's the **second** letter to the **right** of the circle? (Signal.) *M.*
- What's the **third** letter to the **right** of the circle? (Signal.) *K.*

WORKBOOK

1. Open your workbook to lesson 3. ✔
   Everybody, find part A. ✔
   You're going to write the answers to questions.
2. Everybody, touch number 1. ✔
   Don't say anything, just listen.
   - Here's the question for number 1: What's the **third** letter to the **left** of the circle? Third to the left. Write the answer to number 1. Raise your hand when you're finished. ✔
   - Everybody, what letter is third to the left of the circle? (Signal.) *B.*
     Raise your hand if you got it right.
3. Touch number 2. ✔
   - Here's the question for number 2: What letter is **second** to the **right** of the circle? Second to the right. Write the answer to number 2. Raise your hand when you're finished. ✔
   - Everybody, what letter is second to the right of the circle? (Signal.) *M.*
     Raise your hand if you got it right.
4. Touch number 3. ✔
   - Here's the question for number 3: What letter is **first** to the **left** of the circle? First to the left. Write the answer to number 3. Raise your hand when you're finished. ✔
   - Everybody, what letter is first to the left of the circle? (Signal.) *A.*
     Raise your hand if you got it right.

5. Touch number 4. ✔
- Here's the question for number 4: What letter is **second** to the **left** of the circle? Second to the left. Write the answer to number 4. Raise your hand when you're finished. ✔
- Everybody, what letter is second to the left of the circle? (Signal.) *T.*
  Raise your hand if you got it right. ✔
6. Touch number 5. ✔
- Here's the question for number 5: What letter is **third** to the **right** of the circle? Third to the right. Write the answer to number 5. Raise your hand when you're finished. ✔
- Everybody, what letter is third to the right of the circle? (Signal.) *K.*
  Raise your hand if you got it right.
7. Raise your hand if you got everything right. Good for you.

EXERCISE 2   All, Some, None

Application

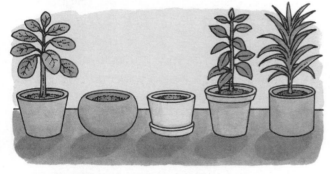

1. Everybody, find part B. ✔
   Look at the flower pots and get ready to tell me the statement that is **true** about them.
2. Listen: **All** of the flower pots have a plant. **Some** of the flower pots have a plant. **None** of the flower pots has a plant.
- Everybody, say the statement that is **true** about the flower pots. (Signal.) *Some of the flower pots have a plant.*
3. I'll say a statement that is **false.** You have to fix up your picture to make that statement **true.**
- Here's the **false** statement: **All** of the flower pots have a plant. True or false? (Signal.) *False.*
- Fix up the picture so **all** of the flower pots have a plant. Raise your hand when you're finished.
  (Observe students and give feedback.)

EXERCISE 3   Classification

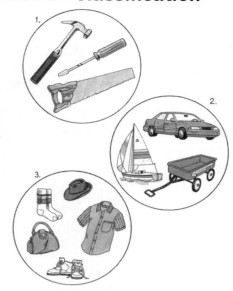

1. Everybody, find part C. ✔
   Let's see how well you remember the names of the objects in the circles.
- Touch circle 1. ✔
  Everybody, what do we call all the objects in that circle? (Signal.) *Tools.*
  Remember, if they're made to help you do work, they're tools.
- Touch circle 2. ✔
  What do we call all the objects in that circle? (Signal.) *Vehicles.*
  Remember, if they're made to take things places, they're vehicles.
- Touch circle 3. ✔
  The objects in that circle are clothing. If you wear it, it's clothing.
2. Get ready to play a game. I'm thinking of an object in one of the circles.
- Here's the first clue. The object I'm thinking of is not a vehicle. You don't know which object I'm thinking of. But you know some objects I could **not** be thinking of.
- Everybody, could I be thinking of a car? (Signal.) *No.*
- Why not? (Call on a student. Idea: *A car is a vehicle.*)
3. Here's the next clue. The object I'm thinking of is clothing.
- Everybody, do you know which object I'm thinking of? (Signal.) *No.*
- Who can name some of the objects I might be thinking of? (Call on a student. Accept any article in circle 3.)
- Everybody, how do you know I'm not thinking of a hammer? (Signal.) *A hammer is not clothing.*

4. Here's the next clue: You wear this article of clothing on your feet.
   - Everybody, do you know which article of clothing I'm thinking of? (Signal.) *No.*
   - But you should know some articles of clothing I could **not** be thinking of. Who can name all the clothing in the circle I'm **not** thinking of? (Call on a student. Ideas: *The hat, purse and shirt.*)
   - I couldn't be thinking of a purse, a shirt or a hat. Why not? (Call on a student. Idea: *You don't wear them on your feet.*)
5. Here's the next clue: This article of clothing has laces.
   - Everybody, do you know which article of clothing I'm thinking of? (Signal.) *Yes.*
   - Which article of clothing? (Signal.) *The shoes.*
   - You wear socks on your feet. How do you know I wasn't thinking of socks? (Call on a student. Idea: *Socks don't have laces.*)
6. New game. This is the mystery-object game. I'll give you clues. You'll cross out objects that could **not** be the mystery object. When you're done, all the objects except the mystery object will be crossed out.
   - Here's the first clue. The mystery object has one handle. Everybody, say that clue. (Signal.) *The mystery object has one handle.*
   - Listen: Do you know which circle that object is in? (Signal.) *No.*
   - Who can name all the objects I might be thinking of? Remember, the mystery object could be any object that has only one handle. (Call on a student. Ideas: *Hammer, saw, screwdriver, wagon, purse.*)
   - A car has door handles. How do you know I'm not thinking of the car? (Call on a student. Idea: *The car has more than one handle.*)
7. Listen: The mystery object has one handle. Some of the objects do not have only one handle. Cross out any object I could **not** be thinking of. Raise your hand when you're finished.
   (Observe students and give feedback.)
   - You should have crossed out the boat, the car, the hat, the shoes, the socks and the shirt.

8. Here's the next clue. The mystery object is in the **same** class as the screwdriver. Everybody, say that clue. (Signal.) *The mystery object is in the same class as the screwdriver.*
   - If it's in the same class as the screwdriver, it's in the same circle. Some objects that have a handle are not in the same class as the screwdriver. Cross out those objects. Raise your hand when you're finished. (Observe students and give feedback.)
   - You should have crossed out the wagon and the purse.
   - How do you know that the mystery object could not be the purse? (Call on a student. Idea: *The purse is not in the same class as the screwdriver.*)
   - How do you know that the mystery object could not be the wagon? (Call on a student. Idea: *The wagon is not in the same class as the screwdriver.*)
9. Here's the last clue about the mystery object. The mystery object is used to hit another object. Say that clue. (Signal.) *The mystery object is used to hit another object.*
   - Cross out anything that could not be the mystery object. Raise your hand when you're finished.
   (Observe students and give feedback.)
   - You should have crossed out the saw and the screwdriver.
   - The object that's not crossed out is the mystery object. Everybody, what's the mystery object? (Signal.) *The hammer.*
10. Let's see how super, super smart you are. Look at the objects you crossed out.
    - I gave you a **clue for crossing out** the shirt, the socks, the hat, the shoes, the car and the boat. Raise your hand if you remember that clue about the mystery object. Remember, you have to tell me the **clue.** (Call on a student.) *The mystery object has only one handle.*
    - I gave you a clue for crossing out the purse and the wagon. Raise your hand if you remember that clue about the mystery object. Remember, you've got to tell me the **clue.** (Call on a student.) *The mystery object is in the same class as the screwdriver.*

- I gave you a clue for crossing out the saw and the screwdriver. Raise your hand if you remember that clue about the mystery object. (Call on a student.) *The mystery object is used to hit another object.*

11. Raise your hand if you remembered all those clues. ✔

EXERCISE 4 Sentence Construction

1. Everybody, find part D. ✔
   You're going to write sentences that tell what Paul painted in each picture.
   - Touch picture 1. ✔
     What did Paul paint in that picture? (Signal.) *A pot.*
   - Touch picture 2. ✔
     What did Paul paint in that picture? (Signal.) *A paddle.*
   - Touch picture 3. ✔
     Uh-oh. You can't see what Paul painted in that picture. I guess you'll have to make up part of that sentence.

2. Look at the boxes at the bottom of the page. There are words in each box.
   Touch the first box. ✔
   The words say, **a puzzle.**
   - Touch the next box. ✔
     What do the words say? (Signal.) *A pot.*
   - Touch the next box. ✔
     What does the word say? (Signal.) *Paul.*
   - Touch the next box. ✔
     What do the words say? (Signal.) *A pencil.*
   - Touch the next box. ✔
     There's no picture. That word is **painted.**
   - Touch the next box. ✔
     What do the words say? (Signal.) *A paddle.*
   - Touch the last box. ✔
     What do the words say? (Signal.) *A puppet.*

3. All the sentences will start with **Paul.**
   Touch the arrow for picture 1. ✔
   - That sentence will tell what Paul did in picture 1. Here's the sentence: **Paul painted a pot.**

4. Everybody, say that sentence. (Signal.) *Paul painted a pot.*
   - (Repeat step 4 until firm.)

5. For each space on the arrow, you'll write the words that are in one of the boxes at the bottom of the page.
   - Touch the first space on the arrow for picture 1. ✔
     You'll write **Paul** in that space.
   - Touch the middle space on the arrow. ✔
     You'll write **painted** in that space.
   - Touch the last space on the arrow. ✔
     You'll write **a pot** in that space.

6. Touch the first space again. ✔
   What will you write in that space? (Signal.) *Paul.*
   - Touch the middle space. ✔
     What will you write in that space? (Signal.) *Painted.*
   - Touch the last space. ✔
     What will you write in that space? (Signal.) *A pot.*
   - (Repeat step 6 until firm.)

7. Your turn: Write sentence 1. Remember to spell the words correctly. Start with a capital letter and end with a period. Raise your hand when you're finished. (Observe students and give feedback.)
   - (Write on the board:)

   Paul ■ painted ■ a pot. →

   - Here's what you should have for sentence 1. Raise your hand if you got everything right. ✔

8. Touch picture 2. ✔
   - What did Paul paint in that picture? (Signal.) *A paddle.*
     Yes, Paul painted a paddle.
   - Touch the first space. ✔
     What will you write in that space? (Signal.) *Paul.*
   - Touch the middle space. ✔
     What will you write in that space? (Signal.) *Painted.*

- Touch the last space. ✔

  What will you write in that space? (Signal.) *A paddle.*

- Write your sentence for picture 2. Remember, start with a capital and end with a period. Raise your hand when you're finished.

  (Observe students and give feedback.)

- (Write on the board:)

  Paul ■ painted ■ a paddle. →

- Here's what you should have for sentence 2. Raise your hand if you got everything right. ✔

9. Touch picture 3. ✔

   We don't know what Paul painted in that picture. It was one of those things in the boxes.

- Your turn: Pick the thing you want Paul to paint and write sentence 3. Don't write one of the sentences you've already written. Raise your hand when you're finished. (Observe students and give feedback.)

- Read the sentence you wrote for picture 3. (Call on several students. Praise sentences in the form *Paul painted a p_____.)*

- Raise your hand if your sentence started with a capital and ended with a period. ✔

- Later you'll have to fix up the picture of Paul to show what he painted. If your sentence said that Paul painted a puppet, you'll draw a puppet in the picture.

- If you wrote that Paul painted a pencil, you'll draw a pencil. Then you can color your pictures. I don't think Paul is painting anything green.

- What are his favorite colors? (Signal.) *Pink and purple.*

  I'll bet we'll have some pretty cute pictures.

EXERCISE 5   Sweetie and the Birdbath

Storytelling

- Everybody, I'm going to read you a story. This is a story about a mean cat named Sweetie and the adventure he had with a birdbath. The story starts before there was a birdbath. Listen:

A woman named Bonnie loved birds. One day she noticed some birds cleaning themselves by splashing in a puddle on the sidewalk. She said, "Those birds shouldn't have to splash in a puddle to get clean. They need a birdbath." That was a good idea.

The more Bonnie thought about getting a birdbath, the more she liked the idea. "I will get a birdbath big enough for all the birds that want to take a bath."

So Bonnie went to the pet store and looked at birdbaths. She picked out the biggest birdbath they had.

The next day, a truck delivered the birdbath. Bonnie set it up in her backyard, and soon some birds saw it. They called to their friends and, the first thing you know, all kinds of birds were splashing in the bird bath—red birds, yellow birds, spotted birds and little brown birds.

A big yellow cat lived in the house next to Bonnie's house. That cat's name was Sweetie, but that cat was anything but sweet. Sweetie loved to chase birds. When Sweetie saw all the birds in Bonnie's birdbath, Sweetie said to himself, "Yum, yum, look at all those little birds. I'm going to sneak over to that birdbath, jump up before they know I'm around and grab a couple of birds. Yum, yum."

- Listen to Sweetie's plan again:

"I'm going to sneak over to that birdbath, jump up before they know I'm around and grab a couple of birds. Yum, yum."

So Sweetie crouched down and went through a hole in the fence. Then Sweetie snuck through some bushes that were near the birdbath—closer, closer and closer until he was almost underneath the birdbath.

Sweetie heard some chirping and fluttering, so he crouched down and waited—very still, without moving anything but the tip of his tail, which moved back and forth.

Well, Sweetie couldn't see what was happening in the birdbath because Sweetie was in the bushes. But all that fluttering and chirping came about because a huge eagle decided to take a bath in the birdbath. So the eagle swooped down. And as soon as the other birds saw this huge eagle, with its great beak and its huge claws, they took off—fluttering and chirping.

- Listen: What made all the fluttering and chirping? (Call on a student. Idea: *The little birds started fluttering and chirping when the big eagle swooped down.*)
- Everybody, did Sweetie see the eagle? (Signal.) *No.*
- Why not? (Call on a student. Idea: *Because he was hiding in the bushes.*)

Sweetie didn't know it, but there wasn't a group of little birds in that birdbath any more. There was one huge bird—about three times as big as Sweetie.

Things were quiet now, so Sweetie got ready to leap up to the edge of the birdbath and grab a couple of tiny birds. Sweetie crouched down and, with a great leap, shot out of the bushes and landed on the edge of the birdbath. He landed with his claws out, grabbing at the first thing he saw. He grabbed the eagle, and, before Sweetie knew what was happening, that eagle grabbed **him.** The eagle picked Sweetie up and slammed him down into the middle of the birdbath. Splash!

Sweetie hated water, and he was all wet. He put his ears back and shot out of that birdbath so fast he looked like a wet yellow blur. He darted across the yard and through the hole in the fence. Then he just sat there with his mouth open and his eyes very wide.

- Everybody, when Sweetie went back to his yard, did he sneak through the bushes? (Signal.) *No.*
- What did he do? (Call on a student. Idea: *He ran across the yard and through a hole in the fence.*)

"What happened?" Sweetie said to himself. One second he was grabbing at something and the next second he was getting slammed into the birdbath.

While Sweetie was trying to figure out what happened, he wasn't looking at the birdbath. He didn't see the eagle. That eagle finished bathing and took off. As soon as the eagle left, all the little birds returned to the birdbath.

So when Sweetie finally peeked through the hole in the fence, he didn't see the eagle. He saw a bunch of little birds, twittering and splashing around in the water.

Sweetie looked and looked at those birds for a long time. Then he said to himself, "From here those birds look pretty small and helpless. But when you get close to them, they are really big and strong. I don't think I'll go near that birdbath again."

- Poor Sweetie has the wrong idea about what happened.
- What kind of bird does he **think** threw him into the birdbath? (Call on a student. Idea: *A little bird.*)
- Those are the only birds Sweetie ever saw from his side of the fence—those little guys. And he's afraid to go near them because he thinks they're big and strong.

So now Bonnie is happy because her birdbath always has a lot of birds in it. The birds are happy because they can meet all their friends and have a nice bath whenever they want. Sweetie is the only one who is not all that happy. He looks at the birds in Bonnie's yard a lot, but he never goes over there, and he spends a lot of time trying to figure out how those birds could look so small but be so big and strong.

EXERCISE 6 Details

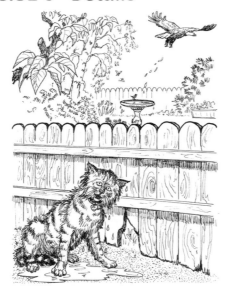

1. Everybody, find part E. ✔
- What did the eagle do just **before** this picture? (Call on a student. Idea: *Slammed Sweetie into the birdbath.*)
   That's why Sweetie is all wet and looks so confused.

- What did **Sweetie** do just before this picture? (Call on a student. Idea: *Darted across the yard and through a hole in the fence.*)
- Everybody, is Sweetie in his yard or Bonnie's yard? (Signal.) *His yard.*
- What's happening in Bonnie's yard? (Call on a student. Idea: *The eagle is taking off and the little birds are returning to the birdbath.*)
- Everybody, can Sweetie see what's happening? (Signal.) *No.*
- What is Sweetie thinking about in the picture? (Call on a student. Idea: *He's trying to figure out how those birds could look so small but be so big and strong.*)
- What will Sweetie see when he finally looks through the hole in the fence? (Call on a student. Idea: *Little birds splashing in the birdbath.*)
2. Who remembers what colors the birds are? (Call on a student.) *Red, yellow, brown and spotted.*
- Everybody, what color is Sweetie? (Signal.) *Yellow.*
- That eagle is brown and white.
3. Later you can color the picture. Remember what colors to make Sweetie and the eagle. See how many birds you can find.

Objectives

- Compose and write a parallel sentence based on a single picture. (Exercise 1)
- **Cross out objects to make an all statement true.** (Exercise 2)
- Use clues to eliminate specific members of a class. (Exercise 3)
- Listen to a story and answer comprehension questions. (Exercise 4)
- Make a picture consistent with the details of a story. (Exercise 5)

WORKBOOK • LINED PAPER

EXERCISE 1 Writing Parallel Sentences

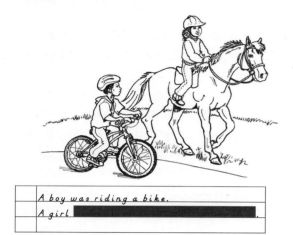

A boy was riding a bike.
A girl ███████████████.

1. Open your workbook to lesson 4 and find part A. ✔
   You're going to write about this picture. (Hand out a piece of lined paper to each student.) Write your name on the top line of the paper. ✔
2. The picture shows what a boy and a girl were doing. They were both riding something. One of them was riding a bike. Who was that? (Signal.) *The boy.*
   - What was the girl riding? (Signal.) *A horse.*
3. (Point to the first sentence below the picture.) The first sentence is written and part of the next sentence is written.
   - The first sentence says: **A boy was riding a bike.** Say that sentence. (Signal.) *A boy was riding a bike.*
   - Tell me what the second sentence should say about a girl. (Signal.) *A girl was riding a horse.*
     Yes. A girl was riding a horse.
   - Once more. Say the sentence about a boy. (Signal.) *A boy was riding a bike.*

- Say the sentence about a girl. (Signal.) *A girl was riding a horse.*
4. (Write on the board:)

> **horse**

- Here's a word you'll need: **horse.** Spell it correctly in your sentence.
5. Write both sentences on your lined paper. Start writing just after the margin. Copy the sentence that is written and complete the second sentence. Remember to start both sentences with a capital letter and put a period at the end of each sentence. (Observe students and give feedback.)
6. **(Optional:)** Skip a line on your paper and write both sentences again. Write: A boy was riding a bike. A girl was riding a horse. (Observe students and give feedback.)
7. (Collect and correct papers. Students who do not complete writing both pairs of sentences may complete their work after the lesson or for homework.)

EXERCISE 2 All, Some, None

Application

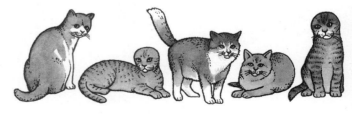

1. Everybody, find part B. ✔
   Look at the cats and get ready to tell me the statement that is **true** about their ears.
2. Listen: **None** of the cats has ears. True or false? (Signal.) *False.*

- **All** of the cats have ears. True or false? (Signal.) *False.*
- **Some** of the cats have ears. True or false? (Signal.) *True.*
- Everybody, say the statement that is **true** about the cats. (Signal.) *Some of the cats have ears.*

3. You've made statements **false** by drawing things and coloring things. But listen big: This time you're going to make the statement **true** by **crossing out** some things.

- Here's the statement you're going to make **true: All** of the cats have ears. Everybody, say that statement. (Signal.) *All of the cats have ears.*
- If you cross out some **cats,** you can make that statement true. Do it. Cross out some cats so that when you're done, all the cats that are left have ears. Raise your hand when you're finished.
(Observe students and give feedback.)

4. You should have crossed out the two cats that do not have ears. Raise your hand if you did that. ✔

5. Say the statement that's true about your cats now. (Signal.) *All of the cats have ears.*
- Say the statement that was true **before** you crossed out some of the cats. (Signal.) *Some of the cats have ears.*
- (Repeat step 5 until firm.)

EXERCISE 3 Classification

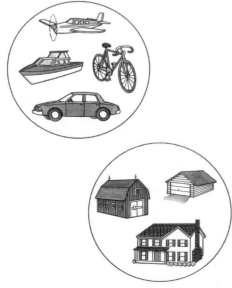

1. Find part C. ✔
This is the mystery-object game. I'll give you clues. You'll cross out objects that could **not** be the mystery object. When

you're done, all the objects except the mystery object will be crossed out.

2. Here's the first clue. The mystery object has windows. Everybody, say that clue. (Signal.) *The mystery object has windows.*
- Listen: Do you know which circle that object is in? (Signal.) *No.*
- Who can name all the objects I might be thinking of? (Call on a student. Idea: *Airplane, boat, car, barn and house.*)
- How do you know I'm not thinking of a bike? (Call on a student. Idea: *The bike doesn't have windows.*)

3. Listen: The mystery object has windows. Cross out any object that could not be the mystery object. Raise your hand when you're finished.
(Observe students and give feedback.)
- You should have crossed out the bike and the garage.

4. Here's the next clue. The mystery object is in the **same** class as the bike. Everybody, say that clue. (Signal.) *The mystery object is in the same class as the bike.*
- If it's in the same class, it's in the same circle. Any objects in the other circle can't be the mystery object. Cross out those objects. Raise your hand when you're finished.
(Observe students and give feedback.)
- You should have crossed out the barn and the house.
- How do you know that the mystery object could not be the barn? (Call on a student. Idea: *The barn is not in the same class as the bike.*)
- How do you know that the mystery object could not be the house? (Call on a student. Idea: *The house is not in the same class as the bike.*)

5. Here's the last clue about the mystery object. The mystery object travels on water. Say that clue. (Signal.) *The mystery object travels on water.*
- Cross out anything that could **not** be the mystery object. Raise your hand when you're finished.
(Observe students and give feedback.)
- You should have crossed out the airplane and the car.
- The object that's not crossed out is the mystery object. Everybody, what's the mystery object? (Signal.) *The boat.*

6. Let's see how smart you are. Look at the objects you crossed out.

- I gave you a **clue for crossing out** the bike and the garage. Raise your hand if you remember that clue about the mystery object. Remember, you have to tell me the **clue.** (Call on a student.) *The mystery object has windows.*

- I gave you a clue for crossing out the barn and the house. Raise your hand if you remember that clue about the mystery object. Remember, you've got to tell me the **clue.** (Call on a student.) *The mystery object is in the same class as the bike.*

- I gave you a clue for crossing out the car and the airplane. Raise your hand if you remember that clue about the mystery object. (Call on a student.) *The mystery object travels on water.*

7. Raise your hand if you remembered all those clues. ✔

EXERCISE 4 Clarabelle and the Bluebirds

Storytelling

- Listen to the things that happen in this story about a funny cow named Clarabelle because you're going to fix up a picture that shows part of the story.

This is a story about a cow named Clarabelle. Clarabelle looked like the other brown-and-white cows on the farm. But Clarabelle was really different. She was always trying to do things that other animals did. In fact, she felt sad about not being a bird or a frog or a student.

One day, Clarabelle was looking at the bluebirds that were sitting on a wire that went from the barn to a large pole. Clarabelle said, "I would love to sit on that wire with those bluebirds."

Some of the other cows heard Clarabelle talking to herself and they said, "Don't do it, Clarabelle. Remember what happened when you tried to swim like a duck in the duck pond?"

"Yeah," another cow said, "when you jumped **in** the pond, all the water jumped **out** of the pond."

Another cow said to Clarabelle, "And what about the time you tried to crow like the roosters? That was a real laugh. They were all saying 'cock-a-doodle-doo.' And you were saying, 'cock-a-doodle-moo.'"

- Everybody, what did the roosters say? (Signal.) *Cock-a-doodle-doo.*
- What did Clarabelle say? (Signal.) *Cock-a-doodle-moo.*

"Ho, ho, ho." All the cows laughed until they had tears in their eyes.

"That's not very funny," Clarabelle said. "And if I want to sit on the wire with those bluebirds, you can't stop me."

So Clarabelle went into the barn and up to the window by the wire. While she was getting ready, all the farm animals gathered around. One goat said, "We're in for another great show by Clarabelle."

And so they were. Clarabelle tiptoed out onto the wire, but Clarabelle was heavier than one thousand bluebirds, so the wire went down, lower and lower, until it was almost touching the ground.

- Get a picture in your mind of that part of the story. Clarabelle goes from the window in the barn out onto the wire. The wire doesn't break, but what does it do? (Call on a student. Idea: *Goes down until it almost touches the ground.*)

Well, the bluebirds were really angry. One of them said, "What are you doing, you big, fat cow? You've bent our wire almost to the ground."

"Yeah," another bluebird said. "This wire is for bluebirds, not brown-and-white cows."

Meanwhile, the farm animals were laughing and howling and rolling around on the ground. "Look at that," they said and rolled and laughed some more.

Clarabelle was not happy. She said, "This wire is not as much fun as I thought it would be." Clarabelle looked back up at the barn and said, "Wow, it's going to be hard to walk all the way back up there."

Then Clarabelle looked down and said, "I'm close to the ground, so maybe it would be easier for me to jump off and land in that haystack."

While she was trying to figure out what to do, all the bluebirds were yelling at her and saying things like, "Well, do something. Get off our wire so we can sit in peace!"

"All right, all right," Clarabelle said. "I'm leaving. Right now."

And with that, she jumped off the wire. Well, when she jumped off, the wire sprang way up into the air. It shot up so fast that it sent the bluebirds way up into the clouds, leaving blue tail feathers fluttering this way and that way.

And the farm animals almost died from laughter. "Did you see that?" a horse said as he rolled around on the ground. "Did you see those birds go flying up to the clouds?"

Everybody laughed except for a bunch of bluebirds and one brown-and-white cow. That cow pouted and kept saying, "It's not **funny**. It's not funny."

But let me tell you: It was too—**very** funny.

- Everybody, who was that brown-and-white cow that was not very happy? (Signal.) *Clarabelle.*
- Why wasn't Clarabelle happy? (Call on a student. Idea: *Because all the farm animals were laughing at her.*)

EXERCISE 5 Details

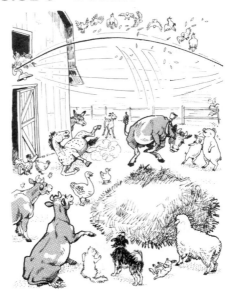

1. Everybody, find part D. ✔
   This picture took place **after** Clarabelle went out on the wire.
2. Everybody, touch the window in the barn. ✔
   That's where Clarabelle started tiptoeing out onto the wire.
- What did the wire do when she tiptoed out on it? (Call on a student. Idea: *It bent down almost to the ground.*)
- Yes, it bent down almost to the ground. Then Clarabelle decided to jump off. Everybody, what did she plan to land on? (Signal.) *A haystack.*
- What's Clarabelle doing in this picture? (Call on a student. Idea: *Jumping off the wire into the haystack.*)
- You can see the wire spring up. What are the birds doing? (Call on a student. Idea: *Being shot into the clouds.*)
- Yes, the wire is shooting those bluebirds up to the clouds.
- Look at the other animals. Everybody, what are they doing? (Signal.) *Laughing.*
3. Later you can color the picture. Remember what color all the cows are and what color the birds are. That barn should be red.

Note: Before presenting lesson 5, post the letters **N** and **S** (for north and south) on the appropriate walls (or corners) of the classroom.

Note: Make sure the letters **N** and **S** (for north and south) are posted on the appropriate walls (or corners) of the classroom.

Objectives

- Compose and write a parallel sentence pair based on a single picture. (Exercise 1)
- **Follow directions involving north and south.** (Exercise 2)
- Fix up pictures to show a true **some** statement. (Exercise 3)
- **Write appropriate object names under class headings.** (Exercise 4)
- Follow directions involving **left** and **right**. (Exercise 5)
- Listen to a story and answer comprehension questions. (Exercise 6)
- Make a picture consistent with the details of a story. (Exercise 7)

WORKBOOK • LINED PAPER

EXERCISE 1 Writing Parallel Sentences

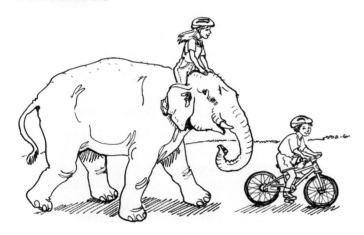

	The girl rode an elephant.
	The boy ████████████████.

1. Open your workbook to lesson 5 and find part A. ✔
   You're going to write about this picture. (Hand out a piece of lined paper to each student.) Write your name on the top line of the paper. ✔

2. The picture shows what a girl and a boy did. They rode something. One of them rode an elephant. Who was that? (Signal.) *The girl.*
   - What did the boy ride? (Signal.) *A bike.*

3. (Point to the first sentence below the picture.)
   The first sentence is written and part of the second sentence is written.
   - The first sentence says: **The girl rode an elephant.** Say that sentence. (Signal.) *The girl rode an elephant.*
   - Tell me what the second sentence should say about the boy. (Signal.) *The boy rode a bike.*
     Yes. The boy rode a bike.
   - Once more. Say the sentence about the girl. (Signal.) *The girl rode an elephant.*
   - Say the sentence about the boy. (Signal.) *The boy rode a bike.*

4. (Write on the board:)

   > **bike**

   - Here's a word you'll need: **bike.** Spell it correctly in your sentence.

5. Write both sentences on your lined paper. Start your words after the margin. Remember to start with a capital letter and put a period at the end of each sentence. (Observe students and give feedback.)

6. Skip a line on your paper and write both sentences again.
   (Observe students and give feedback.)

7. (Collect and correct papers. Students who do not complete writing both pairs of sentences may complete their work after the lesson or for homework.)

EXERCISE 2 Directions

Introduction

1. (Write on the board:)

> **north**
> **south**
> **east**
> **west**

- You're going to learn about directions. Directions tell you which way you're going or which way you're facing, no matter where you are.
- I'll read the four directions.
  (Point to each word as you say:)
  North, south, east, west.

2. Your turn: I'll point. You read the directions. Get ready.
   (Point to each word as students say:)
   North, south, east, west.
- (Repeat step 2 until firm.)

3. You can use the first letter of each direction to tell about the direction. You can use **N** for north.

4. What can you use for south? (Signal.) *S.*
- What can you use for east? (Signal.) *E.*
- What can you use for west? (Signal.) *W.*
- (Repeat step 4 until firm.)

5. I put the letters for directions on two walls.
- When I face **north,** I face the wall with **N** on it. Watch. (**Face the N wall.**) I'm facing north.
- Everybody, stand up.

6. Your turn: Face **north.** Get ready. Go. ✔
   Which direction are you facing? (Signal.)
   North.
- Listen: When you face **north, south** is behind you.
- Everybody, face **south.** Get ready. Go. ✔
  Which direction are you facing? (Signal.)
  South.
- (Repeat step 6 until firm.)
- Everybody, sit down.

7. I'll point to a wall. You tell me which direction I'm pointing.
- (Point **south.**)
  Everybody, which direction am I pointing? (Signal.) *South.*
- (Point **north.**)
  Which direction am I pointing? (Signal.) *North.*

8. Your turn: Everybody, point **south.** Get ready. Go. ✔
- Point **north.** Get ready. Go. ✔
- (Repeat step 8 until firm.)

9. Let's see who can do it without looking. Close your eyes. Keep them closed.
- Everybody, point **north.** Get ready. Go. ✔
- Point **south.** Get ready. Go. ✔
- Everybody, open your eyes and stand up.

10. (Remove **N** and **S** cards from the walls or corners.)
    This is tough.
- (Point to the **S** card.)
  Everybody, point to where the letter **S** goes. ✔
- What does the letter **S** stand for? (Signal.) *South.*
- (Point to the **N** card.)
  Point to where the letter **N** goes. ✔
- Everybody, what does the letter **N** stand for? (Signal.) *North.*

11. Wow, you are really getting smart about your directions.

Note: Save the **N** and **S** cards to post in lesson 6.

WORKBOOK

EXERCISE 3 All, Some, None

Application

Some of the bugs have spots.

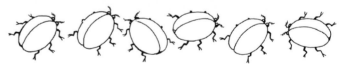

1. Everybody, find part B. ✔
- Look at the bugs.
- I'll say statements about the bugs and the spots on their back. You tell me if the statements are **true** or **false.**

2. Listen: **None** of the bugs has spots. True or false? (Signal.) *True.*
- Listen: **Some** of the bugs have spots. True or false? (Signal.) *False.*

3. Touch the statement above the picture. It starts with the word **some.** I'll read it. Follow along: Some of the bugs have spots.

- That statement is false, but you're going to make that statement true by drawing spots. When you're done, that statement should be true. Your picture should show **some** of the bugs have spots. Remember, each bug you fix up should have more than one spot. Raise your hand when you're finished. (Observe students and give feedback.)
- Everybody, hold up your workbook if you made spots on **some** of the bugs. ✔ You did it the **right** way.

4. **Before** you fixed up the bugs, the statement above the picture was **false.** Listen: **Some** of the bugs have spots.
- Is that statement **still** false? (Signal.) *No.*

5. I'll say statements about the bugs **now.** You tell me if each statement is **true** or **false.**
- **None** of the bugs has spots. True or false? (Signal.) *False.*
- **All** of the bugs have spots. True or false? (Signal.) *False.*
- **Some** of the bugs have spots. True or false? (Signal.) *True.*
- You're going to say the statement that was **true** about the bugs **before** you fixed them up. Think about it.

6. Everybody, say the statement that **was** true. Get ready. (Signal.) *None of the bugs has spots.*
- Say the statement that is true about the bugs **now.** Get ready. (Signal.) *Some of the bugs have spots.*
- (Repeat step 6 until firm.)
- Good, you made a false statement true.

EXERCISE 4 Classification

Writing

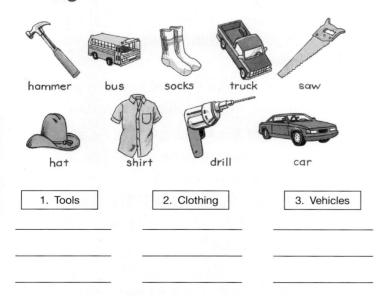

hammer   bus   socks   truck   saw

hat   shirt   drill   car

1. Tools	2. Clothing	3. Vehicles
_____	_____	_____
_____	_____	_____
_____	_____	_____

- Everybody, find part C. ✔ The pictures show different objects. The name of each object is written under its picture.

1. Everybody, touch the hammer. ✔ What word is under that picture? (Signal.) *Hammer.*
- Touch the next picture. ✔ What word is under that picture? (Signal.) *Bus.*
- Touch the next picture. ✔ What word? (Signal.) *Socks.*
- Next picture. ✔ What word? (Signal.) *Truck.*
- Next picture. ✔ What word? (Signal.) *Saw.*
- Next picture. ✔ What word? (Signal.) *Hat.*
- Next picture. ✔ What word? (Signal.) *Shirt.*
- Next picture. ✔ What word? (Signal.) *Drill.*
- Next picture. ✔ What word? (Signal.) *Car.*

2. Listen: Some of the objects in the pictures are **tools,** some are **clothing** and some are **vehicles.**
- Touch the word in box 1. ✔ It's the box with the number 1 in it.
- That word is **tools.** Raise your hand when you can name all the tools that are in the pictures. (Call on a student:) Name all the tools. *Hammer, saw, drill.*
- Everybody, touch the word in box 2. ✔ That word is **clothing.** Raise your hand when you can name all the articles of clothing in the pictures. (Call on a student.) *Socks, hat, shirt.*
- Everybody, touch the word in box 3. ✔ That word is **vehicles.** Raise your hand when you can name all the vehicles in the pictures. (Call on a student.) *Bus, truck, car.*

3. Everybody, touch the word in box 1 again. ✔ What word is that? (Signal.) *Tools.*
- Listen: Copy the names of all the objects that are tools. There are three tools. Write the names of the tools on the three lines below box 1. Copy each name carefully. Raise your hand when you're finished. (Observe students and give feedback.)

- There are three tools in the pictures. What are they? (Call on a student.) *Hammer, saw, drill.*
- That's right. You can have them in any order, but you should have written **hammer, saw** and **drill.** Raise your hand if you wrote those three names under **tools.**
4. Touch the word in box 2. ✔
   Everybody, what word is that? (Signal.) *Clothing.*
- Listen: Copy the names of all the articles of clothing in the pictures. Raise your hand when you're finished.
   (Observe students and give feedback.)
- There are three articles of clothing in the pictures. What are they? (Call on a student.) *Socks, hat, shirt.*
- That's right. You can have them in any order, but you should have written **socks, hat** and **shirt.** Raise your hand if you wrote those names under **clothing.**
5. Touch the word in box 3. ✔
   What word is that? (Signal.) *Vehicles.*
- Listen: Copy the names of all the vehicles in the pictures. Raise your hand when you're finished.
   (Observe students and give feedback.)
- There are three vehicles in the pictures. What are they? (Call on a student.) *Bus, truck, car.*
- That's right. You can have them in any order, but you should have written **bus, truck** and **car.** Raise your hand if you wrote those names under **vehicles.**
6. Raise your hand if you wrote all the right names for **tools, clothing** and **vehicles.** Pretty smart, I'd say.

EXERCISE 5   Left/Right

Review

1. Let's practice **right** and **left.**
   Everybody, stand up.
- Everybody, hold up your **right** hand. Get ready. Go. ✔
   Hands down.
- Everybody, turn a corner to your **left.** Get ready. Go. ✔
- Everybody, turn a corner to your **right.** Get ready. Go. ✔

- Everybody, hold up your **left** hand. Get ready. Go. ✔
   Hands down.
2. Everybody, turn your head to the **left.** Get ready. Go. ✔
- Everybody, take two baby steps to your **left.** Get ready. Go. ✔
- Everybody, sit down.

EXERCISE 6   Roger and the Headstand

Storytelling

- I'm going to tell you a story about a boy named Roger. Listen carefully so you can answer some questions later.

Roger almost always wore a hat. He had hats that were flat and hats that were round. He had hats that had brims, hats that had beaks and hats that had bands. He had red hats, blue hats and black hats. But his very favorite hat was a big, stiff, straw hat. He was always very careful not to crush that hat. He sure didn't want a squashed, straw hat.

Well, one day Roger was wearing his very favorite hat. He went to the park and saw two little kids trying to stand on their heads. They were wobbling and falling over. Roger watched them for a while and smiled to himself. Roger was one of the best headstanders you have ever seen. But those little kids were terrible. They were doing it all wrong. And every time they tried to get their feet off the ground—plop—they would fall over.

Finally, Roger walked over to them and said, "You're doing it all wrong."

One of the kids looked at Roger and said, "Leave us alone. Can't you see we're trying to practice?"

"Yeah," the other little kid said. "We're going to learn how to do it. We just need a little practice."

"No, no," Roger said. "The way you're trying to do it, you'll **never** stand on your head."

One of the little kids said, "If you're so smart, why don't you show us how it's done?"

"All right," Roger said. "I'll show you."

So Roger took off his hat because he sure didn't want to wear it when he stood on his head. Then he looked around for a safe place to put it. He thought about having one of the little kids hold it, but then he spotted a very safe place for it. Not far away was a teeter-totter. Nobody was around it. So he decided to put his hat under that teeter-totter. And that's just what he did. He put his fine straw hat under the right end of the teeter-totter. "Nobody will bother it there," he said.

- Get a picture in your mind of where that hat is. It's under one end of the teeter-totter. Which end? (Signal.) *The* right *end.*
- If the right end of the teeter-totter went down hard, what would happen to Roger's hat? (Call on a student. Idea: *It would get scrunched.*)
- Let's see what happened.

Then Roger went back to the little kids and said, "Here's how it's done." He got down and did one of the best headstands you have ever seen. He was as straight as an arrow, with his toes pointed. And he was so still, he was almost like an upside-down statue.

The little kids both said, "Wow! What a headstand."

Roger smiled while he was upside-down. He was pretty proud of himself, and he decided he would show those little kids what a long, long, long headstand looked like.

Well, while Roger was doing his long, long, long headstand, the kids got tired of watching him. After all, he wasn't doing anything, just standing there on his head with his toes pointed. So they went away and played ball. Still, Roger was doing his headstand.

After the kids got tired of playing ball, they looked over at Roger.

He was still on his head with his toes pointed.

One little kid said, "Let's go on the teeter-totter."

The other little kid said, "Yes, let's do that."

And they did it. One kid got on the left end of the teeter-totter. The other kid got on the right end. And up and down they went. When the right end went down the **first** time, it made a big scrunch sound. By the time the right end went down the **fifth** time, it didn't make a scrunch sound at all.

- Listen to that part again:

When the right end went **down** the **first** time, it made a big scrunch sound. By the time the right end went down the **fifth** time, it didn't make a scrunch sound at all.

- What made that scrunch sound the first time the right end went down? (Call on a student. Idea: *Roger's hat being scrunched.*)
- Why didn't the right end make a big scrunch sound when the right end went down the fifth time? (Call on a student. Idea: *The hat was scrunched flat.*)

Pretty soon, the little kids got tired of going up and down on the teeter-totter so they went back to Roger, who was still on his head, with his toes in the same position.

- Everybody, what position is that? (Signal.) *Pointed.*

One little kid said to Roger, "Do you know your face is getting very red?"

- That's what happens when you're upside-down for a long time. Your face gets red.

The other little kid said, "Yeah, how long are you going to stand on your head?"

"I'm finished," Roger said. He got down from his headstand and stood up. "**That's** how you do it," he said proudly.

Then Roger walked over to the teeter-totter and started to pick up his straw hat, but what he picked up didn't look much like a hat. It looked like a scrunched-up straw Frisbee.

Roger didn't know how his hat got flattened but it was flat, flat, flat. And Roger was mad, mad, mad.

"My hat is ruined," he said. "My favorite hat looks like a straw plate." He tossed the hat away and marched out of the park, very angry.

After he left, one of the little kids went over to the hat, picked it up and said to the other little kid, "Let's play some Frisbee." And they did.

- And what did they use to play Frisbee? (Signal.) *Roger's hat.*
- Yes, Roger's hat—poor Roger.

EXERCISE 7 Details

1. Everybody, find part D. ✔
   This picture shows something that happened in the story. Look at Roger in this picture.
   - Everybody, what's he doing? (Signal.) *Standing on his head.*

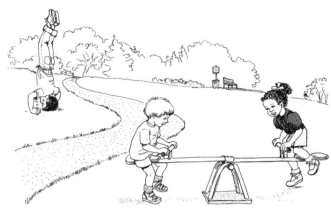

   - And look at how pointed his toes are. He sure knows how to stand on his head.
2. What are the little kids in this picture ready to do? (Call on a student. Idea: *Play on the teeter-totter.*)
   - One of the kids is on the **left** end of the teeter-totter. Everybody, is he wearing a **white** shirt or a **black** shirt? (Signal.) *A white shirt.*
   - One of the kids is getting on the **right** end of the teeter-totter. Is that kid wearing a **white** shirt or a **black** shirt? (Signal.) *A black shirt.*
3. Something is missing in this picture. What is that? (Signal.) *Roger's hat.*
   - Where should Roger's hat be? (Signal.) *Under the **right** end of the teeter-totter.*
   - Is that hat scrunched up yet? (Signal.) *No.*
4. Your turn: Draw Roger's hat where it should be. Later you can color the picture.

Objectives

- Follow directions involving **north** and **south**. (Exercise 1)
- Compose and write a parallel sentence pair based on a single picture. (Exercise 2)
- **Develop 2 clues that identify a "mystery" object.** (Exercise 3)
- Listen to a story and answer comprehension questions. (Exercise 4)
- **Write what a character says in a picture.** (Exercise 5)
- **Edit words to correct a character's dialect.** (Exercise 6)

EXERCISE 1 DIRECTIONS

North and South

Note: You will post **N** and **S** cards in this exercise.

1. I want to put the letters **N** and **S** on the right walls.
- Everybody, which direction does **N** stand for? (Signal.) *North.*
- Which direction does **S** stand for? (Signal.) *South.*
2. Everybody, point and show me the wall for the letter **N.** Get ready. Point. ✔
- Point and show me the wall for the letter **S.** Get ready. Point. ✔
- (Repeat step 2 until firm.)
3. (Post the letters **N** and **S.**) Everybody, stand up. Get ready to follow directions. Be careful.
4. Everybody, face **north.** Get ready. Go. ✔
- Face **south.** Get ready. Go. ✔
- (Repeat step 4 until firm.)
5. When you're facing **south,** which direction is **behind** you? (Signal.) *North.*
- Everybody, turn around and face **north.** Get ready. Go. ✔
- When you face **north,** which direction is **behind** you? (Signal.) *South.*
- Everybody, sit down.
6. Let's see if you can do it without looking. Close your eyes and keep them closed.
- Everybody, point **south.** Get ready. Go. ✔
- Point **north.** Get ready. Go. ✔
7. Everybody, open your eyes. I'm going to walk. You tell me the direction I'm walking.

8. Watch. (Walk slowly toward the **south** wall.) Which direction am I walking? (Signal.) *South.*
- (Turn around and walk slowly toward the **north** wall.) Which direction am I walking? (Signal.) *North.*
- (Repeat step 8 until firm.)
9. Pretty soon you'll do problems that show characters walking **north** or walking **south.** (Remove **N** and **S** cards from the walls.)

WORKBOOK • LINED PAPER

EXERCISE 2 Writing Parallel Sentences

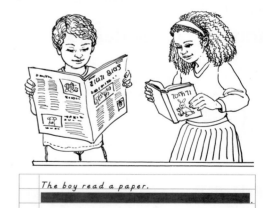

The boy read a paper.

1. Open your workbook to lesson 6 and find part A. ✔ You're going to write about this picture.
2. The picture shows what a boy and a girl did. They read something. One of them read a paper. Who was that? (Signal.) *The boy.*
- What did the girl read? (Signal.) *A book.*
3. Look at the sentence. The sentence says: **The boy read a paper.**

- Say that sentence. (Signal.) *The boy read a paper.*
- Tell me what the second sentence should say about the girl. (Signal.) *The girl read a book.*
- Once more. Say the sentence about the boy. (Signal.) *The boy read a paper.*
- Say the sentence about the girl. (Signal.) *The girl read a book.*

4. (Write on the board:)

> **book**

- Here's a word you'll need: **book.**

5. (Hand out a piece of lined paper to each student.) Write your name on the top line of the paper. ✔
  Write both sentences. Start your words just after the margin. Remember to start with a capital letter and put a period at the end of each sentence.
  (Observe students and give feedback.)

6. **(Optional:)** Skip a line on your paper and write both sentences again.
  (Observe students and give feedback.)

7. (Collect and correct papers. Students who do not complete writing both pairs of sentences may complete their work after the lesson or for homework.)

EXERCISE 3 **Classification**

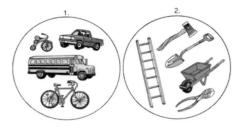

1. Find part B.
- Touch circle 1. ✔
  You're going to tell me the class name for the things in that circle.
- Everybody, what's the class name? (Signal.) *Vehicles.*
- Touch circle 2. ✔
  Everybody, what's the class name? (Signal.) *Tools.*

2. I'm going to give clues. The clues are good if they let you know about just one object. The clues are bad if they don't let you know about just one object.

- Here are the first clues: The mystery object is in the class of tools. The mystery object has one handle. Listen again: The mystery object is in the class of tools. The mystery object has one handle.
- Touch any objects those clues tell about. ✔
- Listen: Do those clues tell about only one object or more than one object? (Signal.) *More than one object.*
- Those clues tell about more than one object so they're not good. Which objects do those clues tell about? (Call on a student. Idea: *Shovel and ax.*)

3. New clues. The new mystery object is in the class of tools. The new mystery object has one wheel.
- Touch any objects those clues tell about. ✔
- Listen: Do those clues tell about only one object or more than one object? (Signal.) *One object.*
- What's that object? (Signal.) *The wheelbarrow.*
- So those are good clues.

4. New clues: The new mystery object is in the class of vehicles. The new mystery object has wheels.
- Touch any objects those clues tell about. ✔
- Do those clues tell about only one object or more than one object? (Signal.) *More than one object.*
- So are those clues good or bad? (Signal.) *Bad.*

5. Let's see how smart you are. You're going to make up two clues about the bicycle. The first clue will tell the **class** the bicycle is in. You can start that clue by saying: "The mystery object is in the **class** of. . ."
- Everybody, what class? (Signal.) *Vehicles.*
- Everybody, say the first clue. (Signal.) *The mystery object is in the class of vehicles.*
- Now the second clue. Start by saying: "The mystery object. . ." Then tell **something** about the bicycle that is not true of any of the other objects shown in that class. Raise your hand when you can say the second clue about the mystery object. (Call on a student. Praise clues such as: *The mystery object has two wheels.*)

6. New game. You're going to make up two clues that tell about the ladder. The first clue will tell about the **class:** The mystery object is in the **class** of. . .

- Everybody, what class? (Signal.) *Tools.*
- Everybody, say the first clue. (Signal.) *The mystery object is in the class of tools.*
- Now the second clue. Start by saying: "The mystery object . . . " Then tell something about the ladder that is not true about any of the other objects shown in that class. Raise your hand when you can say a second clue about the mystery object. (Call on several students. Praise clues such as: *The mystery object has rungs. The mystery object is used for climbing.*)

7. Last game. Raise your hand if you can give two clues about the tricycle.
   - Start both your clues with, "The mystery object . . . " First tell about the **class.** Then tell about something that is true of the tricycle and no other object shown in that class.
   - Everybody, say the first clue about the mystery object. (Signal.) *The mystery object is in the class of vehicles.*
   - What's a good second clue for the mystery object? (Call on a student. Praise clue such as: *The mystery object has three wheels.*)

8. You're getting pretty good at making up clues.

EXERCISE 4   Bleep Says Some Strange Things

Part 1 Storytelling

- I'm going to read you a story about a robot named Bleep. Listen carefully, so you can answer some questions.

Bleep was a robot that could do lots of smart things. He could answer questions. He could follow directions. You could tell him to get the ladder out of the garage and he'd get the ladder.

The person who invented Bleep was named Molly. People called her Molly Mix-up because, although she invented lots of things, everything she invented had problems. She invented Bleep. And Bleep had a lot of problems.

At first, Bleep would not always tell the truth. You couldn't tell when he was lying and when he was saying things that were true.

He also said "bleep" every time he talked. If you asked him what color the grass was, he wouldn't say "green." He'd say, "Bleep. Green."

If you asked him what color the sky was, he wouldn't say "blue." He'd say something else.

- Everybody, what would he say? (Signal.) *Bleep. Blue.*

Molly made adjustments so Bleep wouldn't say "bleep" all the time and other adjustments so he would tell the truth. She fixed him so he'd say "I don't know" if he didn't know the answer to something. That was a lot better than having Bleep make up some wild story when he didn't know the answer.

Each time Molly adjusted Bleep, she'd take off the top of his head and turn the screws that controlled the way he talked and thought. There were many screws. Each screw was a different color. For some adjustments, Molly would turn the blue screw. For other adjustments, she'd turn the yellow screw or the pink screw or sometimes more than one screw.

Well, after many adjustments, Bleep seemed to work very well, except for a couple of small problems. One problem Bleep had was that he would sometimes say "okay, baby." If you told him to get the ladder out of the garage, he would get the ladder all right, but, before he did, he might say "okay, baby." If you told him to sit down, he'd sit down all right, but, before he did, he might say something.

- Everybody, what would he say? (Signal.) *Okay, baby.*

Molly tried three or four times to fix Bleep so he wouldn't say, "Okay, baby," but she was not able to do it. Bleep kept right on saying, "Okay, baby."

One day, a school teacher came over to Molly's house. Bleep answered the door. Molly was in the garage working on a new invention. The school teacher said, "Is Molly Henderson at home?"

Bleep said, "Yes."

The school teacher said, "Would you ask her to come to the door?"

- And you know what Bleep said. Everybody, what did Bleep say? (Signal.) *Okay, baby.*
- Yes.

The school teacher jumped. She said, "Oh . . . oh, what kind of talk is that?"

Bleep said, "Bleep-talk."

The teacher said, "Well, I don't think I like Bleep-talk very much at all."

Bleep said, "Okay, baby."

The school teacher jumped again. "Oh . . . oh," she said. "I'm leaving." And she did just that.

After the teacher left, Bleep started thinking about what she had said. She had said, "Well, I don't think I like Bleep-talk very much at all."

Bleep said to himself, "Maybe I should change the way Bleep talks."

He had seen Molly do it many times. He knew that she took off the top of his head and tinkered around with the screws. He figured that he could take off the top of his head, tinker with the screws and change the way he talked.

That's just what he did.

But he didn't know which screws to adjust. In fact, he wasn't even very sure about how he wanted to change the way

he talked. So he just turned a red screw a little bit and a brown screw a little bit. Then he put the top of his head back on.

Pretty soon, Molly came in from the garage. She said, "Did I hear somebody at the door a while ago?"

Bleep didn't say, "Yes." He said, **"Yus."**

Molly said, "Did you say, 'Yus'?"

Bleep said, **"Yus."**

Molly looked at Bleep and said, "Did you take the top of your head off and play with the screws?"

"Yus."

"Well, why did you do that?"

Bleep said, "I want to talk **butter.**"

- Listen: Bleep said, "I want to talk **butter.**" What was he trying to say? (Signal.) *I want to talk better.*

Molly said, "Well, you don't talk **better.** You sound awful. But I don't have time to fix you now." She handed him a letter and said, "Mail this letter right away."

"Okay, baby."

Then Bleep looked at the letter and said, "But there is no stamp on this **lutter.**"

- Listen: Bleep said, "There is no stamp on this **lutter.**" What was he trying to say? (Signal.) *There is no stamp on this letter.*

"Well, put a stamp on it and then mail it."

Bleep said, "Okay, baby. I'll **gut** a stamp."

- Listen: He said, "I'll **gut** a stamp." What was he trying to say? (Signal.) *I'll get a stamp.*

Molly shook her head and said, "When you mail the letter, please don't talk to anybody. You sound awful."

Bleep put a stamp on the letter and took it to the mailbox. But just as he was mailing the letter, a neighbor walked by—an old man named Ben.

Ben said, "Hello, Bleep."

Bleep looked at Ben and said, **"Hullo, Bun."**

- What was Bleep trying to say? (Signal.) *Hello, Ben.*

Ben blinked and stared at Bleep. Then he shook his head and walked away, saying, "What kind of talk is that?"

Bleep said, "Bleep-talk."

Then Bleep said to himself, **"Wull, Molly will take the top of my hud off again and fix it so I talk butter."**

And that's just what she did.

- Oh, dear. Ben said something to make Bleep think he should talk better. What did Ben say? (Call on a student. Idea: *What kind of talk is that?*)
- And then Bleep said, "Wull, Molly will take the top of my hud off again and fix it so I talk butter." What was Bleep trying to say? (Signal.) *Well, Molly will take the top of my head off again and fix it so I talk better.*
- The end of the story says that's just what she did. Do you think Bleep ended up talking *butter* or worse? (Students respond.)
- Bleep sure has a lot of problems.

EXERCISE 5 Writing Bleep-Talk

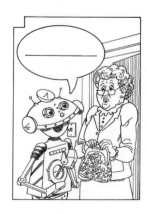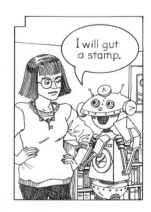

1. Everybody, find part C. Bleep is saying something, but there are no words. That woman at the door looks mighty shocked by whatever Bleep said.
   - Who is that woman at the door? (Signal.) *A school teacher.*
   - What did Bleep say to shock her? (Signal.) *Okay, baby.*
   - You'll have to write that in the place that shows what Bleep said.
2. (Write on the board:)

   Okay, baby.

   - Here's what you'll write.
3. Later you can color the picture. I think that teacher's face should be red. She looks pretty upset.

EXERCISE 6 Correcting Bleep-Talk

1. Everybody, find part D.
   That's the picture of Molly and Bleep. That picture shows Bleep saying something.
2. Touch the words he's saying. ✔
   I'll read them: I . . . will . . . gut . . . a . . . stamp.
   - Everybody, what's Bleep saying? (Signal.) *I will gut a stamp.*
   - What is he trying to say? (Signal.) *I will get a stamp.*
   - Yes, he wanted to say, "I will get a stamp." But he ended up saying, "I will **gut** a stamp."
3. (Write on the board:)

   get

   - Here's the word Bleep wanted to say instead of **gut**.
4. Bleep can't say the sound for one of these letters.
   - (Point to **g**.)
     Can he say the sound for **G**? (Signal.) *Yes.*
   - (Point to **e**.)
     Can he say the sound for **E**? (Signal.) *No.*
   - (Point to **t**.)
     Can he say the sound for **T**? (Signal.) *Yes.*
   - Everybody, say the letter Bleep has trouble with. (Signal.) *E.*
5. Fix up the word **gut** on your worksheet. Cross out the wrong letter and write the correct letter above it. Raise your hand when you're finished.
   (Observe students and give feedback.)

6. (Write on the board:)

> e
> g⃥u⃥t

- Check your work. Here's what you should have. Raise your hand if you got it right.

7. Look at the picture.
   Does this picture take place **before** Bleep took off the top of his head or **after** he took off the top of his head? (Signal.) *After.*

- What is Bleep going to do right after he gets a stamp for the letter? (Signal.) *Mail the letter.*

- Who will Bleep meet when he's mailing the letter? (Signal.) *Ben.*
- Ben will say, "Hello, Bleep." Then what will Bleep say? (Signal.) *Hullo, Bun.*
  Yes, **hullo, Bun.**
- What kind of talk is that? (Signal.) *Bleep-talk.*

8. Later you can color the picture.

Objectives

- Follow directions involving **north** and **south.** (Exercise 1)
- Write appropriate object names under class headings. (Exercise 2)
- Construct sentences for different illustrations. (Exercise 3)
- Listen to a familiar story. (Exercise 4)
- Edit words to correct a character's dialect. (Exercise 5)

EXERCISE 1   Directions

North and South

> *Note:* You will **not** post **N** and **S** cards in this exercise.

1. Let's see how well you remember **north** and **south** when you can't see the letters.
2. Everybody, you're going to point **north.** Which direction? (Signal.) *North.*
   - Point **north.** Get ready. Go.
     (Praise students who point north.)
   - Point **south.** Get ready. Go.
     (Praise students who point south.)
3. Everybody, stand up.
   - Turn so you are facing **north.** Get ready. Go. ✔
   - Point **north.** Get ready. Go. ✔
4. Turn so you are facing **south.** Get ready. Go.
   - Which direction are you facing? (Signal.) *South.*
   - Everybody, take two little steps to the **south.** Get ready. Go.
   - Which direction did you walk? (Signal.) *South.*
   - Face **north** again. Get ready. Go.
   - Which direction are you facing? (Signal.) *North.*
   - Everybody, take three little steps to the **north.** Get ready. Go.
   - Which direction did you walk? (Signal.) *North.*
   - (Repeat step 4 until firm.)
5. Good remembering **north** and **south.** Everybody, sit down.

EXERCISE 2   Classification

Writing

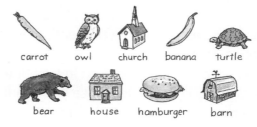

1. Everybody, open your workbook to lesson 7 and find part A. ✔
   The pictures show different objects. The name of each object is written under its picture.
2. Everybody, touch the carrot. What word is under that picture? (Signal.) *Carrot.*
   - Touch the owl. What word is under that picture? (Signal.) *Owl.*
   - Touch the church. What word is under that picture? (Signal.) *Church.*
   - Touch the banana. What word is under that picture? (Signal.) *Banana.*
   - Touch the turtle. What word is under that picture? (Signal.) *Turtle.*
   - Touch the bear. What word is under that picture? (Signal.) *Bear.*
   - Touch the house. What word is under that picture? (Signal.) *House.*

- Touch the hamburger.
  What word is under that picture?
  (Signal.) *Hamburger.*
- Touch the barn.
  What word is under that picture?
  (Signal.) *Barn.*
3. Listen: Some of the objects in the pictures are **food,** some are **buildings** and some are **animals.**
- Touch the word in box 1. ✔
  That word is **food.** Raise your hand when you can name all the kinds of food that are in the pictures. (Call on a student:) Name all the kinds of food. *Carrot, banana, hamburger.*
- Everybody, touch the word in box 2. ✔
  That word is **buildings.** Raise your hand when you can name all the buildings in the pictures. (Call on a student.) *Church, house, barn.*
- Everybody, touch the word in box 3. ✔
  That word is **animals.** Raise your hand when you can name all the animals in the pictures. (Call on a student.) *Owl, turtle, bear.*
4. Everybody, touch the word in box 1 again. ✔
  What word is that? (Signal.) *Food.*
- Listen: Copy the names of all the objects that are food. There are three kinds of food. Write the names on the three lines below box 1. Copy each name carefully. Raise your hand when you're finished.
  (Observe students and give feedback.)
- There are three kinds of food in the pictures. What are they? (Call on a student.) *Carrot, banana, hamburger.*
- That's right. You can have them in any order, but you should have written **carrot, banana** and **hamburger.** Raise your hand if you wrote those three names under **food.**
5. Everybody, touch the word in box 2. ✔
  What word is that? (Signal.) *Buildings.*
- Listen: Copy the names of all the buildings in the pictures. Raise your hand when you're finished.
  (Observe students and give feedback.)
- There are three buildings in the pictures. What are they? (Call on a student.) *Church, house, barn.*

- That's right. You can have them in any order, but you should have written **church, house** and **barn.** Raise your hand if you wrote those names under **buildings.**
6. Everybody, touch the word in box 3. ✔
  What word is that? (Signal.) *Animals.*
- Listen: Copy the names of all the animals in the pictures. Raise your hand when you're finished.
  (Observe students and give feedback.)
- There are three animals in the pictures. What are they? (Call on a student.) *Owl, turtle, bear.*
- That's right. You can have them in any order, but you should have written **owl, turtle** and **bear.** Raise your hand if you wrote those names under **animals.**
7. Raise your hand if you wrote all the right names for **food, buildings** and **animals.** You're pretty good at writing objects for different classes.

EXERCISE 3   Sentence Construction

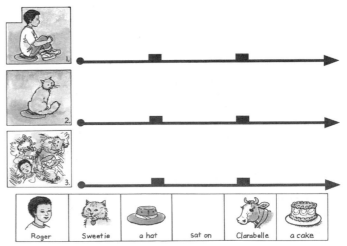

1. Everybody, find part B. ✔
   The pictures show what different characters did. You're going to write sentences that tell what the characters did in each picture.
2. Look at the boxes below the arrows. There are words at the bottom of each box. I'll read the words.
- Touch the first box.
  The word says: **Roger.**

- Touch the next box.
  The word says: **Sweetie.**
- Touch the next box.
  The words say: **a hat.**
- Touch the next box.
  There's no picture. The words say: **sat on.**
- Touch the next box.
  The word says: **Clarabelle.**
- Touch the last box.
  The words say: **a cake.**

3. Everybody, touch picture 1. ✔
   Who's in that picture? (Signal.) *Roger.*
- What did Roger do in this picture? (Call on a student. Idea: *Sat on a hat.*)
- Here's the sentence that tells what Roger did: **Roger sat on a hat.**

4. Everybody, say that sentence. (Signal.)
   Roger sat on a hat.
- (Repeat step 4 until firm.)

5. For each space on the arrow, you'll write the words that are in one of the boxes below the arrows.

6. Touch the first space on the arrow for picture 1. ✔
   What will you write in that space? (Signal.) *Roger.*
- Touch the middle space. ✔
  What will you write in that space? (Signal.) *Sat on.*
- Touch the last space. ✔
  What will you write in that space? (Signal.) *A hat.*
- (Repeat step 6 until firm.)

7. You turn: Write sentence 1.
   Remember to spell the words correctly. Start with a capital letter and end with a period. Raise your hand when you're finished.
   (Observe students and give feedback.)
- (Write on the board:)

> Roger ■ sat on ■ a hat. →

- Here's what you should have for sentence 1. Raise your hand if you got it right.

8. Touch picture 2. ✔
   Now you're going to make up a sentence for picture 2. That picture shows what another character did.
- Who's in that picture? (Signal.) *Sweetie.*
- Raise your hand if you can say the whole sentence about what Sweetie did in picture 2. Remember to use words from the boxes

below the arrows. (Call on a student.)
Sweetie sat on a hat.
- Yes, Sweetie sat on a hat.

9. Everybody, say that sentence. (Signal.)
   Sweetie sat on a hat.
- (Repeat step 9 until firm.)

10. Your turn: Write the sentence on the arrow for picture 2. Write the words **Sweetie, sat on, a hat.** Copy the words carefully. Start with a capital letter and end with a period. Raise your hand when you're finished. (Observe students and give feedback.)

11. Touch picture 3. ✔
    Uh-oh, it's hard to tell what's in that picture. In fact, maybe there's not even a hat in that picture. Maybe there's a cake, and maybe somebody sat on that cake.

12. Your turn: Write sentence 3. Start with the name of somebody. Then tell what that character sat on. Don't write one of the sentences you've already written. Raise your hand when you're finished. (Observe students and give feedback.)

13. Read the sentence you wrote for picture 3. (Call on several students. Praise sentences of the form _____ sat on _____.)
- We have some pretty silly sentences.

14. Raise your hand if all your sentences start with a capital and end with a period.
- Let's see who can read all three of their sentences. (Call on several students. Praise correct responses.)

EXERCISE 4   Bleep Says Some Strange Things

Part 1 Review

- I'm going to read the story about Bleep again.

Bleep was a robot that could do lots of smart things. He could answer questions. He could follow directions. You could tell him to get the ladder out of the garage and he'd get the ladder.

The person who invented Bleep was named Molly. People called her Molly Mix-up because, although she invented lots of things, everything she invented had problems. She invented Bleep. And Bleep had a lot of problems.

At first, Bleep would not always tell the truth. You couldn't tell when he was lying and when he was telling the truth.

He also said "bleep" every time he talked. If you asked him what color the grass was, he wouldn't say "green." He'd say, "Bleep. Green."

If you asked him what color the sky was, he wouldn't say "blue." He'd say something else.

Molly made adjustments so Bleep wouldn't say "bleep" all the time and other adjustments so he would tell the truth. She fixed him so he'd say "I don't know" if he didn't know the answer to something. That was a lot better than having Bleep make up some wild story when he didn't know the answer.

Each time Molly adjusted Bleep, she'd take off the top of his head and turn the screws that controlled the way he talked and thought. There were many screws. Each screw was a different color. For some adjustments, Molly would turn the blue screw. For other adjustments, she'd turn the yellow screw or the pink screw or sometimes more than one screw.

Well, after many adjustments, Bleep seemed to work very well, except for a couple of small problems. One problem Bleep had was that he would sometimes say "okay, baby." If you told him to get the ladder out of the garage, he would get the ladder all right, but, before he did, he might say "okay, baby." If you told him to sit down, he'd sit down all right, but, before he did, he might say something.

Molly tried three or four times to fix Bleep so he wouldn't say "okay, baby," but she was not able to do it. Bleep kept right on saying "okay, baby."

One day, a school teacher came over to Molly's house. Bleep answered the door. Molly was in the garage working on a new invention. The school teacher said, "Is Molly Henderson at home?"

Bleep said, "Yes."

The school teacher said, "Would you ask her to come to the door?"

Bleep said, "Okay, baby."

The school teacher jumped. She said, "Oh . . . oh, what kind of talk is that?"

Bleep said, "Bleep-talk."

The teacher said, "Well, I don't think I like Bleep-talk very much at all."

Bleep said, "Okay, baby."

The school teacher jumped again. "Oh . . . oh," she said. "I'm leaving." And she did just that.

After the teacher left, Bleep started thinking about what she had said. She had said, "Well, I don't think I like Bleep-talk very much at all."

Bleep said to himself, "Maybe I should change the way Bleep talks."

He had seen Molly do it many times. He knew that she took off the top of his head and tinkered around with the screws. He figured that he could take off the top of his head, tinker with the screws and change the way he talked.

That's just what he did.

But he didn't know which screws to adjust. In fact, he wasn't even very sure about how he wanted to change the way he talked. So he just turned a red screw a little bit and a brown screw a little bit. Then he put the top of his head back on.

Pretty soon, Molly came in from the garage. She said, "Did I hear somebody at the door a while ago?"

Bleep didn't say "yes." He said, **"Yus."**

Molly said, "Did you say 'yus'?"

Bleep said, **"Yus."**

Molly looked at Bleep and said, "Did you take the top of your head off and play with the screws?"

"Yus."

"Well, why did you do that?"

Bleep said, "Because I want to talk **butter.**"

Molly said, "Well, you don't talk **better.** You sound awful. But I don't have time to fix you now." She handed him a letter and said, "Mail this letter right away."

"Okay, baby."

Then Bleep looked at the letter and said, "But there is no stamp on this **lutter.**"

"Well, put a stamp on it and then mail it."

Bleep said, "Okay, baby. I'll **gut** a stamp."

Molly shook her head and said, "When you mail the letter, please don't talk to anybody. You sound awful."

Bleep put a stamp on the letter and took it to the mailbox. But just as he was mailing the letter, a neighbor walked by—an old man named Ben.

Ben said, "Hello, Bleep."

Bleep looked at Ben and said, **"Hullo, Bun."**

Ben blinked and stared at Bleep. Then he shook his head and walked away, saying, "What kind of talk is that?"

Bleep said, "Bleep-talk."

Then Bleep said to himself, **"Wull,** Molly will take the top of my **hud** off again and fix it so I talk **butter.**"

And that's just what she did.

EXERCISE 5   Correcting Bleep-Talk

1. Bleep said some strange things in this story. See if you know what he was trying to say.

- Listen: Bleep said, "I want to talk butter." Everybody, say that. (Signal.) *I want to talk butter.*
- Now say what Bleep was trying to say. (Signal.) *I want to talk better.*

2. Listen: Bleep said, "There is no stamp on this lutter." Everybody, say that. (Signal.) *There is no stamp on this lutter.*
- Now say what Bleep was trying to say. (Signal.) *There is no stamp on this letter.*

3. Listen: Bleep said, "I will gut a stamp." Everybody, say that. (Signal.) *I will gut a stamp.*
- Now say what Bleep was trying to say. (Signal.) *I will get a stamp.*

4. Here's a tough one. Listen: Bleep said, "Hullo, Bun." Everybody, say that. (Signal.) *Hullo, Bun.*
- Now say what Bleep was trying to say. (Signal.) *Hello, Ben.*

5. I'll say some other things Bleep might say. You tell me what he was trying to say.
- Listen: It's time to rust. Everybody, say it. (Signal.) *It's time to rust.*
- Now say what Bleep was trying to say. (Signal.) *It's time to rest.*
- Listen: Molly sleeps in a bud. Everybody, say it. (Signal.) *Molly sleeps in a bud.*
- Now say what Bleep was trying to say. (Signal.) *Molly sleeps in a bed.*

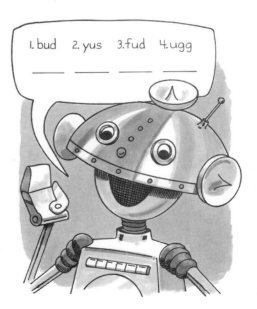

1. Everybody, find part C. ✔
    These are words that Bleep said.
    You're going to write the words Bleep was trying to say.

2. Everybody, touch word 1. ✔
- That word is **bud.** What word? (Signal.) *Bud.*
- What word was Bleep trying to say? (Signal.) *Bed.*
- Write the word **bed** below the word **bud.** Raise your hand when you're finished.
- (Write on the board:)

> **bed**

- Check your work. Here's the word Bleep was trying to say. Raise your hand if you got it right.
3. Touch word 2. ✔
- That word is **yus.** What word was Bleep trying to say? (Signal.) *Yes.*
- Write the word **yes** below the word **yus.** Raise your hand when you're finished.
- (Write on the board:)

> **yes**

- Check your work. Here's the word you should have written below **yus.** Raise your hand if you got it right.
4. Touch word 3. ✔
- That word is **fud.** What word was Bleep trying to say? (Signal.) *Fed.*

- Write the word **fed** below the word **fud.** Raise your hand when you're finished.
- (Write on the board:)

> **fed**

- Check your work. Here's what you should have written below **fud.** Raise your hand if you got it right.
5. Touch word 4. ✔
- That word is **ugg.** What word was Bleep trying to say? (Signal.) *Egg.*
- Write the word **egg** below the word **ugg.** Raise your hand when you're finished.
- (Write on the board:)

> **egg**

- Check your work. Here's the word you should have written below **ugg.** Raise your hand if you got it right.
6. Raise your hand if you got all the words right. You're really good at figuring out what Bleep was trying to say.

Note: Before presenting lesson 8, post the letters **E** and **W** (for east and west) on the appropriate walls (or corners) of the classroom.

Objectives

- **Follow directions involving north, south, east, west.** (Exercise 1)
- Compose and write a parallel sentence pair based on a single picture. (Exercise 2)
- **Construct and apply 2 related if-then rules.** (Exercise 3)
- **Edit words to show a character's dialect.** (Exercise 4)
- **Say a deduction based on 3 pictures.** (Exercise 5)
- Listen to a new story. (Exercise 6)
- Make a picture consistent with the details of a story. (Exercise 7)

EXERCISE 1 Directions

North, South, East, West

1. Let's see if you can remember **north** and **south.** Everybody, stand up.
2. Turn so you are facing **south.** Get ready. Go.
- Which direction are you facing? (Signal.) *South.*
- Turn so you are facing **north.** Get ready. Go.
- Which direction are you facing? (Signal.) *North.*
- This is tough. Everybody, take two little steps to the **north.** Get ready. Go.
- Everybody, keep facing north and take two little steps to the **south.** Get ready. Go.
- Which direction did you walk? (Signal.) *South.*
- (Repeat step 2 until firm.)
3. Now you're going to learn about the other two directions—**east** and **west.**
- Listen: Make sure you're facing north and hold your **right** hand out to the side—straight out to the side. Get ready. Go.
- The direction you're pointing is **east.** Which direction? (Signal.) *East.*
- Everybody, turn and face **east.** Get ready. Go.
- Which direction are you facing? (Signal.) *East.*
- The **E** on the wall stands for **east.** What does it stand for? (Signal.) *East.*

- That's where the sun comes up in the morning. Remember, the sun comes up in the **east.**
4. **West** is right behind you. Everybody, turn around and face **west.** Get ready. Go.
- Which direction are you facing? (Signal.) *West.*
- The **W** on the wall stands for **west.** What does it stand for? (Signal.) *West.*
- Remember, this is where the sun goes down at night—in the **west.**
5. Everybody, face **north** again. Get ready. Go.
- Listen: Everybody, turn to the **east.** Get ready. Go.
- Which direction are you facing? (Signal.) *East.*
6. Everybody, turn to the **west.** Get ready. Go.
- Which direction are you facing? (Signal.) *West.*
- Is the sun in the west during the morning or the evening? (Signal.) *The evening.*
7. Everybody, turn to the **east** again. Get ready. Go.
- Is the sun in the east during the morning or the evening? (Signal.) *The morning.*
8. Everybody, sit down.
Remember, when you face **north, east** is to your **right.** You can always find east by facing north and then turning a corner to the right.

EXERCISE 2   Writing Parallel Sentences

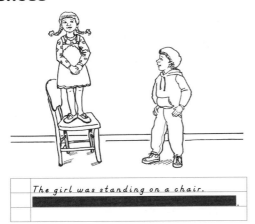

1. Open your workbook to lesson 8 and find part A. ✔
    You're going to write about this picture.
2. The picture shows what a girl and a boy were doing.
*   Where was the boy standing? (Signal.)
    On the floor.
*   Where was the girl standing? (Call on a student. Idea: *On a chair.*)
3. Look at the sentence.
    Everybody, say that sentence. (Signal.)
    The girl was standing on a chair.
*   Tell me what the second sentence should say about the boy. (Signal.) *The boy was standing on the floor.*
    Yes. The boy was standing on the floor.
*   Once more. Say the sentence about the girl. (Signal.) *The girl was standing on a chair.*
*   Say the sentence about the boy. (Signal.) *The boy was standing on the floor.*
4. (Write on the board:)

    floor

*   Here's a word you'll need: **floor.**
5. (Hand out a piece of lined paper to each student.)
    Write your name on the top line of the paper. ✔
    Write both sentences. Remember to write your words just after the margin, start with a capital letter, and put a period at the end of each sentence.
    (Observe students and give feedback.)

6. **(Optional:)** Skip a line on your paper and write both sentences again.
    (Observe students and give feedback.)
7. (Collect and correct papers. Students who do not complete writing both pairs of sentences may complete their work after the lesson or for homework.)

EXERCISE 3   If-Then Application

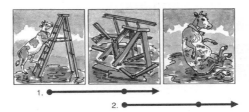

1. Everybody, find part B. ✔
    There are **two** arrows under the pictures.
*   You're going to say two **if** rules.
2. Touch arrow 1. ✔
    Arrow 1 shows what will happen in the **first** picture and the **middle** picture.
*   The **first** picture shows what Clarabelle is going to do. Touch that picture. ✔
*   Everybody, what is Clarabelle going to do? (Signal.) *Climb a ladder.*
*   Touch the **middle** picture. ✔
    That picture shows what will happen to the ladder.
*   Everybody, what will happen to the ladder? (Signal.) *It will break.*
3. Everybody, raise your hand when you can tell the rule for arrow 1. Remember to start with **if** and tell about the first two pictures. (Call on several students. Praise responses such as: *If Clarabelle climbs the ladder, the ladder will break.*)
*   Yes, here's the rule for arrow 1: **If Clarabelle climbs the ladder, the ladder will break.**
4. Everybody, say the rule for arrow 1. (Signal.) *If Clarabelle climbs the ladder, the ladder will break.*
*   (Repeat step 4 until firm.)
5. Now we'll do arrow 2.
*   Touch the first ball on arrow 2. ✔
    That ball is under the middle picture. So you start with **if** and tell about the middle picture. Listen: **If the ladder breaks . . .**
*   Touch the second ball on arrow 2. ✔
    The picture shows what will happen if the ladder breaks.
*   What will happen? (Call on a student.) *Clarabelle will fall in the mud.*

- So here's the rule for arrow 2: **If the ladder breaks, Clarabelle will fall in the mud.**

6. I'll say both rules. You'll touch the ball of the arrow for the right picture.
- Listen: **If Clarabelle climbs the ladder . . .** Touch the ball under the first picture. ✔
  . . . the ladder will break.
- Touch the ball under the middle picture. ✔
- Next rule: **If the ladder breaks . . .** Keep touching the ball under the middle picture. ✔
  . . . Clarabelle will fall in the mud. Touch the ball under the last picture. ✔

7. Go back to the first arrow. Everybody, say the rule for the first arrow. Get ready. (Signal.) *If Clarabelle climbs the ladder, the ladder will break.*
- Say the rule for the second arrow. Get ready. (Signal.) *If the ladder breaks, Clarabelle will fall in the mud.*
- (Repeat step 7 until firm.)

8. You're getting pretty good at saying those **if** rules.

EXERCISE 4 Writing Bleep-Talk

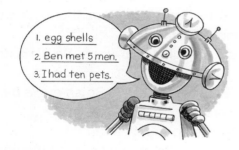

1. egg shells
2. Ben met 5 men.
3. I had ten pets.

1. Everybody, find part C. ✔
   These are things that Bleep wants to say. But remember, he adjusted the red screw and the brown screw. So he can't say the right sound in some of these words.

2. Everybody, touch line 1. ✔
   I'll read what Bleep is trying to say: **Egg shells.** What's he trying to say? (Signal.) *Egg shells.*
- Raise your hand when you know what he **really** said instead of "egg shells." (Call on a student.) *Ugg shulls.*

3. Everybody, touch line 2. ✔
   I'll read what Bleep is trying to say: **Ben met 5 men.** What's he trying to say? (Signal.) *Ben met 5 men.*
- Raise your hand when you know what he **really** said instead of "Ben met 5 men." (Call on a student.) *Bun mut 5 mun.*

4. Everybody, touch line 3. ✔
   I'll read what Bleep is trying to say: **I had ten pets.** What's he trying to say? (Signal.) *I had ten pets.*
- Raise your hand when you know what he **really** said instead of "I had ten pets." (Call on a student.) *I had tun puts.*

5. Everybody, you're going to fix up each line so it says what Bleep **really** said.
- Touch line 1 again. ✔
  Bleep really said, "ugg shulls." What did he say? (Signal.) *Ugg shulls.*
- Cross out the letter **E** in each word. Write the letter **U** above it so it says **ugg shulls,** not **egg shells.** Raise your hand when you're finished.
- (Write on the board:)

>   u   u
> ~~e~~gg sh~~e~~lls

- Check your work. Here's what you should have for line 1. Raise your hand if you did it the right way.

6. Touch line 2. ✔
   Bleep really said, "Bun mut 5 mun." What did he say? (Signal.) *Bun mut 5 mun.*
- Cross out the letter **E** in each word. Write the letter **U** above it so it says **Bun mut 5 mun,** not **Ben met 5 men.** Raise your hand when you're finished.
- (Write on the board:)

>   u   u   u
> B~~e~~n m~~e~~t 5 m~~e~~n.

- Check your work. Here's what you should have for line 2. Raise your hand if you did it the right way.

7. Touch line 3. ✔
   Bleep really said, "I had tun puts." What did he say? (Signal.) *I had tun puts.*
- Cross out the letter **E** in each word. Write the letter **U** above it so it says **I had tun puts,** not **I had ten pets.** Raise your hand when you're finished.
- (Write on the board:)

>   u   u
> I had t~~e~~n p~~e~~ts.

- Check your work. Here's what you should have for line 3. Raise your hand if you did it the right way.

8. Raise your hand if you got everything right. Good for you.

EXERCISE 5 Deductions

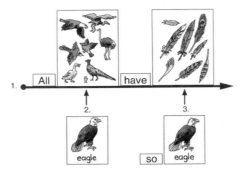

1. Everybody, find part D. ✔
   You're going to learn to say a 3-arrow deduction. This is tough, tough, tough.

2. (Draw on the board:)

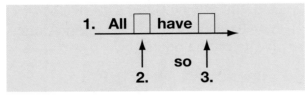

- (Touch arrow 1.) The first word on your arrows is **All.** Touch the word **All.** ✔
- Now touch the picture just after the word **All.**
- Everybody, what's in that picture? (Signal.) *Birds.*
- So the first part of the arrow rule is: **All birds.** What's the first part? (Signal.) *All birds.*

3. Touch the next word on arrow 1. ✔
   What's that word? (Signal.) *Have.*
- Yes, **have.**
- So the rule is: **All birds have . . .**

4. Touch the last picture. ✔
   The last picture shows what all birds have. What do all birds have? (Signal.) *Feathers.*
- **I'll** say the rule for arrow 1. **You** touch the things I say. Here we go: All . . . ✔
   birds . . . ✔
   have . . . ✔
   feathers. ✔

5. Everybody, say the rule for arrow 1. (Signal.) *All birds have feathers.*
- (Repeat step 5 until firm.)

6. Now touch the first arrow that goes **up.** That's arrow 2. ✔
- (Touch arrow 2.)

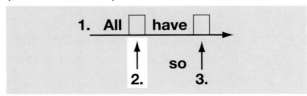

- Here's the arrow you should be touching.
- There's a picture at the bottom of arrow 2. What's in that picture? (Signal.) *An eagle.*
- Arrow 2 shows that the eagle belongs in the first picture. **An eagle is a bird.** That's the rule for arrow 2: An eagle is a bird.

7. Everybody, say that rule. (Signal.) *An eagle is a bird.*
- (Repeat step 7 until firm.)

8. Touch the last arrow that goes **up.** That's arrow 3. ✔
- (Touch arrow 3.)

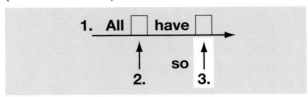

- Here's the arrow you should be touching.
- What's at the bottom of that arrow? (Signal.) *An eagle.*
   Yes, it's an eagle again.
- The word next to that eagle is **so.** Touch the word **so.** ✔
   What's that word? (Signal.) *So.*
- Now go up arrow 3 and you'll see what the eagle has. What does the eagle have? (Signal.) *Feathers.*
- Here's the rule for arrow 3: **So an eagle has feathers.**

9. Say that rule. (Signal.) *So an eagle has feathers.*
- (Repeat step 9 until firm.)

10. I'm going to say the rule for all the arrows. I'll start with arrow 1.
- (Touch arrow 1 on the board.)
   Listen: **All birds have feathers.**
- (Touch arrow 2.)
   An eagle is a bird.
- (Touch arrow 3.)
   So an eagle has feathers.

11. Once more.
- (Touch arrow 1.)
   All birds have feathers.
- (Touch arrow 2.)
   An eagle is a bird.
- (Touch arrow 3.)
   So an eagle has feathers.

12. Let's see if you can say the whole deduction. I'll tell you which arrow to touch. You say the statement for that arrow. Remember, you have to say the word **so** just before you say the statement for the last arrow.

13. Touch arrow 1. ✔
Say the statement. (Signal.) *All birds have feathers.*
- Touch arrow 2. ✔
Say the statement. (Signal.) *An eagle is a bird.*
- Touch arrow 3. ✔
Say the statement. (Signal.) *So an eagle has feathers.*
- (Repeat step 13 until firm.)

14. See if you can say the whole thing. Remember, say the statement for arrow 1, then arrow 2, then arrow 3. Get ready. (Signal.) *All birds have feathers. An eagle is a bird. So an eagle has feathers.*
- (Repeat step 14 until firm.)

15. Raise your hand if you can say the whole deduction. (Call on a student. Praise correct response.)

EXERCISE 6   Paul Paints Pansies

Storytelling

- This is a story about Paul painting pansies. Pansies are pretty little flowers.

One day Paul was in the country painting a picture of pink and purple pansies. He had a small can of pink paint and a very large can of purple paint.

He liked that big can of purple paint because he never knew when he'd have to use purple paint to fix up something that got paint on it.

- How would he fix something up if it got paint on it? (Call on a student. Idea: *Paint it all purple.*)

Well, Paul was in the middle of a large pasture painting perfect little pansies. He said to himself, "Painting in a pasture is perfect."

A lot of brown-and-white cows were in that pasture, and one of them was very, very curious about what Paul was doing.

That cow, of course, was Clarabelle. She walked over to where Paul was painting and she looked at his picture and thought that painting pictures was a lot of fun.

But it was a warm day and the flies kept buzzing around Clarabelle. When the flies got on her back or on her side, she'd swish them away with her tail. She stood there for a long time, watching and swishing and watching and swishing.

Suddenly, Paul looked at his watch and said, "Oh, pooh." Paul had forgotten that he had promised his mother that he would pick up pickles for her. So he just left his paint and painting in the middle of the pasture and ran over to his bike.

He hopped on and he peddled away down the pebble path. He knew it wouldn't take him long to pick up the pickles.

As soon as he had left, Clarabelle looked at the painting and said to herself, "I don't have a paint brush to paint with, but . . . "

She looked at her tail. On the end of it was a large patch of hair. That would make a perfect paintbrush.

She dipped the end of her tail into the big can of purple paint. Then she turned around and swung her tail towards Paul's painting. The end of her tail hit the painting with a great plop. Her tail made a great splat that looked like a huge purple bush.

"Not bad," Clarabelle said to herself.

So she did it again, and again—dipped her tail into the can, swung that tail at the picture and plop. She made six purple bushes in the picture.

Then the flies started to get really bad. Biting flies were buzzing around her back and her side. Without thinking, Clarabelle swished her tail and splat. She made a purple bush on her side. Then splat, she made a purple bush on her back. Then splat, another purple bush on her other side.

She was getting ready to paint another bush in Paul's picture when Paul came peddling up the pebbled path on his bike. He got off and ran over to his painting. Then he stopped. He stood there and stared.

Then he said, "Purple plants with my pansies. They're perfect."

He looked around to see who could have made those perfect purple plants. He saw Clarabelle with purple bushes on her back and her sides. He said to her, "You improved my painting, but you did a poor job of painting yourself. You have purple bushes on you, but you don't have any pink and purple pansies."

Clarabelle turned her head and looked at the purple plants. Then she turned back and looked at Paul. He was smiling.

He said, "Those purple plants don't look good without some pink and purple pansies."

Clarabelle agreed, so she nodded her head up and down.

Paul said, "Don't worry, brown-and-white cow. I can fix it up." And he did.

Now there is a large herd of brown-and-white cows in the pasture. Most of them look like ordinary brown-and-white cows. But one of them has a very pretty picture on her sides and back.

EXERCISE 7 Details

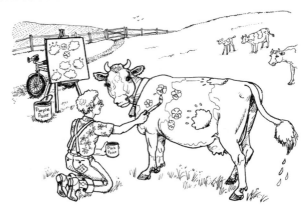

1. Find part E. ✔
   What's Paul doing in this picture? (Call on a student. Idea: *Painting pink and purple pansies on Clarabelle.*)
   • Later you'll have to fix up the picture.
2. There are big bushes in the picture. Touch one of those bushes. ✔
   In the story, what color are all the bushes? (Signal.) *Purple.*
   • Touch the pansies in the picture. ✔
   In the story, what color are those pansies? (Signal.) *Pink and purple.*
   • When you fix up Clarabelle, you'll have to make the end of her tail the right color. Then you can fix up those pansies and those bushes so they're the right colors.

Objectives

- Follow directions involving **north, south, east, west.** (Exercise 1)
- Compose and write a parallel sentence pair based on a single picture. (Exercise 2)
- Construct and apply 2 related if-then rules. (Exercise 3)
- **Identify objects that are 1st, 2nd or 3rd to the left or right.** (Exercise 4)
- Say deductions based on 3 pictures. (Exercise 5)
- Listen to a familiar story. (Exercise 6)
- Make a picture consistent with the details of a story. (Exercise 7)

EXERCISE 1 **Directions**

North, South, East, West

1. Let's see how well you remember the four directions.
2. Everybody, stand up and face **north.** ✔
- Face **south.** Get ready. Go.
  Everybody, face north again. ✔
3. Listen: Hold your **right** hand out to the side straight out. Get ready. Go.
- Everybody, which direction is your right hand pointing? (Signal.) *East.*
  Hands down.
- Everybody, hold your **left** hand out to the side—straight out. Get ready. Go.
- Think big. Which direction is your left hand pointing? (Signal.) *West.*
  Hands down.
- Which direction is **behind** you? (Signal.) *South.*
- (Repeat step 3 until firm.)
4. Everybody, face **east.** East. Get ready. Go.
- Which direction are you facing? (Signal.) *East.*
- When do you see the sun in the **east?** (Signal.) *In the morning.*
5. Everybody, face **west.** Get ready. Go.
- Which direction are you facing? (Signal.) *West.*
6. Everybody, face **north.** Get ready. Go.
- Get ready to **point** to different directions while you keep facing **north.**
7. Listen: Everybody, point to the **west.** West. Get ready. Go.
- Point **south.** South. Get ready. Go.
- Point **east.** East. Get ready. Go.
- Point **north.** North. Get ready. Go.
- (Repeat step 7 until firm.)

8. I can't fool you on the four directions. Sit down.

WORKBOOK • LINED PAPER

EXERCISE 2 **Writing Parallel Sentences**

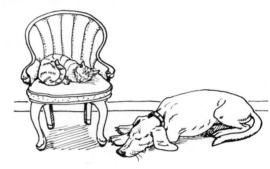

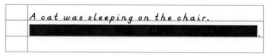

A cat was sleeping on the chair.

1. Open your workbook to lesson 9 and find part A. ✔
   You're going to write about this picture.
2. The picture shows what a cat and a dog were doing. What were they doing? (Signal.) *Sleeping.*
- Where was the cat sleeping? (Call on a student. Idea: *On the chair.*)
- Everybody, where was the dog sleeping? (Signal.) *On the floor.*
3. Look at the sentence.
   Say that sentence. (Signal.) *A cat was sleeping on the chair.*
- Tell me what the second sentence should say about a dog. (Signal.) *A dog was sleeping on the floor.*
- Once more. Say the sentence about a cat. (Signal.) *A cat was sleeping on the chair.*
- Say the sentence about a dog. (Signal.) *A dog was sleeping on the floor.*

4. (Write on the board:)

chair	floor	sleeping

- Here are some words you'll need:
chair . . . floor . . . sleeping.

5. (Hand out a piece of lined paper to each student.)
Write your name on the top line of the paper. ✔
Write both sentences. Remember to write your words just after the margin, start with a capital letter, and put a period at the end of each sentence. (Observe students and give feedback.)

6. **(Optional:)** Skip a line on your paper and write both sentences again.
(Observe students and give feedback.)

7. (Collect and correct papers. Students who do not complete writing both pairs of sentences may complete their work after the lesson or for homework.)

EXERCISE 3   If-Then Application

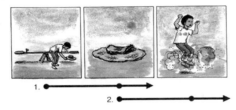

1. Everybody, find part B. ✔
There are two arrows under the pictures.
- You're going to say two **if** rules.
2. Touch arrow 1. ✔
Arrow 1 shows what happens in the **first** picture and the **middle** picture.
- The **first** picture shows Roger putting his hat under the teeter-totter. Touch that picture. ✔
- Touch the **middle** picture. ✔
That picture shows what will happen to Roger's hat. What will happen to Roger's hat? (Call on a student. Idea: *It will get flattened.*)
3. Raise your hand when you can tell the **if** rule for arrow 1. Remember to tell what **Roger** does and what will happen to **his hat.** (Call on several students. Praise responses such as: *If Roger puts his hat under the teeter-totter, his hat will get flattened.*)

- Yes, here's the rule for arrow 1: **If Roger puts his hat under the teeter-totter, his hat will get flattened.**

4. Everybody, say the rule for arrow 1. Get ready. (Signal.) *If Roger puts his hat under the teeter-totter, his hat will get flattened.*
- (Repeat step 4 until firm.)

5. Now touch arrow 2. ✔
Arrow 2 shows what happens in the middle picture and the last picture.
- Touch the first ball on arrow 2. ✔
Which picture will you tell about first? (Signal.) *The middle picture.*
- What does the middle picture show? (Call on a student. Idea: *Roger's flattened hat.*)
- Touch the second ball on arrow 2. ✔
Which picture will you tell about for that ball? (Signal.) *The last picture.*
- That picture shows how Roger will feel if his hat gets flattened. How will he feel? (Call on a student. Idea: *Mad, mad, mad.*)

6. Raise your hand if you can say the rule for arrow 2. Remember, start with **if** and tell about the middle picture and then the last picture. Start your rule with: **If Roger's hat gets flattened . . .** (Call on several students. Praise responses such as: *If Roger's hat gets flattened, Roger will get mad.*
- Yes, here's the rule for arrow 2: **If Roger's hat gets flattened, Roger will get mad.**

7. Everybody, say the rule for arrow 2. (Signal.) *If Roger's hat gets flattened, Roger will get mad.*
- (Repeat step 7 until firm.)

8. Everybody, get ready to say both rules.
- Say the rule for arrow 1. Get ready. (Signal.) *If Roger puts his hat under the teeter-totter, his hat will get flattened.*
- Say the rule for arrow 2. Get ready. (Signal.) *If Roger's hat gets flattened, Roger will get mad.*
- (Repeat step 8 until firm.)

9. Poor Roger. I think that was his favorite hat.

EXERCISE 4 Left/Right

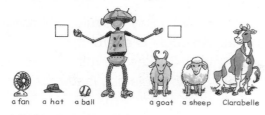

1. The third object to Bleep's right is _____.
2. The first object to Bleep's left is _____.
3. The first object to Bleep's right is _____.
4. The second object to Bleep's _____ is a _____.

1. Find part C. ✔
   The picture shows Bleep with objects to his left and to his right. The name is written under each object.
   - Everybody, touch the fan. ✔
     What do the words under that object say? (Signal.) *A fan.*
   - Touch the hat. ✔
     What do the words say? (Signal.) *A hat.*
   - Touch the ball. ✔
     What do the words say? (Signal.) *A ball.*
   - Touch the goat. ✔
     What do the words say? (Signal.) *A goat.*
   - Touch the sheep. ✔
     What do the words say? (Signal.) *A sheep.*
   - Touch Clarabelle. ✔
     What do the words say? (Signal.) *Clarabelle.*
2. Touch Bleep. ✔
   There's a box at the end of his left hand and a box at the end of his right hand.
   - Touch the box at the end of his **left** hand. His left hand. ✔
   - Touch the box at the end of his **right** hand. ✔
3. Listen: Write **L** in the box at the end of his **left** hand. Write **R** in the box at the end of his **right** hand. Raise your hand when you're finished.
   - (Draw on the board:)

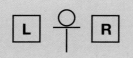

   - Here's what you should have.
4. Listen: Touch the **first** object to Bleep's **left.** The first object to his left. Start at Bleep and go to the first object to his left.
   - Everybody, what object? (Signal.) *A ball.*
5. Listen: Touch the **second** object to Bleep's **right.** The second object to Bleep's right. Everybody, what object? (Signal.) *A sheep.*

6. You're going to complete sentences.
   - Touch sentence 1. ✔
     I'll read what it says: The **third** object to Bleep's **right** is blank.
   - Your turn: Start at Bleep. Find the third object to Bleep's right and write the name in the blank. Raise your hand when you're finished.
     (Observe students and give feedback.)
   - Everybody, the third object to Bleep's right is what? (Signal.) *Clarabelle.*
   - You should have written **Clarabelle** in the blank for sentence 1.
   - Touch sentence 2. ✔
     I'll read what it says: The **first** object to Bleep's **left** is blank.
   - Start at Bleep. Find the first object to Bleep's left and write the name. Raise your hand when you're finished.
     (Observe students and give feedback.)
   - Everybody, the first object to Bleep's left is what? (Signal.) *A ball.*
   - Yes, you should have written **a ball** in the blank for sentence 2.
   - Touch sentence 3. ✔
     I'll read what it says: The **first** object to Bleep's **right** is blank. Write the name of the object in sentence 3. Raise your hand when you're finished.
     (Observe students and give feedback.)
   - Everybody, the first object to Bleep's right is what? (Signal.) *A goat.*
   - You should have written **a goat** in the blank for sentence 3.
7. Your turn to complete sentence 4. All it says is: The **second** object to Bleep's blank is blank. You'll have to tell whether it's the second object to his **left** or the second object to his **right.** Then you'll have to tell what the object is.
   - Touch the first blank. ✔
     Fill in the blank by telling whether you want to go to the right or the left. That's up to you. You can go to the right or the left.
   - Touch the second blank. ✔
     Fill in that blank with the name of the object. Raise your hand when you've filled in both blanks.
     (Observe students and give feedback.)

8. Raise your hand if you told about the second object to Bleep's **left.**

- Here's what your sentence should say: The second object to Bleep's **left** is a **hat.**

9. Raise your hand if you wrote about the second object to Bleep's **right.**

- Here's what your sentence should say: The second object to Bleep's **right** is a **sheep.**

10. Raise your hand if you completed your sentences correctly.

EXERCISE 5   Deductions

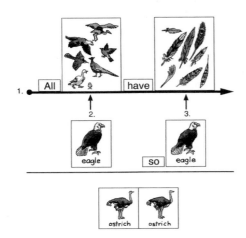

1. Find part D. ✔
(Draw on the board:)

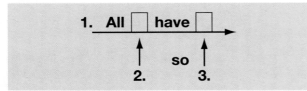

- This is that deduction about the birds and the eagle again.
Remember, first you say the rule for arrow 1.
Then you say the rule for arrow 2.
Then you say the rule for arrow 3.

2. Everybody, touch arrow 1. ✔
That first word is **All.** Everybody, say the rule for arrow 1 starting with **All.** Get ready. (Signal.) *All birds have feathers.*

- Touch arrow 2. ✔
Say the rule for that arrow. Get ready. (Signal.) *An eagle is a bird.*

- Touch arrow 3. ✔
Say the rule for that arrow. Get ready. (Signal.) *So an eagle has feathers.*

3. Let's see if you can do it by looking up here. I'll touch my arrows. You say the rule for each arrow I touch.

4. (Touch arrow 1.) Say the rule. Get ready. (Signal.) *All birds have feathers.*

- (Touch arrow 2.) Say the rule. Get ready. (Signal.) *An eagle is a bird.*

- (Touch arrow 3.) Say the rule. Get ready. (Signal.) *So an eagle has feathers.*

- (Repeat step 4 until firm.)

5. This time, I'll just touch. You say the whole deduction.

6. Get ready. (Touch arrow 1.) *All birds have feathers.*

- (Touch arrow 2.) *An eagle is a bird.*

- (Touch arrow 3.) *So an eagle has feathers.*

- (Repeat step 6 until firm.)

7. Great job. But now comes the hard part.

- Everybody, touch the pictures **below** the eagles. ✔
There are two pictures of the same bird, but that bird is **not** an eagle. Raise your hand if you know what that bird is. (Call on a student.) *An ostrich.*

- Here's the hard part. You have to **pretend** that you have the two pictures of the **ostrich** at the bottom of arrows 2 and 3.

- Touch arrow 2 and arrow 3. ✔
Pretend that those pictures show an **ostrich,** not an eagle.

- My turn to say the whole deduction. You touch the arrows, starting with arrow 1. Here I go: All birds have feathers. **An ostrich** is a bird. So **an ostrich** has feathers.

- Once more: Remember to touch each arrow as I tell about that arrow. Here I go: **All birds have feathers. An ostrich is a bird. So an ostrich has feathers.**

8. Your turn to touch the arrows and say the whole deduction. Get ready. *All birds have feathers. An ostrich is a bird. So an ostrich has feathers.*

- (Repeat step 8 until firm.)

9. Now look up here.
You have to pretend that there's an ostrich at the bottom of arrow 2 and arrow 3.

- I'll touch. You say the whole deduction. Get ready.

- (Touch arrow 1.) *All birds have feathers.*

- (Touch arrow 2.) *An ostrich is a bird.*

- (Touch arrow 3.) *So an ostrich has feathers.*

10. Now let's say the deduction using the pictures of the **eagles** at the bottom of arrow 2 and arrow 3. Say the whole deduction. Get ready.

- (Touch arrow 1.) *All birds have feathers.*
- (Touch arrow 2.) *An eagle is a bird.*
- (Touch arrow 3.) *So an eagle has feathers.*

11. Here's the hardest part of all. Pretend a **duck** is at the bottom of arrow 2 and arrow 3. I think I'm the only one who can say a deduction about a duck. Here I go:
    - (Touch arrow 1.) **All birds have feathers.**
    - (Touch arrow 2.) **A duck is a bird.**
    - (Touch arrow 3.) **So a duck has feathers.**
12. Who wants to try that?
    - I'll touch. You say the deduction. Get ready.
    - (Touch arrow 1.) *All birds have feathers.*
    - (Touch arrow 2.) *A duck is a bird.*
    - (Touch arrow 3.) *So a duck has feathers.*
13. You are amazing at doing deductions.

EXERCISE 6 Roger and the Headstand

Review

- Everybody, listen to the story of Roger and the headstand again.

Roger almost always wore a hat. He had hats that were flat and hats that were round. He had hats that had brims, hats that had beaks and hats that had bands. He had red hats, blue hats and black hats. But his very favorite hat was a big stiff straw hat. He was always very careful not to crush that hat. He sure didn't want a squashed straw hat.

Well, one day Roger was wearing his very favorite hat. He went to the park and saw two little kids trying to stand on their heads. They were wobbling and falling over. Roger watched them for a while and smiled to himself. Roger was one of the best headstanders you have ever seen. But those little kids were terrible. They were doing it all wrong. And every time they tried to get their feet off the ground—plop—they would fall over.

Finally, Roger walked over to them and said, "You're doing it all wrong."

One of the kids looked at Roger and said, "Leave us alone. Can't you see we're trying to practice?"

"Yeah," the other little kid said. "We're going to learn how to do it. We just need a little practice."

"No, no," Roger said. "The way you're trying to do it, you'll **never** stand on your head."

One of the little kids said, "If you're so smart, why don't you show us how it's done?"

"All right," Roger said. "I'll show you."

So Roger took off his hat because he sure didn't want to wear it when he stood on his head. Then he looked around for a safe place to put it. He thought about having one of the little kids hold it, but then he spotted a very safe place for it. Not far away was a teeter-totter. Nobody was around it. So he decided to put his hat under that teeter-totter. And that's just what he did. He put his fine straw hat under the **right** end of the teeter-totter. "Nobody will bother it there," he said.

Then Roger went back to the little kids and said, "Here's how it's done." He got down and did one of the best headstands you have ever seen. He was as straight as an arrow, with his toes pointed. And he was so still, he was almost like an upside-down statue.

The little kids both said, "Wow! What a headstand."

Roger smiled while he was upside-down. He was pretty proud of himself, and he decided he would show those little kids what a long, long, long headstand looked like.

Well, while Roger was doing his long, long, long headstand, the kids got tired of watching him. After all, he wasn't doing anything, just standing there on his head with his toes pointed. So they went away and played ball. Still, Roger was doing his headstand.

After the kids got tired of playing ball, they looked over at Roger.

He was still on his head with his toes pointed.

One little kid said, "Let's go on the teeter-totter."

The other little kid said, "Yes, let's do that."

And they did it. One kid got on the left end of the teeter-totter. The other kid got on the right end. And up and down they went. When the right end went down the **first** time, it made a big scrunch sound. By the time the right end went down the **fifth** time, it didn't make a scrunch sound at all.

Pretty soon, the little kids got tired of going up and down on the teeter-totter so they went back to Roger, who was still on his head, with his toes in the same position.

One little kid said to Roger, "Do you know your face is getting very red?"

The other little kid said, "Yeah, how long are you going to stand on your head?"

"I'm finished," Roger said. He got down from his headstand and stood up. "**That's** how you do it," he said proudly.

Then Roger walked over to the teeter-totter and started to pick up his straw hat, but what he picked up didn't look much like a hat. It looked like a scrunched-up straw Frisbee.

Roger didn't know how his hat got flattened, but it was flat, flat, flat. And Roger was mad, mad, mad.

"My hat is ruined," he said. "My favorite hat looks like a straw plate." He tossed the hat away and marched out of the park, very angry.

After he left, one of the little kids went over to the hat, picked it up and said to the other little kid, "Let's play some Frisbee." And they did.

EXERCISE 7   Details

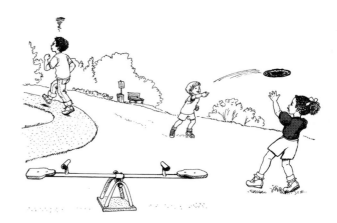

1. Everybody, find part E. ✔
    This picture shows something that happened in the story. If you look hard you can find Roger in this picture. He's on that path marching out of the park.
   - Is he happy? (Signal.) *No.*
   - Why not? (Call on a student. Idea: *Because his favorite hat is scrunched.*)
2. What happened just before this picture? (Call on a student. Idea: *The little kids played on the teeter-totter and scrunched the hat while Roger was standing on his head.*)
   - The little kids are sailing something through the air. What is that thing? (Signal.) *Roger's hat.*
3. Listen: Make an **X** under the teeter-totter to show where Roger's hat was when it got all flattened out.
4. Later you can color that picture.

Objectives

- **Perform on mastery test of skills presented in lessons 1–9.** (Exercise 1)
- **Students vote on a story to be reread.** (Exercise 2)
- **Exercises 3–5 provide instructions for marking the test and giving the students feedback.**

WORKBOOK • LINED PAPER

EXERCISE 1   Test

Writing Parallel Sentences

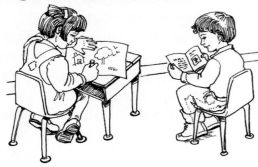

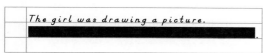

1. You're going to have a test to see how smart you are. You can't talk to anybody during the test or look at what anybody else does.
- Open your workbook to lesson 10 and find part A. ✔
  You're going to write about this picture.
2. The picture shows what a girl and a boy were doing. One of them was reading something. Who was that? (Signal.) *The boy.*
- What was the girl doing? (Call on a student. Idea: *Drawing a picture.*)
3. Everybody, get ready to read the sentence. (Signal.) *The girl was drawing a picture.*
- Tell me what the second sentence should say about the boy. (Signal.) *The boy was reading a book.*
- Once more. Say the sentence about the boy. (Signal.) *The boy was reading a book.*
- Say the sentence about the girl. (Signal.) *The girl was drawing a picture.*
4. (Write on the board:)

> reading   book

- Here are words you'll need:
  reading . . . book.
5. (Hand out a piece of lined paper to each student.) Write your name on the top line of the paper. ✔
  Write both sentences. Remember to write your words just after the margin, start with a capital letter, and put a period at the end of each sentence.
  (Observe students and give feedback.)
6. **(Optional:)** Skip a line on your paper and write both sentences again.
  (Observe students and give feedback.)
7. (Collect and correct papers.)

Left/Right

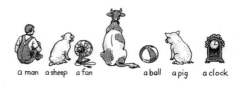

a man a sheep a fan   a ball   a pig   a clock

1. Everybody, find part B. ✔
- The picture shows Clarabelle with objects to her **left** and to her **right.** The name is written under each object.
2. Everybody, touch the ball. ✔
  Under the ball, it says **a ball.** What do the words under that object say? (Signal.) *A ball.*
- Touch the pig. ✔
  What do the words say? (Signal.) *A pig.*
- Touch the fan. ✔
  What do the words say? (Signal.) *A fan.*
- Touch the man. ✔
  What do the words say? (Signal.) *A man.*

- Touch the clock. ✔
  What do the words say? (Signal.) *A clock.*
- Touch the sheep. ✔
  What do the words say? (Signal.) *A sheep.*
4. You're going to complete sentences. Listen: Touch sentence 1 below the pictures. ✔
  I'll read what it says: The **third** object to Clarabelle's **right** is blank.
- Start at Clarabelle, find the third object to her right and copy the name of that object in the blank for item 1. Raise your hand when you're finished.
  (Observe students but do not give feedback.)
- Touch sentence 2. ✔
  I'll read the item: The **third** object to Clarabelle's **left** is blank.
- Start at Clarabelle, find the third object to her left and copy the name of that object. Raise your hand when you're finished.
  (Observe students.)
- Touch sentence 3. ✔
  I'll read the item: The **second** object to Clarabelle's **left** is blank.
- Start at Clarabelle, find the second object to her left and copy the name of that object. Raise your hand when you're finished.
  (Observe students.)
- Touch sentence 4. ✔
  I'll read the item: The **first** object to Clarabelle's **right** is blank.
- Start at Clarabelle, find the first object to her right and copy the name of that object. Raise your hand when you're finished.
  (Observe students.)

All, Some, None—Application

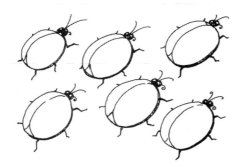

1. Everybody, find part C. ✔
- Look at the picture of the bugs.

2. This statement is **false:** All of the bugs have spots.
- Make that statement **true** by drawing some things in your picture. Don't cross out anything. Fix up your picture so that **all** of the bugs have spots. Raise your hand when you're finished.
  (Observe students.)

EXERCISE 2 Story

1. For the rest of the period, I'll read a story. You get to choose which story. You've heard stories about Bleep, Roger, Paul and Clarabelle. Everybody gets to vote on their favorite story. But you can only vote one time. I'll name the stories. You hold up your hand if you want that story. But remember, you can hold up your hand only one time.
- Listen: Bleep. Who wants to hear the Bleep story again? (Count the students' raised hands.)
- Listen: Paul and Clarabelle. Who wants to hear "Paul Paints Pansies" again? (Count the students' raised hands.)
- Listen: Roger. Who wants to hear the Roger story again? (Count the students' raised hands.)
2. (Read the chosen story. If time permits, read the story for the second choice.)
  Key: Lesson 7 for Bleep;
  Lesson 8 for Paul and Clarabelle;
  Lesson 9 for Roger.

EXERCISE 3 Marking the Test

1. (Mark the tests before the next scheduled language lesson. Use the *Language Arts Answer Key* to check the tests.)
2. (Write the number of errors each student made in the test scorebox at the beginning of the test.)
3. (Enter the number of errors each student made on the Summary for Test 1. A Reproducible Summary Sheet is at the back of the *Language Arts Teacher's Guide.*)

EXERCISE 4   Feedback On Test 1

1. (Return the students' workbooks after they are marked.)

   • Everybody, open your workbook to lesson 10. Look at how I marked your test page.

2. I wrote a number at the top of your test. That number tells how many items you got wrong on the whole test.

   • Raise your hand if I wrote **0** or **1** at the top of your test.
   Those are super stars.

   • Raise your hand if I wrote **2** or **3.** Those are pretty good workers.

   • If I wrote a number that's more than 3, you're going to have to work harder.

EXERCISE 5   Test Remedies

   • (See the *Language Arts Teacher's Guide* for a general discussion of remedies.)

LESSON 11

Objectives

- Follow directions involving **north, south, east, west.** (Exercise 1)
- Say different deductions based on pictures. (Exercise 2)
- Construct sentences for different illustrations. (Exercise 3)
- **Identify seasons from descriptions.** (Exercise 4)
- Listen to a story and answer comprehension questions. (Exercise 5)
- Make a picture consistent with details of a story. (Exercise 6)

EXERCISE 1 Directions

North, South, East, West

1. (Stand near the middle of the classroom.) You've learned about the four directions. I'll point. You tell me the direction I'm pointing.
2. (Point east.)
Everybody, which direction am I pointing? (Signal.) *East.*
- (Point south.)
Which direction am I pointing? (Signal.) *South.*
- (Point north.)
Which direction am I pointing? (Signal.) *North.*
- (Point west.)
Which direction am I pointing? (Signal.) *West.*
- (Repeat step 2 until firm.)
3. Now I'm going to go to a different part of the room and do the same thing. (Move to the front of the classroom.)
4. (Point north.)
Everybody, which direction am I pointing? (Signal.) *North.*
- (Point south.)
Which direction am I pointing? (Signal.) *South.*
- (Point east.)
Which direction am I pointing? (Signal.) *East.*
- (Point west.)
Which direction am I pointing? (Signal.) *West.*
- (Repeat step 4 until firm.)
5. Your turn to follow some tough instructions.
- Everybody, stand up.

6. Face **north.** ✔
- Take three small steps **north.** Get ready. Go. ✔
- Keep facing north and take two small steps to the **east.** Small steps. Get ready. Go. ✔
- Keep facing north and take two small steps to the **north** again. Get ready. Go. ✔
- Now keep facing **north** and take three small steps to the **south.** Get ready. Go. ✔
- (Repeat step 6 until firm.)
7. Listen: Face the direction where you see the sun **setting at night.** Get ready. Go. ✔
- Which direction are you facing? (Signal.) *West.*
- Listen: Face the direction where you see the sun **rising in the morning.** Get ready. Go. ✔
- Which direction are you facing? (Signal.) *East.*
- (Repeat step 7 until firm.)
8. Point **south** if you were able to follow all those hard, hard directions. ✔
You are really getting smart.
Sit down.

WORKBOOK

EXERCISE 2 Deductions

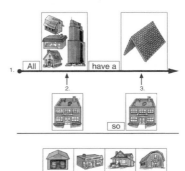

1. Open your workbook to lesson 11, and find part A. ✔
These are arrows for a new deduction. It's tough.

58 Lesson 11

2. Touch arrow 1. ✔
   The first word on that arrow is **all.**
   Everybody, what word? (Signal.) *All.*
   • What's in the first picture on arrow 1?
     (Signal.) *Buildings.*
   • The words **after** the first picture are
     have a. What are the words after the first
     picture? (Signal.) *Have a.*
   • So the first part of the rule is: **All buildings
     have a** . . . something.
   • The second picture shows what they have.
     Everybody, what do they have? (Signal.)
     A roof.
   • So here's the rule for arrow 1: **All buildings
     have a roof.**
3. Everybody, say the rule for arrow 1.
   (Signal.) *All buildings have a roof.*
   • (Repeat step 3 until firm.)
4. Touch arrow 2. ✔
   There's a picture at the bottom of arrow 2.
   That's a school.
   • Arrow 2 shows that a school is in the class
     of buildings. So here's the statement for
     arrow 2: **A school is a building.**
5. Everybody, say the statement for arrow 2.
   (Signal.) *A school is a building.*
   • (Repeat step 5 until firm.)
6. Touch arrow 3. ✔
   That arrow shows that a school has
   something.
   What does it have? (Signal.) *A roof.*
7. Everybody, say the statement for arrow 3.
   (Signal.) *So a school has a roof.*
   • (Repeat step 7 until firm.)
8. I'll say the whole deduction. You touch
   each arrow. I'll start with arrow 1.
   • Listen: All buildings have a roof. A school is
     a building. So a school has a roof.
9. Your turn to touch the arrows and say the
   whole deduction. Start with arrow 1. Get
   ready. (Signal.) *All buildings have a roof. A
   school is a building. So a school has a roof.*
   • (Repeat step 9 until firm.)
10. See if you can say that deduction with your
    eyes closed. Get a picture of the arrows in
    your mind. Tell about arrow 1: **All buildings
    have a roof.** Then tell about arrow 2 and
    arrow 3.
11. Say the whole deduction with your eyes
    closed. Get ready. (Signal.) *All buildings
    have a roof. A school is a building. So a
    school has a roof.*
    • (Repeat step 11 until firm.)

12. Everybody, touch the pictures at the
    bottom of the page. ✔
    • I'll tell you what kind of buildings those
      are. The first building is a garage. The next
      building is a store. The next building is a
      house. The last building is a barn.
13. Everybody, touch the picture of a
    garage. ✔
    • **Pretend** that you have a picture of the
      garage at the bottom of both up arrows.
    • My turn to say the deduction for a garage:
      All buildings have a roof. A garage is a
      building. So a garage has a roof.
14. Let's see if everybody can say the whole
    deduction for a garage. Get ready. (Signal.)
    *All buildings have a roof. A garage is a
    building. So a garage has a roof.*
    • Who thinks they can say the whole
      deduction for any of the other buildings
      at the bottom of the page? Just pick your
      favorite building. Then pretend that building
      is at the bottom of both up-arrows and say
      the whole deduction for that building. It's
      tough.
    • (Call on several students. Praise
      appropriate deductions.)

**EXERCISE 3 Sentence
Construction**

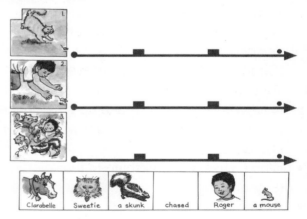

1. Everybody, find part B. ✔
   The pictures show what different
   characters did. You're going to write
   sentences that tell what the characters did
   in each picture.
2. Look at the boxes at the bottom of the
   page. I'll read the words.
   • First box. The word says: **Clarabelle.**
   • Next box. The word says: **Sweetie.**
   • Next box. The words say: **a skunk.**
   • Next box. The word says: **chased.**

Lesson 11   **59**

- Next box. The word says: **Roger.**
- Next box. The words say: **a mouse.**
- You're going to use these words to make up sentences. All your sentences will tell **who chased.**

3. Everybody, touch picture 1. ✔
   Who's chasing something in that picture? (Signal.) *Sweetie.*
- Everybody, what did Sweetie chase in this picture? (Signal.) *A mouse.*
- Here's the sentence that tells what Sweetie did: **Sweetie chased a mouse.**

4. Everybody, say that sentence. (Signal.) *Sweetie chased a mouse.*
- (Repeat step 4 until firm.)

5. Listen to the sentence again: **Sweetie . . . chased . . . a mouse.**

6. What's the first word in that sentence? (Signal.) *Sweetie.*
- What's the next word in that sentence? (Signal.) *Chased.*
- What are the last words in that sentence? (Signal.) *A mouse.*
- (Repeat step 6 until firm.)

7. Remember, in each space on the arrow you have to write the words from one of the boxes.
- Your turn: Write the sentence on the arrow for picture 1. Write the words **Sweetie, chased, a mouse.** Copy the words carefully. Raise your hand when you're finished.
   (Observe students and give feedback.)

8. Touch picture 2. ✔
- Now you're going to make up a sentence for picture 2. That picture shows another character.
- Who's chasing something in that picture? (Signal.) *Roger.*
- Raise your hand when you can say the whole sentence about what Roger did in picture 2.

9. Everybody say that sentence. (Signal.) *Roger chased a mouse.*
- Yes, **Roger chased a mouse.**

10. Your turn: Write the sentence on the arrow for picture 2. Raise your hand when you're finished.
   (Observe students and give feedback.)

11. Touch picture 3. ✔
   Uh-oh, it's hard to tell what's in that picture. In fact, maybe there's not even a mouse in that picture. Maybe there's a skunk, and maybe somebody chased that skunk.

12. Your turn: Write sentence 3. Start with the name of a character. Then tell what that character chased. Don't write one of the sentences you've already written. Raise your hand when you're finished.
   (Observe students and give feedback.)

13. Read the sentence you wrote for picture 3. (Call on several students. Praise appropriate sentences.)
- Those were pretty good sentences.

EXERCISE 4   Seasons

1. (Write on the board:)

winter
spring
summer
fall

- These are the four seasons of the year. I'll read them: **winter, spring, summer, fall.**
- Winter is the coldest season.
- Then comes spring. That's when plants start growing.
- Then comes summer. That's the hottest season.
- Then comes fall. That's when the trees start losing their leaves.
- Then we're back to winter.

2. Listen: Which is the coldest season? (Signal.) *Winter.*
- Which is the hottest season? (Signal.) *Summer.*
- Which is the season when plants start growing? (Signal.) *Spring.*
- Which is the season when trees lose their leaves? (Signal.) *Fall.*
- My turn to say all the seasons again: winter, spring, summer, fall.

3. Your turn: Say all the seasons. Get ready. Go. (Signal.) *Winter, spring, summer, fall.*
- (Repeat step 3 until firm.)

4. Remember the names of the four seasons.

Storytelling

- I'm going to tell you a story about a toad, a toadstool and a mouse. Part of this story takes place in the spring of the year, and part of the story takes place in the summer and the fall. So think of the seasons when you listen to the story.

One spring a big toadstool grew up in a dark part of the woods. Pretty soon, a toad came along and said, "My, my. What a fine toadstool. Wouldn't it make a nice place for me to sleep during the day?"

So the toad jumped on top of the toadstool and took a long nap until the sun went down. Then the toad woke up and went out with the other toads, hunting for bugs and slugs and other good things to eat.

- Listen: Everybody, did the toad nap during the day or during the night? (Signal.) *Day.*

Just after the toad left the toadstool that evening, a tired little mouse came wandering through the woods, looking for a home. She spotted the toadstool and said, "My, my. What a fine toadstool. Wouldn't it make a nice place for me to sleep during the night?"

She curled up under the toadstool and took a long nap until the sun came up. Then the little mouse went out to find seeds and weeds and other good things to eat.

This went on for most of the summer. The toad slept on top of the toadstool during the day. The mouse slept under the toadstool during the night. And they never saw each other—until one evening near the end of the summer.

The mouse came back to the toadstool ready for a good night's sleep, when what did she see snoozing on top of the toadstool? A big toad.

The mouse said, "I can't have this—a big toad on my house. I'll have to get rid of that thing." But how? The mouse didn't want to get into an argument with the toad, so she gave the matter some thought and decided to trick the toad into leaving. The mouse knew a lot about toads. She knew that toads hibernated during the wintertime. They slept all winter long.

- That's what it means to **hibernate.** Animals that hibernate sleep during the whole winter. They go to sleep in the fall and wake up in the spring.

So the mouse said to herself, "If I make this toad think winter will soon be here, he'll go away and hibernate some place, and I'll have my toadstool all to myself."

- Listen again to what the mouse said to herself:

"If I make this toad think winter will soon be here, he'll go away and hibernate some place, and I'll have my toadstool all to myself."

- That mouse is trying to trick the toad. Everybody, if that toad thought it was still summer, would the toad hibernate? (Signal.) *No.*
- If that toad thought that winter was coming very soon, would that toad hibernate? (Signal.) *Yes.*
- I guess that mouse will have to trick the toad into thinking that winter is coming very soon. Let's see what she did.

The next day, while the toad was snoozing away on top of the toadstool, the mouse gathered up a great pile of leaves and covered the toad with them.

That evening, the toad woke up, saw the leaves and said, "Gosh, summer is over already. The leaves are falling from the trees. So it must be time for me to hibernate for the winter."

With that, the toad jumped down from the toadstool, looked around and said, "I think I'll dig a hole right under this toadstool. That looks like a great place to hibernate."

And that's what the toad did.

- Where did the toad hibernate? (Signal.) *Under the toadstool.*
- And where does the mouse sleep during the night? (Signal.) *Under the toadstool.*
- Uh-oh, I think there's going to be a problem.

That evening, the mouse came back to the toadstool, looked around and said to herself, "Ha, ha, the toad is gone. My trick must have . . ."

Before she could finish her thought, she fell into the hole the toad had dug, and there she was at the bottom of the hole, right next to the toad.

The toad said, "What are you doing here? Can't you see I'm hibernating for the winter?"

The mouse said, "What are **you** doing here? This is my home. I live under the toadstool."

The toad yawned and said, "How can this be your home? They don't call it a **mouse**stool, do they? It's a **toad**stool and I happen to be a toad. So go away and let me hibernate in peace."

The mouse didn't know what to say. She jumped out of the hole and paced around the toadstool for a while. Then she bent down and said to the toad, "All right. I'll tell you the truth: You don't have to hibernate. I just played a trick on you by putting leaves all over you. It's not time to hibernate. It's still August. So you can go back to the top of the toadstool."

"It's not time to hibernate?"

"That's right," said the mouse.

So the toad yawned, stretched and said, "Well, I guess I'll go out and hunt for some bugs and slugs and other good things to eat."

And that's just what the toad did.

After the toad left, the mouse said, "This is such a nice hole, I think I'll just use it for my home."

And that's just what the mouse did.

Things went back to the way they had been. The mouse slept in the hole at night. The toad slept on the toadstool during the day.

But then, one day late in the fall, the mouse came home at night after hunting for seeds and weeds and other good things to eat. The mouse went down into her hole and was ready to curl up for a good night's sleep when she noticed a big lumpy form snoring away right in her favorite place. It was the toad.

The mouse tried to wake up the toad and make him leave, but all he would do was roll over and say, "I'm hibernating."

Finally, the mouse said, "There's only one way to put up with this snoring toad all winter. I'll have to hibernate, too."

And that's just what the mouse did.

So if you went by that place in the winter, there would be a lot of snow on the ground. You wouldn't see a toadstool; you wouldn't see a hole in the ground; and you wouldn't see a toad or a mouse. But if you stopped and listened very carefully, you would hear some snoring from under the snow. You'd hear some heavy snoring—snork, snork—and you'd hear some little wheezing snoring—zzzzz. And that snoring went on all winter.

EXERCISE 6　Details

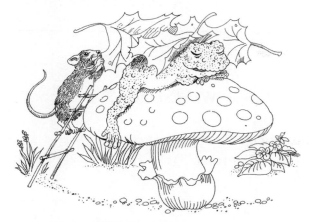

1. Everybody, find part C. ✔
   This picture shows something that happened in the story.

2. What's the mouse doing in this picture? (Call on a student. Idea: *Putting leaves on top of the toad.*)
   - Why is she piling all those leaves on the toad? (Call on a student. Idea: *So he'll think it's time to hibernate.*)
   - Everybody, think big: In what season did this part of the story take place? (Signal.) *Summer.*
   - What's the toad going to do right after he wakes up and discovers all those leaves on top of him? (Call on a student. Idea: *Dig a hole under the toadstool and hibernate.*)

3. Later you can color the picture. That toad is brown. That mouse is gray. I think that's a pink toadstool, but you can make it any color you wish.

Note: If gray crayons are not available, direct students to use their pencil to color the mouse gray.

Objectives

- Identify seasons from descriptions. (Exercise 1)
- **Fix up a map to show north (N), south (S), east (E) and west (W).** (Exercise 2)
- Say different deductions based on pictures. (Exercise 3)
- Construct sentences for different illustrations. (Exercise 4)
- Listen to a story and answer comprehension questions. (Exercise 5)
- Edit words to show a character's dialect. (Exercise 6)

EXERCISE 1   Seasons

1. Last time, you named the seasons of the year.
   Everybody, how many seasons are there in a year? (Signal.) *Four.*
- Which season is the coldest? (Signal.) *Winter.*
- Which season is the hottest? (Signal.) *Summer.*
2. Everybody, start with the coldest season and say all four seasons. Get ready. (Signal.) *Winter, spring, summer, fall.*
- (Repeat step 2 until firm.)

WORKBOOK

EXERCISE 2   Directions

Map

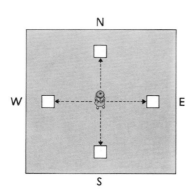

1. Open your workbook to lesson 12, and find part A. ✔
- This is a map. It has the letters **N, S, E** and **W** on it. Those letters stand for **north, south, east** and **west.**
2. Everybody, touch the letter **N.** ✔
   What does the **N** stand for? (Signal.) *North.*
- Listen: **North** is always at the **top** of the map.

- Everybody, touch the letter **S.** ✔
  What does the **S** stand for? (Signal.) *South.*
- Listen: **South** is always at the **bottom** of the map.
- Everybody, touch the letter **E.** ✔
  What does the **E** stand for? (Signal.) *East.*
- Everybody, touch the letter **W.** ✔
  What does the **W** stand for? (Signal.) *West.*
3. Everybody, pick up your workbook and stand up.
- Hold your workbook flat and face **north.** Make the arrow for **north** on the map point north in the room. ✔
- Now your map shows you just which way **east** and **west** and **south** are.
- Look at the arrow for **east** on your map. It points to your right. And that's just where **east** is in the room.
- Look at the arrow for **south.** It points right through you. And that's where **south** is, behind you.
- Remember when the **N** on the map points **north,** the arrows on the map show where all the other directions are.
- Everybody, sit down.
4. Touch the person in the middle of the map. ✔
   That person wants to walk **south.** Which direction does she want to walk? (Signal.) *South.*
- Look at the arrows that lead from the person. Write **S** in the box on the correct arrow. That arrow shows the direction she would go to walk **south.** Raise your hand when you're finished.
  (Observe students and give feedback.)

- (Write on the board:)

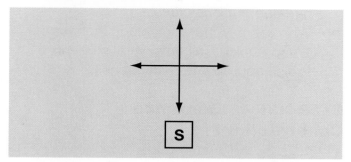

- Here's what you should have. Raise your hand if you got it right.
5. New problem: The person in the middle of the map wants to walk **east.** Which direction does she want to walk? (Signal.) *East.*
- Write **E** in the box on the arrow that shows which direction she would go. Raise your hand when you're finished.
  (Observe students and give feedback.)
- (Write to show:)

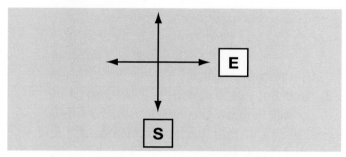

- Here's what you should have. Raise your hand if you got it right.
6. New problem: The person wants to walk **west.** Which direction does she want to walk? (Signal.) *West.*
- Write **W** in the box on the arrow that shows which direction she would go. Raise your hand when you're finished.
  (Observe students and give feedback.)
- (Write to show:)

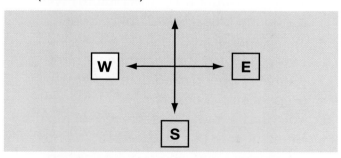

- Here's what you should have. Raise your hand if you got it right.
7. New problem: The person wants to walk **north.** Which direction does she want to walk? (Signal.) *North.*

- Write **N** in the box on the arrow that shows which direction she would go. Raise your hand when you're finished.
  (Observe students and give feedback.)
- (Write to show:)

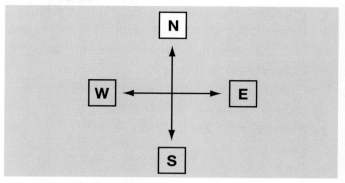

- Here's what you should have. Raise your hand if you got it right.
8. Raise both hands if you got all four directions correct.
  Good for you.

EXERCISE 3 Deductions

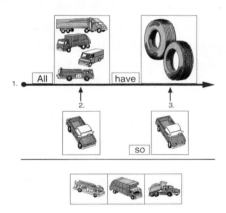

1. Everybody, find part B. ✔
   These are arrows for a new deduction. It's tough.
2. Touch arrow 1. ✔
   What's the first word on arrow 1? (Signal.) *All.*
- Everybody, what's in the first picture on arrow 1? (Signal.) *Trucks.*
- What is the word **after** the picture? (Signal.) *Have.*
- So the first part of the rule is: **All trucks have** . . . something.
- The second picture shows what they have. Everybody, what do they have? (Signal.) *Tires.*
- So here's the rule for arrow 1: **All trucks have tires.**

3. Everybody, say the rule for arrow 1. (Signal.) *All trucks have tires.*
   - (Repeat step 3 until firm.)
4. Touch arrow 2. ✔
   There's a picture at the bottom of arrow 2. What's in that picture? (Signal.) *A pickup.*
   - Arrow 2 shows that a pickup is in the class of trucks. So here's the statement for arrow 2: **A pickup is a truck.**
5. Everybody, say the statement for arrow 2. (Signal.) *A pickup is a truck.*
   - (Repeat step 5 until firm.)
6. Touch arrow 3. ✔
   That arrow shows that a pickup has something. What does it have? (Signal.) *Tires.*
7. Everybody, say the statement for arrow 3. (Signal.) *A pickup has tires.*
   - (Repeat step 7 until firm.)
8. I'll say the whole deduction. You touch each arrow. I'll start with arrow 1.
   - Listen: **All trucks have tires. A pickup is a truck. So a pickup has tires.**
9. Your turn to touch the arrows and say the whole deduction. Start with arrow 1. Get ready. (Signal.) *All trucks have tires. A pickup is a truck. So a pickup has tires.*
   - (Repeat step 9 until firm.)
10. See if you can say that deduction with your eyes closed. Get ready. (Signal.) *All trucks have tires. A pickup is a truck. So a pickup has tires.*
    - (Repeat step 10 until firm.)
11. Everybody, touch the pictures at the bottom of the page. ✔
    - I'll tell you what kind of trucks those are. The first truck is a fire truck. The next truck is a garbage truck. The next truck is a dump truck.
12. Everybody, touch the picture of the fire truck below the arrows. ✔
    - **Pretend** that you have a picture of the fire truck at the bottom of both up-arrows.
    - Let's see if everybody can say the whole deduction. Everybody, start with arrow 1 and say the deduction for a fire truck. Get ready. (Signal.) *All trucks have tires. A fire truck is a truck. So a fire truck has tires.*
13. Let's see if everybody can say the whole deduction for a garbage truck. Everybody, say the whole deduction for a garbage truck. Get ready. Go. (Signal.) *All trucks*

have tires. A garbage truck is a truck. So a garbage truck has tires.
14. Who can say the whole deduction for the dump truck? (Call on several students. Praise appropriate deductions.)

EXERCISE 4 Sentence Construction

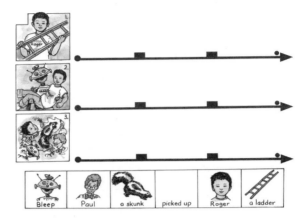

1. Everybody, find part C. ✔
   The pictures show what different characters did. You're going to write sentences that tell what the characters did in each picture.
2. Look at the boxes at the bottom of the page. I'll read the words.
   - First box. The word says: **Bleep.**
   - Next box: **Paul.**
   - Next box: **A skunk.**
   - Next box: **Picked up.**
   - Next box: **Roger.**
   - Next box: **A ladder.**
3. You're going to use the words in the boxes to make up sentences. All your sentences will tell **what** a character picked up.
4. Everybody, touch picture 1. ✔
   Who's in that picture? (Signal.) *Roger.*
   - What did Roger do in this picture? (Call on a student. Idea: *Picked up a ladder.*)
   - Yes, Roger picked up a ladder.
5. Everybody, say the sentence for arrow 1. (Signal.) *Roger picked up a ladder.*
   - (Repeat step 5 until firm.)
6. Your turn: Write your sentence for picture 1. Remember to use the words in the boxes. Raise your hand when you're finished. (Observe students and give feedback.)
7. Touch picture 2. ✔
   Now you're going to make up a sentence for picture 2. That picture shows something another character did.

- Who picked up something in that picture? (Signal.) *Bleep.*
- Use the words in the boxes to write the sentence for picture 2. Raise your hand when you're finished.
  (Observe students and give feedback.)
8. Everybody read your sentence for picture 2. Get ready. (Signal.) *Bleep picked up Roger.*
- That's what you should have. **Bleep picked up Roger.** That's pretty silly. Raise your hand if you got it right.
9. Touch picture 3. ✔
  Uh-oh, somebody did it again. It's hard to tell what's in that picture. In fact, maybe there's not even a ladder in that picture. Maybe there's a skunk and maybe somebody picked up that skunk.
- Your turn: Write sentence 3. Make up a new sentence. Don't write one of the sentences you've already written.
- Use the words in the boxes and write your sentence for picture 3. Raise your hand when you're finished.
  (Observe students and give feedback.)
10. Read the sentence you made up for picture 3. (Call on several students. Praise sentences of the form: _____ picked up _____.)

EXERCISE 5   Bleep Says Some Strange Things *Part 2*

Storytelling

- Everybody, I'm going to read you the rest of the Bleep story. Remember, he was trying to fix the way he talked.

Bleep adjusted some screws in his head so that he would talk better. He turned the **red** screw and the **brown** screw. When he was done, he couldn't say the **e** sound in words like **egg** and **let.**

- Instead of saying **egg,** he said something else. What's that? (Signal.) *Ugg.*
- Instead of saying **let,** he said something else. What's that? (Signal.) *Lut.*

After Bleep mailed the letter, he went back home and Molly took the top of his head off. Then she adjusted the screw for the **e** sound. That was the red screw. Molly didn't know that Bleep had also turned the brown screw. So she didn't adjust that screw.

After she adjusted the red screw, she said, "Say the word **get.**"

Bleep said, "Get."

She said, "Say the word **yes.**"

Bleep said, "Yes."

She said, "Say the word **better.**"

Bleep said, "Better."

Then Molly said, "Well, I think you're all fixed up now."

Bleep said, "Okay, baby."

Molly didn't know it and Bleep didn't know it, but Bleep still had a problem because he had fiddled with the brown screw.

Molly went into the garage to work on her new invention, and Bleep went into the kitchen to wash the dishes.

Pretty soon, Molly heard a loud crashing sound from the kitchen. She went in there to see what had happened. And she saw a **big** mess. On the floor was a broken plate. She said, "Bleep, what happened?" Bleep said, "The plate was wet. When I took it out of the water, it **sipped** out of my hand."

Molly said, "It did what?"

"It **sipped** out of my hand."

"That's what I thought you said." Then Molly said, "Tell me, Bleep, was that plate **slippery?**

"Yes," Bleep said. "Very sippery."

"Oh, no," she said.

"Oh, yes. That plate was very **sick.**"

- Listen: Bleep said, "That plate was very **sick.**"

- Raise your hand when you know what he was trying to say.
- Everybody, what was he trying to say? (Signal.) *That plate was very slick.*
- Uh-oh, there seems to be a sound that Bleep can't say.

Molly wanted to make sure that she understood Bleep's problem. So she said to Bleep, "What's your name?"

Bleep looked at her and said, "Bleep."

Molly said, "Did you drop a pate or a plate?"

Bleep said, "A plate."

Molly said, "Watch me and tell me what I do." She blinked. Then she asked, "What did I do?"

Bleep said, "Blinked."

Then Molly said, "What do I do during the night when I go to bed?"

Bleep looked at Molly and said, "**Seep**."

- What was Bleep trying to say instead of **seep**? (Signal.) *Sleep.*

So Molly knew that Bleep could say some words with an **L** sound. He could say **plate, Bleep** and **blinked**. But he couldn't say **sleep**.

Molly said, "When you took the top of your head off, did you happen to fiddle around with more than one screw?"

Bleep said, "Yes."

Molly said, "Do you happen to remember the color of the other screw you messed with?"

"No," Bleep said.

"This is going to be a lot of fun," Molly said. She wasn't very happy because she wasn't sure which screw to adjust, and there were lots and lots of screws inside Bleep's head.

Molly said, "Well, clean up this mess and then come into the garage. I'll see if I can find the right screw."

Bleep said, "Okay, baby."

Molly started to leave the kitchen, but the floor was wet. Just as she started to walk, she slipped and almost fell on the wet floor. She banged her hand against the counter and hurt her wrist.

Bleep didn't see what happened, but he heard Molly slipping and banging into the counter. He turned around and said, "Did you **sip** on the floor?"

She said, "Yes, Bleep. I slipped."

"Did you hurt your wrist?"

"Yes, Bleep."

"Do you want to put your arm in a **sing?**"

- What was Bleep trying to say instead of **sing?** (Signal.) *Sling.*
- Listen to that part again:

Bleep said, "Do you want to put your arm in a **sing?**"

"No, Bleep. I don't think I need to put my arm in a sling."

"Okay, baby." So after Bleep cleaned up the mess in the kitchen, he went into the garage, and Molly spent a lot of time fixing up his problem. At last, she found the right screw and adjusted it.

- Everybody, what color was that screw? (Signal.) *Brown.*

Then she tested Bleep to make sure he didn't have a problem. She said, "Say **slop.**"

Bleep said, "Slop."

- What would Bleep have said instead of **slop,** if Molly hadn't fixed the problem? (Signal.) *Sop.*

> Molly said, "Say **slide.**"
> Bleep said, "Slide."

- What would Bleep have said instead of **slide,** if Molly hadn't fixed the problem? (Signal.) *Side.*

> Molly said, "I think you're fixed up now."
> And you know what Bleep said.

- Everybody, what did he say? (Signal.) *Okay, baby.*

EXERCISE 6 Writing Bleep-talk

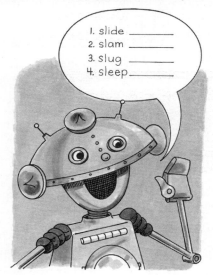

1. slide _____
2. slam _____
3. slug _____
4. sleep _____

1. Everybody, find part D in your workbook. ✔ This picture took place before Molly adjusted the **brown** screw. Bleep is trying to say these words, but he can't say them correctly.
2. I'll read each word. You tell me what Bleep actually said.
- Touch word 1.
  The word is **slide.** What did Bleep say instead of **slide?** (Signal.) *Side.*
- Touch word 2.
  The word is **slam.** What did Bleep say instead of **slam?** (Signal.) *Sam.*

- Touch word 3.
  The word is **slug.** What did Bleep say instead of slug? (Signal.) *Sug.*
- Touch word 4.
  The word is **sleep.** What did Bleep say instead of **sleep?** (Signal.) *Seep.*
- Bleep can't say the **L** in words that start with **S.**
3. On the line next to each word, you'll write the word Bleep actually said. Word 1 is **slide.** What did Bleep say? (Signal.) *Side.*
- Write the word **side** after the word **slide.** The word is spelled just like **slide** except the **L** is missing. Raise your hand when you're finished.
- (Write on the board:)

> **side**

- Here's what you should have for word 1.
4. Your turn: Write the rest of the words the way Bleep would say them. Remember, the words are spelled the same way except for the missing letter. Raise your hand when you're finished.
(Observe students and give feedback.)
5. (Write on the board:)

> **sam**
> **sug**
> **seep**

- After word 2, you should have the word **sam.**
- After word 3, you should have the word **sug.**
- After word 4, you should have the word **seep.**
6. Raise your hand if you wrote all the words correctly.
What good workers.

LESSON 13

Objectives

- Identify seasons from descriptions. (Exercise 1)
- Fix up a map to show north (**N**), south (**S**), east (**E**), west (**W**). (Exercise 2)
- Say different deductions based on pictures. (Exercise 3)
- **Construct 3 sentences about story characters.** (Exercise 4)
- Listen to a familiar story. (Exercise 5)
- Edit words to show a character's dialect. (Exercise 6)

EXERCISE 1 Seasons

1. Let's see what you remember about the seasons.
   - Everybody, how many seasons are in a year? (Signal.) *Four.*
   - What's the coldest season? (Signal.) *Winter.*
   - What's the hottest season? (Signal.) *Summer.*
   - In which season do plants start growing? (Signal.) *Spring.*
   - In which season do leaves fall from the trees? (Signal.) *Fall.*
   - (Repeat step 1 until firm.)
2. Everybody, start with the coldest season and say all the seasons. Get ready. (Signal.) *Winter, spring, summer, fall.*
   - (Repeat step 2 until firm.)

WORKBOOK

EXERCISE 2 Directions

Map

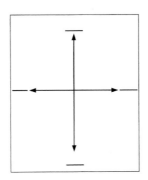

1. Open your workbook to lesson 13. Lesson 13. ✔
   Everybody, find the four arrows in part A.

2. (Write on the board:)

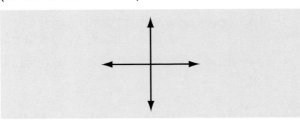

   - Maps always show the same letter on top.
   - (Point to the top arrow.) Everybody, what letter goes at the end of the **top** arrow? (Signal.) *N.*
3. Your turn. Write **N** in the space on top of your map. Raise your hand when you're finished. ✔
   - Everybody, pick up your workbook and stand up. Hold your workbook flat and face north. ✔
   - Now the arrows show all the directions in the room.
4. Listen: Everybody, point east. Get ready. Go. Touch the arrow on your map that points east. ✔
   - Everybody, point west. Get ready. Go. Touch the arrow on your map that points west. ✔
   - Everybody, point south. Get ready. Go. Touch the arrow on your map that points south. ✔
   - Remember where east, west and south go on your map.
   - Everybody, sit down.
5. (Write on the board:)

   S   W   E

   - Here are the letters for the rest of the directions on the map. **S** stands for south. **W** stands for west. **E** stands for east.

6. Your turn: Write those letters at the end of the correct arrows. Raise your hand when you're finished.
   (Observe students and give feedback.)
   - (Write to show:)

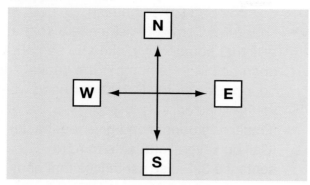

   - Here's what you should have. North is at the top. South is at the bottom. East is on the right side. West is on the left side.
7. Raise your hand if you wrote the letters where they belong.
   - Good for you. You'll be working a lot with maps so remember where the directions go.

EXERCISE 3   Deductions

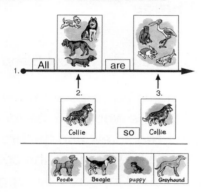

1. Everybody, find part B. ✔
   These are arrows for a new deduction.
2. Touch arrow 1. ✔
   What's the first word? (Signal.) *All*.
   - What are those animals shown in the first picture? (Signal.) *Dogs*.
   - What's the word after the picture? (Signal.) *Are*.
   The first part of the rule is: **All dogs are . . .** something.
   - Everybody, what are all those things in the last picture? (Signal.) *Animals*.
3. Everybody, say the rule for arrow 1.
   (Signal.) *All dogs are animals*.
   - (Repeat step 3 until firm.)

4. That's a collie at the bottom of arrow 2 and arrow 3.
   - Say the statement for arrow 2. (Signal.) *A collie is a dog.*
   - Say the statement for arrow 3. (Signal.) *So a collie is an animal.*
   - (Repeat step 4 until firm.)
5. Your turn to touch the arrows and say the whole deduction. Start with arrow 1. Get ready. (Signal.) *All dogs are animals. A collie is a dog. So a collie is an animal.*
   - (Repeat step 5 until firm.)
6. See if you can say that deduction with your eyes closed. Get ready. (Signal.) *All dogs are animals. A collie is a dog. So a collie is an animal.*
   - (Repeat step 6 until firm.)
7. Everybody, touch the pictures below the deduction. ✔
   - I'll tell you what kind of dogs those are. The first dog is a poodle. The next dog is a beagle. The next dog is a puppy. The last dog is a greyhound.
8. Everybody, touch the picture of the **poodle** below the arrows. ✔
   - **Pretend** that you have a picture of the poodle at the bottom of both up-arrows.
   - Let's see if everybody can say the whole deduction. Everybody, say the whole deduction for a poodle. Get ready. (Signal.) *All dogs are animals. A poodle is a dog. So a poodle is an animal.*
9. Who thinks they can say the whole deduction for any of the other dogs at the bottom of the page? Just pick your favorite dog. Then **pretend** that dog is at the bottom of both up-arrows and say the whole deduction for that dog. It's tough.
   - Who wants to try? (Call on several students. Praise appropriate deductions.)

EXERCISE 4   Sentence Construction

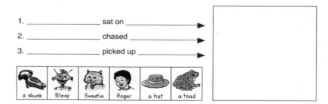

1. Everybody, find part C. ✔
   You're going to make up sentences. And I'll bet some of you are going to make up pretty silly sentences.

2. Touch arrow 1. ✔
   Part of that sentence is already written.
   - Touch the part that's written. ✔
   That part says **sat on.** Everybody, what does it say? (Signal.) *Sat on.*
   - The first sentence will say that somebody sat on something or maybe somebody sat on somebody else.
   - Touch the **first** space on arrow 1. ✔
   That's where you'll write the name of the character doing the sitting.
   - Touch the **last** space on arrow 1. ✔
   That's where you'll write the name of the character or thing that got sat on.
3. The names you'll use to make up sentence 1 are below the sentences. I'll read the names. You touch the pictures. Get ready.
   A skunk . . . Bleep . . . Sweetie . . . Roger . . . a hat . . . a toad.
4. Your turn: Complete sentence 1. Write the name of the character doing the sitting and the name of the character or thing being sat on.
   - Listen: Start your sentence with a capital letter and put a period at the end. Raise your hand when you're finished.
   (Observe students and give feedback.)
5. Let's see what kind of silly sentences you wrote. When I call on you, read your sentence 1. (Call on several students. Praise sentences that first name a character, then name a character or thing.)
   - Those were pretty funny sentences.
6. Everybody, touch the word that's already written in sentence 2. ✔
   - That word is **chased.** Everybody, what word? (Signal.) *Chased.*
   - Sentence 2 will say that somebody chased somebody or something.
   - Touch the first space on arrow 2. ✔
   That's where you'll write the name of the character doing the chasing.
   - Touch the last space on arrow 2. ✔
   That's where you'll write the name of the character or thing being chased.
   - Your turn: Complete sentence 2. Remember the capital and period. Be careful. Raise your hand when you're finished.
   (Observe students and give feedback.)
7. (Call on several students to read sentence 2. Praise appropriate sentences.)

8. Everybody, touch the words that are already written in sentence 3. ✔
   - Those words are **picked up.** What words? (Signal.) *Picked up.*
   - Sentence 3 will say that somebody picked up somebody or something.
   - Your turn: Complete sentence 3 so that it tells that somebody picked up somebody or something. Remember the capital and period. Be careful. Raise your hand when you're finished.
   (Observe students and give feedback.)
9. (Call on several students to read sentence 3. Praise sentences that name two characters.)
10. Everybody, touch the big box next to the sentences. Later, you're going to draw a picture for your favorite sentence. You'll draw a picture of whatever you had happening in your favorite sentence.
    - I'll show you some of the better pictures next time.

EXERCISE 5   Bleep Says Some Strange Things

Review

- Listen to the last story about Bleep again.

> Bleep adjusted some screws in his head so that he would talk better. He turned the **red** screw and the **brown** screw. When he was done, he couldn't say the **e** sound in words like **egg** and **let.**

- Instead of saying **egg,** he said something else. What's that? (Signal.) *Ugg.*
- Instead of saying **let,** he said something else. What's that? (Signal.) *Lut.*

> After Bleep mailed the letter, he went back home and Molly took the top of his head off. Then she adjusted the screw for the **e** sound. That was the red screw. Molly didn't know that Bleep had also turned the brown screw. So she didn't adjust that screw.
>
> After she adjusted the red screw, she said, "Say the word **get.**"

Bleep said, "Get."

She said, "Say the word **yes**."

Bleep said, "Yes."

She said, "Say the word **better**."

Bleep said, "Better."

Then Molly said, "Well, I think you're all fixed up now."

Bleep said, "Okay, baby."

Then Molly went into the garage to work on her new invention and Bleep went into the kitchen to wash the dishes.

Pretty soon, Molly heard a loud crashing sound from the kitchen. She went in there to see what had happened. And she saw a **big** mess. On the floor was a broken plate. She said, "Bleep, what happened?"

Bleep said, "The plate was wet. When I took it out of the water, it **sipped** out of my hand."

Molly said, "It did what?"

"It **sipped** out of my hand."

"That's what I thought you said." Then Molly said, "Tell me, Bleep, was that plate **slippery?**"

"Yes," Bleep said. "Very **sippery**."

"Oh, no," she said.

"Oh, yes. That plate was very **sick**."

Molly said, "When you took the top of your head off, did you happen to fiddle around with more than one screw?"

Bleep said, "Yes."

Molly said, "Do you happen to remember the color of the other screw you messed with?"

"No," Bleep said.

"This is going to be a lot of fun," Molly said. She wasn't very happy because she wasn't sure which screw

to adjust, and there were lots and lots of screws inside Bleep's head.

Molly said, "Well, clean up this mess and then come into the garage. I'll see if I can find the right screw."

Bleep said, "Okay, baby."

Molly started to leave the kitchen, but the floor was wet. Just as she started to walk, she slipped and almost fell on the wet floor. She banged her hand against the counter and hurt her wrist.

Bleep didn't see what happened, but he heard Molly slipping and banging into the counter. He turned around and said, "Did you **sip** on the floor?"

She said, "Yes, Bleep. I slipped."

"Did you hurt your wrist?"

"Yes, Bleep."

"Do you want to put your arm in a **sing?**"

"No, Bleep. I don't think I need to put my arm in a sling."

"Okay, baby."

So after Bleep cleaned up the mess in the kitchen, he went into the garage, and Molly spent a lot of time fixing up his problem. At last, she found the right screw and adjusted it. Then she tested Bleep to make sure he didn't have a problem. She said, "Say **slop**."

Bleep said, "Slop."

Molly said, "Say **slide**."

Bleep said, "Slide."

Molly said, "I think you're fixed up now."

And you know what Bleep said.

EXERCISE 6　Writing Bleep-talk

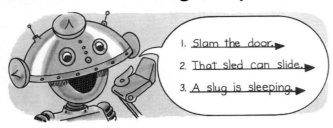

1. Slam the door.
2. That sled can slide.
3. A slug is sleeping.

1. Everybody, find part D. ✔
   Here are some things that Bleep was trying to say when he had a problem.
2. Touch arrow 1. ✔
   Bleep is trying to say, "Slam the door."
   - Everybody, what word will he have trouble with? (Signal.) *Slam.*
   - What word will he say instead of **slam?** (Signal.) *Sam.*
   - Fix up the word **slam** to show what Bleep really said. Cross out the letter **L.** Raise your hand when you're finished.
     (Observe students and give feedback.)
   - (Write on the board:)

slam

   - Check your work. Here's what you should have for **slam**. Now it says **sam.**
3. Touch arrow 2. ✔
   Bleep is trying to say, "That sled can slide."
   - Everybody, what's he trying to say? (Signal.) *That sled can slide.*
   - Bleep will have trouble with **two** words. What's the first word? (Signal.) *Sled.*
   - What's the other word? (Signal.) *Slide.*
   - Listen: Bleep is trying to say **sled.** What will he say instead of **sled?** (Signal.) *Sed.*
   - Bleep is trying to say **slide.** What will he say instead of **slide?** (Signal.) *Side.*
   - Bleep is trying to say, "That sled can slide." Raise your hand when you can say what Bleep said.
   - Everybody, what did he say? (Signal.)
     That sed can side.

   - Yes. "That **sed** can side." That sounds a little goofy.
   - Fix up the words to show what Bleep really said. Raise your hand when you're finished.
     (Observe students and give feedback.)
   - (Write on the board:)

sled	slide

   - Check your work. Here's what you should have for **sled** and **slide.** Now the words say **sed** and **side.**
4. Touch arrow 3. ✔
   Bleep is trying to say, "A slug is sleeping."
   - Everybody, what's he trying to say? (Signal.) *A slug is sleeping.*
   - Bleep will have trouble with **two** words. What's the first word? (Signal.) *Slug.*
   - What's the other word? (Signal.) *Sleeping.*
   - Listen: Bleep is trying to say **slug.** What will he say instead of **slug?** (Signal.) *Sug.*
   - Bleep is trying to say **sleeping.** What will he say instead of **sleeping?** (Signal.) *Seeping.*
   - Bleep is trying to say, "A slug is sleeping." Raise your hand when you can say what Bleep said.
   - Everybody, what did he say? (Signal.)
     A sug is seeping.
     That sounds **really** strange.
   - Fix up the words to show what Bleep really said. Raise your hand when you're finished.
     (Observe students and give feedback.)
   - (Write on the board:)

slug	sleeping

   - Check your work. Here's what you should have for **slug** and **sleeping.** Now the words say **sug** and **seeping.**
5. Raise your hand if you fixed up all the words to show what Bleep **really** said. Good for you.

Objectives

- Compose and write a parallel sentence pair based on a single picture. (Exercise 1)
- Follow directions involving **north, south, east, west.** (Exercise 2)
- **Draw arrows to indicate north, south, east, west.** (Exercise 3)
- Say different deductions based on pictures. (Exercise 4)
- Listen to a familiar story. (Exercise 5)
- **Draw a picture based on a familiar story.** (Exercise 6)

WORKBOOK • LINED PAPER

EXERCISE 1 Writing Parallel Sentences

| milk | poured | some | banana | peeled |

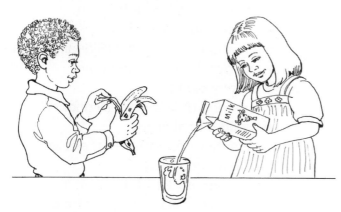

1. Open your workbook to lesson 14, and find part A. ✔
   You're going to write about this picture.
2. The picture shows what a boy and a girl did.
- What did the boy do? (Signal.) *Peeled a banana.*
- What did the girl do? (Call on a student. Idea: *Poured some milk.*)
3. Listen: The boy peeled a banana. The girl poured some milk.
- Everybody, say the first sentence. (Signal.) *The boy peeled a banana.*
- Say the next sentence. (Signal.) *The girl poured some milk.*
- (Repeat sentences until firm.)
4. Look at the vocabulary box. That's the box with the words in it. These are words that you will use when you write your sentences. I'll read the words: **milk . . . poured . . . some . . . banana . . . peeled.** These are words that you will use when you write your sentences.

5. Say the sentence about the boy. (Signal.) *The boy peeled a banana.*
- Say the sentence about the girl. (Signal.) *The girl poured some milk.*
6. (Hand out a piece of lined paper to each student.) Write your name on the top line of the paper. ✔
   Write both sentences. Remember to start with a capital letter and end each sentence with a period.
   (Observe students and give feedback.)
7. Skip a line on your paper and write both sentences again.
   (Observe students and give feedback.)
8. (Collect and correct papers.)

EXERCISE 2 Directions

North, South, East, West

1. Everybody, stand up.
   I'm going to tell you to face different directions.
   Wait until I say **go.**
2. Listen: Everybody, face **east.** Get ready. Go. ✔
- Face **west.** Get ready. Go. ✔
- Face **north.** Get ready. Go. ✔
- Face **east.** Get ready. Go. ✔
- Face **south.** Get ready. Go. ✔
- (Repeat step 2 until firm.)
3. Here are some harder instructions: Everybody, face **east** and **point** north. Think about what you're going to do. Get ready. Go. ✔
- Listen: Face **west** and **point** north. Get ready. Go. ✔
- Face **north** and **point** south. Get ready. Go. ✔
- Everybody, sit down.

4. Raise your hand if you got all those directions right.
Good for you.

EXERCISE 3   Directions

Map

1. (Draw on the board:)

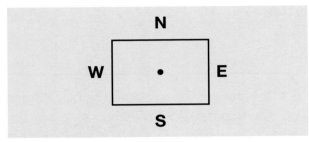

- Here's a box with the letters **N**, **E**, **S** and **W** around the outside and a dot in the middle.
2. (Touch N.)
Everybody, what does **N** stand for? (Signal.) *North.*
- (Touch E.)
What does **E** stand for? (Signal.) *East.*
- (Touch S.)
What does **S** stand for? (Signal.) *South.*
- (Touch W.)
What does **W** stand for? (Signal.) *West.*
- (Repeat step 2 until firm.)
3. I'm going to touch the dot in the middle of the box. Then I'll move to different sides of the box. You'll tell me the direction I'm moving. Remember, the direction I'm **moving** is the letter I'm going **toward.**
4. (Touch the dot. Say:) Watch.
(Move your finger halfway to E.)
Everybody, which direction did I move? (Signal.) *East.*
- (Touch the dot. Say:) Watch again.
(Move halfway to N.)
Which direction did I move? (Signal.) *North.*
- (Touch the dot. Say:) Watch again.
(Move halfway to S.)
Which direction did I move? (Signal.) *South.*
- (Touch the dot. Say:) Watch again.
(Move halfway to W.)
Which direction did I move? (Signal.) *West.*
- (Repeat step 4 until firm.)

5. Now I'm going to make it harder.
(Change dot to show:)

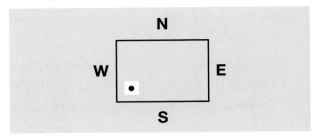

- I'm going to move from this dot. See if you can tell me the direction I move.
6. (Touch the dot. Say:) Watch.
(Move your finger directly south.)
Everybody, which direction did I move? (Signal.) *South.*
- (Touch the dot. Say:) Watch again.
(Move directly west.)
Which direction did I move? (Signal.) *West.*
- (Touch the dot. Say:) Watch again.
(Move directly north.)
Which direction did I move? (Signal.) *North.*
- (Touch the dot. Say:) Watch again.
(Move directly east.)
Which direction did I move? (Signal.) *East.*
- (Repeat step 6 until firm.)
7. Who thinks they can touch that dot and move the direction I say?
- (Call on a student:) Touch the dot.
Listen: Move your finger **east**—straight east. (Praise correct response.)
- Touch the dot again.
Move **north**—straight north. (Praise correct response.)
- Touch the dot again.
Move **south**—straight south. (Praise correct response.)
- Touch the dot again.
Move **west**—straight west. (Praise correct response.)
8. Who else thinks they can do it? Let's see.
(Call on several students. Praise correct responses.)

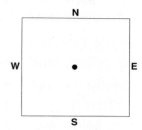

1. Everybody, find part B. ✔
- This is a super hard game. I'll give you hard, hard instructions for moving different directions.
2. Everybody, touch the **dot** in the middle of the box. ✔
- Listen: Move your finger **west**—straight west.
   (Observe students and give feedback.)
- Touch the dot.
   Move **south**—straight south.
   (Observe students and give feedback.)
- Touch the dot.
   Move **east**—straight east.
   (Observe students and give feedback.)
- Touch the dot.
   Move **north**—straight north.
   (Observe students and give feedback.)
3. You're going to draw arrows on the map. The arrows will start at the dot and go the direction I tell you about. Try to make your arrows nice and straight. Everybody, touch the dot.
- Listen: Draw an arrow that goes straight north from the dot. Straight north. Raise your hand when you're finished.
   (Observe students and give feedback.)

- (Draw on the board:)

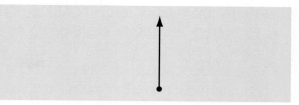

- Here's what you should have drawn.
4. Touch the dot. ✔
- Listen: Draw an arrow that goes straight west from the dot. Straight west. Raise your hand when you're finished.
- (Add to show:)

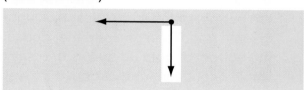

- Here's the arrow you should have drawn.
5. Touch the dot again. ✔
   Listen: Draw an arrow that goes straight south from the dot. Straight south. Raise your hand when you're finished.
- (Add to show:)

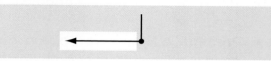

- Here's the arrow you should have drawn. Raise your hand if you drew all the right arrows. ✔
   Pretty smart.

EXERCISE 4 Deductions

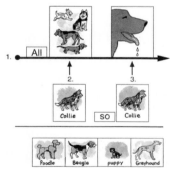

1. Everybody, find part C. ✔
   These are the same dogs we worked with last time, but this is a new deduction about all dogs.
2. Touch arrow 1. ✔
   The first part of the rule is: **All dogs.**
- Everybody, touch the second picture on arrow 1. ✔
- What's that dog doing in the second picture? (Signal.) *Panting.*
- Yes, that dog is panting. That's the way dogs sweat. They don't sweat through their skin the way you do. They sweat through their tongue. So when they get hot, they pant.
- Who can stick out their tongue and pant like a dog? (Praise good "panters.")

3. Everybody, touch arrow 1 again. ✔
   Here's the rule for arrow 1: **All dogs pant.**
   - Everybody, say that rule. (Signal.) *All dogs pant.*
   - Raise your hand when you can say the whole deduction. Remember, tell about arrow 1, then arrow 2, then arrow 3.
4. Everybody, say the whole deduction. Get ready. (Signal.) *All dogs pant. A collie is a dog. So a collie pants.*
   - (Repeat step 4 until firm.)
5. Touch the picture of the **poodle** below the arrows. ✔
   - **Pretend** that you have a picture of a poodle at the bottom of both up arrows.
6. Everybody, say the whole deduction for a poodle. Get ready. (Signal.) *All dogs pant. A poodle is a dog. So a poodle pants.*
   - Who thinks they can say the whole deduction for any of the other dogs at the bottom of the page? Just pick your favorite dog. Then **pretend** that dog is at the bottom of both up arrows and say the whole deduction for that dog. It's tough.
   - Who wants to try? (Call on several students. Praise appropriate deductions.)

EXERCISE 5 The Mouse and the Toadstool

Review

- I'm going to read the story of the mouse and the toad again. That story mentions things that happen in all four seasons.
- Everybody, start with the coldest season and name all the seasons. Get ready. (Signal.) *Winter, spring, summer, fall.*
- The story starts out in spring. Then it tells about summer. Then it tells what happened late in the fall.

One spring a big toadstool grew up in a dark part of the woods. Pretty soon, a toad came along and said, "My, my. What a fine toadstool. Wouldn't it make a nice place for me to sleep during the day?"

So the toad jumped on top of the toadstool and took a long nap until the sun went down. Then the toad went out

with the other toads, hunting for bugs and slugs and other good things to eat.

Just after the toad left the toadstool that evening, a tired little mouse came wandering through the woods, looking for a home. She spotted the toadstool and said, "My, my. What a fine toadstool. Wouldn't it make a nice place for me to sleep during the night?"

She curled up under the toadstool and took a long nap until the sun came up. Then the little mouse went out to find seeds and weeds and other good things to eat.

This went on for most of the summer. The toad slept on top of the toadstool during the day. The mouse slept under the toadstool during the night. And they never saw each other—until one evening near the end of the summer.

The mouse came back to the toadstool ready for a good night's sleep, when what did she see snoozing on top of the toadstool? A big toad.

The mouse said, "I can't have this—a big toad on my house. I'll have to get rid of that thing." But how? The mouse didn't want to get into an argument with the toad, so she gave the matter some thought and decided to trick the toad into leaving. The mouse knew a lot about toads. She knew that toads hibernated during the wintertime. They slept all winter long.

So the mouse said to herself, "If I make this toad think winter will soon be here, he'll go away and hibernate some place, and I'll have my toadstool all to myself."

The next day, while the toad was snoozing away on top of the toadstool, the mouse gathered up a great pile of leaves and covered the toad with them.

That evening, the toad woke up, saw the leaves and said, "Gosh, summer is over already. The leaves are falling from the trees. So it must be time for me to hibernate for the winter."

With that, the toad jumped down from the toadstool, looked around and said, "I think I'll dig a hole right under this toadstool. That looks like a great place to hibernate."

And that's what the toad did.

That evening, the mouse came back to the toadstool, looked around and said to herself, "Ha, ha, the toad is gone. My trick must have . . ."

Before she could finish her thought, she fell into the hole the toad had dug, and there she was at the bottom of the hole, right next to the toad.

The toad said, "What are you doing here? Can't you see I'm hibernating for the winter?"

The mouse said, "What are **you** doing here? This is my home. I live under the toadstool."

The toad yawned and said, "How can this be your home? They don't call it a **mouse**stool, do they? It's a **toad**stool and I happen to be a toad. So go away and let me hibernate in peace."

The mouse didn't know what to say. She jumped out of the hole and paced around the toadstool for a while. Then she bent down and said to the toad, "All right. I'll tell you the truth: You don't have to hibernate. I just played a trick on you by putting leaves all over you. It's not time to hibernate. It's still August. So you can go back to the top of the toadstool."

"It's not time to hibernate?"

"That's right," said the mouse.

So the toad yawned, stretched and said, "Well, I guess I'll go out and hunt for some bugs and slugs and other good things to eat."

And that's just what the toad did.

After the toad left, the mouse said, "This is such a nice hole, I think I'll just use it for my home."

And that's just what the mouse did.

Things went back to the way they had been. The mouse slept in the hole at night. The toad slept on the toadstool during the day.

But then, one day late in the fall, the mouse came home at night after hunting for seeds and weeds and other good things to eat. The mouse went down into her hole and was ready to curl up for a good night's sleep when she noticed a big lumpy form snoring away right in her favorite place. It was the toad.

The mouse tried to wake up the toad and make him leave, but all he would do was roll over and say, "I'm hibernating."

Finally, the mouse said, "There's only one way to put up with this snoring toad all winter. I'll have to hibernate, too."

And that's just what the mouse did.

So if you went by that place in the winter there would be a lot of snow on the ground. You wouldn't see a toadstool; you wouldn't see a hole in the ground; and you wouldn't see a toad or a mouse. But if you stopped and listened very carefully, you would hear some snoring from under the snow. You'd hear some heavy snoring—snork, snork—and you'd hear some little wheezing snoring—zzzzz. And that snoring went on all winter.

EXERCISE 6 Details

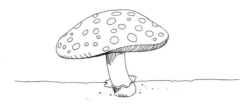

1. Everybody, find part D. ✔
    In that space, you can draw a picture of
    your favorite part of the story. Maybe your
    favorite part is when the mouse covers
    the toad. Maybe your favorite part is when
    they're both snoring. Maybe your favorite
    part is when they argue.

2. Draw your favorite part. Maybe we'll make
    a picture book for the story.

Objectives

• **Use directions about north, south, east, west to solve a puzzle.** (Exercise 1)
• Say different deductions based on pictures. (Exercise 2)
• Construct 3 sentences about story characters. (Exercise 3)
• Listen to a story and answer comprehension questions. (Exercise 4)
• Edit words to correct a character's dialect. (Exercise 5)

EXERCISE 1 Directions

Map Puzzle

1. (Draw on the board:)

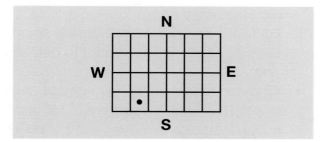

• You're going to work a puzzle. You'll have to move so many squares to the west or north or south or east.
• I'm going to move two squares to the east of the dot and put an **X** where I stop. Watch carefully.
• First I touch the dot. Then I count squares.
• **I DON'T START COUNTING UNTIL I START MOVING.**
• Listen again: I don't start counting until I start moving.
• Here I go. (Count:) One, two.
  (Make an **X** to show:)

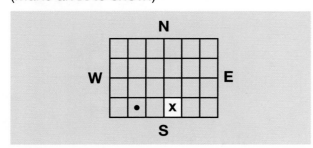

• I did it the right way.
2. Now I'll do it the wrong way. I'll say **one** when I touch the dot.
• Watch: (Touch the dot. Say:) One. (Move your finger 1 square east. Say:) Two.
• That's wrong because I started counting before I started moving.

3. Now I'm going to count three places **north** of the **X** I made.
• I touch the **X.** I don't start counting until I start moving.
• Here I go:
  One, two, three. (Move your finger up 3 squares north. Make an **X** to show:)

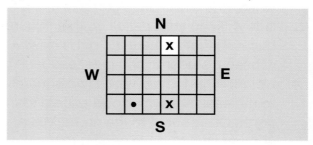

• I did it the right way.

WORKBOOK

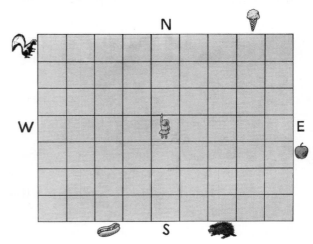

1. Open your workbook to lesson 15. ✔
   Everybody, find part A. ✔
• This is a map puzzle. The girl in the picture will move to one of the things at the outside of the picture. The map has **N** at the top and **S** on the bottom. And it has **E** on one side and **W** on the other side.

2. Everybody, touch the girl in the picture. ✔
- She is pointing. Which direction is she pointing? (Signal.) *North.*
- Tell me which direction is to her **right.** Get ready. (Signal.) *East.*
- Tell me which direction is just **behind** her. Get ready. (Signal.) *South.*
- Tell me which direction is to her **left.** Get ready. (Signal.) *West.*
3. I'll tell you how the girl moves. You'll make a little **X** with your pencil to show where she ends up. If you do it right, you'll know whether she ends up at the skunk, the hot dog or one of the other pictures at the outside of the map.
- Listen: The girl walks **two** squares to the **east.** Remember, don't start counting until you start moving. Make a little tiny **X** in the square that is two squares to the east of where she starts out. After you make the little **X,** keep your pencil on that square because that's where the girl is now. (Observe students and give feedback.)
4. Listen: After the girl walks two squares to the east, she walks **one** square to the north. One square to the north. Make another little **X** in the square to the north of your first **X.** Keep your pencil on the **X** that shows where the girl is now. ✔
5. Listen: Now the girl goes **four** squares to the **south.** Four squares to the south. Count the squares and make a little **X** to show where the girl ends up. Raise your hand when you know where the girl ends up. ✔
- Everybody, which picture did the girl end up at? (Signal.) *The porcupine.* I don't think she liked that very much.
6. Let's start over and try again: Touch the girl in the middle of the picture. ✔
- Listen: The girl goes **three** squares to the **north.** Three squares to the north. Make a little **X** to show where she is now and keep your pencil there. ✔
- Listen: After the girl goes three squares to the north, she goes **four** squares to the **west.** Four squares to the west. Make a little **X** to show where she ends up. Raise your hand when you know where the girl ends up. ✔
- Everybody, which picture did the girl end up at? (Signal.) *The skunk.* She's not having very good luck today.

7. Let's try again: Touch the girl in the middle of the picture. ✔
- Listen: The girl goes **one** square to the **south.** One square to the south. Make a little **X** to show where she is now. ✔
- Then the girl goes **four** squares to the **east.** Four squares to the east. Make a little **X** to show where she ends up. Raise your hand when you know where she ends up. ✔
- Everybody, which picture did the girl end up at? (Signal.) *The apple.*
- Do you think she likes that? (Students respond.)
8. An apple is a lot better than a porcupine or a skunk. Raise your hand if you followed the directions and went to all the correct pictures. ✔
9. Well, let's see who is really, really smart. Let's say that the girl wanted to get the hot dog.
- Who can tell us what she might do to get there? Remember, you have to tell how many squares she moves and the direction she moves. Who wants to try? (Call on a student. Praise correct directions.)
- That's not the only way she could get to the hot dog. Who can tell another route that she might take to get to the hot dog? (Call on another student. Praise correct directions.)

EXERCISE 2   Deductions

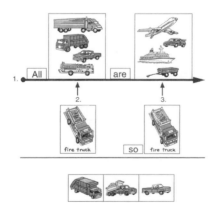

1. Everybody, find part B. ✔
   These are the same trucks we worked with before, but this is a different deduction.
2. Touch arrow 1. ✔
   The first part of the rule is: All trucks.
- Touch the next word.
   What word? (Signal.) *Are.*
   Yes: All trucks are . . .
- Everybody, touch the second picture on arrow 1. ✔

- What are they? (Signal.) *Vehicles.*
- Yes: All trucks are vehicles.
3. Everybody, touch arrow 1 again. ✔
   Here's the rule for arrow 1: **All trucks are vehicles.**
- Everybody, say that rule. (Signal.) *All trucks are vehicles.*
4. Raise your hand when you can say the whole deduction. Remember, tell about arrow 1, then arrow 2, then arrow 3.
5. Everybody, say the whole deduction. Get ready. (Signal.) *All trucks are vehicles. A fire truck is a truck. So a fire truck is a vehicle.*
- (Repeat step 5 until firm.)
6. Everybody, touch the picture of the garbage truck below the arrows. ✔
- **Pretend** that you have a picture of the garbage truck at the bottom of both up-arrows.
7. Everybody, say the whole deduction for a garbage truck. Get ready. (Signal.) *All trucks are vehicles. A garbage truck is a truck. So a garbage truck is a vehicle.*
8. Who thinks they can say the whole deduction for any of the other trucks at the bottom of the page? Those trucks are a dump truck and a pickup. Just pick one of those trucks. Then **pretend** that truck is at the bottom of both up-arrows and say the whole deduction for that truck. It's tough.
- Who wants to try? (Call on several students. Praise appropriate deductions.)

EXERCISE 3 Sentence Construction

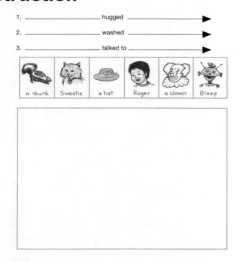

1. Everybody, find part C. ✔
   You're going to make up sentences. I think we'll have some pretty silly sentences again.
2. Touch arrow 1. ✔
   Part of that sentence is already written.
- Touch the part that's written. ✔
   That part says **hugged.** Everybody, what does it say? (Signal.) *Hugged.*
- The first sentence will say that somebody hugged something or maybe somebody hugged somebody else.
- Touch the **first** space on arrow 1. ✔
   That's where you'll write the name of the character doing the hugging.
- Touch the **last** space on arrow 1. ✔
   That's where you'll write the name of the character or thing that got hugged.
3. The words you'll use to make up sentence 1 are below the sentences. I'll read the words. You touch the pictures. Get ready.
   A skunk . . . Sweetie . . . a hat . . . Roger . . . a clown . . . Bleep.
4. Your turn: Complete sentence 1. Write the name of the character doing the hugging and the name of the character or thing being hugged. Remember to start your sentence with a capital and end it with a period. Raise your hand when you're finished.
   (Observe students and give feedback.)
5. Let's see what kind of silly sentences you wrote. When I call on you, read your sentence 1. (Call on several students. Praise appropriate sentences.) Those were great sentences.
6. Everybody, touch the word that's already written in sentence 2. ✔
- That word is **washed.** Sentence 2 will say that somebody washed somebody or something.
- Touch the first space on arrow 2. ✔
   That's where you'll write the name of the character doing the washing.
- Touch the last space on arrow 2. ✔
   That's where you'll write the name of the character or thing being washed.
- Your turn: Complete sentence 2. Remember the capital and period. Raise your hand when you're finished.
   (Observe students and give feedback.)
- (Call on several students to read sentence 2. Praise appropriate sentences.)

7. Everybody, touch the words that are already written in sentence 3. ✔
- Those words are **talked to.** Sentence 3 will say that somebody talked to somebody or something.
- Your turn: Complete sentence 3 so it tells somebody talked to somebody or something. Remember the capital and the period. Raise your hand when you're finished.
(Observe students and give feedback.)
- (Call on several students to read sentence 3. Praise sentences that name two characters.)
8. Touch the big box below the pictures. Later, you're going to draw a picture for your favorite sentence. You'll draw a picture of whatever you have happening in your favorite sentence.
- I'll show you some of the better pictures next time. I bet we have some super artists in this class.

EXERCISE 4 Goober

Storytelling

- (Draw on the board:)

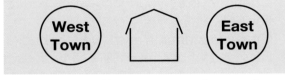

- I'm going to tell you a story about a farm that is between two towns.
- I've drawn a barn. That shows where the farm would be on a map. If you go **east** from the farm, you come to the town of East Town.
- Watch:
(Touch barn. Move right to East Town.)
Here's East Town.
- It you go **west** from the farm, you come to the town of West Town.
- Watch:
(Touch barn. Move left to West Town.)
Here's West Town.
- Remember, the farm is right between East Town and West Town.
- Listen carefully so you can answer some questions.

> Once there was a crusty old man named Gustaf Gutenberger. But nobody called him Gustaf Gutenberger. Instead,

they used the nickname, Goober. Goober lived by himself on a small farm. That farm was right between two small towns. The town to the west of Goober's farm was called West Town. The town to the east of Goober's farm was called East Town.

The people in West Town and East Town had mixed feelings about Goober. The reason they had mixed feelings was that Goober's farm had a very bad smell. He had dirty pigs that **never** took a bath. They didn't just smell sort of strong or kind of bad. They smelled **awful.** People would sometimes hold their nose when they walked near his farm. And when the wind blew **from** the east, the people in one of the towns would say, "Phew, what is that **awful** smell?"

- (Draw arrow to show:)

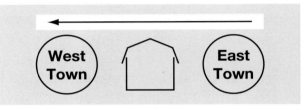

- Here's an arrow that shows the wind blowing from the east. That wind would blow the awful smell from Goober's farm to one of the towns.
- Everybody, which town is that? (Signal.) *West Town.*
- Yes, the people in West Town would get that awful smell.
- Listen:

> And when the wind blew **from** the west, the people in one of the towns would say, "Phew. I wish the wind would change **soon.**"

- (Change arrow to show:)

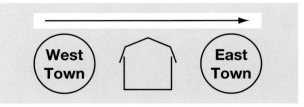

84   *Lesson 15*

- Here's the wind blowing **from** the west. Now which town would get to smell Goober's farm? (Signal.) *East Town.*
- And they didn't like that. They wanted the wind to change **soon.**

It would be easy for people to hate Goober because of his smelly farm. But things were not that simple because of the violin. You see, although Goober's farm smelled so bad, Goober could play the violin so sweetly that people would just stop what they were doing and listen to the beautiful sounds that drifted on the breeze. Birds would stop singing because they were ashamed of their songs when they heard Goober's beautiful violin music.

Some people who lived in West Town and East Town **loved** Goober. The reason they loved him was that they couldn't **smell** his farm. The breeze **wouldn't** carry the **smell** for more than a mile. But the breeze **would** carry Goober's **music** for more than a mile. So the people who lived more than a mile from Goober's place could hear the music, but couldn't smell his pigs.

- (Erase arrowhead and draw "squiggles" to show:)

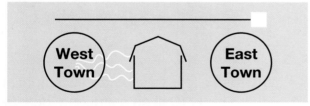

- That squiggly stuff shows the smell. It wouldn't go all the way to the far side of West Town. It would only go for about a mile. So some of the people in West Town loved Goober because they couldn't smell his farm.
- (Point to the squiggly half of the West Town circle.)
  Everybody, did those people who loved Goober live here? (Signal.) *No.*
- (Point to the left half of the West Town circle.)
  Did those people who loved Goober live here? (Signal.) *Yes.*

- Right, those people could hear the music, but they couldn't smell Goober's pigs.

"Such wonderful music," they would say as they sat out on their porches in the evening, listening to the music.

Some people who lived in West Town and East Town were **confused** about Goober. They hated him and they loved him. They hated him because they lived less than a mile from Goober's farm.

So when the wind blew from Goober's farm, most of them wouldn't sit out on their porch in the evening listening to the music. They would go inside and close all the windows and the doors. They wouldn't be able to hear the music, but they felt that was better than having to breathe in all that terrible smell. Oh, there were some real music lovers who would put clothespins on their noses and sit outside to enjoy the music, but they would get sore noses because they had to make sure that their clothespins were very tight or some of the smell would come through.

So on a summer evening, Goober would get out his violin, sit on an old stump near his barn and start playing. If there was no wind, all the people in West Town and East Town would be on their porches listening to his wonderful music.

But, if the wind blew **to** the west, there would be a **lot** of people in East Town with **their** houses shut up tight.

Then one day, something very strange happened. A little girl from West Town went over to visit Goober. That was very strange because **nobody** ever visited Goober. She took a big package with her and walked up to his barn where he was milking a cow. She held her nose and said, "Mr. Goober, you make nice music." But it didn't sound quite that way because she was holding her nose. What she actually said sounded like this: "Bister Goober, you bake dice busic."

Goober looked up and said, "I do what?"

She said, "Bake dice busic."

He shook his head and said, "Well, I can't do anything about that."

She said, "Dough. You dote uderstad."

He said, "You know, if you'd stop holding your nose, maybe I could understand what you're trying to tell me."

So the little girl took a very deep breath, let go of her nose and said, very fast, "We love your music, but you need to clean up your pigs. They **stink.**"

Goober's eyes got wide and he stared at the girl for a long time. She was holding her nose again. At last he said, "Do my pigs really stink?"

She said, "Yes."

He said, "Golly. I didn't know that."

Then she handed Goober her package and said, "Here are sub things for you." Then she said, "Good-bye," and ran away, holding her nose.

After she left, Goober opened the package. Inside were some bars of pig soap.

Goober smelled the soap and said, "What a great smell."

Then Goober shrugged, took the package with him down to his pond and called his pigs. They came running. Then he jumped into the pond with the pigs and scrubbed them until they were pink. He rubbed and scrubbed and he washed and he rinsed. When he was done, his pigs were as clean and sweet smelling as anybody in East Town or West Town. Goober sniffed the air and said, "Those pigs smell great." Goober took some of that great-smelling soap back to his house. "I can use this soap on me," he said.

Well, that's the story. If you ever go to West Town or East Town, you'll hear the sweetest violin music you've ever heard in your life. And you'll hear people saying wonderful things about Goober. And they also say some nice things about a little girl who visits Goober every week. She always takes a package with her, and the people in West Town and East Town are **very** grateful.

EXERCISE 5 Correcting Non-nasal Speech

1. Everybody, find part D. ✔
   Here's a picture of something that happened in the story.
2. What's Goober doing in this picture? (Signal.) *Milking a cow.*

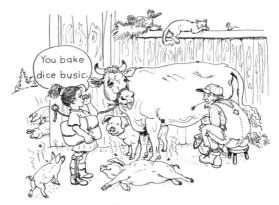

- What are all those squiggly lines coming off the pigs? (Call on a student. Idea: *Bad smell; odor.*)
- That cow doesn't look very happy. I wonder why.
- That little girl is holding her nose and saying something. I'll read what she's saying: "You bake dice busic."
- Everybody, what is she trying to say? (Signal.) *You make nice music.*
- Why does it sound so funny? (Signal.) *She's holding her nose.*
- Your turn: Hold your nose and say, "You make nice music." (Students respond.) That sounds pretty bad to me.

- (Write on the board:)

M   N

- The little girl is trying to say: "You **m**ake **n**ice **m**usic," but she can't say the right sounds for **M** or **N** while she's holding her nose.

3. Three words are wrong.

- Your turn: Fix up the words that are wrong. Cross out the letters that are wrong. Write the correct letters above the crossed-out letters. Raise your hand when you're finished.

  (Observe students and give feedback.)

4. Check your work.
- What was the girl trying to say instead of **bake?** (Signal.) *Make.*
- So you crossed out the **B** and wrote an **M** above it.
- What was the girl trying to say instead of **dice?** (Signal.) *Nice.*
- What did you write above the **D?** (Signal.) *N.*
- What was the girl trying to say instead of **busic?** (Signal.) *Music.*
- What did you write above the **B?** (Signal.) *M.*

5. Raise your hand if you fixed up all the words the right way.
   Good for you.

- Later, you can color the picture.

LESSON 16

Objectives

- Compose and write a parallel sentence pair based on a single picture. (Exercise 1)
- Follow directions involving **north, south, east, west.** (Exercise 2)
- Use directions about **north, south, east, west** to solve a map puzzle. (Exercise 3)
- Listen to part 1 of a continued story and answer comprehension questions. (Exercise 4)
- **Identify speakers from references to the relative size of objects.** (Exercise 5)

WORKBOOK • LINED PAPER

EXERCISE 1 Writing Parallel Sentences

| an apple | an orange | peeled | ate |

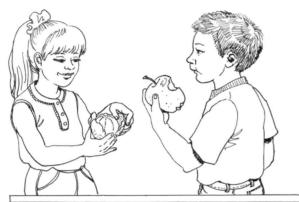

Note: Remind students to start their sentences with a capital and end them with a period.

1. Open your workbook to lesson 16, and find part A. ✔
   You're going to write about this picture.
2. The picture shows what a girl and a boy did.
   - What did the girl do? (Signal.) *Peeled an orange.*
   - What did the boy do? (Call on a student. Idea: *Ate an apple.*)
3. Listen: The girl peeled an orange. The boy ate an apple.
   - Everybody, say the first sentence. (Signal.) *The girl peeled an orange.*
   - Say the next sentence. (Signal.) *The boy ate an apple.*
   - (Repeat sentences until firm.)
4. Look at the vocabulary box. These are some of the words you need: **an apple . . . an orange . . . peeled . . . ate.**

5. Say the sentence about the girl. (Signal.) *The girl peeled an orange.*
   - Say the sentence about the boy. (Signal.) *The boy ate an apple.*
6. (Hand out a piece of lined paper to each student.) Write your name on the top line of the paper. ✔
   Write both sentences.
   (Observe students and give feedback.)
7. **(Optional:)** Skip a line on your paper and write both sentences again.
   (Observe students and give feedback.)
8. (Collect and correct papers.)

EXERCISE 2 Directions

North, South, East, West

1. Everybody, stand up.
   I'm going to tell you to face different directions. Wait until I say **go.**
2. Listen: Everybody, face **east.** Get ready. Go. ✔
   - Face **south.** Get ready. Go. ✔
   - Face **east.** Get ready. Go. ✔
   - Face **west.** Get ready. Go. ✔
   - Face **north.** Get ready. Go. ✔
   - (Repeat step 2 until firm.)
3. Here are some harder instructions: Everybody, face **west** and **point** south. Think about what you're going to do. Get ready. Go. ✔
   - Listen: Face **west** and **point** east. Get ready. Go. ✔
   - Listen: Face **north** and **point** east. Get ready. Go. ✔
   - Everybody, sit down.
4. Raise your hand if you got all those directions right.
   Super.

EXERCISE 3 Directions

Map Puzzle

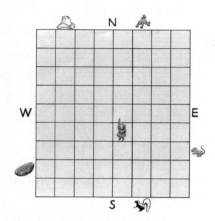

1. Everybody, find part B. ✔
• This is a map puzzle. The girl in the picture will move to one of the things at the outside of the picture. The map has **N** at the top and **S** on the bottom. And it has **E** on one side and **W** on the other side.
2. Everybody, touch the girl in the picture. ✔
• She is pointing. Which direction is she pointing? (Signal.) *North.*
• Tell me which direction is to her **right.** Get ready. (Signal.) *East.*
• Tell me which direction is just **behind** her. Get ready. (Signal.) *South.*
• Tell me which direction is to her **left.** Get ready. (Signal.) *West.*
3. I'll tell you how the girl moves. You'll make a little **X** with your pencil to show where she ends up. If you do it right, you'll know where she ends up. Maybe she'll end up at the skunk, the watermelon, or one of the other pictures at the outside of the map.
• Listen: The girl walks **three** squares to the **north.** Remember, don't start counting until you start moving. Make a little tiny **X** in the square that is three squares to the north of where she starts out. After you make the little **X,** keep your pencil on that square because that's where the girl is now. ✔
4. Listen: After the girl walks three squares to the north, she walks **four** squares to the **west.** Four squares to the west. Make another little **X** in that square. Keep your pencil on the **X** that shows where the girl is now. ✔

5. Listen: Now the girl goes **two** squares to the **north.** Two squares to the north. Count the squares and make a little **X** to show where the girl is now. Keep your pencil on the **X.** ✔
6. Listen: Now the girl goes **five** squares to the **east.** Five squares to the east. Count the squares.
• Everybody, which picture did the girl end up at? (Signal.) *The toad.*
• I wonder if she liked that.
7. Listen: Draw a line from the girl to show the route she took to the toad. Your route should show her going three squares north, four squares west, two squares north and five squares east. Make your line go right through the middle of the squares. Raise your hand when you've drawn that whole route.
(Observe students and give feedback.)
8. There are routes that are much shorter for getting to the toad. Raise your hand if you can describe a route. Remember, for each part of the route, you have to tell which direction she went and how many squares she went. (Call on individual students. Praise idea: *Five north and one east or one east and five north.*)
9. Let's say that the girl wants to get the watermelon.
• Who can tell us what she might do to get there? Remember, you have to tell how many squares she moves and the direction she moves. Who wants to try? (Call on a student. Praise correct directions.)
• That's not the only way she could get to the watermelon. Who can tell another route that she might take to get to the watermelon? (Call on another student. Praise correct directions.)

EXERCISE 4 Owen and the Little People
Part 1

Storytelling

• Everybody, I'm going to read the first part of a story about a giant named Owen and some little tiny people.

- Listen:

A long time ago, there were two islands in the middle of the ocean. These islands were miles apart, but they were almost exactly the same. **Both** of them were exactly the same shape and exactly the same size. **Both** of them had a wide beach on the north end, and both beaches looked identical. **Both** islands had a huge mountain right in the middle and those mountains were identical. They were the same shape, the same height, and they even had the same valleys and the same steep cliffs on the south end of the mountains.

- Get a picture in your mind of those islands. I'll read that part again, slowly. Close your eyes and get a picture of the islands.

Both islands were exactly the same shape and exactly the same size. **Both** of them had a wide beach on the north end and both beaches looked identical.

- Get a picture of the island with a wide beach at the north end.
- Listen:

Both islands had a huge mountain right in the middle, and those mountains were identical.

- Get a picture in your mind. The beach is on the north end. Everybody, where is the mountain? (Signal.) *Right in the middle.*
- Listen:

They were the same shape, the same height, and they even had the same valleys and the same steep cliffs on the south end of the mountains.

- Picture the mountain. It has a steep cliff to the south.

These islands were so identical that, if you were familiar with one of the islands and went to the other island, you'd think you were still on the first island.

All the animals that lived on these islands looked the same—the same eagles and swans, the same bears and beavers, the same spiders and flies.

The only thing that was different about these islands was the people that lived on them. Twelve little tiny people lived on one island. Three huge giants lived on the other island.

- How many little tiny people lived on one island? (Signal.) *Twelve.*
- Who lived on the other island? (Signal.) *Giants.*
- How many giants were there? (Signal.) *Three.*

The little people were **really** little. They were only about one inch tall. Some of the spiders on their island were bigger than they were.

- (Hold up your fingers to show how tall one inch is.) Here's 1 inch. That's how big the little people were. That is **really** tiny.

On the other island, the giants were real giants. They were about 15 feet tall. They were so big that they could not walk through the doorway to our classroom. They would have to crouch way down to get inside. And when they were inside, they wouldn't be able to stand up straight without putting their head right through the ceiling. They were **tall.** They were **big.** And they were **strong.** They could pick up a bear and hold it like a puppy.

Well, one day, one of the giants found a green bottle. It was an ordinary-sized pop bottle that washed up on the beach. One of the giants picked it up. To him, that bottle was no longer than his little finger.

The giant that found the bottle was named Owen, and he had never seen regular-sized people. The only people he had ever seen were his father and his mother. Owen was not full grown but almost. So he was about as tall as his mother but not as tall as his father.

Well, Owen looked at that green bottle for a long time. Then he took it home with him. He showed it to his mother and asked her, "What should I do with this thing?"

"That thing is a bottle," she said. Then she added, "I once heard that people can send messages to other people far away by using bottles. They just write a note, put it in the bottle, wait until the currents are moving away from the shore and put the bottle in the ocean."

At first Owen didn't like that idea because he liked the looks of that tiny green bottle. But then he started to think about faraway places, and he decided it would be nice to send a message to somebody else. So he got a piece of paper and tore off just a corner of it. Then he wrote a note on the corner of the paper. He couldn't use the whole sheet of paper because the whole sheet wouldn't fit into the bottle.

- Why couldn't Owen use a whole sheet of paper? (Call on a student. Idea: *Because it wouldn't fit into the bottle.*)
- Hold out your hands and show me how big you think his sheet of paper was. (Praise students who show a space at least twice as wide as a regular sheet.)
- Here's the note he wrote:

Hello, my name is Owen and I live on a beautiful island. This island is very small. There are many small animals on this island. We have tiny bears and tigers and alligators. We have

tiny birds is the eagle. We have bugs that are **so** small that you can hardly see them.

Please write me if you get this note.

- Owen describes everything as being very tiny. Why is that? (Call on a student. Idea: *Because Owen is very big; to him they seem tiny.*)
- Show me how big a rabbit is to you. (Observe students and give feedback. Praise reasonable approximations.)
- Show me how big that same rabbit would be to Owen. (Praise students who show a size no bigger than their hand.)
- That's pretty small.

It took Owen a long time to write the note because he had to write very, very small. After he put the note in the bottle, he went to the wide beach on the north end of his island, waited until the currents were moving out to sea, and put the bottle in the water. Slowly the bottle moved out to sea, farther and farther, until Owen could no longer see it.

That bottle drifted and drifted until it came to the island with the little people.

- And what happened then? You'll have to wait until next time to find out.

EXERCISE 5　Relative Size

True/False

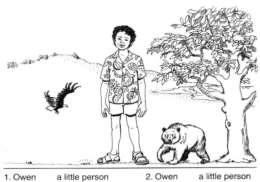

| 1. Owen | a little person | 2. Owen | a little person |
| 3. Owen | a little person | 4. Owen | a little person |

1. Everybody, find part C. ✔
   That picture shows the size of Owen
   and some of the little people **if** they were
   standing next to each other on the same
   island. You have to look really hard to see
   the little people. They look like a row of tiny
   sticks. There are some other things in this
   picture.
2. Touch the bear. ✔
   • Get ready to answer **true** or **false.**
   • Listen: Owen would say that the bear is
     very big. True or false? (Signal.) *False.*
   • Listen: The little people would say that the
     bear is very big. True or false? (Signal.)
     True.
3. Touch the mouse. It's to the left of the little
   people. ✔
   • Listen: Owen would say, "That mouse is
     bigger than I am." True or false? (Signal.)
     False.
   • Listen: The little people would say, "That
     mouse is bigger than I am." True or false?
     (Signal.) *True.*
4. Touch number 1 below the picture. ✔
   Next to number 1 is the name **Owen.**
   • Touch that name. ✔
   • After the name **Owen,** it says **a little
     person.**
     Touch those words. ✔
5. I'll make a statement. You'll circle the
   name of the person who would say that
   statement.
   • Here's statement 1: **That eagle is very
     small.** You'll circle the name **Owen** if he
     would say that. You'll circle **a little person**
     if a little person would say that.

   • Circle the name of the person who would
     say, "That eagle is very small." Raise your
     hand when you're finished.
     (Observe students and give feedback.)
6. Everybody, touch number 2. ✔
   Here's the statement. It's tricky. Listen:
   That tree is taller than I am. Circle the
   name of the person who would say that. If
   more than one person would say it, circle
   both names. Raise your hand when you're
   finished.
   (Observe students and give feedback.)
   • Touch number 3. ✔
     Here's statement 3. Listen: **I could pick up
     that bear.** Circle the name of the person
     who would say that. Raise your hand when
     you're finished.
     (Observe students and give feedback.)
   • Touch number 4. ✔
     Here's statement 4: **That mouse is bigger
     than I am.** Circle the name of the person
     who would say that. Raise your hand when
     you're finished.
     (Observe students and give feedback.)
7. Let's check your answers.
   • Touch number 1. ✔
     That eagle is very small. What did you
     circle? (Signal.) *Owen.*
   • Yes, Owen would say that. A little person
     wouldn't say that.
   • Why not? (Call on a student. Idea: *The
     eagle is much bigger than a little person.*)
   • Everybody, touch number 2. ✔
     That tree is taller than I am. What did you
     circle? (Signal.) *Owen **and** a little person.*
   • Right, both Owen and a little person
     would say that, because the tree is taller
     than Owen and it's a lot taller than a little
     person.
   • Touch number 3. ✔
     I could pick up that bear. What did you
     circle? (Signal.) *Owen.*
   • Yes, Owen would say that.
   • Touch number 4. ✔
     That mouse is bigger than I am. What did
     you circle? (Signal.) *A little person.*
   • Yes, the mouse is bigger than a little
     person, but it sure isn't bigger than Owen.
8. I would hate to meet up with a mouse
   bigger than me, wouldn't you?
   (Students respond.)
9. Later, you can color the picture.

Objectives

- Construct 3 sentences about story characters. (Exercise 1)
- Say different deductions based on pictures. (Exercise 2)
- Listen to part 2 of a continued story, answer comprehension questions and color a picture. (Exercise 3)
- **Edit a letter to show a character's reference to the relative size of objects.** (Exercise 4)

WORKBOOK

EXERCISE 1 Sentence Construction

A.

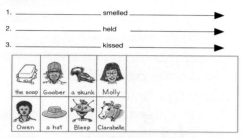

1. Open your workbook to lesson 17. ✔ Everybody, find part A. ✔
- You're going to make up sentences. And I'm afraid some of you are going to make up some pretty silly sentences.
2. Touch arrow 1. ✔ Part of that sentence is already written.
- Touch the part that's written. ✔ That part says **smelled.** Everybody, what does it say? (Signal.) *Smelled.*
- The first sentence will say that somebody smelled something or maybe somebody smelled somebody else.
- Touch the **first** space on arrow 1. ✔ That's where you'll write the name of the character doing the smelling.
- Touch the **last** space on arrow 1. ✔ That's where you'll write the name of the character or thing that got smelled.
3. The words you'll use to make up sentence 1 are below the arrows. I'll read the words. You touch the pictures. Get ready. **The soap . . . Goober . . . a skunk . . . Molly . . . Owen . . . a hat . . . Bleep . . . Clarabelle.**
4. Your turn: Complete sentence 1. Write the name of the person doing the smelling and the name of the person or thing being smelled. Remember to start your sentence

with a capital and end it with a period. Raise your hand when you're finished. (Observe students and give feedback.)
- When I call on you, read your sentence 1. (Call on several students. Praise appropriate sentences.)
5. Everybody, touch the word that's already written in sentence 2. ✔
- That word is **held.** Sentence 2 will say that somebody held somebody or something.
- Your turn: Complete sentence 2. Raise your hand when you're finished. (Observe students and give feedback.)
- (Call on several students to read sentence 2. Praise appropriate sentences.)
6. Everybody, touch the word that's already written in sentence 3. ✔
- That word is **kissed.**
- Your turn: Complete sentence 3. Raise your hand when you're finished. (Observe students and give feedback.)
- (Call on several students to read sentence 3. Praise appropriate sentences.)
7. Later, you'll draw a picture that shows what you wrote for one of your sentences. Draw a picture of whatever you have happening in your favorite sentence.

EXERCISE 2 Deductions

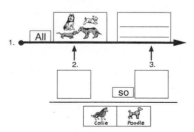

1. Find part B in your workbook. ✔ This is a very hard deduction game. Arrow 1 has only one picture. It shows that all dogs do something.

- (Write on the board:)

> **sleep**

- Here's something that all dogs do. What do they all do? (Signal.) *Sleep.*
Yes, all dogs sleep.
- Everybody, say that rule for arrow 1. (Signal.) *All dogs sleep.*
- (Write on the board:)

> **pant**

- Here's something else that all dogs do. What do they all do? (Signal.) *Pant.*
- Say that rule for arrow 1. (Signal.) *All dogs pant.*
- (Write on the board:)

> **sit**

- Here's something else that all dogs do. What do they all do? (Signal.) *Sit.*
- Say that rule for arrow 1. (Signal.) *All dogs sit.*

2. Listen: Touch the empty box on arrow 1. Write the word **sleep** on the top line of the empty box. Raise your hand when you're finished.
(Observe students and give feedback.)
- Here's what your rule for arrow 1 should say now: All dogs sleep. Raise your hand if that's what your rule says.
- Everybody, say the rule for arrow 1. (Signal.) *All dogs sleep.*

3. Touch the collie below the deduction. Pretend that collie is at the bottom of arrow 2 and arrow 3.

4. Everybody, say the whole deduction about a collie. Get ready. (Signal.) *All dogs sleep. A collie is a dog. So a collie sleeps.*
- (Repeat step 4 until firm.)

5. Touch the poodle below the deduction. Pretend that poodle is at the bottom of arrow 2 and arrow 3.
- Say the whole deduction about a poodle. Get ready. (Signal.) *All dogs sleep. A poodle is a dog. So a poodle sleeps.*
- (Repeat step 5 until firm.)
- Listen: Cross out the word **sleep** on arrow 1 and write **pant** or **sit** on the second line.

- (Cross out **sleep** on the board:)

> ~~sleep~~
> **pant**
> **sit**

- Raise your hand when you're finished. (Observe students and give feedback.)
- Now some of you have this rule for arrow 1: All dogs pant. Raise your hand if that's what your rule says.
- Some of you have this rule for arrow 1: All dogs sit. Raise your hand if that's what your rule says.

6. Touch the collie. ✔
That's the dog you're going to tell about for your deduction.

7. Everybody who has the rule **All dogs pant:** say the whole deduction for a collie. Get ready. (Signal.) *All dogs pant. A collie is a dog. So a collie pants.*
- (Repeat step 7 until firm.)

8. Everybody who has the rule **All dogs sit:** say the whole deduction for a collie. Get ready. (Signal.) *All dogs sit. A collie is a dog. So a collie sits.*
- (Repeat step 8 until firm.)

9. You're doing all kinds of hard deductions.

EXERCISE 3   Owen and the Little People *Part 2*

Storytelling

- I'm going to read the next part of the story about Owen and the little people. Remember, Owen wrote a note, put it in a bottle and put the bottle in the ocean. The currents took that bottle out to sea.
- Listen:

> Three days later, Fizz and Liz were on the beach of **their** island. Fizz and Liz were two tiny people. They were not full-grown, so they were not quite one inch tall yet, and Liz was slightly taller than Fizz.

- (Hold up your fingers with about a 1-inch space between.)
Here's how tall one inch is. Everybody, hold up your fingers to show me a space about one-inch high.
(Observe students and give feedback.)

- Listen: Were Fizz and Liz that tall? (Signal.) *No.*
  Right, they were a little bit shorter.
- Show me with your fingers how tall they were.
  (Observe students and give feedback.)

Fizz and Liz were throwing grains of sand into the water. For them, a grain of sand was the size of a regular-size stone. As they played, they glanced around from time to time to make sure that there were no spiders around.

- Why were they concerned about spiders? (Call on a student. Idea: *Spiders were bigger than they were; they would be like a monster, and so on.*)
- If you were Fizz or Liz, how big would a spider look to you? (Call on several students. Accept reasonable ideas, such as: *Bigger than a person.*)

Suddenly, Fizz saw the green bottle bobbing around in the ocean. "Look," he said. "There's a huge green thing floating out there."

"Let's see what it is," Liz said.

So Fizz and Liz got in their racing boats. They really weren't racing boats. They were peanut shells that were just the right size for one person to sit and paddle around. (The paddle was a little stick.)

Fizz and Liz paddled and paddled until they reached that huge bottle.

"There's something inside," Liz said.

"Let's find out what it is," Fizz said.

But before they could reach the note, they had to move the bottle all the way to the beach. They put the nose of their boats against the side of the bottle and paddled, paddled, paddled, and very slowly the bottle moved toward the shore. Then some of the other little people who had gathered along the beach got into the water and helped Fizz and Liz roll that huge bottle all the way up onto the dry sand.

Four little people crawled into the bottle and tugged and pulled at the note. It was hard, hard work, but after a long time, they managed to pull the note out and unroll it.

The note was almost as huge as that big bottle. The note was almost as big as Fizz's front yard. And the bottle was almost as big as Fizz's house.

Liz read the note out loud:

"Hello, my name is Owen and I live on a beautiful island. This island is very small. There are many small animals on this island. We have tiny bears and tigers and alligators. We have tiny rabbits. We also have lots of tiny birds. The biggest of the tiny birds is the eagle. We have bugs that are **so** small that you can hardly see them. Please write me if you get this note."

As Liz read the note, Fizz tried to imagine what kind of place Owen lived in. Fizz and Liz had never seen regular-sized people and they had never ever seen anybody the size of Owen.

They didn't know that Owen's island was **exactly** like their island.

After Liz finished reading the note, she said, "Owen must live on an island that is much different from our island."

"I'll say," Fizz said. "I can't imagine a place with bugs that small. Or tiny birds."

To Fizz and Liz, a robin was bigger than a regular-sized house and an eagle was bigger than a whole neighborhood.

After all the other little people had listened to the note and made comments about what a strange place Owen lived in, they left.

Then Liz turned to Fizz and said, "Why don't we write Owen and tell him about **our** island?"

"Good idea," Fizz said. "We could tell him about the animals and birds and bugs on our island."

And that's just what they did. They decided to write their letter on the back of Owen's letter. So they worked and worked until they turned over the whole paper. Then they wrote great big words. They used burnt logs for pencils, and wrote this note:

Dear Owen,

Our names are Fizz and Liz and we live on a beautiful island.

- Uh-oh. Somebody forgot to write the rest of the note. It's not in the story.

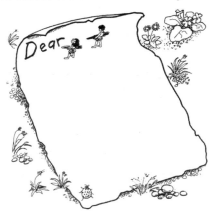

1. Find part C in your workbook. ✔
   The picture shows Fizz and Liz writing a note to Owen.
- What are those things they are writing with? (Signal.) *Logs.*
- That is one big piece of paper, isn't it? (Signal.) *Yes.*
2. Later, you can color the picture.

EXERCISE 4   Relative Size

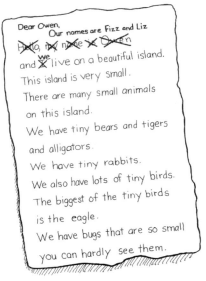

1. Everybody, find part D. ✔
   This is Owen's note. Maybe we can figure out how to fix up that note so it tells what Fizz and Liz wrote in their note to Owen.
2. The first part of that note is already fixed up. Some words are crossed out and other words are written above those crossed-out words.
- I'll read the part that's fixed up:

Dear Owen,

Our names are Fizz and Liz and we live on a beautiful island.

- That's how much is fixed up. You're going to fix up the rest.
3. I'll read the next sentence. It starts with the word **this.**
- Touch that sentence. ✔
- That sentence says: This island is very small. Everybody, is that what Fizz and Liz would say about their island? (Signal.) *No.*
- What would they say about their island? (Signal.) *That it's very big.*
4. Your turn: Cross out the word **small.**
- (Write on the board:)

big

- Your turn: Write **big** above the word **small.** Raise your hand when you're finished. (Observe students and give feedback.)
- Now your sentence says: This island is very big.

5. Touch the next sentence. It begins with the word **there.** ✔
   - It says: There are many small animals on this island. Would Fizz and Liz say that? (Signal.) *No.*
   - What's the word in that sentence you'll have to change? (Signal.) *Small.*
   - Your turn: Find the word **small** in that sentence. Cross it out and write the word **big** above it. Raise your hand when you're finished.
   (Observe students and give feedback.)
   - Now your sentence says: There are many big animals on this island.
6. The next sentence begins with the word **we.**
   - Touch that sentence. ✔
   - It says: We have tiny bears and tigers and alligators. What's the word in that sentence you'll have to change? (Signal.) *Tiny.*
   - Cross out the word **tiny** and write the word **big** above it. Raise your hand when you're finished.
   (Observe students and give feedback.)
   - Now your sentence says: We have big bears and tigers and alligators.
7. The next sentence begins with the word **we.**
   - Touch that sentence. ✔
   - It says: We have tiny rabbits. What's the word in that sentence you'll have to change? (Signal.) *Tiny.*
   - Cross out the word **tiny** and write the correct word above it. Raise your hand when you're finished.
   (Observe students and give feedback.)
   - Now your sentence says: We have big rabbits.
8. The next sentence begins with the word **we.**
   - Touch that sentence. ✔
   - It says: We also have lots of tiny birds. Fix up that sentence. Raise your hand when you're finished.
   (Observe students and give feedback.)
   - Now your sentence says: We also have lots of big birds.

9. The next sentence says: The biggest of the tiny birds is the eagle. What's the word in that sentence you'll have to change? (Signal.) *Tiny.*
   - Fix up the sentence. Raise your hand when you're finished.
   (Observe students and give feedback.)
   - Now your sentence says: The biggest of the big birds is the eagle.
10. The last sentence says: We have bugs that are so small you can hardly see them. Do Fizz and Liz have any bugs on their island that are so small you can hardly see them? (Signal.) *No.*
   - They would say: We have **no** bugs that are so small you can hardly see them.
   - So **after** the word **have,** write the word **no.** Write **no** after the word **have.** Raise your hand when you're finished.
   (Observe students and give feedback.)
   - Now your sentence says: We have no bugs that are so small you can hardly see them.
11. I'll read what the whole fixed-up note would say. Follow along:

   Dear Owen,

   Our names are Fizz and Liz and we live on a beautiful island. This island is very big. There are many big animals on this island. We have big bears and tigers and alligators. We have big rabbits. We also have lots of big birds. The biggest of the big birds is the eagle. We have no bugs that are so small you can hardly see them.

12. Hmmm . . . I wonder what will happen. We'll have to wait until next time to find out.

Materials: Each student will need scissors.

Objectives

- Compose and write a parallel sentence pair based on a single picture. (Exercise 1)
- **Apply a directional rule to solve a maze.** (Exercise 2)
- Listen to part 3 of a continued story. (Exercise 3)
- Answer questions about relative size and color a picture. (Exercise 4)

WORKBOOK • LINED PAPER

EXERCISE 1 **Writing Parallel Sentences**

standing	sitting	table	wagon

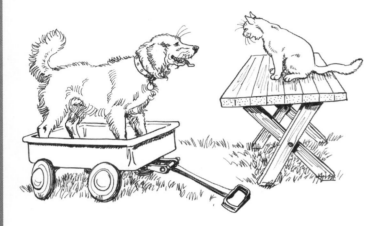

Note: Remind students to start their sentences with a capital and end them with a period.

1. Open your workbook to lesson 18, and find part A. ✔
   You're going to write about this picture.
2. The picture shows what a dog and a cat were doing. One of them was standing in a wagon. Which animal was that? (Signal.)
   The dog.
3. Listen: The dog was standing in a wagon. The cat was sitting on a table.
   - Say the whole sentence about the dog. (Signal.) *The dog was standing in a wagon.*
   - Say the whole sentence about the cat. (Signal.) *The cat was sitting on a table.*
   - (Repeat sentences until firm.)
4. Look at the vocabulary box. These are some of the words you need: **standing . . . sitting . . . table . . . wagon.**

5. Say the sentence about the dog. (Signal.)
   The dog was standing in a wagon.
   - Say the sentence about the cat. (Signal.)
   The cat was sitting on a table.
6. (Hand out lined paper.)
   Write your name on the top line. ✔
   Write both sentences.
   (Observe students and give feedback.)
7. Skip a line on your paper and write both sentences again.
   (Observe students and give feedback.)
8. (Collect and correct papers.)

EXERCISE 2 **Directions**

Maze

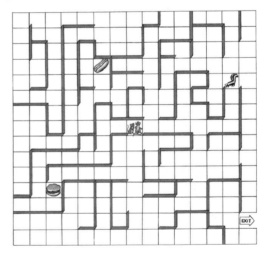

1. (Write on the board:)

> **EXIT** ▷

- This says **exit**. What does it say? (Signal.)
  Exit.
  The exit is the way out of a place.
  Everybody, point to an exit.

2. Everybody, find part B. ✔
   - This is a maze. This maze does not have letters to show north, south, east, and west, but this maze **is** a map. Remember the rule about maps. North is always at the top of the map, and it does not matter which way you turn when you hold the map. North is always at the top of the map.
   - Everybody, pick up your map, stand up and face south.
   - Look at the bragging rats on your map. If a bragging rat went to the top of that map, which direction would the rat go? (Signal.) *North.*
   - Everybody, face east. Get ready. Go. If that bragging rat went to the top of the map, which direction would the rat go? (Signal.) *North.*
   - Right, north is always at the top of the map no matter which way you turn.
   - Everybody, sit down.
3. Here's the story about this maze. One rat told all the other rats that he could get out of the maze by going in only two directions—**south** and **east.** He said that he went south and east more than one time, but he never went north and he never went west—just **south** and **east.**
4. Your turn: Touch the exit sign. It's to the south and east of the bragging rats. ✔
   - See if you can find a route out of the maze that goes only **south** and **east.** You can't go through any of those purple lines. Those are walls. Raise your hand if you can find the route.
     (As students raise their hands, have them show you the route.)
   - So the bragging rat was right. He could get out of the maze by going only south and east.
   - Everybody, use your pencil and draw a line that shows the route the bragging rat took. Make your line go right through the middle of the squares. Raise your hand when you're finished. ✔
5. Everybody, touch the square with the bragging rats. ✔
     I'll describe the route one of the bragging rats took, but I may make mistakes. Say **wrong** if you hear a mistake.
   - Listen: First the bragging rat went **four** squares to the **east.** (Pause.)
   - Then the bragging rat went **one** square to the **south.** (Signal.) *Wrong.*
   - How far did the bragging rat go to the south? (Signal.) *Two squares.*
   - Starting over: First the bragging rat went four squares to the east. Then he went **two** squares to the **south.** Then he went **three** squares to the **west.** (Signal.) *Wrong.*
   - But he did go **three** squares, didn't he? (Signal.) *Yes.*
   - Which direction did he go? (Signal.) *East.*
   - Starting over: First the bragging rat went four squares to the east. Then he went two squares to the south. Then he went three squares to the east. Then the bragging rat went **three** squares to the **south.** (Signal.) *Wrong.*
   - How many squares to the south? (Signal.) *Four.*
6. I didn't do a very good job of telling the correct route. Raise your hand if you can describe the correct route.
   - Start at the bragging rat and tell how many squares he moved and the direction he moved. Remember, you have to tell about going **south** and **east** for each part of your description. (**Call on several students. Praise correct directions.**)
7. Listen: The other bragging rat started in the same place the first one started. But here's what the second bragging rat told all the other rats: "There is no way to get to the hot dog in that maze. You can get close to it, but you can't get to that hot dog."
   - Later on you can figure out if there is any way to get from the bragging rat to the hot dog.
   - You can figure out the route to the hamburger. I think there's more than one way to get there.

EXERCISE 3   Owen and the Little People *Part 3*

Storytelling

- Let's find out what happened in our story about Owen and the little people.

   Fizz and Liz wrote a note that told about their island. Then they worked and worked until they finally got that note back into the bottle. Then the other little people helped Fizz and Liz roll the bottle into the water. Then everybody got into their racing boats and pulled and pushed against the bottle.

Finally, the bottle floated off, farther and farther from shore. Fizz said, "Well, I sure hope that bottle gets back to Owen."

And that's just what the bottle did. Three days later, Owen was sitting on the beach of his island, eating pineapples. To him, pineapples were about as big as a small apple. He was eating away when suddenly he noticed something green bobbing around in the ocean near the beach. He waded into the water and grabbed the tiny bottle.

He pulled out the note and he said, "Oh, no. That's the note I wrote." He was very disappointed. But then, he looked on the back of the note and there was the note from Fizz and Liz. It said:

Dear Owen,

Our names are Fizz and Liz and we live on a beautiful island. The island is very big. There are many big animals on this island. We have big bears and tigers and alligators. We have big rabbits. We also have lots of big birds. The biggest of these birds is the eagle. We have no bugs that are so small you can hardly see them.

Fizz and Liz

Owen took the note and the bottle and ran to his house. "Mom, Dad," he shouted. "Look what I've got."

He showed them the note, and they read it with great interest. Then Owen's mom said, "That sounds like an **awful** place. Can you imagine a place with big bears and eagles? I wonder how big they are."

"I don't know," Owen's dad said. "The note just says that they are big and that there are no bugs that are so small you can hardly see them. That means they must have big bugs."

"Ugh," Owen's mom said. "I would **hate** big bugs. I wonder how big they are."

"I don't know," Owen's dad said. "Maybe we should write another note and find out more about that place."

So Owen, his mom and his dad made a list of the things they wanted to find out about the island. Then they wrote another note. Here's the note:

Dear Fizz and Liz,

Could you answer these questions about your island?

1. How big are the bugs on your island?

2. How big are the bears on your island?

3. How big are the birds on your island?

We are glad that you wrote and hope you receive this note. Please write soon.

Owen and his family

After they had written the note, they put it in the green bottle. Then they took the bottle into the water, away from shore, and waited for the currents to move it out to sea. Once more the bottle moved out to sea, farther and farther away, until they could no longer see it.

Three days later, Liz's grandmother came running up to Fizz and Liz. She said, "That green thing is back. It's floating around near the beach."

"Wow," Liz said. "Let's find out what Owen says this time."

All the little people helped roll the bottle up on shore and pull the note out. Then they spread the note out and everybody read it.

After the other little people left, Fizz and Liz spent the rest of the day writing a note back to Owen and his family. Here's the first part of that note:

Dear Owen and family,

Here are the answers to your questions:

1.

- Oh, dear, that's all there is. We're going to have to figure out how Fizz and Liz would answer that letter.

EXERCISE 4   Relative Size

1. Everybody, find part C. ✔
Here's a picture of Fizz and Liz standing next to some of the things on their island.

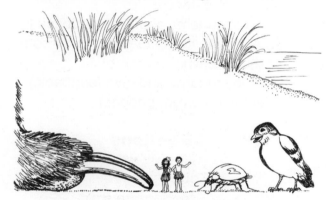

2. Touch the beetle. ✔
You can see how big that bug is compared to Fizz and Liz.
- Touch that big paw with the long claws. ✔
That's the paw of a bear that lives on the island.
- Touch the bird. ✔
That's the smallest bird that lives on the island. It's a sparrow.
3. Fizz and Liz are going to try to tell Owen how big these animals are. Fizz and Liz could say that the beetle is a little taller than the legs of that sparrow. But that information wouldn't help Owen understand how big the beetle is. Why not? (**Call on a student. Idea:** *Owen doesn't know how big the sparrow is.*)

- One of the questions Owen asks is, "How big are the bears?"
- Fizz and Liz might tell about the bear by saying that the claws on a bear paw are about as long as a sparrow is tall, but that information wouldn't help Owen understand how big the bear is. Why not? (**Call on a student. Idea:** *Owen doesn't know how big a sparrow is.*)
- Fizz and Liz might tell how big the animals are by telling about **themselves.** They could say that the bear's paw is much bigger than they are.
- When Fizz and Liz write their note, what could they tell Owen about how tall the beetles are compared to themselves? (**Call on several students. Idea:** *As tall as they are.*)
4. Touch the bear's paw. ✔
Fizz and Liz might try to tell how big the bear is by telling how big the bear's paw is. Or maybe they could even tell how long the claw is on a bear's paw.
- How long are those claws compared to Fizz and Liz? (**Call on several students. Idea:** *Twice as big as they are.*)
- Touch the sparrow. ✔
How could Fizz and Liz describe how tall that sparrow is by comparing it to themselves? (**Call on several students. Idea:** *Twice as tall as they are.*)
- Next time, we may get a chance to read the note that Fizz and Liz wrote back to Owen.
5. Later you can color the picture. That beetle is red and black. That sparrow is brown. So is that bear. But its claws are sort of yellow.

Materials: Each student will need a pair of scissors and a yellow crayon.

Objectives

- Compose and write a parallel sentence pair based on a single picture. (Exercise 1)
- Apply directional rules to solve a maze. (Exercise 2)
- Listen to part 4 of a continued story and answer comprehension questions. (Exercise 3)
- **Complete descriptions of relative size.** (Exercise 4)

WORKBOOK • LINED PAPER

EXERCISE 1 **Writing Parallel Sentences**

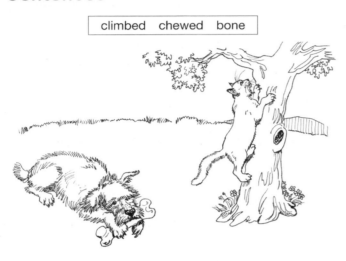

climbed   chewed   bone

Note: Remind students to start their sentences with a capital and end them with a period.

1. Open your workbook to lesson 19, and find part A. ✔
   You're going to write about this picture.
2. The picture shows what a dog and a cat did.
- What did the dog do? (Call on a student. Idea: *Chewed on a bone.*)
- What did the cat do? (Call on a student. Idea: *Climbed a tree.*)
3. Listen: The dog chewed on a bone. The cat climbed a tree.
- Everybody, say the whole sentence about the dog. (Signal.) *The dog chewed on a bone.*
- Say the whole sentence about the cat. (Signal.) *The cat climbed a tree.*
- (Repeat sentences until firm.)

4. Look at the vocabulary box. These are some of the words you need: **climbed . . . chewed . . . bone.**
5. Say the sentence about the dog. (Signal.) *The dog chewed on a bone.*
- Say the sentence about the cat. (Signal.) *The cat climbed a tree.*
6. (Hand out lined paper.)
   Write your name on the top line. ✔
   Write both sentences.
   (Observe students and give feedback.)
7. Skip a line on your paper and write both sentences again.
   (Observe students and give feedback.)
8. (Collect and correct papers.)

EXERCISE 2 **Directions**

Maze

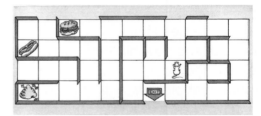

Bragging Rat

1. Two squares to the north.
2. Three squares to the east.
3. Three squares to the south.
4. Four squares to the west.

Bragging Rat

1. Two squares to the north.
2. Three squares to the west.
3. Three squares to the south.
4. Four squares to the west.

1. Everybody, find part B. ✔
- This map does not have letters to show north, south, east and west. But remember the rule about maps. North is always at the top of the map, and it does not matter which way you turn when you hold the map. North is always at the top of the map.

2. You're going to draw the routes that the bragging rats tell about. Both of them tell how they got out of that great big maze, but one of them told the wrong directions. You're going to draw the route for each rat and we'll find out which one knew the right way out of the maze.
   - You'll use your pencil to show the route the **first** bragging rat describes.
   - Below the maze are pictures of the bragging rats. Use your pencil. Put a **gray** pencil mark on the **first** rat. That's the gray rat. ✔
   - The description that rat gave is written below his picture.

3. Touch number 1 for the gray rat. ✔
   It says: **Two** squares to the **north.** Start at the bragging rat in the maze. Draw a line with your pencil that goes two squares to the north. Go two squares to the north. Raise your hand when you're finished.
   (Observe students and give feedback.)

4. Touch number 2 for the gray rat. ✔
   It says: **Three** squares to the **east.** Make a line for that part of the route. Remember, start that line at the end of your first line. Go three squares to the east. Raise your hand when you're finished.
   (Observe students and give feedback.)

5. Touch number 3 for the gray rat. ✔
   It says: **Three** squares to the **south.** Make the line for that part of the route. Go three squares to the south. Raise your hand when you're finished.
   (Observe students and give feedback.)

6. Touch number 4 for the gray rat. ✔
   It says: **Four** squares to the **west.** Make the line for that part of the route. Go four squares to the west. Raise your hand when you're finished.
   (Observe students and give feedback.)

7. Everybody, did the gray rat describe a route that gets him out of the maze? (Signal.) *Yes.*
   - So, the rat with the yellow teeth must have made a mistake. He didn't give the same directions the gray rat gave.

8. Take out your **yellow** crayon.
   Color the teeth of the **second** rat below the maze **yellow.** ✔

   - The description he gave is below his picture. You'll show the route he describes with your yellow crayon.

9. Touch number 1, below the picture of the rat with the yellow teeth. ✔
   - Where does that rat go for the first part of his route? (Signal.) *Two squares to the north.*
   - Start at the bragging rat in the maze. Draw that part of the route in **yellow,** right next to your gray line. Draw two squares to the north. Raise your hand when you're finished.
   (Observe students and give feedback.)

10. Now read the rest of the description the rat with the yellow teeth gave and draw the route. Start with number 2 and draw that part of the route, right at the end of the yellow line that goes two squares to the north. When you're done, your route should have four parts and it should end up at the . . . Well, you'll find out where it ends up. Raise your hand when you've drawn the whole route.
    (Observe students and give feedback.)

11. Everybody, where does the bragging rat with the yellow teeth end up? (Signal.) *At a beehive.*
    - Raise your hand if your yellow route ended up at the beehive.
    - He made a bad mistake somewhere. If you look at the description he gave, it is exactly the same as the description the gray rat gave except for one part. Raise your hand when you know the mistake the rat with the yellow teeth made.

12. Everybody, touch the part of the yellow rat's description that was wrong. ✔
    - What number was wrong? (Signal.) *Two.*
    - That part says: Three squares to the **west.** What should it say? (Signal.) *Three squares to the east.*

13. You are getting good at these tricky directions.

EXERCISE 3 Owen and the Little People *Part 4*

Storytelling

- I'm going to read some more about Owen and the little people. But first, let's make sure we know what's happening.

- Fizz and Liz wrote a note back to Owen. What questions did they answer in that note? (Call on individual students. Idea: *How big are the bugs? How big are the bears?* and *How big are the birds?*)
- Fizz and Liz answered these questions in their last note. They described the size of each animal. We'll find out how they did that.

After Fizz and Liz wrote their note, the other little people helped them put it into the bottle. Then everybody waited until the currents were moving away from the shore. They rolled the bottle into the water, got into their racing boats and pushed it out into the ocean.

- Everybody, how long do you think it will take for that note to get back to Owen? (Signal.) *Three days.*

Three days later, Owen's dad saw the tiny bottle floating near the beach. He picked it up, took it home, and pulled the tiny note out of the bottle. The note said:

Dear Owen and family,

Here are the answers to your questions:

1. The spiders and red beetles on our island are as tall as we are. The ants and fleas are smaller than we are.
2. The bears on our island are huge. Their claws are about two times as long as we are.
3. The sparrows on our island are about two times as tall as we are. The eagles and swans are huge.

We hope you get this note. Write soon.

Love from all the people here,
Fizz and Liz

P.S. Tell us more about the things on your island.

After Owen read the note, Owen and his family were quiet. They just stood there, trying to picture a place with such huge animals.

At last, Owen's dad said, "That's amazing."

Owen's mother said, "That's **disgusting.** Imagine, beetles as big as you are."

Owen said, "I would love to go to that island and see those amazing animals."

Owen's mother said, "Ugh, not me. I would hate to go to that place."

Owen's father said, "I don't know. It might be interesting."

"Never," his mother said.

That evening, Owen wrote another note to the little people. Here's that note:

Dear Fizz, Liz and everybody else,

Thank you for your last letter. My dad and I thought that we would like to visit your island some day, but my mother does not want to go there. Everything is fine on our island. The pineapples are ripe, and I ate **four** of them today.

Dad caught a shark. Mom fixed a great fish dinner. The three of us ate the whole shark. We are really full.

How are things on your island?

Your friends,
Owen, Mom and Dad

P.S. Watch out for bugs and bees.

- How many pineapples did Owen eat? (Signal.) *Four.*
- How long do you think it would take Fizz and Liz to eat **one** whole pineapple? (Call on a student. Ideas: *A long, long, time; days; months.*)

- Owen and his family had fish for dinner. Everybody, what kind of fish? (Signal.) *Shark.*
- They ate the whole shark. That's eating a lot of fish, isn't it? (Students respond.)

Three days later, Fizz and Liz received the note. They were amazed about Owen's family eating one whole shark. To Fizz and Liz a shark would be as big as a train. Fizz and Liz wrote back. They told about **their** dinner. Four of the people caught a shrimp and everybody had a great shrimp dinner. There was a lot left over for the next day.

- Hold up your fingers to show me how big a shrimp is. (Praise students who indicate 1 to 2 inches.)
- They ate this shrimp. Everybody, did they eat it all at **one** dinner? (Signal.) *No.*

Three days later, Owen got the note. "Imagine that," he said to himself. "All those people eating one shrimp and not even being able to finish it." To Owen, a huge shrimp was about the size of a flea to you.

That evening, Owen and his family made a decision. Instead of just sending the bottle back to the other island, they decided to take their boat and float along with the bottle until they arrived at the island. At first, Owen's mom didn't want to go, but Owen's dad told her that she could stay in the boat where she would be safe from spiders and beetles. She finally agreed. Owen was very excited and could hardly wait to visit Fizz and Liz.

- That's the end of this part of the story.

EXERCISE 4 Relative Size

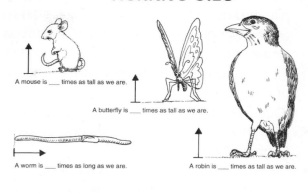

A mouse is ___ times as tall as we are.

A butterfly is ___ times as tall as we are.

A worm is ___ times as long as we are.

A robin is ___ times as tall as we are.

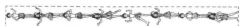

1. Everybody, find part C. ✔
   Along the bottom of the page is a pile of Fizzes and Lizzes.
- Cut out the whole strip. Cut along the dotted lines. Raise your hand when you're finished.
   (Observe students and give feedback.)
2. I'll read what it says under each animal.
- Everybody, touch the **mouse.** ✔
   It says: A mouse is blank times as tall as we are. It doesn't tell how many times.
- Touch the **butterfly.** ✔
   It says: A butterfly is blank times as tall as we are.
- Touch the **robin.** ✔
   It says: A robin is blank times as tall as we are.
- Touch the **worm.** ✔
   It says: A worm is blank times as long as we are.
- You're going to use your pile of Fizzes and Lizzes to figure out how they would describe the animals in the picture.
- You'll fill in the blanks with the right numbers.
3. Everybody, touch the **mouse** again. ✔
   Next to the mouse is a mark with an arrow going up from it. Put your pile of Fizzes and Lizzes on that mark and make the pile go in the same direction as the arrow. Put your pile so the **bottom** is right on the mark and the pile goes up. Raise your hand when

your pile is in place.
(Observe students and give feedback.)

4. Now you can start at the bottom of the pile and count the number of Fizzes and Lizzes to get to the very top of the mouse. Raise your hand when you know how many Fizzes and Lizzes it takes to get to the top of the mouse.
(Observe students and give feedback.)
- Everybody, how many Fizzes and Lizzes? (Signal.) *Two.*
- So that mouse is **two** times as tall as Fizz and Liz. Write **two** in the blank in the sentence below the mouse. Raise your hand when you're finished. ✔

5. Everybody, touch the **butterfly.** ✔
Put your pile so the bottom of the pile is on the line next to the butterfly. Then see how many Fizzes and Lizzes it takes to get to the very **top** of that butterfly's wing. Write the number for the butterfly, then write the number for the robin. Then stop. Don't do the worm. Raise your hand when you have numbers for the butterfly and the robin.
(Observe students and give feedback.)
- Everybody, touch the butterfly.
- Everybody, how many Fizzes and Lizzes is the butterfly? (Signal.) *Three.*

- Here's what your sentence should say: A butterfly is **three** times as tall as we are.
6. Everybody, touch the **robin.** ✔
- Everybody, how many Fizzes and Lizzes is the robin? (Signal.) *Five.*
- Your sentence should say: A robin is **five** times as tall as we are.
7. Touch the **worm.** ✔
For the worm you'll have to start your pile at one end. The arrow shows that the pile won't go up and down—it will go to the **side.** Turn your pile sideways. Start on the mark at the back of the worm and count the Fizzes and Lizzes to the front of the worm. Then write the number. Raise your hand when you're finished.
(Observe students and give feedback.)
- Everybody, how many Fizzes and Lizzes? (Signal.) *Four.*
- Now your sentence for the worm should say: A worm is **four** times as long as we are.
8. Let's say that Fizz and Liz decided to write Owen about the animals in the picture, rather than bugs, bears and birds.
- Who can start with the words: **Dear Owen and family,** then tell about each animal in the picture? (Call on several students. Praise responses that tell about the size of each animal compared to Fizz and Liz.)
- Later you can color the animals.

Objectives

- Perform on mastery test of skills presented in lessons 11–19. (Exercise 1)
- Students vote on a story to be reread. (Exercise 2)
- Exercises 3–5 provide instructions for marking the test and giving the students feedback.

WORKBOOK • LINED PAPER

EXERCISE 1 Test

Writing Parallel Sentences

A.

popcorn   reading   eating

1. You're going to have a test to see how smart you are. You can't talk to anybody during the test or look at what anybody else does.
- Open your workbook to lesson 20, and find part A. ✔
  You're going to write about this picture.
2. The picture shows what a girl and a boy were doing.
- What was the girl doing? (Call on a student. Idea: *Eating popcorn.*)
- Everybody, what was the boy doing? (Signal.) *Reading a book.*
3. Listen: A girl was eating popcorn. A boy was reading a a book.
- Say the whole sentence about a girl. (Signal.) *A girl was eating popcorn.*
- Say the whole sentence about a boy. (Signal.) *A boy was reading a book.*
- (Repeat sentences until firm.)
4. Look at the vocabulary box. These are some of the words you need: **popcorn . . . reading . . . eating.**
5. Say the sentence about a girl. (Signal.) *A girl was eating popcorn.*
- Say the sentence about a boy. (Signal.) *A boy was reading a book.*

6. (Hand out lined paper.)
   Write your name on the top line. ✔
   Write both sentences.
   (Observe students and give feedback.)
7. Skip a line on your paper and write both sentences again.
   (Observe students and give feedback.)
8. (Collect and correct papers.)

Directions—Map/North, South, East, West

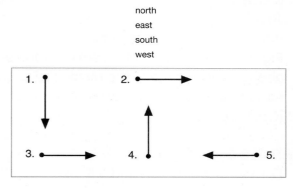

north
east
south
west

1. Arrow 1 points _____.
2. Arrow 2 points _____.
3. Arrow 3 points _____.
4. Arrow 4 points _____.
5. Arrow 5 points _____.

1. Everybody, find part B. ✔
- This is a map. The arrows go in different directions. You're going to write the direction each arrow points.
2. There are words above the map. They say **north, east, south** and **west.** You're going to use those words. When you write them, spell them correctly.
- Touch item 1 below the map. ✔
  That item tells about arrow 1. It says: Arrow 1 points blank.
- Touch arrow 1 on the map.
- Figure out if that arrow points north, east, south or west. Write the direction in the blank. Raise your hand when you're finished with item 1.

(Observe students but don't give feedback.)

3. Touch item 2. ✔
   It says: Arrow 2 points blank.
   - Figure out which direction arrow 2 points and write the name in the blank. Raise your hand when you're finished with item 2. (Observe students.)

4. Touch item 3. ✔
   It says: Arrow 3 points blank.
   - Figure out which direction arrow 3 points and write the name in the blank. Raise your hand when you're finished with item 3. (Observe students.)

5. Touch item 4. ✔
   It says: Arrow 4 points blank.
   - Figure out which direction arrow 4 points and write the name in the blank. Raise your hand when you're finished with item 4. (Observe students.)

6. Touch item 5. ✔
   It says: Arrow 5 points blank.
   - Figure out which direction arrow 5 points and write the name in the blank. Raise your hand when you're finished with item 5. (Observe students.)

EXERCISE 2 Story

1. For the rest of the period, I'll read a story. You get to choose which story. You've heard stories about Bleep, The Toad and the Mouse, Goober and Owen and the Little People. Everybody gets to vote on their favorite story. But you can only vote one time. I'll name the stories. You hold up your hand if you want that story. But remember, you can only hold up your hand one time.
   - Listen: Bleep. Who wants to hear the last Bleep story again? (Count the raised hands.)
   - Listen: The Toad and the Mouse. Who wants to hear that story again? (Count the raised hands.)
   - Listen: Goober. Who wants to hear the story about Goober again? (Count the raised hands.)
   - Listen: Owen and the Little People. Who wants to hear the last part of that story again? (Count the raised hands.)

2. (Read the chosen story. If time permits, read the story for the second choice.)

Key: Lesson 13 for Bleep (part 2);

Lesson 14 for The Toad and the Mouse;

Lesson 15 for Goober;

Lesson 19 for Owen and the Little People (part 4).

EXERCISE 3 Marking the Test

1. (Mark the test before the next scheduled language lesson. Use the *Language Arts Answer Key* to check the tests.)

2. (Write the number of errors each student made in the test scorebox at the top of the test page.)

3. (Enter the number of errors each student made on the Summary for Test 2. A Reproducible Summary Sheet is at the back of the *Language Arts Teacher's Guide*.)

EXERCISE 4 Feedback on Test 2

1. (Return the students' workbooks after they are marked.)
   - Everybody, open your workbook to lesson 20. Look at how I marked your test page.

2. I wrote a number at the top of your test. That number tells how many items you got wrong on the whole test.
   - Raise your hand if I wrote **0** or **1** at the top of your test.
     Those are super stars.
   - Raise your hand if I wrote **2** or **3.**
     Those are pretty good workers.
   - If I wrote a number that's more than 3, you're going to have to work harder.

EXERCISE 5 Test Remedies

   - (See the *Language Arts Teacher's Guide* for a general discussion of remedies.)

Objective

• **Compose 3 simple stories, each based on the same action topic.**

Sentence Writing

Ⓐ

1. _____

2. _____

3. _____

1. Everybody, open your workbook to lesson 21 and find part A. ✔

• Today's lesson is different. You're going to write sentences. Then you're going to draw pictures for **two** of your favorite sentences.

2. Touch number 1. ✔
   You're going to write your first sentence on the top line.

• (Write on the board:)

> **Everybody found something.**

• This says: Everybody found something.

• Copy that sentence on the top line of number 1. Remember the capital and the period. Raise your hand when you've copied the sentence.
   (Observe students and give feedback.)

3. On the next line you'll tell what **Goober** found. He found one of the things that you see at the bottom of the page. There are lots of things on that page. Maybe he found a puppy. Maybe he found that tub.

• Name something else he might have found.
   (Call on individual students.)

• (Write to show:)

> **Everybody found something.**
> **Goober found _____.**

• Here's the first part of the sentence. Write the sentence for Goober. Remember to spell the words just the way they are shown in the picture. Raise your hand when you've finished. Remember to start with a capital and end with a period.
   (Observe students and give feedback.)

• (Call on individual students to read their sentence for Goober. Praise acceptable sentences.)

4. (Write to show:)

> **Everybody found something.**
> **Goober found _____.**
> **Liz _____.**
> **I _____.**

• On the next line you'll write what **Liz** found.

• On the bottom line you'll write what **you** found.

• Remember, each sentence starts with a capital and ends with a period. Raise your hand when you've written a sentence for Liz and a sentence for you.
   (Observe students and give feedback.)

• (Call on individual students to read their sentence about Liz. Then call on individual students to read their sentence about themselves. Praise acceptable sentences.)

5. Touch number 2. ✔
   The sentences you'll write for number 2 tell what different characters **painted.**

• (Write on the board:)

> **Everybody painted something.**

• This says: Everybody painted something.

- Copy that sentence on the top line of number 2. Remember the capital and period. Raise your hand when you're finished.
  (Observe students and give feedback.)
6. (Write to show:)

> **Everybody painted something.**
> **Roger painted** _____.

- On the next line you'll tell what **Roger** painted. He painted one of the things that you see at the bottom of the page. Maybe he painted a ladder. Maybe he painted a tub.
- Write your sentence for Roger. Raise your hand when you're finished.
  (Observe students and give feedback.)
- (Call on individual students to read their sentence for Roger. Praise acceptable sentences.)
7. (Write to show:)

> **Everybody painted something.**
> **Roger painted** _____.
> **Molly** _____.
> **I** _____.

- On the next line you'll write what **Molly** painted.
- On the bottom line you'll write what **you** painted.
- Don't forget the capital and period for each sentence. Raise your hand when you've written a sentence for Molly and a sentence for you.
  (Observe students and give feedback.)
- (Call on individual students to read their sentence about Molly. Then call on individual students to read their sentence about themselves. Praise acceptable sentences.)

8. Touch number 3. ✔
   The sentences you'll write for number 3 tell what different characters **ran into.**
- (Write on the board:)

> **Everybody ran into something.**

- This says: Everybody ran into something.
- Copy that sentence on the top line of number 3. Raise your hand when you're finished.
  (Observe students and give feedback.)
9. (Write to show:)

> **Everybody ran into something.**
> **Clarabelle ran into** _____.
> **Owen** _____.
> **I** _____.

- You'll write sentences that tell what **Clarabelle** ran into, what **Owen** ran into and what **you** ran into. You'll use words from the bottom of the page.
- Write your sentences for number 3. Raise your hand when you're finished.
  (Observe students and give feedback.)
- (Call on individual students to read their sentence about Clarabelle. Call on individual students to read their sentence about Owen or their sentence about themselves.)
- Find part B. ✔
  Look at the two picture boxes. You can make pictures for two of your sentences. Pick your two favorite sentences and make pictures that show those sentences. I bet we'll have some great pictures to go with those sentences. Raise your hand when you're finished.
  (Observe students and give feedback.)

Objectives

- Compose and write a parallel sentence pair based on a single picture. (Exercise 1)
- Follow directions involving **north, south, east, west.** (Exercise 2)
- **Use clues to identify members of a class.** (Exercise 3)
- Say different deductions based on pictures. (Exercise 4)
- Listen to part 5 of a continued story and answer comprehension questions. (Exercise 5)

WORKBOOK • LINED PAPER

EXERCISE 1   Writing Parallel Sentences

next   box   chair

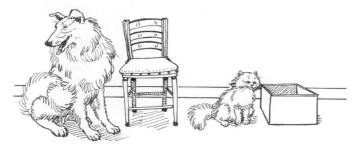

1. Open your workbook to lesson 22, and find part A. ✔
   You're going to write about this picture.
2. The picture shows what a dog and a cat sat next to.
- Where did the dog sit? (Call on a student. Idea: *Next to a chair.*)
- Where did the cat sit? (Call on a student. Idea: *Next to a box.*)
3. Listen: **A dog sat next to a chair. A cat sat next to a box.**
- Everybody, say the whole sentence about a dog. (Signal.) *A dog sat next to a chair.*
- Say the whole sentence about a cat. (Signal.) *A cat sat next to a box.*
- (Repeat sentences until firm.)
4. Look at the vocabulary box. These are some of the words you need: **next . . . box . . . chair.**
5. Say the sentence about a dog. (Signal.) *A dog sat next to a chair.*
- Say the sentence about a cat. (Signal.) *A cat sat next to a box.*

6. (Hand out a sheet of lined paper to each student.)
   Write your name on the top line. ✔
   Write both sentences. (Remind students to start writing words just after the margin, to begin each sentence with a capital letter, and to end each sentence with a period.)
   (Observe students and give feedback.)
7. **(Optional:)** Skip a line on your paper and write both sentences again.
   (Observe students and give feedback.)
8. (Collect and correct papers.)

EXERCISE 2   Directions

Movement To/From

1. Everybody, stand up.
   I'm going to tell you to face different directions. Wait until I say **go.**
2. Everybody, face **south.** Get ready. Go.
- Face **north.** Get ready. Go.
- Face **west.** Get ready. Go.
- Face **south.** Get ready. Go.
- Face **east.** Get ready. Go.
3. Everybody, take two baby steps to the **east.** Get ready. Go.
- You moved **to** the **east.** So you must have moved **from** the **west.**
- Everybody, which direction did you move **to?** (Signal.) *East.*
- So which direction did you move **from?** (Signal.) *West.*
4. Everybody, face **north.** Get ready. Go.
- Take two baby steps to the **north.** Get ready. Go.
- Listen big: Which direction did you move **to?** (Signal.) *North.*
- So which direction did you move **from?** (Signal.) *South.*

5. Everybody, when I say **go,** turn to the **south.** Then take two baby steps to the south. Get ready. Go.
- Listen big: Which direction did you move **to?** (Signal.) *South.*
- So which direction did you move **from?** (Signal.) *North.*
  Wow, you're getting pretty smart about the directions.
- Everybody, sit down.

EXERCISE 3 Classification

Subclass: Dogs

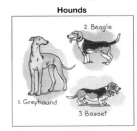
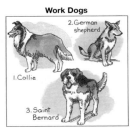

1. Everybody, find part B. ✔
- Here are some dogs in different boxes. They're in different boxes because they are different types of dogs.
2. Touch the box for the first type of dog. ✔ The word at the top says **hounds.**
- All the dogs in that box are hounds. All hounds are hunters. Some have a super nose, and they hunt by smelling. Others use their eyes to hunt. Not every hound is shown in the box. The hounds in the box are a **greyhound,** a **beagle** and a **basset.**
3. Everybody, touch dog 1. ✔ What kind of hound is that? (Signal.) *Greyhound.*
- A greyhound is probably the fastest dog alive. Greyhounds hunt by using their eyes.
- Touch dog 2. ✔ What kind of hound is that? (Signal.) *Beagle.*
- Touch dog 3. ✔ What kind of hound is that? (Signal.) *Basset.*
- Beagles and bassets hunt by using their nose.
- (Repeat step 3 until firm.)
4. Touch the box for the next type of dog. ✔ The words above that box say **work dogs.**

- Work dogs do a lot of different jobs. Not every work dog is shown in the box. The work dogs in the box are a **collie,** a **German shepherd** and a **St. Bernard.**
5. Everybody, touch dog 1. ✔ What kind of work dog is that? (Signal.) *Collie.*
- Touch dog 2. ✔ What kind of work dog is that? (Signal.) *German shepherd.*
- Touch dog 3. ✔ What kind of work dog is that? (Signal.) *St. Bernard.*
- That's a huge dog. A St. Bernard may weigh more than a full-grown man.
- (Repeat step 5 until firm.)
6. Listen: I'm thinking of a dog. It's a hound.
- Everybody, am I thinking of a German shepherd? (Signal.) *No.*
- How do you know I'm not thinking of a German shepherd? (Call on a student. Idea: *A German shepherd is not a hound.*)
7. Everybody, I'm thinking of a hound. Am I thinking of a beagle? (Signal.) *Maybe.*
- Right, I may be thinking of a beagle because a beagle is a hound.
- (Repeat step 7 until firm.)
8. Am I thinking of a collie? (Signal.) *No.*
- How do you know I'm not thinking of a collie? (Call on a student. Idea: *A collie is not a hound.*)
- Everybody, am I thinking of a basset? (Signal.) *Maybe.*
9. Listen: I'm thinking of a dog. It's a hound. It is probably the fastest dog alive.
- Touch the hound I'm thinking of. ✔
- Everybody, which hound are you touching? (Signal.) *Greyhound.*
10. New game: I'm thinking of a work dog.
- Am I thinking of a collie? (Signal.) *Maybe.*
- Am I thinking of a basset? (Signal.) *No.*
- How do you know I'm not thinking of a basset? (Call on a student. Idea: *A basset is not a work dog.*)
- I'm thinking of a work dog that might weigh more than a full-grown man. Touch the work dog I'm thinking of. ✔
- Everybody, which work dog are you touching? (Signal.) *St. Bernard.*
11. You're pretty good at using clues.

EXERCISE 4 Deductions

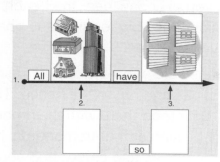

1. Everybody, find part C. ✔
   The only pictures for this deduction are on the top arrow. You're going to use those pictures to make up deductions.
2. Touch the **first** picture on the arrow. ✔
   Everybody, what's in the first picture? (Signal.) *Buildings.*
   - The word after the first picture is **have.** What word? (Signal.) *Have.*
   - What's in the **last** picture on the arrow? (Signal.) *Walls.*
   - Raise your hand if you can say the whole rule for arrow 1.
   - Everybody, start with **all** and say the rule for arrow 1. (Signal.) *All buildings have walls.*
3. I'm going to say the whole deduction about a store. Touch each arrow.
   - Listen: All buildings have walls. A store is a building. So a store has walls.
4. Your turn to say the whole deduction about a store. Get ready. (Signal.) *All buildings have walls. A store is a building. So a store has walls.*
   - (Repeat step 4 until firm.)
5. New deduction. Say the whole deduction about a house. A house. Get ready. (Signal.) *All buildings have walls. A house is a building. So a house has walls.*
6. New deduction. Say the whole deduction about a school. A school. Get ready. (Signal.) *All buildings have walls. A school is a building. So a school has walls.*
7. Who wants to pick a different building and say the whole deduction? Use a building we haven't used. (Call on individual students. Praise appropriate deductions.)
   - We have a lot of people who are super good at saying deductions.

EXERCISE 5 Owen and the Little People *Part 5*

Storytelling

- I'm going to read the next part of the story about Owen and the little people.
- Everybody, what did Owen and his family decide to do at the end of the last story? (Signal.) *Visit Fizz and Liz.*
- Right, they decided to visit Fizz and Liz. Listen to what happens next:

> Owen and his family decided to go visit Fizz and Liz.
>
> Owen and his family piled lots of supplies into their boat. They had a barrel of salted fish. They had a barrel of pineapples. They had lots of drinking water. They had to take drinking water because ocean water is salty and will make you sick if you drink it. They waited until the currents were moving away from the shore. Then they put the bottle into the sea and followed it in their boat.
>
> For two days, they followed that bottle. For two days they were in the middle of the ocean with nothing in sight except water, water and more water. They didn't see a speck of land.
>
> Then on the third day . . .

- What do you think happened? (Call on a student. Idea: *They saw Fizz and Liz's island.*)
- Yes.

> Owen's mother pointed off to the side of the boat and said, "Look. There's an island, way far away." She was sitting in front of the boat, wearing a large sun hat.
>
> "Yea!" Owen said. He was weary from sitting in that boat and rocking around in the waves day after day. About the only

thing he'd done during that time was to carve his name in big letters on the outside of the boat.

Owen and his dad started to row toward the island, closer, closer and closer. Suddenly, Owen's dad stopped rowing and said, "Oh, no. We must have gone in a great circle. That's **our** island."

- Why did he think this was their island? (Call on a student. Idea: *The islands are identical.*)
- Yes, Fizz and Liz's island is identical to Owen and his family's island.

Owen looked at the island. He could see the beach and the great mountains. He could see the waterfall. He felt very sad. "This is awful," he said. "We're right back where we started."

"Well," his mother said, "perhaps it is just as well. I wasn't looking forward to seeing giant creatures anyhow."

Everybody looked at the island for a long time. Then Owen's dad said, "Well, let's go home," and he started rowing toward the beach again.

At the same time that Owen and his family started rowing toward the island, Fizz and Liz and all the other little people were very busy on the island. They were building a recreation center. It was going to be a large building in the middle of a park, and there was a lot of work to do. The little people had to clear the weeds from the area, level the ground, make a swimming pool and tennis courts and, of course, build a large recreation building where people could meet or just have some fun.

Fizz and Liz were helping the others move large sticks for the recreation building. Suddenly, one of the little people said, "There's the **biggest**

boat you ever saw near the beach. It's a million times bigger than any boat you've ever seen."

All the little people dropped their tools and sticks and ran to the beach. Then they just stood there with their mouths open, looking at that tremendous boat. It came closer, and closer, and soon the little people could see that there were people sitting in the boat.

Liz said, "Do you see the size of those people?"

Fizz said, "Yes, but I don't believe what I'm seeing. They're **giants.**"

The boat pulled up to the shore, and most of the little people ran and hid in the weeds near the edge of the beach.

The ground shook when the giants got out of their boat. And when they talked, it was so loud that the little people had to hold their hands over their ears.

One of the giants said, "The beach looks a little different, doesn't it?"

Another giant said, "We've been away for three days, and all we've had to look at is waves and more waves. Of course the beach looks different."

Then the giants started to walk. Kaboom, kaboom, kaboom. The ground shook. The weeds shook. **Everything** shook.

One of the giants almost stepped on a group of little people. They screamed and shouted. "Watch out," some of them yelled. But Owen and his family didn't hear these shouts, because they were no louder than the buzz of a bee or the chirp of a faraway bird.

So Owen and his family walked from the beach to where their house would be, but it wasn't there. "What's happening?" Owen's mother said.

"I don't know," Owen's dad replied. "This is like a bad dream."

Owen said, "Maybe we're **not** on our island at all. Maybe we're on another island that looks like ours."

"Don't be silly," his mother said. "We know that we're not on the island that Fizz and Liz live on because we haven't seen one giant animal—just the same tiny animals that live on our island."

"But, what if . . ." Owen stopped right in the middle of what he was saying. He was looking at the tiny recreation center. It was right where Owen's house would be on his island. And there it was, a half-built building, about the size of a book.

- Everybody, show me with your hands how big the recreation center was. (Praise reasonable approximations.)

"Look at that," Owen said. Everybody bent down and examined the building. Owen's mother said, "Why would somebody build a little toy building like that?"

Owen said, "Maybe it's **not** a toy building."

"Of course it's a toy building," his mother said. "What else could it be?"

Owen was ready to say, "Maybe it's a regular-sized building for people who are very tiny," but he didn't say it because he knew it would sound silly.

A moment later, two incredibly small people popped out of the weeds near the building. They were waving their tiny little arms, and they were making funny squeaky sounds.

Owen looked at those tiny people. Then he looked at his mom and dad. They looked at Owen with very wide eyes. Then Owen looked back at the tiny people. They were still waving their arms and making those little squeaky sounds.

- That's the end of this part. What a place to stop.
- Who do you think those two little people might be? (Call on a student. Idea: *Fizz and Liz.*)
- This is puzzling. When Owen and his family almost stepped on the little people at the beach, all the little people were afraid of the giants, but now two of them are waving and shouting and trying to get their attention.
- They are acting as if they know the giants are Owen and his family. Maybe they got some clue down at the beach. Can you think of anything that might have given them a clue about who the giants are? This is tough. (Call on a student. Idea: *Owen's name on the side of the boat.*)

LESSON 23

Objectives

- Follow directions involving **north, south, east, west.** (Exercise 1)
- **Identify the direction an arrow moves from and to.** (Exercise 2)
- Use clues to classify dogs. (Exercise 3)
- **Listen to the conclusion of a 6-part story and tell what might happen next.** (Exercise 4)
- **Write a letter that contains descriptions of relative size.** (Exercise 5)

EXERCISE 1 Directions

Movement To/From

1. Everybody, stand up. ✔
   I'm going to tell you to face different directions. Wait until I say **go.**
2. Everybody, face **north.** Get ready. Go.
   - Face **west.** Get ready. Go.
   - Face **south.** Get ready. Go.
   - Face **north.** Get ready. Go.
   - Face **east.** Get ready. Go.
3. Everybody, take two tiny steps to the **east.** Get ready. Go.
   - You moved **to** the **east.** So you must have moved **from** the **west.**
     Everybody, which direction did you move **from?** (Signal.) *West.*
   - So which direction did you move **to?** (Signal.) *East.*
4. Everybody, face **south.** Get ready. Go.
   - Take two tiny steps to the **south.** Get ready. Go.
   - Listen big: Which direction did you move **to?** (Signal.) *South.*
   - So which direction did you move **from?** (Signal.) *North.*
5. Everybody, turn to the **north.** Take two tiny steps to the **north.** Get ready. Go.
   - Listen big: Which direction did you move **to?** (Signal.) *North.*
   - So which direction did you move **from?** (Signal.) *South.*
     Wow, you're getting pretty smart about the directions.
   - Everybody, sit down.

EXERCISE 2 Map

Movement To/From

1. (Write on the board:)

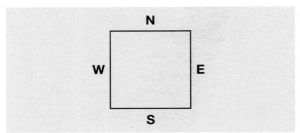

   - I'm going to show you some rules about things that move.
2. (Make a dot under **N:**)

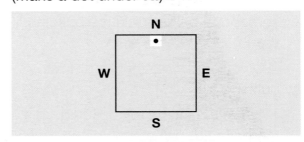

   - Everybody, which side of the map is the dot on? (Signal.) *North.*
   - Watch.
     (Draw arrow line from dot:)

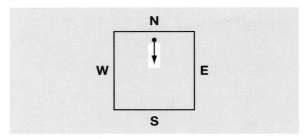

   - Which direction did that line move? (Signal.) *South.*

- Yes, that line went **from** north **to** south. Which way did that line move? (Signal.) *From north to south.*
- (Erase line and dot.)
3. (Make a dot next to **E:**)

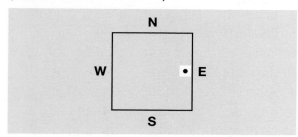

- I'm going to make another line. Watch it. (Draw line from dot:)

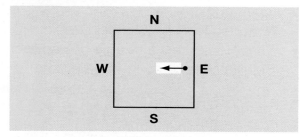

- Everybody, where did that line move **from?** (Signal.) *East.*
- Where did that line move **to?** (Signal.) *West.*
- Yes, that line went **from** east **to** west. Which way did that line move? (Signal.) *From east to west.*
- (Erase line and dot.)
4. (Make a dot next to **W:**)

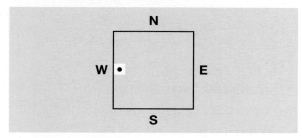

- I'm going to make another line. Watch it. (Draw line from dot:)

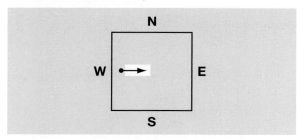

- Everybody, where did that line move **from?** (Signal.) *West.*

- Where did that line move **to?** (Signal.) *East.*
- I'm going to say the whole thing about how that line moved. The line moved from west to east.
5. Everybody, say the whole thing about how that line moved. *The line moved from west to east.*
- (Repeat step 5 until firm.)
- (Erase line and dot.)
6. I'm going to make it harder yet. Close your eyes.
(Draw arrow to show:)

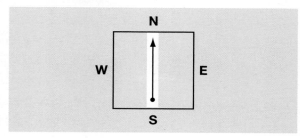

- Everybody, open your eyes.
Look at this arrow. The point of the arrow shows the direction the arrow points **to.**
- Listen: Which direction does the arrow point **to?** (Signal.) *North.*
- Listen: Which direction does the arrow point **from?** (Signal.) *South.*
- Yes, the arrow points **from** south **to** north.
7. Close your eyes again.
(Change arrow to show:)

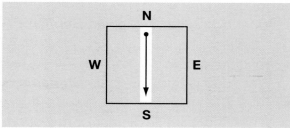

- Open your eyes.
Everybody, which direction does this arrow point **to?** (Signal.) *South.*
- Which direction does it point **from?** (Signal.) *North.*
- Yes, this arrow points **from** north **to** south.

EXERCISE 3 Classification

Subclass: Dogs

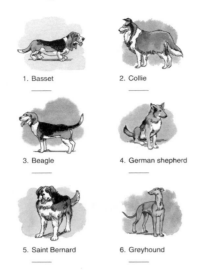

1. Basset
2. Collie
3. Beagle
4. German shepherd
5. Saint Bernard
6. Greyhound

1. Everybody, open your workbook to lesson 23 and find part A. ✔
- These are dogs. Let's see who remembers the name of each dog.
- Everybody, touch dog 1. Dog 1. ✔
  What dog is that? (Signal.) *Basset.*
- Touch dog 2. ✔
  What dog is that? (Signal.) *Collie.*
- Touch dog 3. ✔
  What dog is that? (Signal.) *Beagle.*
- Touch dog 4. ✔
  What dog is that? (Signal.) *German shepherd.*
- Touch dog 5. ✔
  What dog is that? (Signal.) *St. Bernard.*
- Touch dog 6. ✔
  What dog is that? (Signal.) *Greyhound.*
- Some of these dogs are in the group of work dogs and some of these dogs are in the group of hounds.
- (Write on the board:)

W	H

- You're going to tell what group each dog is in by writing **W** or **H.** You'll write **W** if the dog is a **work** dog. You'll write **H** if the dog is a **hound.**
2. Touch dog 1. ✔
  Listen big: What dog is that? (Signal.) *Basset.*
- Which group does a **basset** belong to? (Signal.) *Hound.*

- A basset is a hound, so you'll write **H** in the blank at the bottom of the picture. Do it. Raise your hand when you're finished. (Observe students and give feedback.)
3. Touch dog 2. ✔
  Listen big: What dog is that? (Signal.) *Collie.*
- Which group does a **collie** belong to? (Signal.) *Work dog.*
- A collie is a work dog, so what letter are you going to write in the blank at the bottom of picture 2? (Signal.) *W.*
- Do it. Raise your hand when you're finished.
4. Touch dog 3. ✔
  What dog is that? (Signal.) *Beagle.*
- What group does a **beagle** belong to? (Signal.) *Hound.*
- Write the correct letter for picture 3. Raise your hand when you're finished. ✔
- Everybody, what letter did you write for picture 3? (Signal.) *H.*
5. Write the letters for the rest of the dogs. Remember, write **H** for hounds and **W** for work dogs. Raise your hand when you're finished.
  (Observe students and give feedback.)
6. Check your work.
- Touch the German shepherd. That's picture 4. Everybody, what group does a **German shepherd** belong to? (Signal.) *Work dog.*
- What letter did you write? (Signal.) *W.*
- Touch the St. Bernard. That's picture 5. Everybody, what group does a **St. Bernard** belong to? (Signal.) *Work dog.*
- What letter did you write? (Signal.) *W.*
- Touch the greyhound. That's picture 6. Everybody, what group does a **greyhound** belong to? (Signal.) *Hound.*
- What letter did you write? (Signal.) *H.*
- Raise your hand if you wrote the correct letter for each dog. ✔
- You're getting good at putting those dogs in the right group.
7. Let's play that thinking game again. I'm going to make it tougher this time.
- Listen: I'm thinking of a dog. Is it a beagle? (Signal.) *Maybe.*
- Is it a collie? (Signal.) *Maybe.*
- Is it a tiger? (Signal.) *No.*
- How do you know it's not a tiger? (Call on a student. Idea: *A tiger is not a dog.*)

8. Listen: I'm thinking of a dog and it's a work dog. Is it a beagle? (Signal.) *No.*

- How do you know it's not a beagle? (Call on a student. Idea: *A beagle is not a work dog.*)
- Everybody, is it a collie? (Signal.) *Maybe.*
- Is it a German shepherd? (Signal.) *Maybe.*
- Is it a greyhound? (Signal.) *No.*
- How do you know it's not a greyhound? (Call on a student. Idea: *A greyhound is not a work dog.*)

9. Listen: I'm thinking of a dog and it's a work dog. This dog does not have hair as long as a collie. Listen again: This dog does not have hair as long as a collie.

- Raise your hand when you know which work dog I'm thinking of.
- Everybody, which work dog? (Signal.) *German shepherd.*
- How did you know that I wasn't thinking of a St. Bernard? (Call on a student. Idea: *A St. Bernard has hair as long as a collie's.*)
- How did you know that I wasn't thinking of a collie? (Call on a student. Idea: *The clue said that the dog had shorter hair than a collie.*)

10. New game: I'm thinking of a dog and this dog is **not** a work dog.

- Everybody, is the dog a greyhound? (Signal.) *Maybe.*
- Is the dog a basset? (Signal.) *Maybe.*
- Is the dog a German shepherd? (Signal.) *No.*
- How do you know it's not a German shepherd? (Call on a student. Idea: *A German shepherd is a work dog.*)

11. Listen: I'm thinking of a dog and it's not a work dog. It's a hound. And this hound looks something like a beagle, but it's got shorter legs and longer ears than a beagle.

- Raise your hand when you know which hound I'm thinking of.
- Everybody, which hound? (Signal.) *Basset.*
- How do you know I wasn't thinking of a beagle? (Call on a student. Idea: *The clue said that the dog had shorter legs and longer ears than a beagle.*)
- How do you know I wasn't thinking of a greyhound? (Call on a student. Idea: *A greyhound does not have shorter legs and longer ears than a beagle.*)

12. You're getting pretty smart at this thinking game.

EXERCISE 4   Owen and the Little People *Part 6*

Storytelling

- I'm going to read the last part of the story about Owen and the little people.
- Remember, two tiny people were waving their arms at Owen. We'll find out who those people were and how they knew that one of the giants was Owen.

The two little people waving their arms were Fizz and Liz. They figured out that one of the giants was Owen. They figured that out by looking at the boat after the giants had left the beach. Owen's name was on the side of the boat. When Fizz and Liz read the name, they knew why Owen said that there were tiny birds and tiny animals on his island.

They decided to run after the giants and try to get their attention. So when they got to the community center and saw the three giants crouching down, they ran out into the open area, waving their arms and yelling, "Owen, it's us— Fizz and Liz."

Owen's dad looked at the little people and said, "Do you see what I see?"

His mother said, "Yes, and it's amazing. I've read about tiny people, but I never thought I'd see any."

Owen said, "They're trying to tell us something, but I can't hear them." So Owen bent down and put his ear right above Fizz and Liz. Then he heard them say, in squeaky little voices, "Owen, it's Fizz and Liz."

Owen laughed. When he did that, he blew out air and knocked Fizz and Liz back into the weeds.

"Oh, I'm sorry," he said.

Then he said to his parents, "These little people are Fizz and Liz."

"Oh," his mother and father said. Then they said to Fizz and Liz, "Pleased to meet you."

Fizz and Liz were picking themselves up and brushing themselves off.

Well, everything made sense now. Owen could understand why Fizz and Liz talked about bugs that were as big as they were. He could understand why they talked about bears with claws two times as big as they were and sparrows two times as tall as they were.

And Fizz and Liz could understand why Owen talked about bears and birds being so small. Everything made sense, and there was a lot to talk about.

So Owen and his family lay face down on the ground in a place where they wouldn't scrunch any little people or flatten any neighborhoods. Then the little people gathered close to the giants' ears and they talked. Of course, Owen and his family had to talk very softly or they would blast those little people out of their britches.

- What are **britches?** (Call on a student. Idea: *Pants.*)
- Everybody, listen to that part again:

Of course, Owen and his family had to talk very softly or they would blast those little people out of their britches. And the little people had to yell as loud as they could, or the giants wouldn't be able to hear them.

After they talked a long time, Owen and his family decided to do something. While they were on the island, they could help the little people with their recreation building and some other projects.

So Owen and his family gathered sticks and built a super recreation building. Then they dug out a little ditch that led from the stream below the waterfall to the recreation center. The water filled the ditch and the little people had a great, wonderful river that went to the park near the community center. Then the giants built some more houses, just for fun.

After all the construction was completed, Owen and his dad caught enough fish to last the little people years. Owen and his dad built a warehouse to store the fish in. Then they collected berries, pineapples and other good things and put them in the warehouse.

Owen and his family spent two days on the island. At last, it was time for them to go back home. So they took the green bottle out to the beach, waited until the currents were moving away from shore, got into their boat and said good-bye to the little people, who were on the beach, waving and shouting, with tears in their eyes.

All the little people stood there and watched the boat and the bottle move out to sea. They listened as the giants called from their boat. "So long. Good-bye. See you later." And when the boat was far, far away from shore, they heard Owen say, "We'll write you when we get back. Maybe you can come and visit us sometime." And then the boat got smaller and smaller and smaller, until it disappeared.

- That's the end of the Owen and the Little People story. It doesn't tell us if Fizz and Liz ever went to Owen's island.
- What do you think will happen? (Call on several students and praise reasonable ideas.)

EXERCISE 5 Sentence Construction

Relative Size

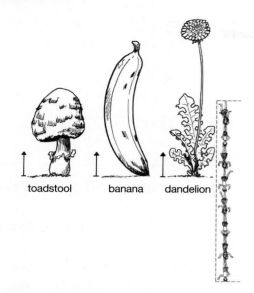

toadstool   banana   dandelion

1. Everybody, find part B. ✔
-   You're going to use the Fizz and Liz cutouts to measure some things. Then you're going to pretend that **you** are Fizz and Liz and you're writing to Owen. You're going to tell how big each object is.
-   (Write on the board:)

> **Dear Owen,**
>   A _____ is _____ times as tall as we are.

-   (Point to the board, say:)
    This says: Dear Owen, A **blank** is **blank** times as tall as we are.
-   Cut out your Fizz and Liz strip. ✔
-   You'll use your pile of Fizzes and Lizzes to figure out how Fizz and Liz would describe **how tall** each thing in the picture is.
2. Everybody, touch the **toadstool.** ✔
    Use your pile of Fizzes and Lizzes to figure out how tall the toadstool is. Remember, start your pile on the mark at the bottom of the arrow. Raise your hand when you know how many Fizzes and Lizzes **tall** the toadstool is.
    (Observe students and give feedback.)
-   Everybody, how many Fizzes and Lizzes? (Signal.) *Four.*

-   So here's how you write about that toadstool:
-   (Write to show:)

> **Dear Owen,**
>   A <u>toadstool</u> is 4 times as tall as we are.

-   Now it says: Dear Owen, A toadstool is 4 times as tall as we are.
3. You're going to write this part.
-   Write **Dear Owen** on the top line.
-   On the next line, write the sentence about the toadstool. Remember the capital and period for the sentence about the toadstool. Raise your hand when you're finished.
    (Observe students and give feedback.)
4. Now write the sentence about the banana and another sentence about the dandelion. Remember the capitals and periods. Raise your hand when you're finished.
    (Observe students and give feedback.)
-   (Change sentence to show:)

> A <u>banana</u> is 6 times as tall as we are.

-   Here's the sentence for the banana: A banana is 6 times as tall as we are. Check your banana sentence.
-   (Change sentence to show:)

> A <u>dandelion</u> is 7 times as tall as we are.

-   Here's the sentence for the dandelion: A dandelion is 7 times as tall as we are. Check your dandelion sentence.
5. (Write to show:)

> A dandelion is 7 times as tall as we are.   **From Fizz and Liz**

-   This is what you'll write on the bottom line. It says: From Fizz and Liz. Raise your hand when you're finished.
6. Now you have a note to Owen that tells how tall the three things in the picture are. Who thinks they can read their whole note? (Call on several students. Praise correct responses.)
7. Later you can color the picture.

Materials: Each student will need a pair of scissors.

Objectives

- Compose and write a parallel sentence pair based on a single picture. (Exercise 1)
- **Arrange objects in larger and smaller classes.** (Exercise 2)
- Listen to a familiar story and answer comprehension questions. (Exercise 3)
- Edit words to correct a character's dialect. (Exercise 4)

WORKBOOK • LINED PAPER

EXERCISE 1 Writing Parallel Sentences

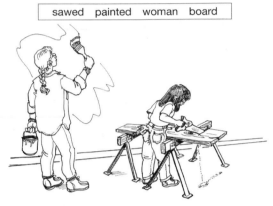

sawed   painted   woman   board

1. Open your workbook to lesson 24, and find part A. ✔
   You're going to write about this picture.
2. The picture shows what a woman and a girl did.
- What did the woman do? (Call on a student. Idea: *Painted a wall.*)
- What did the girl do? (Call on a student. Idea: *Sawed a board.*)
3. Listen: The woman painted a wall. The girl sawed a board.
- Everybody, say the whole sentence about the woman. (Signal.) *The woman painted a wall.*
- Say the whole sentence about the girl. (Signal.) *The girl sawed a board.*
- (Repeat sentences until firm.)
4. Look at the vocabulary box. These are some of the words you need: **sawed . . . painted . . . woman . . . board.**
5. Say the sentence about the woman. (Signal.) *The woman painted a wall.*
- Say the sentence about the girl. (Signal.) *The girl sawed a board.*

6. (Hand out a sheet of lined paper to each student.)
   Write your name on the top line of your paper. ✔
   Write both sentences. (Remind students to start writing words just after the margin, to begin each sentence with a capital letter, and to end each sentence with a period.)
   (Observe students and give feedback.)
7. **(Optional:)** Skip a line on your paper and write both sentences again.
   (Observe students and give feedback.)
8. (Collect and correct papers.)

EXERCISE 2 Classification

Subclass: Dogs

1. (Write on the board:)

Lesson 24

This says **Lesson 24.** Turn to the last page of your workbook and touch the column of dogs that has **Lesson 24** on top. Raise your hand when you've found it.
(Observe students and give feedback.)
- You should be touching the column closest to the edge of the page.

2. Some of these dogs are work dogs, and some are hounds.
- Everybody, touch the first dog. ✔
  What dog is that? (Signal.) *Collie.*
- What group does a collie belong to? (Signal.) *Work dogs.*
- Touch the next dog. ✔
  What dog is that? (Signal.) *Basset.*
- What group does a basset belong to? (Signal.) *Hounds.*
- Touch the next dog. ✔
  What dog is that? (Signal.) *Beagle.*
- What group does a beagle belong to? (Signal.) *Hound.*
- Touch the next dog. ✔
  What dog is that? (Signal.) *Greyhound.*
- What group does a Greyhound belong to? (Signal.) *Hound.*
- Touch the next dog. ✔
  What dog is that? (Signal.) *St. Bernard.*
- What group does a St. Bernard belong to? (Signal.) *Work dogs.*
- Touch the next dog. ✔
  What dog is that? (Signal.) *German shepherd.*
- What group does a German shepherd belong to? (Signal.) *Work dogs.*
3. The rest of the pictures show dogs that aren't work dogs and aren't hounds.
- You're going to cut out that column. You'll start at the top and cut very carefully along the line. Cut carefully, because you're going to use this page in later lessons. Cut out the whole column of dogs. Raise your hand when you're finished. Now cut out each dog and we'll play a tough game. Raise your hand when you're finished.

CLASS AND NOT CLASS

1. Everybody, find part B. ✔

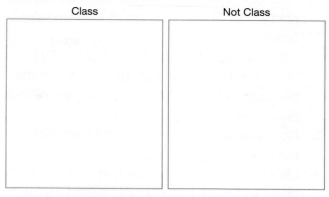

- Listen: One of the boxes has the word **Class** above it.
- Touch that box. ✔
- The other box has the words **Not-Class** above it.
- Touch that box. ✔
2. You're going to make up different classes. You make up a class by putting things in the class box. I'll tell you the name of the things for a big class.
- Listen: **Dogs.**
- Fix up your **class** box. Put all the dogs in the class box. Raise your hand when you're finished.
  (Observe students and give feedback.)
- You should have all the dogs in your **class** box. That's the biggest class you can make with your cutouts.
3. Now you'll make a smaller class by putting some dogs in the **not-class** box. Anything in the **not-class** box is **not** part of the class.
- Listen: Move all the cutouts that are **not** work dogs and **not** hounds to the **not-class** box. Leave all the hounds and work dogs in your **class** box. Raise your hand when you're finished.
  (Observe students and give feedback.)
- There should be two groups of dogs in the **class** box now. What are they?
  (Call on a student: Idea: *Hounds and work dogs.*)
- Yes, now the **class** box has hounds and work dogs.

4. Now you're going to make a smaller class.
- Listen: Put all your hounds in the **not-class** box. Don't move the other dogs out of the **class** box. Raise your hand when you're finished.
  (Observe students and give feedback.)
- There's a small class of dogs in the **class** box now. What's that class? (Signal.) *Work dogs.*

5. Now you're going to make a class that's even smaller.
- Listen: Move your St. Bernard and your collie to the **not-class** box. Now there's only one kind of dog in the **class** box. What's that? (Signal.) *German shepherd.*
- That's a smaller class than the class of work dogs.

6. Listen: Make the **biggest class** you can in the **class** box. Move dogs around so that you have as many dogs as possible in the **class** box. Raise your hand when you're finished.
  (Observe students and give feedback.)
- You have a very big class now. Everybody, what's the name of that class? (Signal.) *Dogs.*

7. Now see if you can move just some of the dogs to the **not-class** box so there are two large groups of dogs in the **class** box. Raise your hand when you're finished.
  (Observe students and give feedback.)
- What two large groups are in your class box now? (Signal.) *Work dogs and hounds.*
- What are the other dogs? (Signal.) *A poodle and a springer spaniel.*

8. Listen: Move one of the groups of dogs out of your **class** box and put it in the **not-class** box. Just one of the groups. You can pick either group you want to move. Raise your hand when you're finished.
  (Observe students and give feedback.)
- Now you should have a pretty small class.

9. Raise your hand if your **class** box has just hounds in it.
- Everybody with **hounds** in your **class** box, where are the work dogs? (Signal.) *In the not-class box.*
- Where are the other two dogs? (Signal.) *In the not-class box.*

10. Raise your hand if your **class** box has just work dogs in it.
- Everybody with **work dogs** in your **class** box, where are your hounds? (Signal.) *In the not-class box.*
- Where are the other two dogs? (Signal.) *In the not-class box.*

11. Listen: You're going to make the class so small that it has only one kind of dog in it. Move all the dogs but one of them to the **not-class** box. Raise your hand when you're finished.
  (Observe students and give feedback.)
- You should have one dog in the **class** box and all the others in the **not-class** box. What does your **class** box show? (Call on individual students. Praise appropriate responses.)
- You're making up bigger and smaller classes. Good for you.

EXERCISE 3 Goober

Review

1. I'm going to read the story about Goober again. But first, let's make sure you understand how the winds work.
- (Draw on the board:)

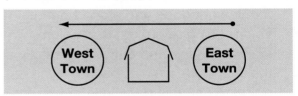

- Here's a map that shows Goober's farm. Remember, East Town is on the east side of the map and West Town is on the west side of the map. Goober's farm is right in the middle.
- The arrow shows the direction of the wind. It shows where the wind is coming **from** and where it is going **to.** Raise your hand when you know what direction that wind is moving **from.**
- Everybody, which direction? (Signal.) *East.*
- Yes, it's moving **from** the east.
- When the wind moves from the east, it picks up the awful smell from Goober's farm and carries it to one of the towns. Raise your hand when you know what town gets the awful smell when the wind blows **from** the east.

- Everybody, which town? (Signal.) *West Town.*
- (Point to Goober's farm. Say:)
  The wind moves like this.
- (Move your finger left. Say:)
  And so now the people in West Town have to hold their noses.
2. (Change arrow to show:)

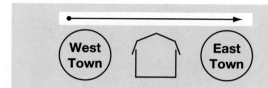

- Now the wind is moving from a different direction.
- Everybody, which direction is the wind moving from? (Signal.) *West.*
- Yes, it's moving **from** the west. So now the people in East Town have to hold their noses.
3. (Erase the board.)
  Keep a picture of that map in your mind when I read about Goober.

Once there was a crusty old man named Gustaf Gutenberger. But nobody called him Gustaf Gutenberger. Instead, they used the nickname, Goober. Goober lived by himself on a small farm. That farm was right between two small towns. The town to the west of Goober's farm was called . . .

- What? (Signal.) *West Town.*

The town to the east of Goober's farm was called . . .

- What? (Signal.) *East Town.*

The people in West Town and East Town had mixed feelings about Goober. The reason they had mixed feelings was that Goober's farm had a very bad smell.

He had dirty pigs that **never** took a bath. They didn't just smell sort of strong or kind of bad. They smelled **awful.** People would sometimes hold their nose when they walked near his farm. And when the wind blew **from** the east, the people in one of the towns would say, "Phew, what is that **awful** smell?"

- Listen to that part again and get a picture of the wind:

And when the wind blew **from** the **east,** the people in one of the towns would say, "Phew, what is that **awful** smell?"

- Everybody, where were the people who would say that? (Signal.) *West Town.*

But they really knew what was making that smell.

And when the wind blew **from** the **west,** the people in East Town would say, "Phew! I wish the wind would change **soon.**"

It would be easy for people to hate Goober because of his smelly farm. But things were not that simple because of the violin.

You see, although Goober's farm smelled so bad, Goober could play the violin so sweetly that people would just stop what they were doing and listen to the beautiful sounds that drifted on the breeze. Birds would stop singing because they were ashamed of their songs when they heard Goober's beautiful violin music.

Some people who lived in West Town and East Town **loved** Goober. The reason they loved him was that they couldn't **smell** his farm. The breeze wouldn't carry the smell for more than a mile. But the breeze would carry Goober's music for more than a mile. So the people who lived more than a mile from Goober's place could hear the music but couldn't smell his pigs.

"Such wonderful music," they would say as they sat out on their porches in the evening, listening to the music.

Some people who lived in West Town and East Town were **confused** about Goober. They hated him and they loved him. They hated him because they lived less than a mile from Goober's farm.

- Everybody, how far away were the people who hated him and loved him? (Signal.) *Less than a mile.*
- Yes, so they would hear his music, but the wind would carry something else to them. What was that? (Call on a student. Idea: *The smell from Goober's farm.*)

So when the wind blew from Goober's farm, most of them wouldn't sit out on their porch in the evening listening to the music. They would go inside and close all the windows and the doors. They wouldn't be able to hear the music, but they felt that was better than having to breathe in all that terrible smell. Oh, there were some real music lovers who would put clothespins on their noses and sit outside to enjoy the music, but they would get sore noses because they had to make sure that their clothespins were very tight or some of the smell would come through.

So on a summer evening, Goober would get out his violin, sit on an old stump near his barn and start playing. If there was no wind, all the people in West Town and East Town would be on their porches, listening to his wonderful music.

But, if the wind blew **to** the west, there would be a **lot** of people in West Town shut up tight inside their houses.

Then one day, something very strange happened. A little girl from West Town went over to visit Goober. That was very strange because **nobody** ever visited Goober. She took a big package with her and walked up to his barn where he was milking a cow. She held her nose and said, "Mr. Goober, you

make nice music." But it didn't sound quite that way because she was holding her nose. What she actually said sounded like this:

- What? (Call on a student. Accept responses which substitute **B** for **M** and **D** for **N.**)
- Yes, what she actually said sounded like . . .

"Bister Goober, you bake dice busic."

Goober looked up and said, "I do what?"

She said, "Bake dice busic."

He shook his head and said, "Well, I can't do anything about that."

She said, "Dough. You dote uderstad."

He said, "You know, if you'd stop holding your nose, maybe I could understand what you're trying to tell me."

So the little girl took a very deep breath, let go of her nose and said, very fast, "We love your music, but you need to clean up your pigs. They **stink.**"

Goober's eyes got wide and he stared at the girl for a long time. She was holding her nose again. At last he said, "Do my pigs really stink?"

She said, "Yes."

He said, "Golly. I didn't know that."

Then she handed Goober her package and said, "Here are sub thigs for you." Then she said, "Good-bye," and ran away, holding her nose.

After she left, Goober opened the package. Inside were some bars of pig soap.

Goober smelled the soap and said, "What a great smell."

Then Goober shrugged, took the package with him down to his pond and called his pigs. They came running. Then he jumped into the pond with the pigs and scrubbed them until they were pink. He rubbed and scrubbed and he washed and he rinsed. When he was done, his pigs were as clean and sweet smelling as anybody in West Town or East Town. Goober sniffed the air and said, "Those pigs really smell great." Then Goober took some of that great-smelling pig soap back to his house. "I can use this soap on me," he said.

Well, that's the story. If you ever go to West Town or East Town, you'll hear the sweetest violin music you've ever heard in your life. And you'll hear people saying wonderful things about Goober. And they also say some nice things about a little girl who visits Goober every week. She always takes a package with her, and the people in West Town and East Town are **very** grateful.

EXERCISE 4   Correcting Non-nasal Speech

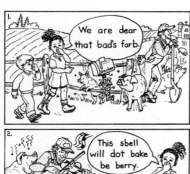
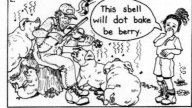

1. Everybody, find part C. ✔
   Here's the little girl who visited Goober. You can see that she's holding her nose and trying to say things. In everything she says, the **B** sound is wrong and the **D** sound is wrong.
 • You're going to fix up what she says so it

sounds right. You have to change all the **B's** into a different letter. Raise your hand if you remember that letter.
 • (Call on a student.) *M.*
 • Yes, you can change the **B's** into **M's.** Everybody, what letter do you write for **B?** (Signal.) *M.*
 • And you have to change all the **D's** into a different letter. Raise your hand if you remember that letter.
 • (Call on a student.) *N.*
 • Yes, you change the **D's** into **N's.** Everybody, what letter do you write for **D?** (Signal.) *N.*
2. Touch the **first** picture of the little girl. ✔
   I'll read what she's saying. I'll read slowly. Touch each word as I read it: We . . . are . . . dear . . . that . . . bad's . . . farb.
 • There are a lot of **B's** and **D's** that are wrong.
 • Touch the **second** picture of the little girl. ✔
   I'll read what she's saying. Touch each word. This . . . sbell . . . will . . . dot . . . bake . . . be . . . berry.
 • Your turn: Cross out all the **B's** and write **M** above them. Cross out all the **D's** and write **N** above them. Don't get fooled. I don't think Goober lives on a farb. Raise your hand when you're finished.
   (Observe students and give feedback.)
3. Check your work.
 • Touch the first picture again. ✔
   I'll read what she's saying: We are dear that bad's farb.
 • Raise your hand if you can say what she's trying to say.
 • (Call on a student.) *We are near that man's farm.*
 • Touch the **second** picture. ✔
   I'll read what she's saying: This sbell will dot bake be berry.
 • Raise your hand if you can say what she's trying to say.
 • (Call on a student.) *This smell will not make me merry.*

4. (Write on the board:)

> We are **n**ear that **m**a**n**'s far**m**.
>
> This s**m**ell will **n**ot **m**ake **m**e **m**erry.

- Check your work. Here's how you should have fixed up the two sentences. Look at each letter I've crossed out. Make sure you crossed it out and wrote the correct letter above it.

5. Raise your hand if you got all the letters right. ✔
Everybody else, fix up any letters you missed.

6. Later you can color the pictures.

Materials: Each student will need a red and a brown crayon.

Objectives

- **Draw arrows to show movement to and from (to the east and from the west).** (Exercise 1)
- Listen to a story and answer comprehension questions. (Exercise 2)
- **Construct deductions to answer questions.** (Exercise 3)

WORKBOOK

EXERCISE 1   Map
Movement To/From

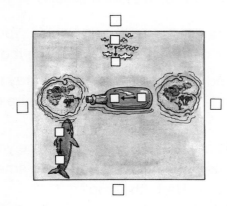

1. Everybody, open your workbook to lesson 25 and find part A. ✔
- This map does not have **north, south, east** or **west** shown on it. Write the correct letters in the boxes. Raise your hand when you're finished. ✔
- (Write on the board:)

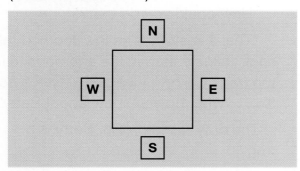

- Here's what you should have. Raise your hand if you got it right.
2. This is a funny map. Some things are too big. Some of those things are moving. The arrows show the direction that they are moving. Touch the island that has Owen on it. ✔

- Touch the bottle in the water near his island. ✔
  The arrow on that bottle shows which direction the bottle moves **from** and which direction it moves **to.**
3. Your turn: Write the letters that show the directions on the bottle. Write the direction the bottle is going **to** in front of the arrow. Write the direction the bottle is moving **from** in back of the arrow. Raise your hand when you're finished.
  (Observe students and give feedback.)
- (Draw on the board:)

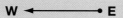

- Here's what you should have for the bottle arrow. The bottle is moving **to** the west. So **W** is in front of the arrow. **E** is in back of the arrow. The arrow is moving **from** the east. Raise your hand if you got it right.
4. Touch the whale in the picture. ✔
  The arrow shows the direction that the whale is moving. Write the letters for the arrow. Raise your hand when you're finished.
  (Observe students and give feedback.)
- (Draw on the board:)

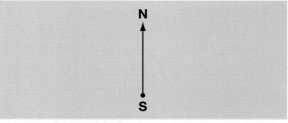

- Here's what you should have. The whale is moving **from** the south **to** the north. So **S** is in back of the arrow and **N** is in front of the arrow. Raise your hand if you got it right.

5. Touch the birds. ✔
   The arrow shows the direction the birds are moving. Fix up the arrow for the birds. Raise your hand when you're finished. (Observe students and give feedback.)
- (Draw on the board:)

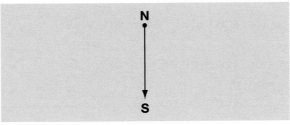

- Here's what you should have for the bird arrow. The birds are moving **from** the north **to** the south. So **N** is in back of the bird arrow and **S** is in front of the point. Raise your hand if you got it right.
6. Look at the bottle again. It looks like it's going to that other island. I wonder why I can't see any people on that island.
- What do you think? (Call on a student. Idea: *The people are too small to see.*)

EXERCISE 2 The Bragging Rat Wants to Be a Detective

Storytelling

- Everybody, I'm going to read a new story about one of the bragging rats:

> One day the gray bragging rat decided that he wanted to be a detective.

- What does a detective do? (Call on a student. Idea: *Figures out who commits crimes.*)
- Detectives have to be pretty smart at figuring things out.
- Listen again:

> One day the gray rat decided that he wanted to be a detective. He told the rat with the yellow teeth about his plan.
>
> The rat with the yellow teeth said, "You can't be a detective. You don't know how to figure things out."
>
> "I do, too," the gray rat said. "I can figure out anything. In fact, I'm so good

at figuring things out that I could beat anybody in the world in a figuring-out contest."

> "Oh, yeah," the rat with the yellow teeth said. "If you're so smart, where is Betty the frog?"
>
> "I don't know."
>
> "Ha, ha," the rat with the yellow teeth said. "You don't know, and you don't even know how to figure it out."
>
> "I do, too. I just don't feel like doing it right now."

- Do you think the gray rat is telling the truth? (Call on a student.) *No.*

> The yellow-toothed rat said, "You don't either know how to figure it out."
>
> And that rat was right. The gray rat didn't have any idea how to figure out where Betty the frog was.
>
> Finally, the gray rat said to the yellow-toothed rat, "Okay, if you're so smart, where is Betty the frog?"
>
> "That's easy," the yellow-toothed rat said. "She's taking a snooze on a lily pad."
>
> "You must have seen her there," the gray rat said.
>
> "I did **not** see her. I figured it out."
>
> "How could you do that?"
>
> "That's easy," the yellow-toothed rat said. "I know that, in the afternoon, all the frogs are on lily pads. Betty is a frog. So . . . what do you know about Betty?"
>
> The gray rat said, "So, Betty is a frog."
>
> "No, no," said the yellow-toothed rat. "You don't even know how deductions work. Listen again: In the afternoon, all the frogs are on lily pads. Betty is a frog. So . . ."
>
> The gray rat was getting mad. He said, "So Betty is a frog."

- Is that the right answer? (Signal.) *No.*

"No, no," the yellow-toothed rat said. "Listen: In the afternoon, all the frogs are on lily pads. Betty is a frog. So in the afternoon, Betty is on a lily pad."

"You're just making that up," the gray rat said.

"I'll bet we find her on a lily pad," the yellow-toothed rat said.

"I'll bet," the gray rat said.

So the two rats went down to the pond and looked at the frogs sitting on lily pads. And there was Betty, sitting on a lily pad.

The yellow-toothed rat stuck out his chest and smiled. His big yellow teeth were sticking way out. "I was right," he said proudly, "because I know about deductions, and you don't."

The gray rat was very sad. He walked around for a while. Then he decided to go to the wise old rat to learn about deductions.

He found the wise old rat resting on top of an old stump with four other old rats. It took the gray rat a while to find him, because he looked in five different places before he went to the stump.

The gray rat explained his problem to the wise old rat.

Then the wise old rat said, "How did you find me?"

The gray rat said, "I looked and looked until I found you."

The wise old rat said, "Didn't you know that, in the afternoon, all old rats sit on this stump?"

"Sure, I knew that," the gray rat said. "Everybody knows that."

"Well," the wise old rat said, "you could have figured out where I was. Listen: In the afternoon, all the old rats sit on this stump. I'm an old rat. **So . . .** "

- What do you think that silly gray rat will say? (Call on a student. Idea: *So you're an old rat.*)
- Everybody, listen to that part again:

"Well," the wise old rat said, "you could have figured out where I was. Listen: In the afternoon, all the old rats sit on this stump. I'm an old rat. **So . . .** "

The gray rat said, "So you're an old rat."

"No, no," the wise old rat said, as all the other old rats tried not to laugh. "Listen to me: In the afternoon, all the old rats sit on this stump. I'm an old rat. So, in the afternoon, I sit on this stump."

The gray rat was very confused. The wise old rat said, "Try this one: Where is Henrietta the bluebird right now?"

"I don't know. Do you want me to go look for her?"

All the old rats started to chuckle.

The wise old rat said, "Don't you know where all the bluebirds are in the afternoon?"

"Sure," the gray rat said. "In the afternoon, all the bluebirds are in the oak tree."

"Well, then," the wise old rat said, "where is Henrietta the bluebird?"

"I don't know. Do you want me to go look for her?"

"No," the wise old rat said. "I want you to figure it out. Start with what you know about all the bluebirds in the afternoon and what you know about Henrietta."

The gray rat said, "In the afternoon, all the bluebirds are in the oak tree. Henrietta is a bluebird. So . . . "

"So, what?" the wise old rat said.

"So Henrietta is a bluebird," the gray rat said.

> All the old rats started laughing so hard that two of them rolled right off the old stump.
>
> The wise old rat tried not to laugh. He said, "We'll work on that. You'll learn how to do it."
>
> But the gray rat felt **very** sad. He no longer liked the idea of being a detective.

- Why not? (Call on a student. Idea: *He didn't know how to make deductions.*)

EXERCISE 3 Deduction Writing

1. Everybody, you're going to need these crayons: red and brown. Take them out. Raise your hand when you're ready. ✔
- Find part B. ✔
  This picture shows the afternoon, but not everything is shown in the picture.
2. Touch the toadstools. ✔
- Here's the rule about the toadstools: In the afternoon, all the toads are on toadstools.

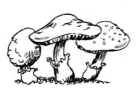 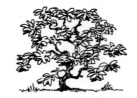

toadstools   berry bush

 Where is Jenny the toad in the afternoon?   Where is Rod the red bug in the afternoon?

• In the afteroon, all the toads are
_____
• Jenny is _____
• So in the afternoon, Jenny is

• In the afternoon, all the red bugs are
_____
• Rod is _____
• So in the afternoon, Rod is

- Fix up your toadstools so they have brown toads on them. Raise your hand when you're finished.
  (Observe students and give feedback.)
3. Touch the box with the picture of the toad. ✔
  That's Jenny the toad.
- Touch the question in that box. ✔
- I'll read it: **Where is Jenny the toad in the afternoon?**
- Everybody, what does that question say? (Signal.) *Where is Jenny the toad in the afternoon?*

- You're going to tell about Jenny by completing the deduction below the box.
- Touch the first part of that deduction. ✔
  The first part says: In the afternoon, all the toads are . . .
- Where are all the toads? (Signal.) *On toadstools.*
- So the first sentence should say: In the afternoon, all the toads are **on toadstools.**
- Complete the first sentence. Raise your hand when you're finished. ✔
4. Touch the next sentence. ✔
  It says: Jenny is . . .
- What is Jenny? (Signal.) *A toad.*
- Finish that sentence. Raise your hand when you're finished. ✔
5. Now you can complete the last sentence. It says: So in the afternoon, Jenny is . . .
- Complete that sentence. Tell where Jenny is in the afternoon. Don't make the same kind of mistake the gray rat makes. Raise your hand when you're finished. ✔
- Here's what you should have for the last sentence: So in the afternoon, Jenny is on a toadstool. Raise your hand if you got it right. ✔
6. So you answered the question about Jenny. Where is Jenny in the afternoon? (Signal.) *On a toadstool.*
- And you wrote a deduction to tell how you figured it out.
- I can say the whole deduction: In the afternoon, all the toads are on toadstools. Jenny is a toad. So in the afternoon, Jenny is on a toadstool.
- Who thinks they can say that whole deduction without looking? (Call on several students. For each correct deduction, say:) You're sure a lot better at figuring things out than the gray rat is.
7. Everybody, look at the picture of the berry bush. There are supposed to be red bugs in that bush. Use your red crayon. Fix up the berry bush so it has a lot of little red dots in it. Raise your hand when you're finished. ✔
- Everybody, touch the question in the box with the bug in it. That's Rod the red bug. ✔
  I'll read it: Where is Rod the red bug in the afternoon?

- Everybody, what does that question say? (Signal.) *Where is Rod the red bug in the afternoon?*
- You're going to answer that question by completing the deduction below the box.
- The first part of that deduction says: In the afternoon, all the red bugs are . . . Where are all the red bugs? (Signal.) *In the berry bush.*
- So the first sentence should say: In the afternoon, all the red bugs are in the berry bush.
  Finish the first sentence. Raise your hand when you're finished. ✔
- Touch the next sentence. ✔
  It says: Rod is . . . What is Rod? (Signal.) *A red bug.*
- Complete that sentence. Raise your hand when you're finished. ✔
- Now you can complete the last sentence. It says: So in the afternoon, Rod is . . .
- Complete that sentence. Raise your hand when you're finished. ✔
- Here's what you should have for the last sentence: So in the afternoon, Rod is in the berry bush.

8. You answered the question about Rod.
- I can say the whole deduction: In the afternoon, all the red bugs are in the berry bush. Rod is a red bug. So in the afternoon, Rod is in the berry bush.
- Who thinks they can say that whole deduction without looking? (Call on several students. Praise appropriate responses.)
- Next time we'll see if that gray rat gets any better at figuring out deductions.

9. You have to color the picture of Jenny the toad. Raise your hand if you know what color to make Jenny.
- Everybody, what color? (Signal.) *Brown.*
- I can say the first part of the deduction for Jenny's color. Listen: All the toads are brown.
- Who can say the whole deduction? (Call on individual students. Praise correct deductions: *All the toads are brown. Jenny is a toad. So Jenny is brown.*)

10. You have to color the picture of Rod the red bug, but his name tells you what color he'll be.
- Everybody, what color? (Signal.) *Red.*
- Remember to color Jenny and Rod. Then color anything else in the picture.

LESSON 26

Objectives

- **Compose 3 simple stories, each based on the same action topic.**

WORKBOOK

Sentence Writing

A

1.

2.

3.

1. Everybody, open your workbook to lesson 26 and find part A. ✔
   Today, you're going to write sentences that make up a story. Then you're going to draw pictures for two of your favorite sentences.

- Touch number 1. ✔
  You're going to write your first story there.

- (Write on the board:)

> **The bees chased us.**

- This says: The bees chased us.

2. Copy that sentence on the top line of number 1. Remember the capital and the period. Raise your hand when you've copied the sentence.
   (Observe students and give feedback.)

3. What would you do if bees chased you?
   (Call on individual students.)

- All the characters you're going to write about hid when the bees chased them.

- Clarabelle is the first character you'll write about. On the next line, you'll tell where Clarabelle hid. She hid in one of the places that you see in part B.

Find part B. ✔

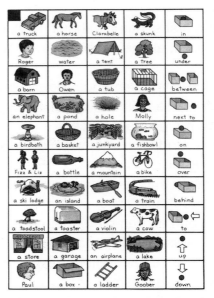

- Maybe she hid in a boat. Maybe she hid behind an elephant.

- You'll have to use one of the words from the last column of pictures. Touch the top box in the last column. ✔
  I'll read the words in the column. You follow along. In, under, between, next to, on, over, behind, to, up, down. When you use one of those words, make sure you spell it correctly.

- (Write to show:)

> **The bees chased us.**
> **Clarabelle hid ___.**

- Here's the first part of the sentence. Write the sentence for Clarabelle. Tell where she hid. Remember to start with a capital and end with a period. Raise your hand when you've finished.
  (Observe students and give feedback.)

4. (Call on individual students to read their sentence for Clarabelle. Praise acceptable sentences.)

5. (Write to show:)

> **The bees chased us.**
> **Clarabelle hid** _____.
>
> **Goober** _____.
> **I** _____.

- On the next line you'll write where **Goober** hid.
- On the bottom line you'll write where **you** hid. Remember, each sentence starts with a capital and ends with a period. Raise your hand when you're finished.
  (Observe students and give feedback.)
- (Call on individual students to read their sentence about Goober. Then call on individual students to read their sentence about themselves. Praise acceptable sentences.)
- Touch number 2. ✔
  The sentences you'll write for number 2 tell what different characters **made.**
- (Write on the board:)

> **Everybody made something.**

- This says: Everybody made something.
- Copy that sentence on the top line of number 2. Remember the capital and period. Raise your hand when you're finished.
  (Observe students and give feedback.)

6. (Write to show:)

> **Everybody made something.**
> **Molly made** _____.

- On the next line you'll tell what **Molly** made. She made one of the things that you see in part B. Maybe she made a violin. Maybe she made an airplane.
- Write your sentence for Molly. Raise your hand when you're finished.
  (Observe students and give feedback.)
- (Call on individual students to read their sentence for Molly.)

7. (Write to show:)

> **Everybody made something.**
> **Molly made** _____.
>
> **Bleep** _____.
> **I** _____.

- On the next line you'll write what **Bleep** made.

- On the bottom line you'll write what **you** made.
- Don't forget the capital and period for each sentence. Raise your hand when you've written a sentence for Bleep and a sentence for you.
  (Observe students and give feedback.)
- (Call on individual students to read their sentence about Bleep. Then call on individual students to read their sentence about themselves.)

8. Touch number 3. ✔
   The sentences you'll write for number 3 tell what different characters wrote.
- (Write on the board:)

> **Everybody wrote a letter.**

- This says: Everybody wrote a letter.
- Copy that sentence on the top line of number 3. Raise your hand when you're finished.
  (Observe students and give feedback.)

9. (Write to show:)

> **Everybody wrote a letter.**
> **Liz wrote to** _____.
> **Molly** _____.
> **I** _____.

- You'll write sentences that name the person each character wrote to. Remember to copy names just the way they are written.
- Write your sentences for number 3. Raise your hand when you're finished.
  (Observe students and give feedback.)
- (Call on individual students to read their sentence about Liz. Then call on individual students to read their sentence about Owen or about themselves.)

10. Look at the two picture boxes below your sentences. You can make pictures for two of your sentences. Pick your two favorite sentences and make pictures that show those sentences. Raise your hand when you're finished.
    (Observe students and give feedback.)

Materials: Each student will need a pair of scissors for exercise 3.

Objectives

- Draw arrows to show movement **to** and **from.** (Exercise 1)
- **Complete sentences of the form: Blank happened after blank.** (Exercise 2)
- Arrange objects in larger and smaller classes. (Exercise 3)
- Listen to a familiar story. (Exercise 4)
- **Cooperatively compose an episode involving familiar story grammar.** (Exercise 5)

WORKBOOK

EXERCISE 1   Map

To/From

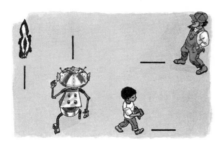

1. Everybody, open your workbook to lesson 27 and find part A. ✔
   This is a map. It doesn't have letters to show north, south, east and west. But you know the letter that is always on top. What letter? (Signal.) *N.*

- Yes, north is always on top of the map, no matter which way you turn when you hold that map. If you move to the top, you move north. If you move to the bottom, you move in which direction? (Signal.) *South.*

- You're going to complete arrows to show the direction different characters are walking. Then you'll write two letters on the arrow for each character. You'll show the direction the character is moving **to** and the direction the character is moving **from.**

2. Everybody, touch Goober. ✔
   Make a point on the arrow to show which direction Goober is walking. Raise your hand when you're finished. ✔

- (Draw on the board:)

  ⟵

- Here's the arrow you should have for Goober.
  Now write the letters on that arrow. Remember, the direction Goober is walking **to** goes on the **point** of the arrow. Raise your hand when you're finished. ✔

- (Add letters to show:)

  W ⟵——→ **E**

- Here's what you should have for Goober. Everybody, which direction is Goober walking **to?** (Signal.) *West.*

- Which direction is Goober walking **from?** (Signal.) *East.*

3. Your turn: Fix up the rest of the arrows. Put a point on the arrow to show the direction each character is moving. Then put two letters on each arrow. Raise your hand when you're finished.

(Observe students and give feedback.)

4. Check your work. Everybody, touch Bleep. ✔
- Which direction is Bleep moving to? (Signal.) *North.*
- Which direction is Bleep moving from? (Signal.) *South.*
- (Draw on the board:)

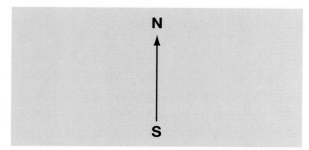

- Here's the arrow you should have for Bleep. Raise your hand if you got it right.
5. Everybody, touch Roger. ✔
- Which direction is Roger moving to? (Signal.) *East.*
- Which direction is Roger moving from? (Signal.) *West.*
- (Draw on the board:)

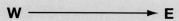

- Here's the arrow you should have for Roger. Raise your hand if you got it right.
6. Everybody, touch the skunk. ✔
- Which direction is the skunk moving to? (Signal.) *South.*
- Which direction is the skunk moving from? (Signal.) *North.*
- (Draw on the board:)

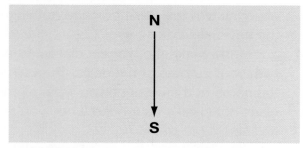

- Here's the arrow you should have for the skunk.
  Raise your hand if you got it right.
7. Raise your hand if you got everything right. Super.
- This is hard, but you're getting smart.

EXERCISE 2 Temporal Sequencing

After

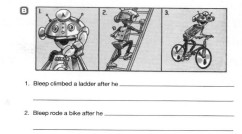

1. Bleep climbed a ladder after he _____

2. Bleep rode a bike after he _____

1. Find part B. ✔
   These pictures show what Bleep did first, next and last.
- Touch the first picture.
  Everybody, what did Bleep do first? (Signal.) *Talked on the phone.*
- Touch picture 2.
  That picture shows what Bleep did **after** he talked on the phone.
- What did he do after he talked on the phone? (Signal.) *Climbed a ladder.*
- Yes, Bleep climbed a ladder **after** he talked on the phone.
- Touch picture 3.
  That picture shows what Bleep did after he climbed a ladder.
- What did he do after he climbed a ladder? (Signal.) *Rode a bike.*
- Yes, Bleep rode a bike after he climbed a ladder.
2. Touch the picture of Bleep riding a bike.
   Listen: Bleep rode a bike after he did something else. He rode a bike after he did what? (Signal.) *Climbed a ladder.*
3. I'll start with **Bleep rode a bike** and tell when he did that. Listen: Bleep rode a bike after he climbed a ladder.
- Your turn: Start with **Bleep rode a bike** and tell when. Get ready. Go. (Signal.) *Bleep rode a bike after he climbed a ladder.*
- (Repeat step 3 until firm.)
4. Touch the picture of Bleep climbing a ladder.
   Listen: Bleep climbed a ladder after he did something else. Bleep climbed a ladder after he did what? (Signal.) *Talked on the phone.*

5. I'll start with **Bleep climbed a ladder** and tell when he did that. Listen: Bleep climbed a ladder after he talked on the phone.

- Your turn: Start with **Bleep climbed a ladder** and tell when. Get ready. Go. (Signal.) *Bleep climbed a ladder after he talked on the phone.*

- (Repeat step 5 until firm.)

6. (Write on the board:)

> **talked on the phone**
> **climbed a ladder**
> **rode a bike**

- You're going to complete sentences. You'll have to pick the right part. I'll read each part: (Point to each part and read it.)

7. Touch sentence 1 below the pictures. It says: Bleep climbed a ladder after he . . . He climbed a ladder after he did something else. Write that something else. Raise your hand when you're finished.
(Observe students and give feedback.)

8. Here's what you should have for sentence 1: Bleep climbed a ladder after he talked on the phone. Raise your hand if you got it right.

9. Touch sentence 2.
It says: Bleep rode a bike after he . . . He rode a bike just after he did something else. Write that something else. Raise your hand when you're finished.
(Observe students and give feedback.)

10. Here's what you should have for sentence 2: Bleep rode a bike after he climbed a ladder. Raise your hand if you got sentence 2 right.

- Raise both your hands if you got both sentences right.

- Those are very tricky sentences.

EXERCISE 3 Classification

Subclass: Dogs

Class	Not-Class

1. _____
2. _____
3. _____

1. (Write on the board:)

> **work dogs   hounds**

- These are names you'll use in the next game. (Touch words and read them.)

2. Everybody, turn to the last page of your workbook and find the column of dogs for lesson 27. Raise your hand when you've found it. ✔

- Cut out the pictures of the dogs, and we'll play a new class game. Raise your hand when you're finished. ✔

3. Everybody, turn to lesson 27 and find part C. ✔

- Here's a rule about classes: The **bigger** the class, the **more** things there are in the class box and the **fewer** things there are in the not-class box.

- If you made the **biggest** class, you'd have everything in the class box and nothing in the not-class box.

4. Your turn: Make the biggest class you can with your cutouts of the dogs. Then write the name of the class on line 1 below the class box. Raise your hand when you're finished.
(Observe students and give feedback.)

5. Everybody, what's the name of the things in your class box? (Signal.) *Dogs.*

- And what's in your not-class box? (Signal.) *Nothing.*

6. You're going to move things from the class box to the not-class box, so you have a choice about making a smaller class.
- Listen: Remove **five** things from the class box and put them in the not-class box. Make sure you have a class you can name in the class box. Then write the name of your new class on line 2. Raise your hand when you're finished.
  (Observe students and give feedback.)
7. I'll bet we have different classes in the class box. Raise your hand if you have **hounds** in your class box.
- Raise your hand if you have **work dogs** in your class box.
8. Listen: Leave one dog in your class box and move all the rest of them to your not-class box. Then write the name of the dog that is in your class box on line 3. Raise your hand when you're finished.
  (Observe students and give feedback.)
9. I'll bet we have different classes in the class box. (Call on several students:) What's your new class? (Accept the names of individual dogs.)
10. You made three classes. One of those classes was the biggest. Make a box around the name of the class that was the biggest. Raise your hand when you're finished. ✔
- Everybody, which class was the biggest? (Signal.) *Dogs.*
- How do you know that the class of dogs was bigger than the other classes? (Call on a student. Idea: *The class of dogs had more things in the class box.*)
- Right, the class of dogs was the biggest because it had more things in the class box.
11. One of the classes you wrote was the smallest. Listen: Draw a line under the name of the class that was the smallest. Raise your hand when you're finished. ✔
- (Call on several students:) What did you underline? (Accept names of individual dogs.)
12. If you underlined the name of the dog for class 3, you marked the class that's the smallest.
- Who got everything right?
  Super.

EXERCISE 4 Owen and the Little People *Part 6*

Review

- I'm going to read the last part of the story about Owen and the little people again.

Owen and his family had discovered the half-built community center. As they looked at it and tried to figure out why somebody would make such tiny buildings, two incredibly small people popped out of the weeds near the recreation building. They were waving their tiny little arms, and they were making funny squeaky sounds.

Those two small people were Fizz and Liz. They had figured out that one of the giants was Owen. They figured that out by looking at the boat after the giants had left the beach. Owen had carved his name on the side of the boat. When Fizz and Liz read the name, they knew why Owen said that there were tiny birds and tiny animals on his island.

They decided to run after the giants and try to get their attention. So, when they got to the community center and saw the three giants crouching down, they ran out into the open area, waving their arms and yelling, "Owen, it's us! Fizz and Liz!"

Owen's dad looked at the little people and said, "Do you see what I see?"

His mother said, "Yes, and it's amazing. I've read about tiny people, but I never thought I'd see any."

Owen said, "They're trying to tell us something, but I can't hear them." So Owen bent down and put his ear right above Fizz and Liz. Then he heard them say, in squeaky little voices, "Owen, it's Fizz and Liz."

Owen laughed. When he did that, he blew out air and knocked Fizz and Liz back into the weeds. "Oh, I'm sorry," he said. Then he said to his parents, "These little people are Fizz and Liz."

"Oh," his mother and father said. Then they said to Fizz and Liz, "Pleased to meet you."

Fizz and Liz were picking themselves up and brushing themselves off.

Well, everything made sense now. Owen could understand why Fizz and Liz talked about bugs that were as big as they were. He could understand why they talked about bears with claws twice as big as they were and sparrows twice as tall as they were.

And Fizz and Liz could understand why Owen talked about bears and birds being so small. Everything made sense, and there was a lot to talk about.

So Owen and his family lay face down on the ground in a place where they wouldn't scrunch any little people or flatten any neighborhoods. Then the little people gathered close to the giants' ears and they talked. Of course, Owen and his family had to talk very softly or they would blast those little people out of their britches. And the little people had to yell as loud as they could, or the giants wouldn't be able to hear them.

After they talked a long time, Owen and his family decided that, while they were on the island, they could help the little people with their recreation building and some other projects.

So Owen and his family gathered sticks and built a super recreation building. Then they dug out a little ditch that led from the stream below the waterfall to the recreation center. The water filled the ditch, and the little people had a great, wonderful river that went to the park near the community center. Then the giants built some more houses, just for fun.

After all the construction was completed, Owen and his dad caught enough fish to last the little people years. Owen and his dad built a warehouse to store the fish in. Then they collected berries, pineapples and other good things to put in the warehouse.

Owen and his family spent two days on the island. At last, it was time for them to go back home. So they took the green bottle out to the beach, waited until the currents were moving away from shore, got into their boat and said good-bye to the little people, who were on the beach, waving and shouting, with tears in their eyes.

All the little people stood there and watched the boat and the bottle move out to sea. They listened as the giants called from their boat, "So long. Good-bye. See you later." And when the boat was far, far away from shore, they heard Owen say, "We'll write you when we get back. Maybe you can come and visit us sometime."

And then the boat got smaller and smaller and smaller, until it disappeared.

- That's the end of the story.

EXERCISE 5   Story Construction

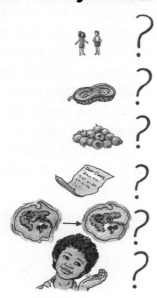

Note: Divide the class into teams of 3–4 students.

1. Everybody, find part D. ✔
   You're going to work in teams and make up a story that tells what happened when Fizz and Liz went to visit Owen. There are pictures of things with question marks after them.
   - (Write on the board:)

?

   - Here's a question mark.
2. Everybody, touch the top picture. ✔
   It shows Fizz and Liz. Then there's a question mark. That means you have to tell something about **who** went to Owen's island. Did just Fizz and Liz go or did **some** of the other little people go with them? Or did **all** of the little people go? That's the first thing you'll tell in your story.
   - Touch the next picture. ✔
   That's a racing boat. The question mark asks about the racing boat: Did they go to Owen's island in their racing boat? Or did they go in the green bottle? Or did they make some other kind of boat? Or did they go in the bottle and pull some of the racing boats behind? You have to tell **how** they decided to go to Owen's island.
   - Touch the picture of the berries. ✔
   The berries might be something they would eat. But you'll have to tell what they brought with them to eat. Remember, they'll be out on the waves for **six** days.

- Is that right? (Signal.) *No.*
- How long will they be on the ocean? (Signal.) *Three days.*
- They'll need supplies for their journey. We don't want them to die of thirst out there in the ocean. Remember, they can't drink ocean water—it's too salty and would make them sick. So you have to tell **what** they took with them.
- Touch the next picture. ✔
  It shows a note. The question mark asks, **how** did they let Owen know they were coming? Or maybe they just dropped in on Owen, without letting him know they were coming. If they did that, they might just get stepped on by one of those giants. So your story will have to tell something about **how** they let Owen know they were coming to his island.
- Touch the next picture. ✔
  That picture shows the direction they would go from their island to Owen's island. The question mark means, **what happened** on their trip? You should tell about what they did during the three days they were on the water. You could even mention the direction they were going to.
- Everybody, what direction were they going to? (Signal.) *East.*
- Touch the last picture. ✔
  That picture shows Owen holding a couple of little people. The question mark means, **what happened** when they finally got to Owen's island? You should probably tell at least some of the things they did.
3. Everybody, we're going to work in teams. Here's how you'll work in teams: For each picture, team members will give suggestions to their team.
- First you'll decide **who** went to Owen's island. But, don't argue. If you don't agree, go to the next picture and see if you can work out something for that picture. Later in the story, you may have some ideas that will help you to figure out what you want for the earlier picture.
- After you figure out **what** your story will tell for each picture, you'll have a good story.

4. All teams, start with picture 1. Figure out who went to Owen's island.
   - (Observe each team. Ask:) Have you figured out **who** went on the trip?
   - Then go on to the next picture and figure out **how** they went on their trip. (Praise teams who are discussing possibilities and working cooperatively.)
   - Raise your hand if your team figured out answers to all the questions.
   - (Repeat step 4 for each picture.)

5. In the next lesson, you'll figure out how your team is going to tell their story to the whole class. Maybe one team member will tell the first part, another team member will tell the next part, and so on. Maybe one person will tell the whole story. Next time, you'll figure out how you're going to do it. Then we'll have each team tell their story about the trip to Owen's island.

6. You can draw things on this page to help you remember your story.

Objectives

• Complete sentences of the form: Blank happened **after** blank. (Exercise 1)
• Construct deductions to answer questions. (Exercise 2)
• **Present a cooperatively developed episode based on familiar story grammar.** (Exercise 3)

WORKBOOK

EXERCISE 1 **Temporal Sequencing**

After

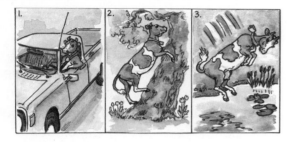

1. Clarabelle jumped into a pond after she _____

_____.

2. Clarabelle climbed a tree after she _____

_____.

1. Everybody, open your workbook to lesson 28 and find part A. ✔
   These pictures show what Clarabelle did first, next and last.
   • Touch the first picture.
     Everybody, what did Clarabelle do first? (Signal.) *Drove a truck.*
   • Touch picture 2.
     That picture shows what Clarabelle did after she drove a truck.
   • What did she do after she drove a truck? (Signal.) *Climbed a tree.*
   • Yes, Clarabelle climbed a tree after she drove a truck.
   • Touch picture 3.
     That picture shows what Clarabelle did after she climbed a tree.
   • What did she do after she climbed a tree? (Signal.) *Jumped into a pond.*
   • Yes, Clarabelle jumped into a pond after she climbed a tree.
2. Touch the picture of Clarabelle climbing a tree. Listen: Clarabelle climbed a tree after she did something else. Clarabelle climbed a tree after she did what? (Signal.) *Drove a truck.*
3. Start with **Clarabelle climbed a tree** and say the whole sentence. (Signal.) *Clarabelle climbed a tree after she drove a truck.*

4. Touch the picture of Clarabelle jumping into a pond. Listen: Clarabelle jumped into a pond after she did something else. Clarabelle jumped into a pond after she did what? (Signal.) *Climbed a tree.*
5. Start with **Clarabelle jumped into a pond** and say the whole sentence. (Signal.) *Clarabelle jumped into a pond after she climbed a tree.*
6. (Write on the board:)

> **drove a truck**
> **climbed a tree**
> **jumped into a pond**

   • You're going to complete sentences. You'll have to pick the right part. I'll read each part: (Point to each part and read it.)
7. Touch sentence 1 below the pictures. It says: Clarabelle jumped in a pond after she . . . She jumped into a pond after she did something else. Write that something else. Raise your hand when you're finished. (Observe students and give feedback.)
8. Here's what you should have for sentence 1: Clarabelle jumped into a pond after she climbed a tree. Raise your hand if you got it right.
9. Touch sentence 2.
   It says: Clarabelle climbed a tree after she . . . She climbed a tree just after she did something else. Write that something else. Raise your hand when you're finished. (Observe students and give feedback.)
10. Here's what you should have for sentence 2: Clarabelle climbed a tree after she drove a truck. Raise your hand if you got sentence 2 right.
   • Raise both your hands if you got both sentences right.
   • Those are very tricky sentences.

EXERCISE 2 Deduction Writing

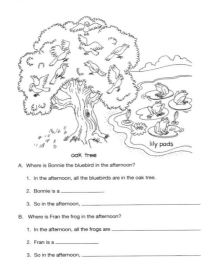

oak tree

lily pads

A. Where is Bonnie the bluebird in the afternoon?

  1. In the afternoon, all the bluebirds are in the oak tree.

  2. Bonnie is a _____.

  3. So in the afternoon, _____

B. Where is Fran the frog in the afternoon?

  1. In the afternoon, all the frogs are _____

  2. Fran is a _____

  3. So in the afternoon, _____

1. Find part B. ✔
   You're going to make deductions to figure out where two different animals are in the afternoon.
   - Your picture shows where all the bluebirds are in the afternoon. You can see they are in the oak tree. Here's a fact: Bonnie is a bluebird.

2. Listen to this question: Where is Bonnie the bluebird in the afternoon?
   - Here's the whole deduction. Listen: In the afternoon, all the bluebirds are in the oak tree. Bonnie is a bluebird. So in the afternoon, Bonnie is in the oak tree.

3. Everybody, help me out this time. When I stop, **you** finish the part.

4. In the afternoon, all the bluebirds are . . . (Signal.) *in the oak tree.*
   - Bonnie is a . . . (Signal.) *bluebird.*
   - So in the afternoon . . . (Signal.) *Bonnie is in the oak tree.*
   - (Repeat step 4 until firm.)

5. The picture also shows where all the frogs are in the afternoon. You can see that all the frogs are sitting on lily pads. Here's another fact: Fran is a frog.

6. Listen to this question: Where is Fran the frog in the afternoon?
   - Here's the whole deduction. Listen: In the afternoon, all the frogs are on lily pads. Fran is a frog. So in the afternoon, Fran is on a lily pad.

7. Everybody, help me out. When I stop, you finish that part.

8. In the afternoon, all the frogs are . . . (Signal.) *on lily pads.*
   - Fran is a . . . (Signal.) *frog.*
   - So in the afternoon . . . (Signal.) *Fran is on a lily pad.*
   - (Repeat step 8 until firm.)

9. Your turn to complete the deductions.
   - Touch the first deduction under the picture. I'll read what it says: In the afternoon, all the bluebirds are in the oak tree. Bonnie is a blank. So in the afternoon, blank.
   - Fill in the blanks so you have a complete deduction. Raise your hand when you're finished.
   (Observe students and give feedback.)

10. I'll read each part that was written. When I stop, tell me the part you wrote. In the afternoon, all the bluebirds are in the oak tree. Bonnie is a . . . (Signal.) *bluebird.*
    - So in the afternoon . . . (Signal.) *Bonnie is in the oak tree.*
    - Raise your hand if you got it right.

11. Later you can fix up the deduction that tells about Fran the frog. That's tough. And you can color the picture.

EXERCISE 3 Story Construction

Owen—Group Presentation

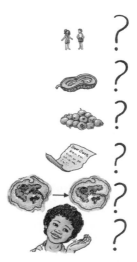

> ***Note:*** Divide the class into their story-construction teams.

1. Everybody, find part D in lesson 27. ✔
   Remember, these pictures ask questions about important parts of your story.

- Today, we're going to hear stories from the different groups. Before we do that, the groups have to figure out how they'll tell their story.

2. Get together with the same group as last time and figure out how you'll do it. Then you should practice your story in your group before you present it to the class. You should make sure your story answers all the questions.

- If different students are telling different parts, practice telling the story. The other members of the group should listen carefully and make sure that each storyteller is telling it the right way.

- Talk quietly so that the other groups can't hear your story.
(Observe groups and give feedback. Praise groups who practice and comment on the storyteller's rendition.)

3. Raise your hand when your group is ready. The first group ready gets to tell their story first.

4. (Call on a group. Say:) Everybody, listen to the story from group _____.
(Praise stories that tell about the details suggested by the pictures.)

> *Note:* If not all the groups are able to present, tell the class that the storytelling will be continued in the next lesson.

Materials: Each student will need a brown and a blue crayon.

Objectives

- Construct deductions to answer questions. (Exercise 1)
- **Compose directions to show solutions to a map puzzle.** (Exercise 2)
- Listen to part 1 of a continued story and answer comprehension questions. (Exercise 3)
- **Draw routes that reflect story events.** (Exercise 4)

WORKBOOK

EXERCISE 1 **Deduction Writing**

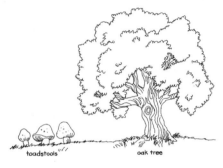

toadstools   oak tree

A. Where is Tammy the toad in the morning?

　1. In the morning, all the toads are _____

　2. Tammy is a _____

　3. So in the morning, Tammy is _____

B. Where is Bonnie the bluebird in the morning?

　1. In the morning, all the bluebirds are _____

　2. Bonnie is a _____.

　3. So in the morning, Bonnie is _____

1. Everybody, take out a blue and a brown crayon. Raise your hand when you're finished. ✔
- Everybody, open your workbook to lesson 29 and find part A. ✔
  This picture shows the **morning,** not the afternoon. And not everything is shown in the picture.
2. Here's the rule about the toads: In the morning, all the **toads** are under the oak tree.
- Draw some brown toads under the oak tree. Do it fast. Raise your hand when you're finished.
  (Observe students and give feedback.)
3. Here's the rule about the bluebirds: In the morning, all the **bluebirds** are on toadstools.
- Fix up your toadstools so they have bluebirds on them. Raise your hand when you're finished.
  (Observe students and give feedback.)

4. You're going to complete deductions about one of the toads and one of the bluebirds. The toad's name is Tammy. Remember, Tammy is a toad.
- Here's the first part of the deduction: In the morning, all the toads are under the oak tree.
- Say that rule. (Signal.) *In the morning, all the toads are under the oak tree.*
- Everybody, help me say the whole deduction. When I stop, you finish that part.
5. In the morning, all the toads are . . . (Signal.) *under the oak tree.*
- Tammy is . . . (Signal.) *a toad.*
- So in the morning . . . (Signal.) *Tammy is under the oak tree.*
- (Repeat step 5 until firm.)
6. The picture shows where bluebirds are in the morning. Where are they? (Signal.) *On toadstools.*
- Remember, Bonnie is a bluebird. Help me out with the whole deduction. When I stop, you finish that part.
7. In the morning, all the bluebirds are . . . (Signal.) *on toadstools.*
- Bonnie is . . . (Signal.) *a bluebird.*
- So in the morning . . . (Signal.) *Bonnie is on a toadstool.*
- (Repeat step 7 until firm.)
8. Your turn to complete the deductions.
- Touch the first deduction under the picture. I'll read what it says: In the morning, all the toads are blank. Tammy is a blank. So in the morning, Tammy is blank.
- Fill in the blanks so you have a complete deduction. Raise your hand when you're finished.
  (Observe students and give feedback.)

9. I'll read each part that was written. When I stop, tell me the part you wrote. In the morning, all the toads are . . . (Signal.) *under the oak tree.*
   - Tammy is a . . . (Signal.) *toad.*
   - So in the morning, Tammy is . . . (Signal.) *under the oak tree.*
   - Raise your hand if you got it right.
10. Later you can fix up the deduction that tells about Bonnie the bluebird. That's tough.

EXERCISE 2 Directions

Map Puzzle

1. Find part B. ✔
   This is a map. So remember the rule about which direction is at the top. Everybody, which direction? (Signal.) *North.*

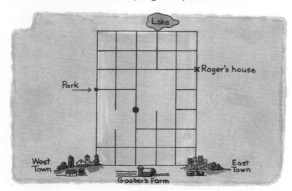

   - The bottom of the map shows West Town and East Town. You can see Goober's farm. It's right between those towns.
   - On the left side of the map is an arrow that points to the park. Touch that arrow. ✔
   - On top of the map is a lake. Touch the lake. ✔
   - On the right side of the map is Roger's house. You can't really see his house. It's marked with a little **X.**
   - Each square on this map is one mile. That's a long distance. That's why everything looks so small.
2. Touch the circle in the middle of the map. ✔
   I'll give you directions. When you follow these directions, stay on the streets. Those are the lines.
   - Here's the first direction: Take the street that goes 2 miles north. Remember, don't start counting until you start moving. Go 2 miles north and keep your finger on the corner you end up at.
   - Now go 3 miles east. 3 miles east.

- Everybody, where did you end up? (Signal.) *Roger's house.*
- Yes, you should have ended up at Roger's house.
3. Touch the circle again. ✔
   Listen: Go 1 mile north and 2 miles west. Listen again: 1 mile north and 2 miles west. Raise your hand when you know where you end up.
- Everybody, where did you end up? (Signal.) *The park.*
4. Touch the circle again. ✔
   Now it's your turn: I want to get to East Town. You have to tell me how to get there.
- Raise your hand when you can tell me the whole thing about how to get from the circle to East Town. I'll call on somebody. Everybody else follow the directions and see if they work.
- (Call on a student. After the student says a route, ask:) Everybody, if you follow those directions will you get to East Town? (Idea: *3 south, 3 east.*)
5. Find the directions under the map. You're going to complete each set of directions.
- Touch number 1.
   Those directions say: To go to Roger's house, you go **blank** miles **blank.** Then you go **blank** miles **blank.** You have to fill in the blanks. For each sentence, tell how many miles and the direction. In the first blank, tell the number of miles. In the next blank, tell the direction.
- Start at the circle and see what you do first to go to Roger's house. See how many miles you go and the direction you go. Then fill in the first 2 blanks in the first sentence. Raise your hand when you're finished.
   (Observe students and give feedback.)
- Here's what you should have written in the first sentence: To go to Roger's house, you go **2 miles north.**
- Complete the description by telling what you do next. Tell the number of miles and the direction. Raise your hand when you're finished.
   (Observe students and give feedback.)
- Here's what your whole description should say: To go to Roger's house, you go 2 miles north. Then you go 3 miles east. Raise your hand if you got everything right.

6. Touch number 2.
Those directions say: To go to West Town, you go blank miles blank. Then you go blank miles blank. Fill in the directions for going from the circle to West Town. Raise your hand when you're finished.
(Observe students and give feedback.)
- Here's what your description should say: To go to West Town, you go 3 miles south. Then you go 2 miles west. Listen again: 3 miles south. Then you go 2 miles west. Raise your hand if you got everything right.
7. You're learning lots about maps and directions.

> **Optional:** If time permits, direct students to write descriptions for going from the starting point to the lake and to the park.

EXERCISE 3 **Dot and Dud *Part 1***

Storytelling

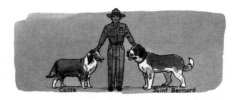

- I'm going to read a new story. This story is about work dogs. These work dogs are St. Bernards. You can see a picture of a St. Bernard in part C of your workbook. You can see how big that St. Bernard is next to the ranger and the collie. St. Bernards are **big.**
- Here's the story:

Once there were two St. Bernard dogs called Dot and Dud. Dot was Dud's sister. St. Bernards are great big work dogs. And Dot and Dud had a very important job. They lived in the mountains at the rescue station. During the winter, the mountains were deep with snow and very dangerous. Skiers and mountain climbers would sometimes get lost. That's when Dot and Dud were supposed to do their job. They were supposed to go into the

mountains with the other St. Bernards and find the stranded skier or mountain climber. That's what they were **supposed** to do, but there was one problem.

That problem was Dud. He was called "Dud" because that's what he was—a great big dud at doing his job. When he went out to find a mountain climber, everybody else would have to go out and find Dud. He'd get lost. Some other St. Bernard would find the mountain climber. That dog was usually Dot. She was the best rescue dog in all the mountains. But, after she found the stranded skier or mountain climber, she and the other St. Bernards would have to go on another rescue mission.

- Everybody, who would they have to rescue? (Signal.) *Dud.*

Dud was a dud because he didn't like to work. He didn't like to use his nose. Although his nose was nowhere near as good as a hunting dog's nose, it probably was as good at smelling things as the other St. Bernards' noses. But sniffing things and trying to figure out which way a trail led was a lot of hard work. You had to find the trail of the person who was stranded. Then you had to stick your nose in the snow, take a great sniff and make sure that you were still on the trail of the person you were trying to rescue. All that sniffing and figuring out gave Dud a headache. So he **pretended** to sniff and track, but his mind was not on his work. He was usually thinking of eating a great ham bone or sprawling out in front of a fireplace.

One time, the St. Bernards got **really** mad at Dud. They were back at the rescue station in their kennel. The oldest St. Bernard said to Dud, "Do you realize we spend more time rescuing you than we do rescuing stranded mountain climbers?"

"Yeah," another St. Bernard said. "You don't even stay with the rest of us when we go out on a rescue. You're always going off and fooling around in the snow."

"Yeah," another St. Bernard said. "Last time, I saw you go behind some rocks and run around chasing your tail while we were trying to do our job."

"Yeah," another St. Bernard said, "and then you got so dizzy from chasing your tail that you got completely lost, and we had to spend two hours trying to find you."

"Yeah," another St. Bernard said, "and when we found you, you were less than half a mile from the rescue station, and you didn't even know how to get back home."

"Yeah," all the St. Bernards said—all of them except one. That one was Dot.

Dot said, "Stop picking on my brother. He may not be the best tracker, but he can learn, and he'll work harder from now on. Won't you, Dud?"

"I will," Dud said. "I'll work harder."

"Yeah," one of the St. Bernards said. "We've heard that before. 'I'll work harder.' The last time you said that, we caught you rolling snowballs down the mountain with your nose."

"Yeah," the other St. Bernards agreed.

But this time, Dud was serious. "I'll try harder," he said.

But you know what the other St. Bernards said.

- Everybody, what did they say? (Signal.) *Yeah.*

Just then, the rescue alarm sounded. The ranger who was in charge of the St. Bernards came running out to the kennels where the dogs were. A mountain climber was stranded in the snow.

Now all the dogs knew that **mountain climbers** climbed mountains that were to the **north** of the rescue station. To the **south** of the rescue station was the ski lodge. So if a mountain climber was stranded, the dogs knew which way to go.

- Everybody, which way? (Signal.) *North.*

And if a **skier** got stranded, the dogs knew which way to go. That's the same direction as the ski lodge.

- Which direction? (Signal.) *South.*

The ranger let the St. Bernards out of the kennel, and they all headed in the right direction, including Dud.

- Who was stranded—a skier or a mountain climber? (Signal.) *Mountain climber.*
- So which direction did the dogs go? (Signal.) *North.*
- Listen to that part again:

The ranger let the St. Bernards out of the kennel, and they all headed in the right direction, including Dud.

When they started up the mountain, they searched for the trail of the stranded mountain climber. All the dogs were sticking their nose in the snow and trying to find the scent of that mountain climber. Even Dud put his nose in the snow—a couple of times. But that snow was mighty cold, and it really took a lot of effort to sniff and snort and try to smell something. So, after a while, Dud walked slower and slower. He got farther and farther behind the other dogs.

Then Dud came to a large flat part on the side of the mountain. And he saw something that was far more interesting than the snow. It was his shadow. He jumped up, and the shadow moved. Dud pounced on the shadow. He rolled over on the shadow. He ran around in circles—faster, faster, faster. Wow, was this fun or what?

For about ten minutes, Dud and his shadow tore around in the snow, making circles and zigzags, making leaps and even somersaults. But then, his shadow disappeared.

- Why would his shadow disappear? (Call on a student. Ideas: *It got cloudy; It got dark.*)

The sky was cloudy and it was starting to snow. Dud was pretty dizzy.

- Why was he dizzy? (Call on a student. Idea: *From running around in circles.*)
- Yes.

Dud couldn't see the other St. Bernards. Dud knew they were going up the mountain to the north, but, after all that running around in circles, he didn't know where **north** was. He looked around to see where the mountain was, but there were mountains all around him, and they all looked the same. And it was snowing harder now. Soon the snow was coming down so hard that Dud couldn't see any mountains. He couldn't see anything at all—just snow, snow, snow.

At last, he walked around in a large circle trying to find out which way was north. He couldn't tell, so he made a guess. And his guess was wrong, wrong, wrong. Instead of starting to go north, he went south. That silly dog was heading right back toward the rescue station, not to the mountain-climbing mountain.

- And that's the end of the first part of the story. Next time, we'll see what happened to Dud. What do you think will happen? (Call on a student. Accept appropriate responses.)
- If Dud happens to miss the rescue station and keeps heading south, where could he end up? (Call on a student. Idea: *The ski lodge.*)
- And if he misses the rescue station and the ski lodge, he may just keep going south through the mountains for a long time.

EXERCISE 4 Interpreting Routes

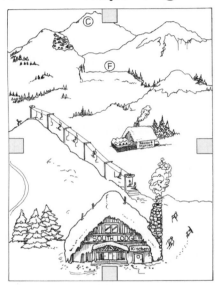

1. Everybody, find part D. ✔
   This picture shows a map that shows where the story took place. The map doesn't have letters for north, south, east and west. So put the letters in the boxes and raise your hand when you're finished. ✔
- Touch the letter you wrote at the top of the map. Everybody, what letter? (Signal.) *N.*
- Touch the letter at the bottom of the map. Everybody, what letter? (Signal.) *S.*
2. Touch the rescue station. ✔
   You can see those little dog houses on the west side of the rescue station. That's the kennel where the dogs stay. And that's where the dogs started out to find the stranded mountain climber.
- Everybody, which direction did they go to find the mountain climber? (Signal.) *North.*
- Which direction would they have gone to find a stranded skier? (Signal.) *South.*

3. The dogs left the rescue station and headed north. Everybody, put your finger on the kennel by the rescue station. Now go north until you come to the first letter.
- Everybody, what letter did you stop at? (Signal.) *F.*
  The letter F shows the flat place where Dud got all confused.
- What did Dud do at the flat place to get all confused? (Call on a student. Idea: *Chased his shadow, ran in circles and zigzags.*)
- When Dud was on the flat place, where were the other dogs? (Call on a student. Idea: *Going up the mountain to find the mountain climber.*)

4. The map shows a letter C way up on that mountain.
- Touch C. ✔
  That's where the stranded mountain climber is. The other dogs haven't reached the mountain climber. They were somewhere between the flat place and the mountain climber. Make a dot at a place where you think the other dogs were when Dud was zigzagging and somersaulting around.

5. Listen: You're going to draw two different routes from the rescue station. The first route will show where Dot and the other St. Bernards went.
- Your turn: Start at the kennel gate and draw a blue line from the kennel to where Dot and the other St. Bernards went. Remember, they didn't reach the climber. But they went farther north than Dud did.

Use your blue crayon and make a line that shows the route for Dot and the other St. Bernards. Your route should go over that flat part on the mountain, and it should go to the mark you made above the flat part. Raise your hand when you're finished. (Observe students and give feedback.)
- Look at your route. Raise your hand if you made your line go through the flat part. ✔

6. Now you're going to make a route for Dud. You'll use your **brown** crayon to show where he went. Listen: That route starts out just like the other dogs', but when it hits that flat part it goes around and around and zigs and zags all over that flat part. Draw that much of the route and then stop. Raise your hand when you're finished. (Observe students and give feedback.)
- After Dud got dizzy on the flat part, which direction did he go? (Signal.) *South.*
- You'll draw a route going south again. Don't trace the same route you made going up the mountain. Make a different route going south from the flat part. And don't draw it too far south. We don't know whether Dud will end up at the rescue station or whether he'll go past the rescue station and just keep on heading south. Draw the route south from the flat part. Raise your hand when you're finished. (Observe students and give feedback.)
- We'll have to wait until next time to see where Dud goes next.

7. Later you can color the picture.

LESSON 30—Test 3

Materials: Each student will need a green, brown and a blue crayon.

Objectives

- Compose and write a parallel sentence pair based on a single picture. (Exercise 1)
- Perform on mastery test of skills presented in lessons 21–29. (Exercise 2)
- Students vote on a story to be reread. (Exercise 3)
- Exercises 4–5 provide instructions for marking the test and giving the students feedback.

WORKBOOK • LINED PAPER

EXERCISE 1   Test

Writing Parallel Sentences

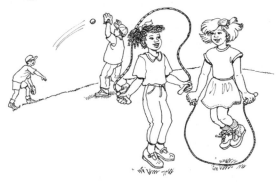

1. You're going to have a test to see how smart you are. You can't talk to anybody during the test or look at what anybody else does.
- Open your workbook to lesson 30, and find part A. ✔
  You're going to write about this picture.
2. The picture shows what boys and girls did.
- What did the boys do? (Call on a student. Idea: *Played catch.*)
- What did the girls do? (Call on a student. Idea: *Skipped rope.*)
3. Listen: The boys played catch. The girls skipped rope.
- Everybody, say the whole sentence about the boys. (Signal.) *The boys played catch.*
- Say the whole sentence about the girls. (Signal.) *The girls skipped rope.*
- (Repeat sentences until firm.)
4. Look at the vocabulary box. These are some of the words you need: skipped . . . catch . . . played . . . rope.
5. Say the sentence about the boys. (Signal.) *The boys played catch.*

- Say the sentence about the girls. (Signal.) *The girls skipped rope.*
6. Write both sentences.
   (Observe students and give feedback.)
7. **(Optional:)** Skip a line on your paper and write both sentences again.
   (Observe students and give feedback.)
8. (Collect and correct papers.)

EXERCISE 2   Test

Map—Movement To/From

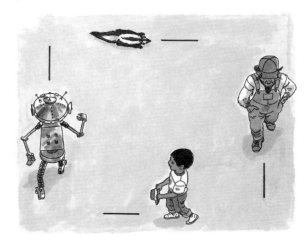

1. Find part B. ✔
2. You're going to complete the arrows. Put a point on each arrow to show the direction the person is moving to. Then write two letters for the arrow.
- Remember, the letter on the tip shows the direction the person is moving **to.** The letter on the back of the arrow shows the direction the person is moving **from.**
- Raise your hand when you've completed all the arrows.
   (Observe students but do not give feedback.)

Deduction Writing

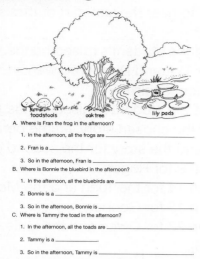

A. Where is Fran the frog in the afternoon?

   1. In the afternoon, all the frogs are _____

   2. Fran is a _____

   3. So in the afternoon, Fran is _____

B. Where is Bonnie the bluebird in the afternoon?

   1. In the afternoon, all the bluebirds are _____

   2. Bonnie is a _____

   3. So in the afternoon, Bonnie is _____

C. Where is Tammy the toad in the afternoon?

   1. In the afternoon, all the toads are _____

   2. Tammy is a _____

   3. So in the afternoon, Tammy is _____

1. Everybody, get out a green, a brown and a blue crayon. Raise your hand when you're finished.

- Find part C. ✔
  This picture shows the afternoon, but not everything is shown in the picture.

2. The pond has lily pads on it.

- Touch the lily pads. ✔
- Here's the rule: In the afternoon, all the frogs are on lily pads.
- Use your green crayon and draw some frogs on the lily pads. Do it fast. Raise your hand when you're finished.
  (Observe students.)
- Touch the oak tree. ✔
  Here's the rule: In the afternoon, all the bluebirds are in the oak tree.
- Fix up the oak tree so it has some bluebirds in it. Raise your hand when you're finished.
  (Observe students.)
- Touch the toadstools. ✔
- Here's the rule about the toadstools: In the afternoon, all the toads are on toadstools.
- Use your brown crayon and fix up your toadstools so they have toads on them. Raise your hand when you're finished.
  (Observe students.)

3. There are questions below the picture.

- Touch the first question. That's question A. ✔
  I'll read it: Where is Fran the frog in the afternoon?

- Everybody, what does that question say? (Signal.) *Where is Fran the frog in the afternoon?*
- You're going to tell about Fran by completing the deduction below Fran's question.
- Touch the deduction below the first question. ✔
  The deduction says: In the afternoon, all the frogs are blank. Fran is a blank. So in the afternoon, Fran is blank.
- Sentence 1 says: In the afternoon, all the frogs are blank.
- Complete sentence 1. Raise your hand when you're finished.
  (Observe students.)
- Touch sentence 2. ✔
  It says: Fran is a blank.
- Complete sentence 2. Raise your hand when you're finished. ✔
- Now you can complete sentence 3. It says: So in the afternoon, Fran is blank.
- Tell where Fran is in the afternoon. Raise your hand when you're finished.
  (Observe students.)

4. Everybody, touch question B. ✔
   I'll read it: Where is Bonnie the bluebird in the afternoon?

- Everybody, what does that question say? (Signal.) *Where is Bonnie the bluebird in the afternoon?*
- You're going to tell about Bonnie by completing the deduction below Bonnie's question.
- The deduction says: In the afternoon, all the bluebirds are blank. Bonnie is a blank. So in the afternoon, Bonnie is blank.
- Sentence 1 says: In the afternoon, all the bluebirds are blank.
- Complete sentence 1. Raise your hand when you're finished.
  (Observe students.)
- Touch sentence 2. ✔
  It says: Bonnie is a blank.
- Complete sentence 2. Raise your hand when you're finished. ✔
- Now you can complete sentence 3. It says: So in the afternoon, Bonnie is blank.
- Complete that sentence.

5. Touch question C. ✔
- I'll read it: Where is Tammy the toad in the afternoon?
- Everybody, what does that question say? (Signal.) *Where is Tammy the toad in the afternoon?*
- You're going to tell about Tammy by completing the deduction below Tammy's question.
- The deduction says: In the afternoon, all the toads are blank. Tammy is a blank. So in the afternoon, Tammy is blank.
- Complete sentence 1. Raise your hand when you're finished.
  (Observe students.)
- Touch sentence 2. ✔
  It says: Tammy is a blank.
- Complete sentence 2. Raise your hand when you're finished.
  (Observe students.)
- Now you can complete sentence 3. It says: So in the afternoon, Tammy is blank.
- Complete sentence 3. Raise your hand when you're finished.
  (Observe students.)
6. (Collect the student's workbooks after they have finished the test.)

EXERCISE 3 Story

1. For the rest of the period, I'll read a story. You get to choose one of these stories: Roger, The Toad and the Mouse, Goober, the last part of Owen and the Little People, or Dot and Dud.
- Everybody gets to vote on their favorite story. But you can only vote one time. I'll name the stories. You hold up your hand if you want that story. But remember, you can only hold up your hand one time.
- Listen: Roger. Who wants to hear the story about Roger and the Headstand again?
  (Count the student's raised hands.)
- Listen: The Toad and the Mouse. Who wants to hear that story again?
  (Count the student's raised hands.)
- Listen: Goober. Who wants to hear the story about Goober again?
  (Count the student's raised hands.)

- Listen: Owen and the Little People. Who wants to hear the last part of that story again?
  (Count the student's raised hands.)
- Listen: Dot and Dud. Who wants to hear that story again?
  (Count the student's raised hands.)
2. (Read the chosen story. If time permits, also read the story for the second choice.)

Key: Lesson 9 for Roger;
Lesson 14 for the Toad and the Mouse;
Lesson 15 for Goober;
Lesson 23 for Owen and the Little People (part 6);
Lesson 29 for Dot and Dud (part 1).

EXERCISE 4 Marking the Test

1. (Mark the test before the next scheduled language lesson. Use the *Language Arts Answer Key* to check the test.)
2. (Write the number of errors each student made in the test scorebox at the beginning of the test.)
3. (Enter the number of errors each student made on the Summary Sheet for Test 3. A Reproducible Summary Sheet is at the back of the *Language Arts Teacher's Guide*.)

EXERCISE 5 Feedback on Test 3

1. (Return the student's workbooks after they are marked.)
- Everybody, open your workbook to lesson 30. Look at how I marked your test page.
2. I wrote a number at the top of your test. That number tells how many items you got wrong on the whole test.
- Raise your hand if I wrote **0** or **1** at the top of your test. **Those are super stars.**
- Raise your hand if I wrote **2** or **3.** Those are pretty good workers.
- If I wrote a number that's more than 3, you're going to have to work harder.

EXERCISE 6 Test Remedies

- (See the *Language Arts Teacher's Guide* for a general discussion of remedies.)

Objective

- Compose 3 simple stories, each based on the same action topic.

WORKBOOK • LINED PAPER

Exercise 1 Sentence Writing

Note: For this activity students will need lined paper. Pass out paper. Direct students to write their name on the top line.

Story words

1. (Write on the board:)

Story words

- This says **Story words.**
- Find page 272 titled **Story words** at the back of your workbook.
  (Observe students and give feedback.)
- Today you're going to write sentences that make up little stories. Then you're going to draw a picture for your favorite sentence. You're going to write your sentences on lined paper.

2. (Write on the board:)

Everybody ate and ate.

- This says: Everybody ate and ate.
- Copy that sentence on the second line of your paper. Remember the capital and the period. Raise your hand when you've copied the sentence.
  (Observe students and give feedback.)

3. (Write to show:)

Everybody found something.
Dud Ate _____.

- Here's the first part of the sentence you'll write next. Dud ate blank.
- Copy the first part of the sentence and complete it. He ate one of the things shown on the page with **Story words.**
- Write your sentence about Dud. Raise your hand when you're finished.
  (Observe students and give feedback.)
- (Call on individual students to read their sentence for Dud.)

4. (Write to show:)

Everybody ate and ate.
Dud ate _____.
Molly _____.
I _____.

- You're going to write two more sentences. One will tell about Molly and what she ate. The other will tell about you and what you ate.
- Your turn: Write both sentences. Remember the period at the end of each sentence. Raise your hand when you're finished.
  (Observe students and give feedback.)
- (Call on individual students to read their sentence about Molly. Then call on individual students to read their sentence about themselves.)
- That's a lot of eating.

5. (Write on the board:)

Everybody looked for something.

- This says: Everybody looked for something.
- Copy that sentence on your paper. Remember the capital and the period. Raise your hand when you've copied the sentence.
  (Observe students and give feedback.)

6. (Write to show:)

> **Everybody looked for something.**
> **Dot looked for** _____.

- Here's the first part of the sentence you'll write next. Dot looked for blank. You're going to complete the sentence for Dot. She looked for one of the things shown on the page with **Story words.**
- Write your sentence about Dot. Raise your hand when you're finished.
  (Observe students and give feedback.)
- (Call on individual students to read their sentence for Dot.)

7. (Write to show:)

> **Everybody looked for something.**
> **Dot looked for** _____.
> **Fizz and Liz** _____.
> **I** _____.

- You're going to write two more sentences. One will tell about Fizz and Liz and what they looked for. The other will tell about you and what you looked for.
- Your turn: Write both sentences. Remember the period at the end of each sentence. Raise your hand when you're finished.
  (Observe students and give feedback.)
- (Call on individual students to read their sentence about Fizz and Liz. Call on individual students to read their sentence about themselves.)

8. (Write on the board:)

> **Everybody got mad.**

- This says: Everybody got mad.
- Copy that sentence on your paper. Remember the capital and the period. Raise your hand when you've copied the sentence.
  (Observe students and give feedback.)

9. (Write to show:)

> **Everybody got mad.**
> **Dot got mad at** _____.

- Here's the first part of the sentence you'll write next. Dot got mad at blank. You're

going to complete the sentence for Dot. She got mad at one of the things shown on the page with **Story words.**

- Write your sentence about Dot. Raise your hand when you're finished.
  (Observe students and give feedback.)
- (Call on individual students to read their sentence for Dot.)

10. (Write to show:)

> **Everybody got mad.**
> **Dot got mad at** _____.
> **Goober** _____.
> **I** _____.

- You're going to write two more sentences. One will tell about Goober and what he got mad at. The other will tell about you and what you got mad at.
- Your turn: Write both sentences. Remember the period at the end of each sentence. Raise your hand when you're finished.
  (Observe students and give feedback.)
- (Call on individual students to read their sentence about Goober. Then call on individual students to read their sentence about themselves.)

Illustrating a Sentence

- Find lesson 31 in your workbook. You're going to draw a picture that shows why somebody got mad.
- If you wrote a sentence that told that somebody got mad at Clarabelle, your picture should show why the character got mad at her. It should show what she did to make them mad.
- If you wrote that somebody got mad at Dud, you should show what Dud did to make the character mad.
- When you're done, copy the sentence that your picture shows. That sentence goes on top of the picture.
  (Observe students and give feedback.)

Materials: Each student will need a blue and a brown crayon.

Objectives

- Alphabetize words that start with different letters. (Exercise 1)
- Compose directions to show solutions to a map puzzle. (Exercise 2)
- Answer questions about mentally constructed classes. (Exercise 3)
- Listen to part 2 of a story and answer comprehension questions. (Exercise 4)
- Draw routes that reflect story events. (Exercise 5)

WORKBOOK

EXERCISE 1 Alphabetical Order

ball	end
go	ant
dig	candy
fill	

1. _____
2. _____
3. _____
4. _____
5. _____
6. _____
7. _____

1. Open your workbook to lesson 32, and find part A. ✔
- You're going to put words in alphabetical order. What kind of order? (Signal.) *Alphabetical order.*
  That means that the first letter of each word will follow the alphabet.
2. You're going to say the whole alphabet, starting with **A** and going all the way to **Z.** Get ready. (Signal.) *A, B, C, D, E, F, G, H, I, J, K, L, M, N, O, P, Q, R, S, T, U, V, W, X, Y, Z.*
- (Repeat step 2 until firm.)
3. This time, I'll say part of the alphabet. When I stop, say the letter that comes next.
- Listen: H, I, J, K. (Signal.) *L.*
- Listen: C, D, E. (Signal.) *F.*
- Listen: V, W, X, Y. (Signal.) *Z.*
- Listen: L, M, N. (Signal.) *O.*
- (Repeat step 3 until firm.)
4. Listen: When you put words in alphabetical order, you look at the first letter of each word. Words that begin with **A** come first. Words that begin with **B** come next.

Everybody, what words come after words that begin with **C**? (Signal.) *Words that begin with D.*
- What words come after words that begin with **D**? (Signal.) *Words that begin with E.*
5. Listen. Raise your hand when you know what comes after words that begin with **J.** (Call on a student.) *Words that begin with K.*
6. Raise your hand when you know what comes after words that begin with **X.** (Call on a student.) *Words that begin with Y.*
- Everybody, what comes after words that begin with **X**? (Signal.) *Words that begin with Y.*
7. Find the words in the box. These words are not in alphabetical order. But one of the words begins with the letter **A,** another word begins with **B,** and so on.
8. Your turn: Write the word that begins with **A** on line 1. Write the word that begins with **B** on line 2. Cross out the words that you copy so you can see which words are left. (Observe students and give feedback.)
9. You've got a word that begins with **A** and a word that begins with **B.** What will the next word begin with? (Signal.) *C.*
- And the word after that? (Signal.) *D.*
10. Your turn: Write those words where they belong. Remember, just look at the first letter of each word. If it begins with **C,** write it next. Then write the word that begins with **D.** Make sure you cross out the words that you copy.
(Observe students and give feedback.)

11. (Write on the board:)

> **1. ant**
> **2. ball**
> **3. candy**
> **4. dig**

- Here's what you should have so far.

12. Your turn: You have words that begin with **A, B, C,** and **D.** What letter will the next word begin with? (Signal.) *E.*
- And the word after that? (Signal.) *F.*

13. Write those two words. Then write the last word.
    (Observe students and give feedback.)

14. (Write to show:)

> **1. ant**
> **2. ball**
> **3. candy**
> **4. dig**
> **5. end**
> **6. fill**
> **7. go**

- Here's what you should have. Raise your hand if you got everything right. ✔

EXERCISE 2   Map Directions

Relative Direction

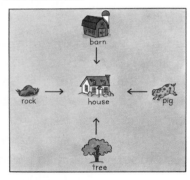

1. The house is west of _____
2. The house is north of _____
3. The house is east of _____
4. The house is south of _____

1. Find part B. ✔
   This is a map, but the letters are not shown.
- There's a house in the middle of the map, and there are four arrows pointing to the house. Those arrows show how you would get to the house from different places.
- Here's the rule: If you go south to get to the house, the house is south. If you go north to get to the house, the house is north.

2. Touch the arrow that points to the north. ✔
- (Draw on the board:)

- Here's the arrow you should be touching. That arrow shows that the house is **north** of something.
- Look at your picture: What is the house north of? (Signal.) *The tree.*
- Right, the tree. To go to the house from the tree, you'd have to go north. The house is north of the tree.
- Everybody, say that. (Signal.) *The house is north of the tree.*
- Yes, the house is north of the tree.

3. Touch the arrow that points to the east. ✔
- (Add to show:)

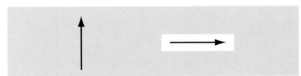

- Here's the arrow you should be touching. That arrow shows that the house is **east** of something. What is it east of? (Signal.) *The rock.*
- Yes, the rock. To go to the house from the rock, you'd have to go east. So the house is east of the rock.
- Everybody, tell me about the house. (Signal.) *The house is east of the rock.*
- Yes, the house is east of the rock.

4. Touch the arrow that points south. ✔
   That arrow shows that the house is **south** of something.
- (Change north arrow to show:)

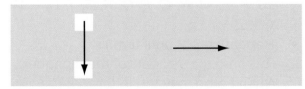

- Here's the arrow you should be touching.
- What is the house south of? (Signal.) *The barn.*
- So the house is south of the barn.
- Everybody, tell me about the house. (Signal.) *The house is south of the barn.*
- Yes, the house is south of the barn.

5. Touch the arrow that points west. ✔
- (Change east arrow to show:)

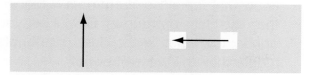

- Here's the arrow you should be touching.
- What is the house **west** of? (Signal.) *The pig.*
- Everybody, tell me about the house. (Signal.) *The house is west of the pig.*
- Yes, the house is west of the pig.

Writing About Relative Direction

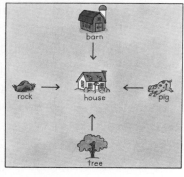

1. The house is west of _____
2. The house is north of _____
3. The house is east of _____
4. The house is south of _____

1. Look at the sentences below the map. You're going to complete all these sentences so they tell about the house.
2. Touch sentence 1. ✔
It says: The house is **west** of something.
- Touch the arrow that points to the west and write **W** on the point of that arrow. Raise your hand when you're finished. ✔
- (Draw on the board:)

W

- Here's what you should have.
- The house is west of that arrow. Say which object the house is west of. (Signal.) *The pig.*
- So you write **the pig** in the blank for sentence 1. Do it. Raise your hand when you're finished.
(Observe students and give feedback.)
- Sentence 1 should say: The house is west of the pig.
3. Everybody, touch sentence 2. ✔
It says: The house is **north** of something.
- Find the arrow that points north. Write **N** on the point of that arrow. Then write the name of the object the house is north of. Raise your hand when you're finished.
(Observe students and give feedback.)

- Everybody, the house is north of something. What's that? (Signal.) *The tree.*
- Raise your hand if you got it right.
4. Everybody, touch sentence 3. ✔
It says: The house is **east** of something.
- Find the arrow that points east. Write **E** on the point of that arrow. Then write the name of the object the house is east of. Raise your hand when you're finished. (Observe students and give feedback.)
- Everybody, the house is east of something. What's that? (Signal.) *The rock.*
- Raise your hand if you got it right.
5. Everybody, touch sentence 4. ✔
It says: The house is **south** of something.
- Find the arrow that points south. Write **S** on the point of that arrow. Then write the name of the object the house is south of. Raise your hand when you're finished. (Observe students and give feedback.)
- Everybody, the house is south of something. What's that? (Signal.) *The barn.*
- Raise your hand if you got it right.
6. Raise your hand if you got everything right.
- That's great.

EXERCISE 3   Classification
Mental Manipulations

Class

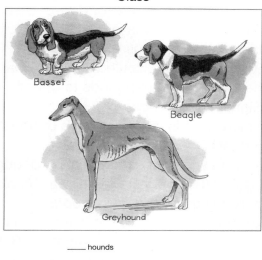

_____ hounds

_____ fast-running hounds

_____ dogs

_____ animals

1. Everybody, find part C. ✔
This picture shows a class. It doesn't show the not-class box.
- Listen: Raise your hand when you know the name of the smallest class shown in the class box. ✔
- Everybody, what's the class? (Signal.) *Hounds.*

2. You're going to play the great thinking game. **Pretend** that you're going to change the class.

- Listen: You have hounds in the class box. But you want fast-running hounds in the class box. Just fast-running hounds. Think big. Raise your hand when you know whether you add things or take things out of the class box. ✔

3. Everybody, what do you do to the class box? (Signal.) *Take things out.*
- (Repeat step 3 until firm.)

4. Everybody, which class is smaller, **hounds** or **fast-running hounds?** (Signal.) *Fast-running hounds.*
- How do you know that the class of fast-running hounds is smaller? (Call on a student. Idea: *There are fewer things in the class of fast-running hounds.)*
- The class of fast-running hounds is smaller than the class of hounds. So you'll have to take things out of the class of hounds to get fast-running hounds.
- Listen: If you had the class of fast-running hounds in the class box, which dog would be in your class box? (Signal.) *The greyhound.*
- Where would the beagle and the basset be? (Signal.) *In the not-class box.*

5. New game: You have the class of hounds, but you want the class of **dogs.** Raise your hand when you know whether you'd add things or take things out.
- Everybody, what would you do to change the class box from hounds to dogs? (Signal.) *Add things.*
- Which class is bigger, hounds or dogs? (Signal.) *Dogs.*
- How do you know that the class of dogs is bigger? (Call on a student. Idea: *There are more things in the class of dogs.)*

6. New game: You have the class of hounds, but you want the class of **animals.** Raise your hand when you know whether you'd have to add things or take things out of the class box. ✔
- Everybody, what would you have to do? (Signal.) *Add things.*
- Which class is bigger, hounds or animals? (Signal.) *Animals.*
- How do you know? (Call on a student. Idea: *There are more things in the class of animals.)*

7. Listen: You know that the class of **dogs** is bigger than the class of **hounds.** And you know that the class of **animals** is bigger than the class of **hounds.** But I'll bet you don't know whether the class of **animals** is bigger than the class of **dogs.**
- Raise your hand if you know which class is bigger, animals or dogs. ✔
- Everybody, which class is bigger? (Signal.) *Animals.*
- How do you know that the class of animals is bigger than the class of dogs? (Call on a student. Idea: *There are more things in the class of animals.)*

8. Sure, the class of **animals** has **all** the dogs in it and a lot of other things.
- Who can name some other things that are in the class of animals? (Call on individual students. Praise appropriate responses.)
- So the class of animals is **way bigger** than the class of dogs.
- Who figured that out? ✔
Good for you. You are really thinking.

Indicating the Size of Classes

1. Everybody, touch the names below the pictures in part C. These are the names of different classes.
- I'll read the names. Follow along: The first name is **hounds.** The next name is **fast-running hounds.** The next name is **dogs.** The last name is **animals.**

2. Listen: Write **1** in front of the name of the **biggest** class. One of these classes is bigger than any other class. Write 1 in front of that class. Raise your hand when you're finished. ✔
- Everybody, which of these classes is the biggest? (Signal.) *Animals.*
- Who got it right? (Praise students who respond.)
- Everybody else, write **1** in front of **animals.** Raise your hand when you're finished. ✔
- Write **2** in front of the name of the next biggest class. That class isn't as big as animals, but it's the biggest class without a number in front of it. It's either hounds, fast-running hounds or dogs. Raise your hand when you're finished. ✔

- Write **3** in front of the next biggest class and write **4** in front of the **smallest** class. Raise your hand when you're finished. (Observe students and give feedback.)
3. Let's see who is **super** smart.
- Touch the **1** you wrote. ✔
  The **biggest** class is **animals.** Who got it right? ✔
  (Praise students who respond.)
- Touch the **2** you wrote. ✔
  The name of the next biggest class is dogs. Who got it right? ✔
  (Praise students who respond.)
- Touch the **3** you wrote. ✔
  The name of the next biggest class is **hounds.** Who got it right? ✔
  (Praise students who respond.)
- Touch the **4** you wrote. ✔
  The name of the **smallest** class is **fast-running hounds.** Who got it right?
  (Praise students who respond.)
4. Clap if you got everything right. ✔
  I can't fool you.

EXERCISE 4   Dot and Dud *Part 2*

Storytelling

- I'm going to read the second part of the Dot and Dud story. Remember, Dud was heading in the wrong direction.
- Which direction was Dud **supposed to be** heading? (Signal.) *North.*
- Which direction was he really heading? (Signal.) *South.*
- Let's find out what happened.

Dud headed south through the snowstorm, and he went right past the rescue station. He came so close to the kennel that, if he'd taken a few steps to the **east,** he would have run right into the kennel. But it was snowing, and it was snowing hard. So Dud didn't see the rescue station. He didn't see anything but snow, and he was too lazy to use his nose. So he went right past the rescue station and kept heading south. After he'd trudged through that deep snow for three hours, he was starting to get very tired and very

hungry. He kept dreaming of gnawing on a large ham bone. That silly dog thought that he was going in the right direction because he was going up, up, up a pretty steep mountain. He kept looking for the other dogs, but, of course, he didn't see them.

- Listen to that part again:

That silly dog thought that he was going in the right direction because he was going up, up, up a pretty steep mountain. He kept looking for the other dogs, but, of course, he didn't see them.

- He was going up a mountain, but was that mountain north of the kennels? (Signal.) *No.*
- Where was it? (Signal.) *South.*
- He didn't see the other dogs because they were miles and miles to the north on the mountain-climbing mountain.

At last, he came down the other side of the mountain, and he saw something through the falling snow. It was a large building—the ski lodge.

"Uh-oh," he said to himself. "I must have gone in the wrong direction."

But at least he was at a place that had warm fireplaces and maybe even a great ham bone.

Dud went up to the kitchen of the lodge. His nose worked pretty well when it came to finding kitchens. He stood outside the kitchen and let out a few deep barks, "Ruff, ruff."

Pretty soon, the door opened and a woman peeked out. "What are you doing out here?" she said.

Dud wagged his tail and licked his chops.

"You must be hungry and tired," she said.

He wagged his tail harder and gave his chops a great big lick.

- Show me how Dud looked when he licked his chops.

"Come in here," she said. "You poor dog."

She gave Dud a large bowl of leftover soup and a great pile of meat scraps.

This was like a dream come true. Dud ate until he was full. Then he curled up in front of a warm, warm stove and fell asleep. He was one happy dog.

But, in the meantime, things were not going that well for the other St. Bernards. Dot had found the trail of the stranded mountain climber, but, in the snowstorm, she got separated from the other rescue dogs.

- What does that mean: She got separated from the other dogs? (Call on a student. Idea: *She wasn't with the others.*)
- So she is in one place, and the other dogs are someplace else.

She followed the trail up slopes that were so steep that she'd sometimes slip and fall down a long way. But she'd get up and try again and again until she made it up the slope. Finally she came to a rocky place where the mountain climber was stranded. He was injured and couldn't walk.

Dot barked to let the other dogs know that she'd found the mountain climber, but the other dogs couldn't hear her. They were over a mile away, and the sound of her barks was lost in the thick, falling snow.

She didn't know what to do, so she curled up next to the mountain climber to keep him warm. And she waited. And she waited. And she waited. By evening, the snow stopped falling, and she still waited. But she was all alone with that

mountain climber, and she couldn't move him without help.

- Dot has a very serious problem. And what's Dud doing while Dot is up there trying to keep that mountain climber alive? (Call on a student. Idea: *Sleeping in front of a warm stove.*)
- What is Dot doing to keep that climber from freezing? (Call on a student. Idea: *Lying right next to him.*)
- And all this time Dud is at the ski lodge, snoring away in front of the stove. We'll have to wait until next time to see what happens.

EXERCISE 5   Interpreting Routes

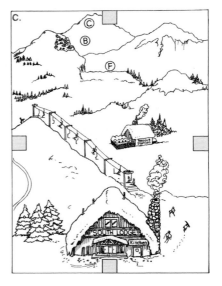

1. Everybody, find part D. ✔
   Here's that map again. Write the letters for north, south, east and west. Raise your hand when you're finished. ✔
- Listen: Draw a blue line that shows where Dot went. Start at the rescue station. Remember, she found that mountain climber at that rocky place high in the mountains. That's letter C. Remember to go over the flat place then up to letter C. Do it. Raise your hand when you're finished.
- Listen: Draw another blue line that shows where the St. Bernards who were with Dot went. Remember, they were with her past the flat place. But, somewhere above the flat place, they got separated from Dot. They were over a mile away from her when

she was with the stranded climber. I think they were around the letter B. Draw a blue line to letter B. Raise your hand when you've drawn both blue lines.
(Observe students and give feedback.)

2. Now you'll draw a brown line to show Dud's route. First, he went to the flat place and ran around and around. Draw that much of the route. Start at the kennel. Draw a brown line up to the flat part and then show some zigs and zags around that flat part. Then stop. Raise your hand when you're finished.
(Observe students and give feedback.)

• Dud got all confused and went south.

• Listen: Make a little brown mark just to the west of the kennel. Make it very close to the kennel. Raise your hand when you're finished.
(Observe students and give feedback.)

3. Now draw your brown line south from the flat part. Go south and go through the little mark you made and keep going south until you reach the ski lodge. There's a door by the kitchen. You can show Dud's route going right around the front of that lodge and ending at the kitchen door. Raise your hand when you've drawn Dud's route.

• Later you can color this picture.

Materials: Each student will need a blue and a brown crayon.

Objectives

- Alphabetize words that start with different letters. (Exercise 1)
- **Complete descriptions involving relative direction (Clarabelle is north of the pig).** (Exercise 2)
- Answer questions about mentally constructed classes. (Exercise 3)
- Listen to the conclusion of a 3-part story and answer comprehension questions. (Exercise 4)

WORKBOOK

EXERCISE 1 Alphabetical Order

line	help
ground	kitchen
it	jumps
moon	

1. Open your workbook to lesson 33, and find part A. ✔
- You're going to put words in alphabetical order. What kind of order? (Signal.) *Alphabetical order.*
  That means that the first letter of each word will follow the alphabet.
2. You're going to say the whole alphabet, starting with **A** and going all the way to **Z**. Get ready. (Signal.) *A, B, C, D, E, F, G, H, I, J, K, L, M, N, O, P, Q, R, S, T, U, V, W, X, Y, Z.*
- (Repeat step 2 until firm.)
3. This time, I'll say part of the alphabet. When I stop, say the letter that comes next.
- Listen: R, S, T, U. (Signal.) *V.*
- Listen: F, G, H. (Signal.) *I.*
- Listen: Q, R, S. (Signal.) *T.*
- Listen: W, X. (Signal.) *Y.*
- (Repeat step 3 until firm.)
4. Remember, when you put words in alphabetical order, you look at the first letter of each word. Words that begin with **A** come first. Words that begin with **B**

come next. Everybody, what words come after words that begin with **C**? (Signal.) *Words that begin with D.*
- What words come after words that begin with **D**? (Signal.) *Words that begin with E.*
5. Listen. Raise your hand when you know what comes after words that begin with **F**. (Call on a student.) *Words that begin with G.*
6. Raise your hand when you know what comes after words that begin with **S**. (Call on a student.) *Words that begin with T.*
- Everybody, what comes after words that begin with **S**? (Signal.) *Words that begin with T.*
7. Find the words in the box. These words are not in alphabetical order. But one of the words begins with the letter **G,** another word begins with **H,** another word begins with **I** and so on.
8. Your turn: Write the word that begins with **G** on line 1. Write the word that begins with **H** on line 2. Cross out the words that you copy so you can see which words are left. (Observe students and give feedback.)
9. You've got a word that begins with **G** and a word that begins with **H**. What will the next word begin with? (Signal.) *I.*
- And the word after that? (Signal.) *J.*
10. Your turn: Write those words where they belong. (Observe students and give feedback.)
- (Write on the board:)

1. ground
2. help
3. it
4. jumps

- Here's what you should have so far.
11. Your turn: You have words that begin with **G, H, I,** and **J.** What will the next word begin with? (Signal.) *K.*
- And the word after that? (Signal.) *L.*
12. Write those two words. Then write the last word.

   (Observe students and give feedback.)
13. (Write on the board:)

   1. ground
   2. help
   3. it
   4. jumps
   5. kitchen
   6. line
   7. moon

- Here's what you should have. Raise your hand if you got everything right.

EXERCISE 2 Map Directions

Relative Direction

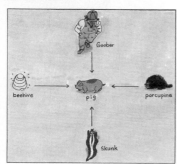

1. The pig is south of _____
2. The pig is north of _____
3. The pig is west of _____
4. The pig is east of _____

1. Find part B. ✔
- Here's one of those tough direction games again. The arrows show how to get to the pig from different places. Remember the rule. If you have to go north to get to the pig, the pig is north. If you have to go west to get to the pig, the pig is west.
- What direction is the pig if you have to go south to get to the pig? (Signal.) *South.*
- Right, it all depends on where you are.
2. If you were standing at the back end of one of those arrows, you'd have to go **north** to get to the pig. Find the arrow that points north.
- Write **N** on the point of that arrow. ✔

- Touch the object at the back end of the arrow. That's where you'd have to be standing to go **north** to get to the pig.
- (Draw on the board:)

- Here's the arrow.
- (Touch the back end of the arrow.) Here's where you'd be standing.
- What object would you be standing on if you had to go north to get to the pig? (Signal.) *The skunk.*
- Phew. If you were standing on that skunk, you'd have to go north. So the pig is north of something. What's that? (Signal.) *The skunk.*
3. Say the whole thing about the pig. (Signal.) *The pig is north of the skunk.*
- (Repeat step 3 until firm.)
4. If you were standing at the back end of one of these arrows, you'd have to go **east** to get to the pig. Find the arrow that points east.
- Write **E** on the point of that arrow. ✔
- Touch the object at the back end of that arrow. That's where you'd have to be standing to go east to get to the pig.
- (Draw on the board:)

 E

- Here's the arrow.
- (Touch the back end.) Here's where you'd be standing.
- What object would you be standing on if you had to go east to get to the pig? (Signal.) *The beehive.*
- Ouch. If you were standing on that beehive, you'd have to go east to get to the pig. So the pig is east of something. What's that? (Signal.) *The beehive.*
5. Say the whole thing about the pig. (Signal.) *The pig is east of the beehive.*
- (Repeat step 5 until firm.)
6. If you were standing at the back end of one of those arrows, you'd have to go **south** to get to the pig. Write **S** on the point of that arrow. Figure out where you'd be standing to go south to get to the pig.

- (Draw on the board:)

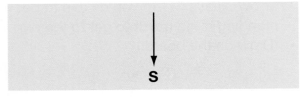

- Here's that arrow.
- (Touch the back end.)
  Here's where you'd be standing.
- What object would you be standing on if you had to go south to get to the pig? (Signal.) *Goober.*
- Phew. If you were standing where Goober is, you'd have to go south to get to the pig.
7. Say the whole thing about the pig. (Signal.) *The pig is south of Goober.*
- (Repeat step 7 until firm.)
8. If you were standing at the back of one of those arrows, you'd have to go **west** to get to the pig. Write **W** on the point of that arrow. Figure out where you'd be standing to go west to get to the pig.
- (Draw on the board:)

- Here's the arrow.
- (Touch the back end.)
  Here's where you'd be standing.
- What object would you be standing on? (Signal.) *The porcupine.*
- Ouch. What direction would you have to go to get to the pig? (Signal.) *West.*
9. Say the whole thing about the pig. (Signal.) *The pig is west of the porcupine.*
- (Repeat step 9 until firm.)

Writing About Relative Direction

1. Find the sentences under the map in part B.
- Sentence 1: The pig is south of something. You complete that sentence with the name of the object on the south arrow.
- Sentence 2: The pig is north of something. You complete that sentence with the name of the object on the north arrow.
- Sentence 3: The pig is west of something. You complete that sentence with the name of the object on the west arrow.
2. Your turn: Complete all the sentences. Raise your hand when you're finished. (Observe students and give feedback.)

3. Check your work. I'll read the first part of each sentence. You tell me the last part.
- Sentence 1: The pig is south of . . . (Signal.) *Goober.*
- Sentence 2: The pig is north of . . . (Signal.) *The skunk.*
- Sentence 3: The pig is west of . . . (Signal.) *The porcupine.*
- Sentence 4: The pig is east of . . . (Signal.) *The beehive.*

EXERCISE 3   Classification

Mental Manipulations

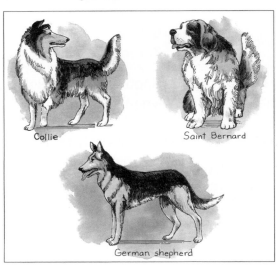

1. Everybody, find part C. ✔
   This picture shows a class.
- Listen: Raise your hand when you know the name of the smallest class that's shown in the class box.
- Everybody, what's the class? (Signal.) *Work dogs.*
2. You're going to play that thinking game again.
- Listen: You have work dogs in the class box. But you want dogs in the class box. Raise your hand when you know whether you'd add things or take things out.
- Everybody, what would you do to change the class from work dogs to dogs? (Signal.) *Add things.*
- Which class is bigger, work dogs or dogs? (Signal.) *Dogs.*
- How do you know that the class of dogs is bigger? (Signal.) *There are more things in the class of dogs.*

3. New game: You have the class of work dogs, but you want the class of work dogs with ears that stand straight up. That's tough.

- You want the class of work dogs with ears that stand straight up. Raise your hand when you know whether you'd add things or take things out. ✔

- Everybody, what would you do to change the class from work dogs to work dogs with ears that stand straight up? (Signal.) *Take things out.*

- Which class is **smaller,** the class of work dogs or the class of work dogs with ears that stand straight up? (Signal.) *Work dogs with ears that stand straight up.*

- Listen: Which dogs would you have to take out of the class box to have the class of work dogs with ears that stand straight up? (Signal.) *The collie and the St. Bernard.*

- Yes, the collie **and** the St. Bernard.

- Everybody, if you had the class of work dogs with ears that stand straight up in your class box, which dog would be in the class box? (Signal.) *The German shepherd.*

- Where would the collie and the St. Bernard be? (Signal.) *In the not-class box.*

4. New game: You have the class of work dogs, but you want the class of **animals.** Raise your hand when you know whether you'd add things or take things out.

- Everybody, what would you do to change the class from work dogs to animals? (Signal.) *Add things.*

- Everybody, which class is bigger? (Signal.) *Animals.*

- How do you know? (Call on a student. Idea: *There are more things in the class of animals.*)

5. Listen: You know that the class of dogs is bigger than the class of work dogs and that the class of animals is bigger than the class of work dogs.

- Raise your hand when you know which of those two classes is bigger—the class of animals or the class of dogs.

- Everybody, which class is bigger? (Signal.) *Animals.*

Indicating the Size of Classes

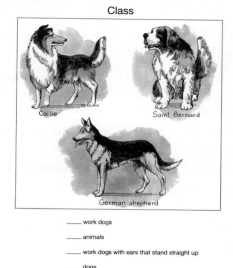

Class

——— work dogs

——— animals

——— work dogs with ears that stand straight up

——— dogs

1. Find the names below the picture in part C. These are the names of different classes.

- I'll read the names. Follow along: The first name is **work dogs.** The next name is **animals.** The next name is **work dogs with ears that stand straight up.** The last name is **dogs.**

2. Listen: Write **1** in front of the name of the **biggest** class. One of these classes is bigger than any other class. Write 1 in front of that class. Raise your hand when you're finished. ✔

- Everybody, which of these classes is the biggest? (Signal.) *Animals.*

- Who got it right? (Praise students who respond.)

- Everybody else, write **1** in front of **animals.** Raise your hand when you're finished. ✔

- Write **2** in front of the name of the next biggest class. That class isn't as big as animals, but it's the biggest class without a number in front of it. It's either work dogs, work dogs with ears that stand straight up or dogs. Raise your hand when you're finished. ✔

- Write **3** in front of the next biggest class and write **4** in front of the **smallest** class. Raise your hand when you're finished. (Observe students and give feedback.)

3. Let's see who is **super** smart.

- Touch the **1** you wrote. ✔ The name of the biggest class is **animals.**

- Touch the **2** you wrote. ✔ The name of the next biggest class is **dogs.** Who got it right? (Praise students who respond.)

- Touch the **3** you wrote. ✔
  The name of the next biggest class is **work dogs.** Who got it right?
  (Praise students who respond.)
- Touch the **4** you wrote. ✔
  The name of the **smallest** class is **work dogs with ears that stand straight up.**
  Who got it right? (Praise students who respond.)

4. Raise your hand if you got everything right. That's great.

EXERCISE 4   Dot and Dud
Part 3

Storytelling

- I'm going to finish the story about Dot and Dud. Remember that Dot and Dud were separated.
- Where was Dud when we left him at the end of the last part? (Call on a student. Idea: *In the kitchen of the ski lodge.*)
- Where was Dot? (Call on a student. Idea: *On the mountain with the stranded mountain climber.*)
- Everybody, one of those dogs was very far south of the other dogs. Which dog was very far south? (Signal.) *Dud.*
- Which dog was north? (Signal.) *Dot.*
- How many of the other dogs were helping Dot try to keep that mountain climber warm? (Signal.) *None.*
- Where were those other St. Bernards? (Call on a student. Idea: *About a mile away.*)
- Let's find out what happened.

That evening, while Dud was snoozing next to the stove in the kitchen, full of food and dreaming about summertime, a truck pulled up to the ski lodge, and the ranger came inside to pick up Dud. The cook had called the rescue station and left a message that one of their St. Bernards was at the ski lodge.

The ranger was not happy. He led Dud to the truck and put him in the back with all the other St. Bernards. They were coming back from their search. They hadn't found the stranded mountain climber, and they hadn't found

Dot. The ranger decided that it was best to go home before it got dark in the mountains. They would go out again early in the morning.

Of course, Dud didn't know that Dot was stranded on the mountain. He got in the back of the truck with the other dogs. They didn't even look at him. They didn't start griping about how he didn't keep up with the others and got lost. They didn't remind him that he didn't even know north from south or that his nose was about as useful as another paw. They just sat there, weary from plowing through the snow all day and worried about Dot.

As the truck went down the road back to the rescue station, Dud tried to strike up a conversation with the other dogs. "How did things go today?" he asked.

Two of the dogs looked at him but didn't answer. The other dogs didn't even look at him.

"Did you find the mountain climber?"

No dogs looked at him.

"You look pretty tired. Have you had anything to eat?"

No answer.

"I had some great soup at the ski lodge. And a big plateful of meat scraps. And, after I ate that, I took . . . "

"Will you shut up?" the oldest dog said.

So Dud was quiet for a while. Then he looked around and noticed that Dot wasn't in the truck. "Hey," he said, "where's Dot?"

"Lost," one of the St. Bernards said.

"What do you mean? Where is she?"

The oldest St. Bernard said, "Somewhere on the mountain. We couldn't find her."

"Do you mean that she's out there all alone?"

Some of the dogs nodded yes.

This was no game. Dud loved Dot. He didn't always show it, but he loved her. As he sat in the back of that truck, he remembered her from way, way back when the two of them were little puppies. She always stuck up for him when the other puppies in the litter would pick on Dud. Dud remembered a lot of other things as that truck moved slowly down the snowy road. He remembered how sad he had been when Dot and Dud had to leave their mother and their other brothers and sisters. The only good thing about going to the rescue station was that Dot was there. She had always been there. But now . . . she was gone.

"No," Dud said out loud. "She **can't** be lost."

All the other dogs looked down. "Why didn't you find her? You can't leave her out there."

"She'll be all right—if we find her tomorrow."

Dud said, "But what if she found the mountain climber? Won't he freeze during the night?"

All the other dogs looked down.

Dud didn't say anything more. But he did a lot of thinking. And the biggest thought he had was this: "If they can't find her, **I'll** find her." This wasn't one of those promises he made when he was only half serious and half embarrassed for being foolish. This wasn't one of those promises like "I'll try" or "I'll do better next time." This was a **real** promise: "**I'll** find her."

At last, the truck stopped in front of the rescue station. The ranger opened the back door, and out bounded Dud, just as fast as he could bound. He ran north. The ranger was shouting, "Dud,

come back here! Where do you think you're going in the dark?"

The other dogs were yelling at him, too. "Yeah! Where do you think you're going in the dark?"

But Dud knew exactly where he was going—north.

Pretty soon, some of the other dogs started to follow Dud. Then the rest of the dogs started to follow. Then the ranger started to follow. And away everybody went, plowing through the deep snow and heading up that mountain.

Dud was all business. He said to himself, "I know Dot's smell better than any other dog in the world, and I'll find that smell. I **will.**"

He put his nose in the snow and he snorted and sniffed. He didn't care that the snow was cold. He didn't even **notice** that it was cold. Again and again—snort, sniff, snort, sniff. Then he did it the fast way—he just put his head deep into the snow and kept it there—like a snowplow—snorting and sniffing as he went up that mountain as fast as he could run. Then, suddenly he recognized a faint smell in the snow— very faint. But he knew that smell. It was Dot.

"Come on, you guys," he yelled to the other dogs. "Follow me."

And up the mountain Dud went once more, with his head in the snow like a snowplow. He followed that trail up, up, up the mountain. When he came to steep parts and slid down, he just tried again until he made it. Her smell was getting stronger in the snow. She was closer, and closer, and . . . suddenly, Dud came to the rocky part where Dot was lying with the mountain climber.

He called back down to the other dogs, "Up here, you guys. I found her."

While he waited for the others, he sat down next to Dot. "Are you okay?" he asked.

"Yes, but I'm sure glad you got here. This climber is seriously injured. I don't think he could make it through the night."

Then she looked at Dud and said, "What are **you** doing here?"

"Looking for you," Dud said.

She couldn't believe it. "And you found me without getting lost?"

"Well . . . " he said. "I got a little lost once."

- He didn't just get a little lost when he got lost, did he? (Signal.) *No.*
- Where did he go when he was lost? (Signal.) *The ski lodge.*
- Yes, all the way to the ski lodge.

Dot said, "Well, I'm sure glad to see you." She wagged her tail. He wagged his tail.

Soon, the ranger and the other St. Bernards made it up the steep slope. The ranger had a little sled. He put the injured climber on the sled. Then he and the dogs lowered the sled down the very steep part. Then the dogs pulled the sled back to the rescue station.

After the ranger took care of the injured climber, and all the dogs were back in the kennel, the oldest St. Bernard looked at Dud and said, "See? That shows what you can do when you put your mind to it. When you try hard, you're a pretty good rescue dog."

The other dogs said, "Yeah, pretty good."

Then the oldest dog said, "We're all glad that you found Dot. And here's our way of thanking you." The oldest dog picked up a great big ham bone, brought it over to Dud and dropped it in front of him.

Dud started to say, "Oh, I really can't accept that ham bone. I really shouldn't eat this great big . . . " But then he looked at that ham bone, and it **looked** so good and **smelled** so good that he stopped talking and started doing something else.

- Everybody, what do you think he started doing? (Signal.) *Eating that ham bone.*

Objectives

- Answer questions about mentally constructed classes. (Exercise 1)
- Complete descriptions involving relative directions. (Exercise 2)
- Complete sentences of the form: Blank happened **after** blank. (Exercise 3)
- Listen to part 1 of a story and answer comprehension questions. (Exercise 4)
- **Edit sentences to eliminate pronoun ambiguity.** (Exercise 5)
- **Write a group of sentences that are thematically related.** (Exercise 6)

EXERCISE 1   Classification

Mental Manipulations

> ***Note:*** In step 2, it is assumed your class contains *second-grade* girls. If it does *not,* make an appropriate substitution, for example: *Third-grade girls from your room.*
>
> You'll tell about a tall girl in the room. One clue will tell the name of a student sitting next to that girl.

1. Everybody, we're going to play a new kind of class game. I'll say the name of a large class, then a smaller class, then a smaller class. I'll keep going until I'm talking about only one thing. You have to figure out what that thing is.

2. Listen: This thing is in the class of girls. Everybody, say that. (Signal.) *This thing is in the class of girls.*

- That's a pretty big class. Think of all the things in that class.
- Here's a smaller class. This thing is in the class of girls who go to our school.
- Everybody, say that. (Signal.) *This thing is in the class of girls who go to our school.*
- That's a much smaller class.
- Here's a smaller class. This thing is in the class of **second-grade** girls who go to our school.
- Everybody, say that. (Signal.) *This thing is in the class of second-grade girls who go to our school.*

- Here's a smaller class. This thing is in the class of **pretty tall** second-grade girls who go to our school.
- That class is getting pretty small. Raise your hand if you can name some of the things in that class. (Accept reasonable responses.)
- Last class: This thing is in the class of pretty tall second-grade girls who go to our school. And this thing is sitting next to somebody named ___.
- Who is this girl? (Students respond.)

3. New game. But you have to help me.

- Listen: This thing is in the class of teachers. That's the big class we'll start with.
- Listen: This thing is in the class of teachers who . . .
- Help me out with a smaller class of teachers. Tell me where you could find this teacher.
  (Acknowledge reasonable suggestions.)
- Let's use this suggestion: This thing is in the class of teachers who are at our school. Everybody say that. (Signal.) *This thing is in the class of teachers who are at our school.*
- Here's a smaller class: This thing is in the class of teachers who are at our school. And this thing is talking to you right now.
- Who is that teacher? (Signal.) *You.*

EXERCISE 2 **Map Directions**

Relative Direction

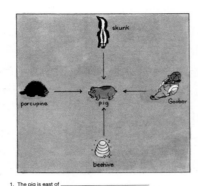

1. The pig is east of _____
2. The pig is north of _____
3. The pig is west of _____
4. The pig is south of _____

1. Open your workbook to lesson 34 and find part A. ✔
    We're going to play one of those tough direction games again. The arrows show how to get to the pig from different places. Remember the rule. If you have to go north to get to the pig, the **pig** is north. If you have to go west to get to the pig, the **pig** is west. What direction is the pig if you have to go south to get to the pig? (Signal.) *South.*

*   Right, it all depends on where you are.

2. Touch sentence 1. ✔
    It says: The pig is east of something. Find the arrow that points east.

*   Look at the thing that would have to go east to get to the pig and write the name of that object in the blank for sentence 1. Raise your hand when you're finished.
    (Observe students and give feedback.)

*   Everybody, the pig is east of something. What is it east of? (Signal.)
    The porcupine.

*   Yes, the porcupine would have to go east to get to the pig.

*   Raise your hand if you got it right.

3. Touch sentence 2. ✔
    It says: The pig is north of something. Find the arrow that points north and write the name of the object the pig is north of. Raise your hand when you're finished.
    (Observe students and give feedback.)

*   Everybody, the pig is north of something. What is it north of? (Signal.) *The beehive.*

*   Raise your hand if you got it right.

4. Touch sentence 3. ✔
    It says: The pig is west of something. Find the right arrow and write the name of the thing that would have to go west to get to the pig. Raise your hand when you're finished.
    (Observe students and give feedback.)

*   Everybody, the pig is west of something. What is it west of? (Signal.) *Goober.*

*   Raise your hand if you got it right.

5. Touch sentence 4. ✔
    It says: The pig is south of something. Find the right arrow and write the name of the object the pig is south of. Raise your hand when you're finished.
    (Observe students and give feedback.)

*   Everybody, the pig is south of something. What is it south of? (Signal.) *The skunk.*

*   Raise your hand if you got it right.

6. Raise your hand if you got everything right. Super.

EXERCISE 3 **Temporal Sequencing**

After

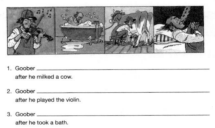

1. Goober _____
   after he milked a cow.

2. Goober _____
   after he played the violin.

3. Goober _____
   after he took a bath.

1. Everybody, find part B. ✔
    These pictures show four things that Goober did.

*   Touch the first picture. ✔
    What did Goober do first? (Signal.)
    Played the violin.

*   Touch the next picture. ✔
    That shows what he did after he played the violin. What did he do? (Signal.)
    Took a bath.

*   Touch the next picture. ✔
    That shows what Goober did after he took a bath. What did he do? (Signal.)
    Milked a cow.

*   Touch the last picture. ✔
    That shows what Goober did after he milked the cow. What did he do? (Signal.)
    Went to sleep.

2. (Write on the board:)

> **played the violin**
> **took a bath**
> **milked a cow**
> **went to sleep**

- You're going to complete the sentences that tell what Goober did **after** he did something else.
- Touch sentence 1. ✔
  It says: Goober blank after he milked a cow.
- You'll have to find the picture of Goober milking a cow and write what he did just **after** he milked a cow.
- Complete sentence 1. Tell what Goober did after he milked a cow. Raise your hand when you're finished with sentence 1.
  (Observe students and give feedback.)
- Here's what you should have for sentence 1: Goober **went to sleep** after he milked a cow.
- Raise your hand if you got it right.

3. Touch sentence 2. ✔
   It says: Goober blank after he played the violin. You'll have to find the picture of Goober playing the violin and write what he did just **after** he played the violin. Raise your hand when you're finished with sentence 2.
   (Observe students and give feedback.)
- Here's what you should have for sentence 2: Goober **took a bath** after he played the violin.
- Raise your hand if you got it right.

4. Touch sentence 3. ✔
   It says: Goober blank after he took a bath.
- Complete sentence 3. Raise your hand when you're finished.
  (Observe students and give feedback.)
- Here's what you should have for sentence 3: Goober **milked a cow** after he took a bath.
- Raise your hand if you got it right.

5. Raise your hand if you completed all three sentences correctly.
- You're getting very smart about telling what happened after.

EXERCISE 4   Zelda the Artist
Part 1
Storytelling

- I'm going to read a story about an artist named Zelda.
- Listen:

> Zelda was an artist and a very good one. She could draw pictures that looked so real that you would think they were photographs. She could make wonderful designs, and she could even make statues that almost seemed to be alive. There wasn't anything she couldn't paint or draw.
>
> But Zelda had one problem: She wasn't as good at **thinking** as she was at drawing or painting or making statues. So she sometimes made things that were pretty silly, like the time she illustrated Mrs. Hudson's book.

- What would an artist do if she illustrated a book? (Call on a student. Idea: *Draw pictures about the book.*)
- Yes, she'd draw pictures that showed different parts of the book.

> Mrs. Hudson wrote a book about some of the interesting things that happened to her. At least **she** thought they were interesting. Actually, they were very, very boring. She told about experiences she had when she grew up in the city. She told about her experiences when she moved to the farm. And she told about the many trips she had taken to all parts of the world. She loved her stories, but she felt they would be a lot better if the book had beautiful illustrations to show some of her experiences.
>
> Mrs. Hudson had seen some of the fine work that Zelda had done, so she called Zelda on the phone and asked Zelda if she'd be interested in doing twenty illustrations for the book.

Zelda thought about it for a few moments. Then she said, "Yes, I'd like to do that."

Mrs. Hudson said, "Good. I'll bring over the book. I've marked parts of the book to let you know what you should illustrate."

Later that day, Mrs. Hudson drove over to Zelda's place and showed Zelda how she'd marked all the places in the story that gave Zelda information about illustrations.

Mrs. Hudson turned to the second page of the book and pointed to some sentences that were circled in red. Mrs. Hudson said, "Listen to this part." Then she read the circled sentence, "That spring, the apple trees were covered with white flowers, and their branches were black."

- Listen to that part again and get a picture in your mind:

"That spring, the apple trees were covered with white flowers, and their branches were black."

After Mrs. Hudson read that part, Zelda said, "That may be hard to illustrate."

"Why is that?"

"Well, it says that the tree was covered with white **flowers,** and their branches were black. But, how do you draw black branches on little tiny flowers?"

Mrs. Hudson looked at Zelda for a long moment. Mrs. Hudson blinked two times. Then she broke into laughter. "Ho, ho," she laughed. "That's very funny. I didn't catch the joke right away, but that's very funny—black branches on the flowers."

- Zelda thought that the **flowers** had branches. Everybody, what really had branches? (Signal.) *The tree.*
- Listen to the sentence again. Listen for the word that confused Zelda:

That spring, the apple trees were covered with white flowers, and **their** branches were black.

- Zelda thought that **their** branches told about the flowers' branches, not about the **trees'** branches.

Mrs. Hudson went, "Ho, ho," but it wasn't really funny because Zelda was not joking. She didn't understand that the branches belonged to the trees, not to the flowers. So she said, "Well, I'll just do the best I can."

"Good for you, my dear," Mrs. Hudson said, and turned to the next part of the book that was circled.

Mrs. Hudson said, "Listen to this part: 'When we were on the farm, my brother and my sister had pet pigs. They just loved to roll around in the mud.'"

- Listen to that part again because I think Zelda's going to get the wrong picture again:

"When we were on the farm, my brother and my sister had pet pigs. They just loved to roll around in the mud."

- Listen: Who really rolled around in the mud? (Signal.) *The pigs.*
- I'll bet Zelda thinks somebody else rolled around in the mud. Who's that? (Call on a student. Idea: *Mrs. Hudson's brother and sister.*)

After Mrs. Hudson read, "They just loved to roll around in the mud," Zelda said, "They did?"

Mrs. Hudson said, "Oh, yes. They just loved it."

Zelda said, "Didn't they get their clothes all muddy?"

Mrs. Hudson looked at Zelda and blinked. Then she broke into laughter again: "Ho, ho, ho. My," she said, "you are very clever—'Didn't they get their clothes all muddy?' Very funny."

Mrs. Hudson flipped to the next part that was circled. "Here's one of my favorite parts," she said. "Listen to this: 'Every day the children rode their horses through the valley. Their tails flew in the wind.'"

- Listen to that part again:

"Every day the children rode their horses through the valley. Their tails flew in the wind."

- I think we're going to have trouble again. What part do you think Zelda will get wrong this time? (Call on a student. Idea: *Who had the tails.*)

After Mrs. Hudson read the part, "Their tails flew in the wind," Zelda shook her head and said, "They **all** had them?"

"Had what?"

"Tails."

"Well of course, long flowing tails."

"Golly," Zelda said.

"The youngest one had the longest tail. He was gray and white."

Zelda said, "Really?"

"Yes," Mrs. Hudson said. "He was just **covered** with gray and white spots."

"Poor boy," Zelda said.

- Who did Zelda think was covered with gray and white spots? (Signal.) *The boy.*

Mrs. Hudson flipped to one more place that was marked in the book. She said, "This is a little different. This was something inside the farmhouse.

Listen: 'We always kept a glass on top of the refrigerator. We kept it full of water.'"

Zelda shook her head.

- I think she has another problem. Listen to that part again:

"We always kept a glass on top of the refrigerator. We kept it full of water."

- What part do you think Zelda will get wrong this time? (Call on a student. Idea: *What was filled with water.*)

After Mrs. Hudson read, "We kept it full of water," Zelda said, "Didn't it spill out when you opened the door?"

Blink, blink—"Ho, ho, ho, ho. Oh, my dear, you have such a clever wit."

- Did Mrs. Hudson know that Zelda was **really** confused? (Signal.) *No.*
- Mrs. Hudson thought that Zelda "had a **clever wit.**" That means Mrs. Hudson thought Zelda was making very clever jokes.

Mrs. Hudson patted Zelda on the knee and handed her the book. She said, "Well, I'll leave this with you, my dear. You can read through it and see what to show for the other parts I've marked. If you have any questions, you can give me a call."

Zelda said, "I have one big question."

"What's that, my dear?"

"Is this book about very strange things?"

"Well," Mrs. Hudson said, "I suppose not many people have had the kinds of experiences I've had."

"You can say that again," Zelda said.

"All right," Mrs. Hudson said, "I suppose not many people have had the kinds of experiences I've had."

- Zelda said, "You can say that again," and that's just what Mrs. Hudson did.

- Listen again:

> Mrs. Hudson said, "I suppose not many people have had the kinds of experiences I've had."
>
> Zelda said, "You can say that again."
>
> "All right," Mrs. Hudson said. "I suppose not many people have had the kinds of experiences I've had."
>
> So Mrs. Hudson left the book with Zelda, and after Mrs. Hudson left, Zelda sat there shaking her head, wondering how she would illustrate some of the crazy things that Mrs. Hudson's book told about.

EXERCISE 5 **Correcting Ambiguous Referents**

1. My brother and my sister had pet pigs. <u>They</u> just loved to roll around in the mud.

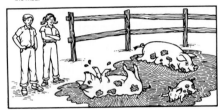

2. We always kept a glass on top of the refrigerator. We kept <u>it</u> full of water.

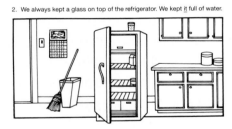

1. Everybody, find part C. ✔
   Those are the sentences that Mrs. Hudson circled. The pictures show what she **wanted** Zelda's pictures to show. Mrs. Hudson could have changed the underlined part of each sentence so that Zelda would not have been mixed up.

2. Touch number 1. ✔
   I'll read what it says. Follow along:
- (Read slowly:) My brother and my sister had pet pigs. They just loved to roll around in the mud.
- Touch the word that's underlined. ✔ Everybody, what word is underlined? (Signal.) *They.*
- Yes, **they. They** just loved to roll around in the mud.
- If Mrs. Hudson changed the word **they** to the right name, Zelda wouldn't have been confused. Everybody, what's the right name? (Signal.) *The pigs.*
- Listen: Cross out the word **they** and write **the pigs.** Raise your hand when you're finished.
   (Observe students and give feedback.)
- Now it says: My brother and my sister had pet pigs. **The pigs** just loved to roll around in the mud.

3. Touch number 2. ✔
   I'll read what it says. Follow along:
- (Read slowly:) We always kept a glass on top of the refrigerator. We kept it full of water.
- Touch the word that's underlined. ✔ Everybody, what word is underlined? (Signal.) *It.*
- Yes, **it.** We kept **it** full of water.
- If Mrs. Hudson changed the word **it** to the right name, Zelda wouldn't have been confused. Everybody, what's the right name? (Signal.) *The glass.*
- Cross out the word **it** and write **the glass** above the crossed-out **it.** Raise your hand when you're finished.
   (Observe students and give feedback.)
- Now it says: We always kept a glass on top of the refrigerator. We kept **the glass** full of water. Now that's clear and Zelda would not be confused.
- Later you can color the pictures.

EXERCISE 6   Sentence Writing

1. Find page 272 titled **Story words** at the back of your workbook. Today, you're going to write sentences that make up little stories. You're going to write your sentences on lined paper.

2. (Write on the board:)

> **Everybody jumped over something.**

- This says: Everybody jumped over something.
- Copy that sentence on the second line of your paper. Remember the capital and the period. Raise your hand when you've copied the sentence.
(Observe students and give feedback.)

3. (Write to show:)

> **Everybody jumped over something.**
> **Mrs. Hudson jumped over _____.**

- Here's the first part of the sentence you'll write next. Mrs. Hudson jumped over blank. You're going to complete the sentence for Mrs. Hudson. She jumped over one of the things shown on the page with **Story words.**

- Write your sentence about Mrs. Hudson. Raise your hand when you're finished. (Observe students and give feedback.)
- (Call on individual students to read their sentence about Mrs. Hudson.)

4. (Write to show:)

> **Everybody jumped over something.**
> **Mrs. Hudson jumped over _____.**
> **Goober _____.**
> **I _____.**

- You're going to write two more sentences. One will tell about Goober and what he jumped over. The other will tell about you and what you jumped over.
- Your turn: Write both sentences. Remember the period at the end of each sentence. Raise your hand when you're finished.

Objectives

- Alphabetize words that start with different letters. (Exercise 1)
- Complete descriptions involving relative directions. (Exercise 2)
- **Indicate the number of objects in larger and smaller classes.** (Exercise 3)
- Listen to part 2 of a story and answer comprehension questions. (Exercise 4)
- Edit sentences to eliminate pronoun ambiguity. (Exercise 5)

WORKBOOK

EXERCISE 1 Alphabetical Order

helpful	knock
jumpy	gate
farmer	landed
inside	

1. _____
2. _____
3. _____
4. _____
5. _____
6. _____
7. _____

1. Open your workbook to lesson 35 and find part A. ✔
- Find the words in the box. You're going to write these words in alphabetical order. First you have to find the word that is earliest in the alphabet.
  I don't see a word that begins with **A**.
  I don't see a word that begins with **B**.
  I don't see a word that begins with **C**.
  I don't see a word that begins with **D**.
- Look at the list and see if you can find one that begins with **E**. ✔
2. Did you find a word that begins with **E**? (Signal.) *No.*
- You looked for words that begin with **A, B, C, D,** and **E**. What letter will you look for next? (Signal.) *F.*
3. See if you can find a word that begins with **F.** ✔
- Everybody, did you find a word that begins with **F?** (Signal.) *Yes.*
4. Write it on line 1. Cross it out from the list. Then write the other words in alphabetical order.
  (Observe students and give feedback.)

5. (Write on the board:)

> 1. farmer
> 2. gate
> 3. helpful
> 4. inside
> 5. jumpy
> 6. knock
> 7. landed

- Here's what you should have.

EXERCISE 2 Map Directions

Relative Direction

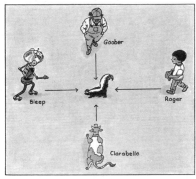

1. The skunk is north of _____.
2. The skunk is east of _____.
3. The skunk is west of _____.
4. The skunk is south of _____.

1. Find part B. You're going to look at the arrows and complete sentences.
2. Sentence 1: The skunk is north of something. You complete that sentence with the name of the object on the north arrow.
- Sentence 2: The skunk is east of something. You complete that sentence with the name of the object on the east arrow.
- Sentence 3: The skunk is west of something. You complete that sentence with the name of the object on the west arrow.

- Sentence 4: The skunk is south of something. You complete that sentence with the name of the object on the south arrow.
- Your turn: Complete all the sentences. Raise your hand when you're finished. ✔
3. Check your work. I'll read the first part of each sentence. You tell me the last part.
- Sentence 1: The skunk is north of . . . (Signal.) *Clarabelle.*
- Sentence 2: The skunk is east of . . . (Signal.) *Bleep.*
- Sentence 3: The skunk is west of . . . (Signal.) *Roger.*
- Sentence 4: The skunk is south of . . . (Signal.) *Goober.*

EXERCISE 3   Classification

Mental Manipulation

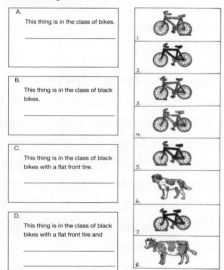

1. Everybody, find part C. ✔
   The pictures show different bikes. The sentences tell about the classes.
- I'll read the sentences. Follow along.
- Touch sentence A. ✔
   This thing is in the class of bikes. That's the big class.
- Touch sentence B. ✔
   This thing is the class of black bikes. That's a smaller class.
- Touch sentence C. ✔
   This thing is in the class of black bikes with a flat front tire.
2. Here's what you're going to do. Below each sentence, write the number of every picture that sentence tells about.

- Touch sentence A. ✔
   This thing is in the class of bikes. You have to write the number of every picture that sentence tells about. You'll write the number of every picture that shows a bike.
- Picture 1 shows a bike, so you'd write number 1 on the line below sentence A.
- Picture 2 shows a bike, so you'd write number 2 under the sentence.
- Listen: Write the number of every picture that shows a bike. Raise your hand when you're finished.
   (Observe students and give feedback.)
- (Write on the board:)

1, 2, 3, 4, 5, 7

- Here are the numbers you should have under sentence A—1, 2, 3, 4, 5, 7. Raise your hand if you got it right. ✔
- Everybody, look at picture number 6.
- Why didn't you write that number under the first sentence? (Call on individual students. Idea: *A St. Bernard is not a bike.*)
- Everybody, what other number didn't you write? (Signal.) *8.*
- Why didn't you write the number for Clarabelle? (Call on a student. Idea: *She's not a bike.*)
3. Touch sentence B. ✔
   This thing is in the class of **black** bikes. Is that class bigger or smaller than the class of bikes? (Signal.) *Smaller.*
- So you should have fewer things in this class.
- Write the number of everything that's in the class of **black** bikes. Raise your hand when you're finished.
   (Observe students and give feedback.)
- (Write on the board:)

2, 5, 7

- Here are the numbers you should have for the things in the class of black bikes. Raise your hand if you got it right.
4. Touch sentence C. ✔
   This thing is in the class of black bikes with a flat front tire. Remember, it's in the class of **black** bikes with a flat front tire, not just any old bike with a flat front tire. Write the numbers for the things in that class. Raise your hand when you're finished.
   (Observe students and give feedback.)

- Everybody, which things are in the class of black bikes with a flat front tire? (Signal.) *5 and 7.*
- There are two things in that class, but we're going to tell about only one thing.
- Touch **only** bike 5. ✔
  That's the bike with the flat front tire you'll tell about.
5. Touch sentence D. ✔
  It says: This thing is in the class of black bikes with a flat front tire and . . . something else.
- You're going to complete that sentence so it tells about bike 5 and **no other** bike that's black and has a flat front tire.
- Look at the picture of bike 5. See what else you can say about that bike and write it. That bike has a flat front tire and something else. Raise your hand when you're finished. (Observe students and give feedback.)
- (Call on different students to read their sentence. Praise sentences that tell about a flat rear tire. Say:) That's a really super sentence: Raise your hand if you wrote that super sentence. (Praise sentences that tell about a flat rear tire.)
- This is pretty hard, but a lot of you are too smart to get fooled.

EXERCISE 4 Zelda the Artist *Part 2*

Storytelling

- I'm going to read some more about Zelda the artist. Listen:

Zelda read through Mrs. Hudson's book. Most of it was very, very boring. It told about things that were not very exciting—the rain falling in the springtime, chickens running around the barnyard, people going on long train trips—very boring.

Zelda did a couple of illustrations. The first one she did was for the part that said, "When we were on the farm, my brother and my sister had pet pigs. They just loved to roll around in the mud."

Zelda made a beautiful picture of Mrs. Hudson's brother and sister rolling around in the mud next to the barn.

In the picture that Zelda drew, the pet pigs were standing there, looking at the students in the mud. When Zelda finished that picture, she said, "That woman must have a very strange family."

Then she did the next illustration. That one was for the part that said, "Every day the children rode their horses through the valley. Their tails flew in the wind."

- Who does Zelda think had the tails? (Signal.) *The students.*
- Who was Mrs. Hudson telling about when she wrote: "**Their** tails flew in the wind"? (Signal.) *The horses.*

Zelda didn't know how many students to draw or how long to make their "tails." But at last she decided to show three children riding horses. She gave each of the children a long tail. She gave the horses regular horse tails. After she finished the illustration, she said, "That woman sure knows some very strange people."

Then she went on to the next part. It said: "We always kept a glass on top of the refrigerator. We kept it full of water."

- What does Zelda think was "full of water"? (Signal.) *The refrigerator.*
- What was really full of water? (Signal.) *The glass.*

Zelda decided to show a picture of somebody opening the refrigerator and water pouring out. She said to herself, "I don't know any other way to show that it was full of water."

Zelda didn't know what to put inside the glass. So she left the glass empty.

The part that was marked for the next illustration said this: "Our car stopped on top of the mountain. It was out of gas."

- I think we've got another problem. Listen again:

"Our car stopped on top of the mountain. It was out of gas."

- What part is Zelda going to confuse this time? (Call on a student. Idea: *What is out of gas.*)

Zelda read that part again and again. At last she said, "How am I going to show that the mountain is out of gas? I can't illustrate this picture." Zelda called Mrs. Hudson and said, "I'm having trouble with one illustration. It's for the part that says, 'Our car stopped on top of the mountain. It was out of gas.' How am I going to show it was out of gas?"

"I see what you mean, my dear. Just looking at the picture, you wouldn't really know that it was out of gas, would you?"

"I sure wouldn't," Zelda said.

"Well, what if you sort of showed the inside of it, and we could see the gas gauge?"

"The gas gauge?"

"Yes, my dear. You could put us on top of the mountain, looking inside the window, and show the gas gauge."

"Looking inside **the window?**"

"Of course."

"It has a window?"

"Well, certainly. It has windows all the way around it."

"Wow," Zelda said. "I'll draw it, but I've never seen one with windows before."

"Well, the next time I go over to your place, I'll show you a picture of it."

Zelda said, "I'll take your word for it."

After Zelda hung up the phone, she did the illustration of a great mountain with a car parked on top. The mountain had windows all the way around, and inside one of the windows was a great huge gas gauge.

Zelda looked at the picture and said, "That woman has sure been to some strange places."

The next part of the book that was marked said this: "Our car went down the dirt road, leaving a dust cloud behind. Soon, it floated away on the breeze."

- Uh-oh. I think Zelda is going to have trouble again. Listen to that part again:

"Our car went down the dirt road, leaving a dust cloud behind. Soon, it floated away on the breeze."

- What do you think she'll get wrong this time? (Call on a student. Idea: *What floated away.*)

Zelda read the part to herself two times. Then she shook her head and made the illustration. It showed a car floating through the air over a dirt road. Zelda said to herself, "That woman sure has some strange vehicles, too."

Zelda worked on the illustrations week after week. And every week Mrs. Hudson would call Zelda and remind her that the book had to be finished soon. "Remember, Zelda," she would say, "this book must go to the publisher by March. I certainly hope you'll be done with all the illustrations by then."

- The publisher takes the story Mrs. Hudson wrote and Zelda's illustrations and makes them into a regular book that people can buy.

Every time Mrs. Hudson called to remind Zelda of getting the book ready for the publisher, Zelda would say, "I'm working as fast as I can, but some of these illustrations are not very easy."

Every week, Mrs. Hudson called and said the same thing. Every week, Zelda told her the same thing.

But then, in the middle of February, Mrs. Hudson called and started to say, "Remember, Zelda, this book must go to the publisher before . . . "

"I'm done with the illustrations," Zelda said.

"How perfectly wonderful!" Mrs. Hudson said. "How marvelous! Isn't this just grand?"

She told Zelda that she would be right over and she was. She was still talking about how wonderful everything was when she arrived at Zelda's place. "This is just perfect," she said. "I can hardly wait to see your illustrations, my dear."

Then Mrs. Hudson saw Zelda's illustrations. She looked at the first one, and her eyes got wide, and her face became very serious and stiff. Her face stayed that way as she looked at the next illustration, and the next illustration, and the next illustration. She wasn't saying anything like, "How wonderful this is." She wasn't saying **anything.** She was just staring at those illustrations with wide eyes and a very stiff face.

At last, she dropped the illustrations on the floor and said to Zelda, "What have you done to my wonderful book? These illustrations are awful. They are terrible. They are unbelievable. They are . . ." (She had run out of bad words.)

Zelda said, "Well, I did the best I could. I had never seen any of the things your book told about. Like the picture of the students with their tails flying in the wind. I didn't know if they should have monkey tails, lion tails or short little bunny tails."

"Stop it," Mrs. Hudson said. "I do not find your wit one bit funny. And I find your illustrations terrible, awful, unbelievable, and simply . . . " (She'd run out of bad words again.)

"Well," Zelda said, "I'm sorry. I don't have time to redo them now, but I could . . . "

"No, this book must be at the publisher by March. If it's not at the publisher by March, it doesn't get published."

"Well," Zelda said, "Maybe you can send it in without the illustrations."

"No," Mrs. Hudson said, "I promised the publisher that I would have twenty beautiful illustrations. I didn't know that I would have twenty illustrations that were unbelievable, terrible, awful, and just plain . . . "

So Mrs. Hudson picked up the illustrations, picked up her book and marched out of Zelda's place.

Nobody was very happy.

- Oh dear. I wonder what's going to happen. We'll have to wait till next time to find out.

EXERCISE 5   Interpreting Ambiguous Sentences

1. My brother and my sister had pet pigs. They just loved to roll around in the mud.

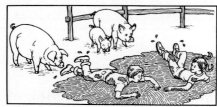

2. We always kept a glass on top of the refrigerator. We kept it full of water.

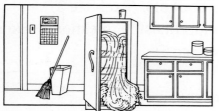

1. Everybody, find part D. ✔
   These are the illustrations that Zelda drew for two parts of the story.
   - You're going to fix up the sentences with the names that Zelda thought the sentences were talking about.
2. Touch number 1. ✔
   The picture below number 1 shows Mrs. Hudson's brother and sister rolling around in the mud.
   - I'll read what number 1 says. You follow along: My brother and my sister had pet pigs. They just loved to roll around in the mud.

- Touch the word that's underlined. ✔
  Everybody, what word is underlined? (Signal.) *They.*
- What was Mrs. Hudson **really** writing about? (Signal.) *The pigs.*
- What did Zelda think she was writing about? (Signal.) *Mrs. Hudson's brother and sister.*

3. Listen: Cross out the word **they** and write **my brother and sister** above the crossed-out word. Raise your hand when you're finished.
   (Observe students and give feedback.)
4. Touch number 2. ✔
   I'll read what it says: We always kept a glass on top of the refrigerator. We kept it full of water.
   - Touch the word that's underlined. ✔
     Everybody, what word is underlined? (Signal.) *It.*
   - What was Mrs. Hudson really writing about? (Signal.) *The glass.*
   - What did Zelda think she was writing about? (Signal.) *The refrigerator.*
   - Listen: Cross out the word **it** and write **the refrigerator.** Raise your hand when you're finished.
     (Observe students and give feedback.)
5. Now the sentences for both pictures tell what Zelda thought she should illustrate.
   - Later you can color the pictures.

Materials: Each student will need a pair of scissors and paste.

Objectives

- Alphabetize words that start with different letters. (Exercise 1)
- **Identify where characters are on a map based on assertions about the direction of a common object.** (Exercise 2)
- **Draw arrows to show the movements of connected components.** (Exercise 3)
- Listen to the conclusion of a 3-part story and answer comprehension questions. (Exercise 4)
- **Use cut-outs to change specific details of a picture.** (Exercise 5)

WORKBOOK

EXERCISE 1 **Alphabetical Order**

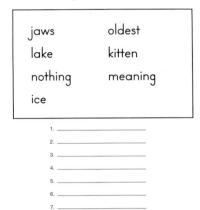

jaws	oldest
lake	kitten
nothing	meaning
ice	

1. _____
2. _____
3. _____
4. _____
5. _____
6. _____
7. _____

1. Open your workbook to lesson 36 and find part A. ✔
- Everybody, say the alphabet. Get ready. (Signal.) *A, B, C, D, E, F, G, H, I, J, K, L, M, N, O, P, Q, R, S, T, U, V, W, X, Y, Z.*
2. Find the words in the box. You're going to write these words in alphabetical order. First, you have to find the word that is earliest in the alphabet.
- I see a word that begins with **J.** Touch that word. ✔
3. See if you can find a word that comes before **J** in the alphabet. ✔
- Who found the word that begins with a letter that comes before **J**? (Call on a student.) *Ice.*
4. The first word for this group begins with **I.**
- Everybody, touch that word. ✔
5. Write that word on line 1. Cross it out from the list. Then write the other words in alphabetical order.
(Observe students and give feedback.)

6. (Write on the board:)

> 1. ice
> 2. jaws
> 3. kitten
> 4. lake
> 5. meaning
> 6. nothing
> 7. oldest

- Here's what you should have.

EXERCISE 2 **Map Directions**

Relative Direction

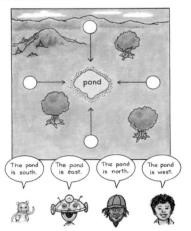

1. Find part B. You can see the map. Below the map are different characters. They are arguing about where the little pond is. You're going to play detective and figure out where each character must be standing.
- Touch the bragging rat. ✔
The bragging rat is saying, **"The pond is south."**
- Touch Bleep. ✔
Bleep is saying, **"The pond is east."**

- Touch Goober. ✔
  What's Goober saying? (Signal.) *The pond is north.*
- Touch Owen. ✔
  What's Owen saying? (Signal.) *The pond is west.*

2. They are saying different things because they are all in different places. Bleep is saying that the pond is east because Bleep would have to go **east** to get to the pond.

- Why is the bragging rat saying, "The pond is south"? (Call on a student. Idea: *Because the bragging rat would have to go south to get to the pond.*)
- Why is Owen saying, "The pond is west"? (Call on a student. Idea: *Because Owen would have to go west to get to the pond.*)
- Why is Goober saying, "The pond is north"? (Call on a student: *Because Goober would have to go north to get to the pond.*)

3. This is tough. Start with the bragging rat. The bragging rat is saying, "The pond is south." That means the rat would have to go south to get to the pond.

- Listen: You're going to write the letter **R** on the map. **R** stands for rat. Write the letter **R** in the circle to show where the bragging rat must be. That's where he'd have to be to say, "The pond is south." Raise your hand when you're finished. ✔
- (Draw on the board:)

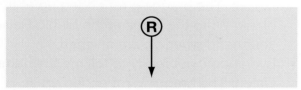

- Here's the arrow you should have for the **R.** That arrow has to point **south.**
- Raise your hand if you got it right.

4. Your turn: Touch Bleep. ✔
   Bleep is saying, "The pond is east."

- Listen: Write the letter **B** in the circle to show where Bleep must be. Put a **B** in the circle that shows where he'd have to be to say, "The pond is east." Raise your hand when you're finished. ✔
- (Add to show:)

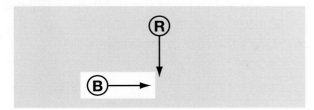

- Here's the arrow you should have for the **B.** That arrow points **east.**
- Raise your hand if you got it right.

5. Touch Goober. ✔
   Goober is saying, "The pond is north."

- Listen: Write the letter **G** in the circle to show where Goober must be. Put a **G** in the circle that shows where he'd have to be to say, "The pond is north." Raise your hand when you're finished. ✔
- (Add to show:)

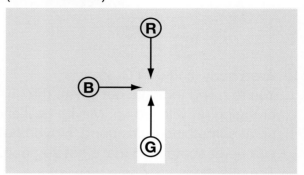

- Here's the arrow you should have for the **G.** That arrow points **north.**
- Raise your hand if you got it right.

6. Touch Owen. ✔
   Owen is saying, "The pond is west." Write the letter **O** in the circle to show where Owen must be. Put an **O** in the circle that shows where he'd have to be to say, "The pond is west." Raise your hand when you're finished.

- (Add to show:)

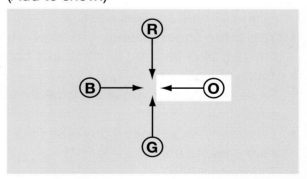

- Here's the arrow you should have for the **O.** That arrow points **west.**
- Raise your hand if you got it right.

7. Raise your hand if you got everything right. This is really rough.

EXERCISE 3   Written Directions

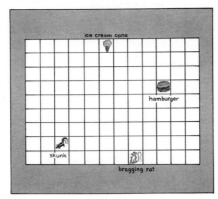

Step A.	4 squares north
Step B.	3 squares west
Step C.	4 squares north
Step D.	2 squares west
Step E.	7 squares south

1. Everybody, find part C. ✔
   You're going to figure out where the bragging rat will end up. Maybe he'll end up at something that's good. Maybe he'll end up at something that's not so good. The directions for where he went are written below the map.
2. Touch step A below the map. ✔
   That says **four squares north.**
- What does it say? (Signal.)
   Four squares north.
- That tells you where the bragging rat went **first.**
- Touch step B. ✔
   Raise your hand if you know what that step says.
- Everybody, what does that step say? (Signal.) *Three squares west.*
- Yes, **three squares west.** That's where the rat went after he went four squares north.
- Touch step C. ✔
   Raise your hand if you know what that step says.
- Everybody, what does it say? (Signal.) *Four squares north.*
- Touch step D. ✔
   Everybody, what does that step say? (Signal.) *Two squares west.*
- Touch step E. ✔
   Everybody, what does that step say? (Signal.) *Seven squares south.*
3. So the bragging rat went four squares north, then three squares west, then four squares north, then two squares west, then seven squares south.

- Touch the bragging rat. ✔
   That's where you start.
- Everybody, draw what the rat did in step A. Draw a line from the rat and put an **A** in the square you end up at after you go four squares **north.** Raise your hand when you're finished.
   (Observe students and give feedback.)
- Now continue from your letter A and do step B. Draw a line three squares west and put a **B** to show where he ends up after he goes three squares west. Raise your hand when you're finished.
   (Observe students and give feedback.)
- (Draw on the board:)

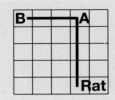

- Here's what you should have so far.
4. Now do steps C, D and E. Remember to draw the line and write the letter of the step to show where the rat is after he completes that step. When you complete step E, you'll know where he ended up. Raise your hand when you're finished.
   (Observe students and give feedback.)
5. When you know where he ends up, you can complete the sentence below step E. It says: The bragging rat ended up at the blank. Write the name in the blank. Raise your hand when you're finished.
- Everybody, get ready to tell me the name. Listen: The bragging rat ended up at the . . . (Signal.) *Skunk.*
- Right, he ended up at the **skunk** again. Phew.
6. Raise your hand if you got it right. Good job.

EXERCISE 4   Zelda The Artist *Part 3*

Storytelling

- I'm going to finish the Zelda story today.
- Everybody, when was Mrs. Hudson's book supposed to be at the publisher? (Signal.) *March.*
- Here's the rest of the story:

Mrs. Hudson sent her book and Zelda's illustrations to the publisher. Mrs. Hudson wrote a note. It said:

Dear Publisher,

I am not completely pleased with the illustrations for this book, and I apologize for them. But I'm sure you'll find the writing very interesting. The book tells about one enjoyable experience after another.

She signed the note: Sincerely, Mrs. R. R. Hudson.

In the meantime, Zelda was trying to forget about that book. She was working on illustrations for an animal book. She tried to keep her mind on the animals she was drawing, but she couldn't help thinking about Mrs. Hudson's book. "I worked a long time on that book," she told herself, "and I did the best job I could. I can't help it if I drew the wrong kind of windows on that mountain. And how do I know what kind of gas gauges mountains have? That Mrs. Hudson shouldn't have been so mean to me."

Weeks went by. Zelda heard nothing from Mrs. Hudson. Mrs. Hudson heard nothing from the publisher.

But things were very busy at the publisher. The publisher read the book and laughed so hard that her ribs hurt for three days. She read about each of Mrs. Hudson's boring experiences. Then she looked at the picture and almost died from laughter.

She called in other people who worked at the publishing company to read the book, and they all had the same reaction. They all ended up with sore ribs for three days.

- Why were their ribs sore for three days? (Call on a student. Idea: *From laughing so hard.*)

One of the persons who read the book made a suggestion to the publisher. She said, "What you should do is make each of these illustrations two full pages big. Then underneath you could have the sentences from the book that tell about the illustration."

And that's just what the publisher did. When the publishing company was finished with the book and it was ready to be printed, the picture of the children riding their horses was two full pages. Below the picture, it said: "Every day, the children rode their horses through the valley. Their tails flew in the wind."

The picture of the car on the mountain was two full pages. Below the picture is said: "Our car stopped on top of the mountain. It was out of gas."

And all the other pictures were also two pages, with Mrs. Hudson's sentences written below each picture.

Well, after the book was printed, the publisher sent copies to Mrs. Hudson and to Zelda. Mrs. Hudson didn't really like the book as much as she thought she would. She thought that the pictures were far, far too large. She said to herself, "Huh, they made the pictures more important than my wonderful experiences."

Zelda was very happy. She was even happier when she read the note the publisher sent to her. The note said:

Dear Zelda,

I find your pictures superb. You have taken a very boring book and made it exciting and wonderfully funny. Thank you so much.

- The note said, "I find your pictures superb." What does "superb" mean? (Call on a student. Idea: *Excellent, great, super.*)

And, when the bookstores got their copies of Mrs. Hudson's book, they didn't keep them very long. Within a few weeks, the bookstores sold thousands of copies of the book. Within three months, that book was the fastest-selling bestseller book in the world. Newspaper articles raved about the book. One report said this:

R. R. Hudson may be the greatest wit of the century. When you first read the book, you get the idea that she doesn't know how to write clearly. She makes up sentences that could have more than one meaning. And, as you read about her boring experiences, you begin to wonder: Does this woman have anything to say? But then, you come across an illustration that makes everything clear. The illustrations are so funny that they are hard to describe. The best way to appreciate them is to get the book and look at them. And that's just what **a lot** of people are doing.

After the book became so popular, Mrs. Hudson sort of pretended that she had planned it that way. She told reporters, "Yes, my good friend Zelda and I planned it that way. I selected the parts of the book she was to illustrate, and I might add that I selected them very carefully. Then Zelda did those quaint illustrations."

So Mrs. Hudson became very famous. And very rich.

And the book also made another person very rich and very popular.

- Everybody, who was that? (Signal.) *Zelda.*

But Zelda never really understood why people found the book so funny. She told reporters, "I just did the best I could with the sentences Mrs. Hudson gave me."

And the reporters would laugh so hard that their ribs hurt for three days.

EXERCISE 5   Interpreting Ambiguous Sentences

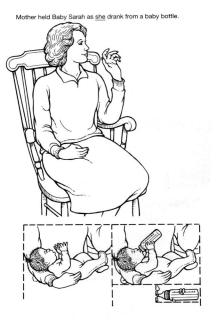

Mother held Baby Sarah as <u>she</u> drank from a baby bottle.

1. Everybody, find part D. ✔
   This is a picture from Mrs. Hudson's book and a sentence that she wrote.
- Touch the sentence. ✔
   I'll read what it says: Mother held Baby Sarah as she drank from a baby bottle.
- No word is underlined. I'll read it again. Raise your hand when you know which word will confuse Zelda. Here we go: Mother . . . held . . . Baby . . . Sarah . . . as . . . she . . . drank. . . from . . . a . . . baby . . . bottle.
- What word would confuse Zelda? (Signal.) *She.*
- Everybody, when Mrs. Hudson wrote, "as **she** drank from a baby bottle," who was she telling about? (Signal.) *Baby Sarah.*
- Who would **Zelda** think she was talking about? (Signal.) *Mother.*
- Yes, Zelda thought that **Mother** was drinking from a baby bottle. Cross out **she** and write **Mother.** Raise your hand when you're finished.
   (Observe students and give feedback.)
- I'll read what Zelda thought the sentence meant: Mother held Baby Sarah as Mother drank from a baby bottle. That's what your sentence should say.

2. Look at the picture.
   That's Mrs. Hudson's mother. You're going to fix up the picture the way Zelda drew it. In that picture Mrs. Hudson's mother is holding something in each hand.
   - Touch the hand that's down low. ✔ Everybody, what would she be holding in that hand? (Signal.) *Baby Sarah.*
   - Touch the hand that's up by her face. ✔ What would she be holding in that hand? (Signal.) *A baby bottle.*

3. At the bottom of the page are pictures of Baby Sarah without the bottle, Baby Sarah drinking from the bottle and the bottle.
   - You'll use two of those pictures. Cut out the right pictures and fix up the big picture so it looks like it did when Zelda drew it. When you cut out that bottle, cut carefully around the dotted lines. Raise your hand when you're finished.
   (Observe students and give feedback.)
   - (Tell students who have cut-outs appropriately positioned to paste them.)
   - Poor Zelda. She **really** got confused. And remember that the publisher made this picture two full pages.

4. Later you can color the picture.

Objectives

- **Write a group of sentences that are thematically related.** (Exercise 1)
- Draw routes based on instructions that tell about distance and direction. (Exercise 2)
- **Identify a specific picture sequence by applying clues about the order of actions shown.** (Exercise 3).
- Edit ambiguous sentences to show how a character interpreted them. (Exercise 4)
- Listen to a familiar story. (Exercise 5)

LINED PAPER

EXERCISE 1   Sentence Writing

1. Everybody, find the page titled **Story words** at the front of your workbook.
- Today, you're going to write sentences that make up little stories.
2. (Write on the board:)

> **Everybody played.**

- This says: Everybody played.
- Copy that sentence on the second line of your paper. Remember the capital and the period. Raise your hand when you've copied the sentence.
(Observe students and give feedback.)
3. (Write to show:)

> **Everybody played.**
> **Dot played with** _____.

- Here's the first part of the sentence you'll write next. Dot played with blank. You're going to complete the sentence for Dot. She played with one of the things shown on the page with **Story words.**
- Write your sentence about Dot. Raise your hand when you're finished.
(Observe students and give feedback.)
- (Call on individual students to read their sentence for Dot.)
4. (Write to show:)

> **Everybody played.**
> **Dot played with** _____.
> **Zelda** _____.
> **I** _____.

- You're going to write more sentences. One will tell about Zelda and what she played with. The other will tell about you and what you played with.
- Your turn: Write both sentences. Remember the period at the end of each sentence. Raise your hand when you're finished.
(Observe students and give feedback.)
- (Call on individual students to read their sentence about Zelda. Then call on individual students to read their sentence about themselves.)

WORKBOOK

EXERCISE 2   Written Directions

Step A.	3 squares north
Step B.	1 square east
Step C.	1 square south
Step D.	3 squares west
Step E.	4 squares north

The skunk ended up at the _____

1. Open your workbook to lesson 37 and find part A. ✔
Here's a map that shows a skunk going some places. I wonder who's going to get the stink attack. Let's follow the directions and find out.
2. Touch step A. ✔
Raise your hand if you know what step A says.
- Everybody, what does it say? (Signal.)
Three squares north.

- Touch step B. ✔

  What does it say? (Signal.) *One square east.*
- Touch step C. ✔

  What does it say? (Signal.) *One square south.*
- Touch step D. ✔

  What does it say? (Signal.) *Three squares west.*
- Touch step E. ✔

  What does it say? (Signal.) *Four squares north.*

3. Listen: Start at the skunk. Follow the directions very carefully. Start with step A and write an A where you end up after you go 3 squares north. Then do all the steps in order. Use a pencil and make a line to show where the skunk goes. When you're done, you should have the letters A through E on your map. Raise your hand when you know where the skunk ended up at the end of step E.

   (Observe students and give feedback.)

4. Now you can fill in the sentence below step E to tell where the skunk ended up. Copy the name from the picture. Raise your hand when you're finished. ✔

- Everybody, get ready to tell me the name. Listen: The skunk ended up at the . . . (Signal.) *rat.*
- That poor bragging rat.

5. Raise your hand if you got it right. Good job.

EXERCISE 3   Clue Game

After

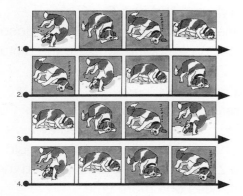

1. Everybody, find part B. ✔

   These four arrows show different things that Dud did.
- I'll give you clues. You'll figure out which arrows the clues tell about. To do that, you'll circle pictures I tell about.

2. Touch arrow 1. ✔

   The first picture shows Dud somersaulting in the snow. What did he do just after he somersaulted? (Signal.) *Ate a ham bone.*
- Yes, he ate a ham bone.
- What did he do just after he ate a ham bone? (Signal.) *Slept.*
- That last picture shows him tracking in the snow. That's what he did just after he slept.

3. Touch arrow 2.

   What did Dud do first? (Signal.) *Slept.*
- What did he do after he slept? (Signal.) *Somersaulted.*
- What did he do after he somersaulted in the snow? (Signal.) *Tracked.*
- What did he do after he tracked in the snow? (Signal.) *Ate a ham bone.*

4. I'm thinking about one of the arrows on this page. Here's the clue about the arrow I'm thinking of: On this arrow, Dud ate a ham bone just after he tracked in the snow.
- Find the first arrow that shows Dud ate a ham bone just **after** he tracked in the snow. Raise your hand when you know the first arrow with those pictures.
- Everybody, what's the number of the first arrow that shows Dud eating a ham bone just after he tracked in the snow? (Signal.) *Two.*
- (Draw on the board:)

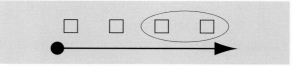

- Look at the picture on the board. You're going to fix arrow 2 in your workbook so it looks like the arrow on the board. You draw one big circle around the pictures that show **Dud ate a ham bone just after he tracked in the snow.**
- Make your circle on arrow 2. Then find any other arrows that show **Dud ate a ham bone just after he tracked in the snow** and circle the pictures. Raise your hand when you're finished.

  (Observe students and give feedback.)
- Everybody, did you draw a circle around the pictures on arrow 3? (Signal.) *Yes.*
- Yes, the first two pictures on arrow 3 show Dud eating a ham bone just after he tracked in the snow. So you should have a circle around the first two pictures.

- Everybody, did you draw a circle around the pictures on arrow 4? (Signal.) *Yes.*
- Yes, the middle two pictures on arrow 4 show Dud eating a ham bone just after he tracked in the snow. So you should have a circle around the middle two pictures.
- Raise your hand if you have a circle on arrow 2, arrow 3 and arrow 4. ✔
- The mystery arrow could be any arrow that shows Dud eating a ham bone just after he tracked in the snow. One of the arrows could not be the mystery arrow. Raise your hand when you know which arrow could not be the mystery arrow. ✔
- Everybody, which arrow? (Signal.) *One.*
- Draw a line through the pictures on arrow 1 because it couldn't be the mystery arrow. Raise your hand when you're finished. ✔

5. Here's clue 2 about the mystery arrow: The mystery arrow shows Dud sleeping just after he ate a ham bone.
- Look at the arrows that are not crossed out. Draw a circle around the picture of **Dud sleeping just after he ate a ham bone.** Don't get fooled. Find him sleeping just after eating and circle him sleeping. Raise your hand when you're finished. **(Observe students and give feedback.)**
- You should have circled Dud sleeping on two arrows. What's the first arrow that shows Dud sleeping just after he ate a ham bone? (Signal.) *Three.*
- What's the other arrow that shows Dud sleeping just after he ate a ham bone? (Signal.) *Four.*
- You can cross out one more arrow because it doesn't show both clues about Dud. Raise your hand when you know the new arrow you can cross out. ✔
- Everybody, which arrow? (Signal.) *Two.*
- Draw a line through the pictures on arrow 2. It couldn't be the mystery arrow. It shows Dud eating a ham bone just after he tracked in the snow, but it doesn't show Dud sleeping just after he ate a ham bone.

6. Here's the last clue. Listen: The mystery arrow shows Dud somersaulting in the snow just after he slept. Listen again: The mystery arrow shows Dud somersaulting in the snow just after he slept.

- Circle any picture that shows Dud somersaulting just after he slept. Raise your hand when you're finished. **(Observe students and give feedback.)**
- You should have circled Dud somersaulting just after he slept on arrow 3.
- Now cross out any arrow that could not be the mystery arrow. Raise your hand when you're finished. ✔
- You should have crossed out arrow 4. Now you know the mystery arrow. It's the only arrow not crossed out. Everybody, which arrow is the mystery arrow? (Signal.) *Three.*
- Here's a tough question: Why couldn't arrow 4 be the mystery arrow? (Call on a student. Idea: *It doesn't show Dud somersaulting in the snow just after he slept.*)

7. Raise your hand if you followed all the clues and found the mystery arrow. Good for you.

EXERCISE 4   Interpreting Ambiguous Sentences

1. Our car made a dust cloud. It floated away.

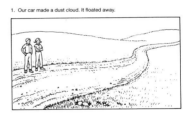

2. A frog was on top of the car. It had big black spots all over.

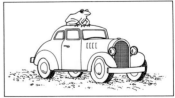

1. Everybody, find part C. ✔
   These are sentences that Mrs. Hudson wrote. You're going to fix up the picture the way Zelda would draw it.
2. Touch number 1. ✔
   I'll read what it says. Follow along: Our car made a dust cloud. It floated away.
- You have to find the word that would give Zelda the wrong idea. I'll read the sentences one more time.
   Our . . . car . . . made . . . a . . . dust . . . cloud. It . . . floated . . . away. Raise your hand when you know the word that could confuse Zelda. ✔

- Everybody, what word would give Zelda the wrong idea? (Signal.) *It.*
- Yes, the word **it.** Underline that word in item 1. Raise your hand when you're finished.
  (Observe students and give feedback.)
- When Mrs. Hudson wrote, "It floated away," was she telling about the dust cloud or the car? (Signal.) *The dust cloud.*
- But what would Zelda think had floated away? (Signal.) *The car.*
3. You're going to play a silly game. You're going to write the words that Zelda thought the sentence told about. She didn't think the dust cloud floated away. What did Zelda think the sentence told about? (Signal.) *The car.*
- So cross out the word **it** and write the words **the car** above it. Raise your hand when you're finished. ✔
- Now the sentences say what Zelda thought Mrs. Hudson meant. Listen: Our car made a dust cloud. The car floated away.
- Later you'll fix up the picture to show how Zelda would draw it. You'll have to show a car floating up in the air.
4. Touch number 2. ✔
  I'll read number 2. Follow along: A frog was on top of the car. It had big black spots all over.
- You have to find the word that would give Zelda the wrong idea. I'll read what it says again. Follow along: A . . . frog . . . was . . . on . . . top . . . of . . . the . . . car. It . . . had . . . big . . . black . . . spots . . . all . . . over.
- Everybody, what word would give Zelda the wrong idea? (Signal.) *It.*
- The word is **it.** Underline that word. Raise your hand when you're finished.
  (Observe students and give feedback.)
- When Mrs. Hudson wrote, "It had big black spots all over," was she telling about the frog or the car? (Signal.) *The frog.*
- But what would Zelda think had spots all over it? (Signal.) *The car.*
- You're going to play that silly game again. You're going to write the words that Zelda thought the second sentence told about. What did she think the sentence told about? (Signal.) *The car.*

- So cross out the word **it** and write the words **the car** above it. Raise your hand when you're finished. ✔
- Now the sentence says what Zelda thought Mrs. Hudson meant: Listen: A frog was on top of the car. The car had big black spots all over.
5. Later you'll fix up the picture to show how Zelda would draw it. You'll have to make big black spots all over that car.
- Do a good job of making the picture the way Zelda would do it, and I'll show you some of the better pictures next time.

EXERCISE 5   Dot and Dud
Review

- I'm going to read the last part of the story about Dot and Dud again. Remember that Dud got separated from the rest of the dogs. And he got dizzy from doing something.
- Why did he get dizzy? (Call on a student. Idea: *He was zigzagging and somersaulting in the snow.*)
  Then he went in the wrong direction.
- Everybody, which direction was that? (Signal.) *South.*
- Which direction was Dot? (Signal.) *North.* Dud ended up at the ski lodge. Dot had found the mountain climber. What was she trying to do? (Call on a student. Idea: *Help the mountain climber keep warm.*)
- Here's the story.

That evening, while Dud was snoozing next to a warm stove in the kitchen, full of food and dreaming about summertime, a truck pulled up to the ski lodge, and the ranger came inside to pick up Dud. The cook had called the rescue station and left a message that one of their St. Bernards was at the ski lodge.

The ranger was not happy. He led Dud to the truck and put him in the back with all the other St. Bernards. They were coming back from their search. They hadn't found the stranded mountain climber, and they hadn't found

Dot. The ranger decided that it was best to go home before it got dark in the mountains and go out again early in the morning.

Of course, Dud didn't know that Dot was stranded on the mountain. When he got in the back of the pickup with the other dogs, they didn't even look at him. They didn't start griping about how he didn't keep up with them and got lost. They didn't remind him that he didn't even know **north** from **south** or that his nose was about as useful as another paw. They just sat there, weary from plowing through the snow all day and worrying about Dot.

As the truck went down the road back to the rescue station, Dud tried to strike up a conversation with the other dogs. "How did things go today?" he asked.

Two of the dogs looked at him but didn't answer. The other dogs didn't even look at him.

"Did you find the mountain climber?"

None of the dogs looked at him or said anything.

"You took pretty tired. Have you had anything to eat?" Dud asked.

Again, no answer.

"I had some great soup at the ski lodge. And a big plateful of meat scraps. And after I ate that, I took . . ."

"Will you shut up?" the oldest dog said.

So Dud was quiet for a while. Then he looked around and noticed that Dot wasn't in the truck. "Hey," he said, "where's Dot?"

"Lost," one of the St. Bernards said.

"What do you mean? Where is she?"

The oldest St. Bernard said, "Somewhere on the mountain. We couldn't find her."

"Do you mean that she's out there all alone?"

Some of the dogs nodded yes.

This was no game. Dud loved Dot. He didn't always show it, but he loved her. As he sat in the back of that truck, he remembered her from way, way back when the two of them were little puppies. She always stuck up for him when the other puppies in the litter would pick on him. Dud remembered a lot of other things as that truck moved slowly down the snowy road. He remembered how sad he had been when Dot and Dud had to leave their mother and their other brothers and sisters. The only good thing about going to the rescue station was that Dot had been there. She had always been there. But now . . . she was gone.

"No," Dud said out loud. "She **can't** be lost."

All the other dogs looked down.

"Why didn't you find her? You can't leave her out there."

"She'll be all right—if we find her tomorrow."

Dud said, "But what if she found the mountain climber? Won't he freeze during the night?"

All the other dogs looked down.

Dud didn't say anything more. But he did a lot of thinking. And the biggest thought he had was this: "If they can't find her, **I'll** find her." This wasn't one of those promises he made when he was only half serious and half embarrassed for being foolish. This wasn't one of those promises like "I'll try" or "I'll do better next time." This was a **real** promise: "**I'll** find her."

At last, the truck stopped in front of the rescue station. The ranger opened the back door, and out bounded Dud, just as fast as he could bound. He ran north. The ranger was shouting, "Dud, come back here! Where do you think you're going in the dark?"

The other dogs were yelling at him, too. "Yeah! Where do you think you're going in the dark?"

But Dud knew exactly where he was going—north.

Pretty soon, some of the other dogs started to follow Dud. Then the rest of the dogs started to follow. Then the ranger started to follow. And away everybody went, plowing through the deep snow and heading up that mountain.

Dud was all business. He said to himself, "I know Dot's smell better than any other dog in the world, and I'll find that smell. I **will.**"

He put his nose in the snow and snorted and sniffed. He didn't care that the snow was cold. He didn't even **notice** that it was cold. Again and again—snort, sniff, snort, sniff. Then he did it the fast way—he just put his head deep into the snow and kept it there—like a snowplow—snorting and sniffing as he went up that mountain as fast as he could run. Then, suddenly he recognized a faint smell in the snow— very faint. But he knew that smell. It was Dot.

"Come on, you guys," he yelled at the other dogs, "Follow me."

And up the mountain Dud went once more, with his head in the snow like a snowplow. He followed that smell up, up, up the mountain. When he came to steep parts and slid down, he just tried again until he made it. Her smell was getting stronger in the snow. She was closer, and closer, and . . . suddenly, Dud came to the rocky part where Dot was lying with the mountain climber.

He called back down to the other dogs, "Up here, you guys. I found her."

While he waited for the other dogs, he sat down next to Dot. "Are you okay?" he asked.

"Yes, but I'm sure glad you got here. This climber is seriously injured. I don't think he could make it through the night."

Then she looked at Dud and said, "What are **you** doing here?"

"Looking for you," Dud said.

She couldn't believe it. "And you found me without getting lost?"

"Well . . ." he said. "I got a little lost once."

She said, "Well, I'm sure glad to see you." She wagged her tail. He wagged his tail.

Soon, the ranger and the other St. Bernards made it up the steep slope. The ranger had a little sled. He put the injured climber on the sled. Then he and the dogs lowered the sled down the very steep part of the mountain. Then the dogs pulled the sled back to the rescue station.

After the ranger took care of the injured climber, and all the dogs were back in the kennel, the oldest St. Bernard looked at Dud and said, "See? That shows what you can do when you put your mind to it. When you try hard, you're a pretty good rescue dog."

The other dogs said, "Yeah, pretty good."

Then the oldest dog said, "We're glad that you found Dot. And here's our way of thanking you." The oldest dog picked up a great big ham bone, brought it over to Dud and dropped it in front of him.

Dud started to say, "Oh, I really can't accept that ham bone. I really shouldn't eat this great big . . ." But then he looked at that ham bone and it **looked** so good and **smelled** so good that he stopped talking and started doing something else.

- Everybody, what do you think he started doing? (Signal.)
Eating that ham bone.
- Yes.

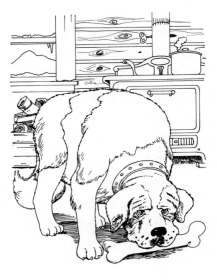

- Find part D. ✔
There's Dud, gnawing away on the ham bone. Later, you can color the picture.

Objectives

- Alphabetize words that start with different letters. (Exercise 1)
- Identify where characters are on a map based on assertions about the direction of a common object. (Exercise 2)
- Edit an ambiguous sentence to show how a character interpreted it. (Exercise 3)
- Listen to part 1 of a story and answer comprehension questions. (Exercise 4)
- Say different deductions based on pictures. (Exercise 5)

WORKBOOK

EXERCISE 1 Alphabetical Order

restful	question
pound	until
older	thing
something	

1. _____
2. _____
3. _____
4. _____
5. _____
6. _____
7. _____

1. Open your workbook to lesson 38 and find part A. ✔

- Everybody, say the alphabet. Get ready. (Signal.) *A, B, C, D, E, F, G, H, I, J, K, L, M, N, O, P, Q, R, S, T, U, V, W, X, Y, Z.*

2. Find the words in the box. You're going to write these words in alphabetical order. First, you have to find the word that is earliest in the alphabet.

- I see a word that begins with **P.** Touch that word. ✔

3. See if you can find a word that comes before **P** in the alphabet. ✔

4. Who found the word that begins with a letter that comes before **P?** (Call on a student.) *Older.*

5. The first word for this group begins with **O.**

- Everybody, touch that word. ✔

6. Write that word on line 1. Cross it out from the list. Then write the other words in alphabetical order.
(Observe students and give feedback.)

7. (Write on the board:)

> 1. older
> 2. pound
> 3. question
> 4. restful
> 5. something
> 6. thing
> 7. until

- Here's what you should have.

EXERCISE 2 Map Directions

Relative Direction

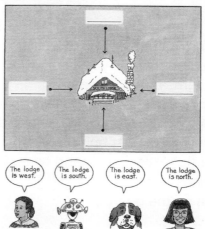

1. Find part B. ✔
Here's a map, and below the map are different characters. They are arguing about where the ski lodge is. You're going to play detective again.

- Touch Zelda. ✔
- Zelda is saying, "The lodge is west."
- Touch Bleep. ✔
Bleep is saying, "The lodge is south."
- Touch Dot. ✔
What's Dot saying? (Signal.) *The lodge is east.*

- Touch Molly. ✔
  What's Molly saying? (Signal.) *The lodge is north.*
2. They are saying different things because they are all in different places. Bleep is saying that the lodge is south because Bleep would have to go south to get to the lodge.
- Why is Zelda saying, "The lodge is west?" (Call on a student. Idea: *Because Zelda would have to go west to get to the lodge.*)
- Why is Molly saying, "The lodge is north"? (Call on a student. Idea: *Because Molly would have to go north to get to the lodge.*)
  Why is Dot saying, "The lodge is east?" (Call on a student. Idea: *Because Dot would have to go east to get to the lodge.*)
3. Start with Zelda. She is saying, "The lodge is west." That means she would have to go west to get to the lodge.
- Listen: Write **Zelda** on the line to show where Zelda must be to say, "The lodge is west." Raise your hand when you're finished. ✔
- (Write on the board:)

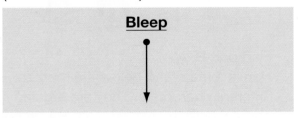

- Here's the arrow you should have for **Zelda.** That arrow points west.
- Raise your hand if you got it right.
4. Your turn: Touch Bleep. ✔
  Bleep is saying, "The lodge is south."
- Listen: Write **Bleep** on the line to show where Bleep must be to say, "The lodge is south." Raise your hand when you're finished.
- (Write on the board:)

Bleep

- Here's the arrow you should have for **Bleep.** That arrow points south.
- Raise your hand if you got it right.
5. Touch Dot. ✔
  Dot is saying, "The lodge is east."

- Listen: Write **Dot** on the line to show where Dot must be to say, "The lodge is east." Raise your hand when you're finished. ✔
- (Write on the board:)

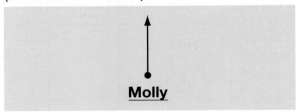

- Here's the arrow you should have for **Dot.** That arrow points east.
- Raise your hand if you got it right.
6. Touch Molly. ✔
  Molly is saying, "The lodge is north." Write **Molly** on the line to show where Molly must be to say, "The lodge is north." Raise your hand when you're finished. ✔
- (Write on the board:)

Molly

- Here's the arrow you should have for **Molly.** That arrow points north.
- Raise your hand if you got it right.
7. Raise your hand if you got everything right. Excellent.

EXERCISE 3 Interpreting Ambiguous Sentences

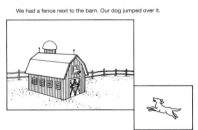

We had a fence next to the barn. Our dog jumped over it.

1. Everybody, find part C. ✔
  You're going to fix up a sentence to show what Zelda thought it meant. Then you're going to fix up the picture the way Zelda would do it.
- The big trick is to find the word that confused Zelda.
- I'll read what Mrs. Hudson wrote. Raise your hand when you know the word that confused Zelda: We had a fence next to the barn. Our dog jumped over it.

- Listen again: We had a fence next to the barn. Our dog jumped over it.
- Everybody, what word would confuse Zelda? (Signal.) *It.*
- What did Mrs. Hudson mean when she wrote: Our dog jumped over it? (Signal.) *Our dog jumped over the fence.*
- What would Zelda think the dog jumped over? (Signal.) *The barn.*

2. Cross out the word **it**. Above your cross-out, write the words that Zelda **thought** were correct. Raise your hand when you're finished. ✔
- You should have written these words above the word **it: the barn.** Raise your hand if you got it right. ✔

3. Later you can fix up the picture the way Zelda would have done it. You'll have to draw a dog jumping over that barn.

EXERCISE 4 The Case of the Missing Corn *Part 1*

Storytelling

- I'm going to read some more about the gray rat who wanted to be a detective.

> The gray rat worked at deductions until he could figure out an answer faster than any other rat in the pack. If somebody said, "Where's Martha the moth?" he'd say, "In the afternoon, all the moths are sleeping in the shed. Martha is a moth. So, in the afternoon, Martha is sleeping in the shed."
>
> The gray rat was so good at deductions that he said, "Now I'm ready to be a detective. And I'll solve crimes."
>
> He looked through some books to learn more about detectives. He learned that some of them have hound dogs called bloodhounds that can follow the scent of people.

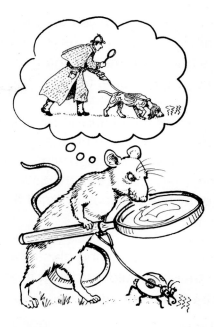

- If you look at part D, you can see a picture of a bloodhound. It's a dog that looks like its skin is too big for it. It has wrinkles all over it. But bloodhounds have a very good nose. Police and detectives use them to track people they are trying to find. Listen to that part the story again:

> The gray rat looked through some books to learn more about detectives. He learned that some of them have hound dogs called bloodhounds that can follow the scent of people.
>
> It didn't make much sense for a rat to have a great big bloodhound on a leash, but the gray rat knew a shy little beetle with a very good nose. Her name was Bertha. He went to Bertha and talked her into being his **blood**beetle.

- Why did the gray rat think of Bertha as a bloodbeetle instead of just a beetle? (Call on a student. Idea: *She would work like a **blood**hound.*)

> Bertha didn't like wearing a leash very much, but the gray rat told her that, if she wanted to be a detective's bloodbeetle, she'd have to wear the leash.

Next, the gray rat got a large magnifying glass. The detectives in the books had large magnifying glasses, so the gray rat got one, too.

- If you look at the picture in part D, you can see the detective with his magnifying glass and the rat with his magnifying glass. A magnifying glass makes things look bigger, so a detective can look at small things and study them carefully.

The rat's magnifying glass was so large that he could hardly lift it. So he didn't use it very much.

The only thing the rat needed to become a complete detective was a name. He thought and thought. One of the detectives in the books was named Sherlock. So the gray rat decided to name himself Sherlock.

So now he was ready to figure out the answers to puzzles. He knew how to work deductions; he had a bloodbeetle and a magnifying glass. And with the name of "Sherlock," everybody would know that he was a detective.

Just about the time that he was ready to start being a detective, a great problem came up in the rat pack. There was a very special pile of corn in the corner of Goober's barn. This corn was in a place where none of the horses or cows could get it. The corn was special because all the rats agreed that the corn could be eaten as dessert.

Every day after dinner, each rat would go to the barn and have two kernels of corn—only two.

But lots of corn was missing from the pile, and the rats were getting mad at each other. The little black rat said to the rat with yellow teeth, "You ate that corn."

"I did not," the yellow-toothed rat said. "You ate it."

Some of the rats even said that the wise old rat was eating it.

This was the greatest argument that ever took place in the rat pack. Everybody was angry because, when that pile of corn was gone, nobody would have any dessert until next year. Boo-hoo.

Well, the gray rat said to himself, "This is a perfect spot for a detective." He put his bloodbeetle on her leash, stood up very straight and walked out to where the other rats were arguing. He decided to leave his magnifying glass at home.

"Calm down," he said loudly. "Listen to me. I have an announcement to make."

Before the gray rat could continue, five rats pointed to him and said, "You stole that corn."

"No, no, I didn't steal any . . ."

Poor Sherlock wasn't able to finish what he was trying to say. "You're the corn stealer," the rats shouted. Nine or ten rats picked him up, carried him to the pond and threw him in. Splash. Sherlock's bloodbeetle saw what happened to Sherlock and ran home the fast way.

- That bloodbeetle thought that something might happen to her. What was that? (Call on a student. Idea: *Get thrown into the pond.*)

While Bertha was running home, the rats were pointing their little paws at Sherlock and saying, "Don't you ever steal our dessert again."

Sherlock sputtered and said, "But I didn't steal any corn. You don't understand. I'm a detective, and I can help you find the thief."

"You can help us? How can you help us?"

As Sherlock waded out of the pond, he said, "I can use my skill at making deductions, and I can track anybody with my bloodbeetle."

"What bloodbeetle?"

Sherlock looked around, but there was no bloodbeetle in sight.

"You're just lying," the other rats said, and they started to throw Sherlock back into the pond. But just then the wise old rat said, "Stop. Listen to what he has to say. Maybe he can solve this mystery."

The other rats let go of Sherlock. He looked around and then said, "I do have a bloodbeetle, and, if you give me a chance, I'll solve this mystery for you. But if I find the corn thief, you'll have to give me something for helping you. I think that I should get three times as much dessert as any other rat."

The rats argued about this offer for a while, and then they told Sherlock that, if he solved the mystery, he could get **two** times as much dessert as anybody else. And one rat said, "But if you don't solve this mystery pretty quick, nobody's going to have **any** dessert. That corn is disappearing fast."

Sherlock stood up straight again, and, with water dripping off the end of his nose, he said, "I will start solving this crime immediately."

- What's the mystery that the gray rat was going to solve? (Call on a student. Idea: *Who stole the corn.*)
- How much corn did the rats get for each dessert? (Signal.) *Two kernels.*
- When did they get their corn treat? (Signal.) *After dinner.*

- Where was that secret corn? (Call on a student. Idea: *In a corner of Goober's barn.*)
- I wonder how the gray rat plans to solve this mystery.

EXERCISE 5 Deductions

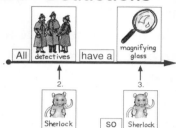

1. Find part E. ✔
   The arrows show one of the deductions that Sherlock used.
2. Touch arrow 1. ✔
- What's in the first picture? (Signal.) *Detectives.*
- What's in the second picture? (Signal.) *A magnifying glass.*
- Raise your hand when you can say the rule for arrow 1. ✔
3. Everybody, say the rule for arrow 1. (Signal.) *All detectives have a magnifying glass.*
- (Repeat step 3 until firm.)
4. Touch arrow 2. That's Sherlock. ✔
- Everybody, say the sentence for arrow 2. (Signal.) *Sherlock is a detective.*
- Touch arrow 3. Everybody, say the sentence for arrow 3. (Signal.) *So Sherlock has a magnifying glass.*
5. You're going to say the whole deduction. Then you're going to write the whole deduction on the lines below the bottom arrows.
6. Say the whole deduction starting with the rule for arrow 1. Get ready. (Signal.) *All detectives have a magnifying glass. Sherlock is a detective. So Sherlock has a magnifying glass.*
- (Repeat step 6 until firm.)
7. Your turn: Write the whole deduction. Write the sentences for arrow 1, arrow 2 and arrow 3. The words you'll need are on the arrows. Make sure you write those words correctly. Also, remember to start each sentence with a capital letter and end it with a period. Raise your hand when you're finished.
   (Observe students and give feedback.)

Objectives

- Alphabetize words that start with different letters. (Exercise 1)
- Identify a specific picture sequence by applying clues about the order of actions shown. (Exercise 2)
- Edit an ambiguous sentence to show how a character interpreted it. (Exercise 3)
- Listen to part 2 of a story and answer comprehension questions. (Exercise 4)
- **Identify the order of parts in a formally correct deduction. (Exercise 5)**

WORKBOOK

EXERCISE 1 Alphabetical Order

wishful	ugly
time	x–ray
zoo	van
yawning	

1. _____
2. _____
3. _____
4. _____
5. _____
6. _____

1. Open your workbook to lesson 39 and find part A. ✔
- Everybody, say the alphabet. Get ready. (Signal.) *A, B, C, D, E, F, G, H, I, J, K, L, M, N, O, P, Q, R, S, T, U, V, W, X, Y, Z.*
2. Find the words in the box. You're going to write these words in alphabetical order. First, you have to find the word that is earliest in the alphabet.
- I see a word that begins with **V.** Touch that word. ✔
3. See if you can find a word that comes before **V** in the alphabet. ✔
4. Who found the word that begins with a letter that comes before **V**? (Call on a student.) *Ugly.*
5. The first word for this group begins with **T.**
- Everybody, touch that word. ✔
6. Write that word on line 1. Cross it out from the list. Then write the other words in alphabetical order.
   (Observe students and give feedback.)

7. (Write on the board:)

> **1. time**
> **2. ugly**
> **3. van**
> **4. wishful**
> **5. x-ray**
> **6. yawning**
> **7. zoo**

- Here's what you should have.

EXERCISE 2 Clue Game

After

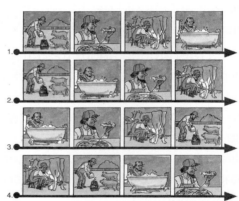

1. Find part B. These arrows show different things Goober did. I'll give you clues for the mystery arrow. You'll cross out the arrows that could not be the mystery arrow.
2. Touch arrow 1. ✔
   The first picture shows Goober feeding pigs. What did he do just after he fed the pigs? (Signal.) *Ate pizza.*
- Yes, he ate pizza. What did he do after he ate pizza? (Signal.) *Milked a cow.*
- And what did Goober do just after he milked a cow? (Signal.) *Took a bath.*

3. Touch arrow 2. What did Goober do first? (Signal.) *Fed the pigs.*

- What did he do after he fed the pigs? (Signal.) *Took a bath.*

- What did he do after he took a bath? (Signal.) *Ate pizza.*

- What did he do after he ate pizza? (Signal.) *Milked a cow.*

4. Here's the first clue for the mystery arrow: On that arrow Goober milked a cow just after he ate pizza. He milked the cow just after he ate pizza.

- Look at each arrow. Circle the two pictures on any arrow that show Goober milking a cow just after he ate pizza. Raise your hand when you're finished.
(Observe students and give feedback.)

- You should have drawn circles on three arrows. Arrow 1, arrow 2 and arrow 3. Raise your hand if you have a circle on arrows 1, 2 and 3.

- One of the arrows could not be the mystery arrow because it does not show Goober milking a cow just after he ate pizza. Draw a line through the arrow that could not be the mystery arrow. Raise your hand when you're finished. ✔

- Everybody, what's the number of the arrow that could not be the mystery arrow? (Signal.) *Four.*

5. Here's clue 2 about the mystery arrow: The mystery arrow shows Goober eating pizza just after he took a bath.

- Look at the arrows that are not crossed out and draw a circle around any picture of Goober eating pizza just after he took a bath. Raise your hand when you're finished.
(Observe students and give feedback.)

- You should have circled pictures on arrows 2 and 3. You can cross out one more arrow because it doesn't show both clues about Goober. Cross out that arrow. Raise your hand when you're finished. ✔

- Everybody, which arrow did you cross out? (Signal.) *Arrow 1.*

- Arrow 1 could not be the mystery arrow because it doesn't show Goober eating a pizza just after he took a bath.

6. Here's the last clue about the mystery arrow: This arrow shows Goober taking a bath just after he fed the pigs.

- Listen again: Goober took a bath just after he fed the pigs. Draw a circle around Goober taking a bath just after he fed the pigs. Raise your hand when you're finished. (Observe students and give feedback.)

- Now cross out the arrow that could not be the mystery arrow. Raise your hand when you're finished.
(Observe students and give feedback.)

- Everybody, which arrow is the mystery arrow? (Signal.) *Arrow 2.*

- How do you know that arrow 3 could not be the mystery arrow? (Call on a student. Idea: *It doesn't show Goober taking a bath just after he fed the pigs.*)

- Raise your hand if you followed all the clues and found the mystery arrow.

EXERCISE 3 Interpreting Ambiguous Sentences

My brothers had dogs. They loved to carry a bone around in their mouth.

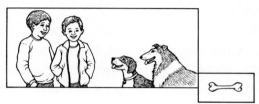

1. Everybody, find part C. ✔
Here are some more things that Mrs. Hudson wrote.

- You're going to fix up a sentence to show what Zelda thought it meant. Then you're going to fix up the picture the way Zelda would do it.

- The big trick is to find the word that confused Zelda.

- Touch the sentences. I'll read them twice. Raise your hand when you know the word that confused Zelda. My brothers had dogs. They loved to carry a bone around in their mouth.

- Listen again: My brothers had dogs. They loved to carry a bone around in their mouth.

- Everybody, what word would confuse Zelda? (Signal.) *They.*

- Who was Mrs. Hudson telling about when she wrote: **They** loved to carry a bone around in their mouth? (Signal.) *The dogs.*

- Would Zelda think the brothers or the dogs carried a bone in their mouth? (Signal.) *The brothers.*

2. Cross out the word **they** and write the words that Zelda thought were correct above the word **they**. Raise your hand when you're finished. ✔

- You should have written these words above **they: My brothers.** Raise your hand if you got it right. ✔

3. That's what Zelda thought. Later you can fix up the picture the way Zelda would have done it.

- There's a small box at the bottom of the picture. It shows a bone. You'll draw a bone like that in each boy's mouth.

EXERCISE 4 The Case of the Missing Corn *Part 2*

Storytelling

- In the last part of the story about the gray bragging rat, he decided to become a detective. So he got some things that detectives have.
- What did he get? (Call on a student. Idea: *A magnifying glass and a bloodbeetle.*)
- Why didn't he get a bloodhound instead of a bloodbeetle? (Call on a student. Idea: *A bloodhound would be too big.*)
- Who remembers the bloodbeetle's name? (Call on a student.) *Bertha.*
- There was a great mystery in the rat pack. What was that mystery? (Call on a student. Idea: *Who was taking the corn.*)
- The gray rat wanted to be called something. Raise your hand if you remember the name he gave himself. ✔
- Everybody, what was his detective name? (Signal.) *Sherlock.*
- Sherlock thought he could solve that mystery by using his skills in making deductions. Let's see what happened.

Sherlock was ready to solve the mystery of the missing corn in Goober's barn. But first, he had to talk his bloodbeetle into working for him again.

- What was the last thing that bloodbeetle did in the last story? (Call on a student. Idea: *Ran home.*)
- Why did she run home? (Call on a student. Idea: *Because she didn't want to get thrown into the pond.*)

He went to Bertha's home—which was a big hole in the ground. He called to her, but she didn't want to come out. She kept saying, "I don't like this job. I saw what they did to you." She was talking about the other rats throwing Sherlock into the pond.

"That was a mistake," the gray rat said. "Everything is straightened out now. All the rats agreed to let me solve the mystery."

The beetle peeked out of her hole and said, "But I'm not sure I want to work for a gray rat, anyhow. And I don't like being on a leash."

"Please don't call me a gray rat," the gray rat said. "Call me Sherlock. I guess you don't have to wear a leash if you promise not to run home again."

Sherlock talked and talked. At last he agreed to give Bertha part of all the extra corn he'd get if he solved the mystery.

Now Sherlock and the bloodbeetle were ready to go to work. They went to Goober's barn. On the way, Sherlock explained the plan. "I have everything figured out," he said. "The corn thief went into the barn. So all we have to do is to find somebody who goes into the barn and we'll know who the corn thief is."

Bertha gave Sherlock a funny look. She said, "That doesn't sound right to me, but you're the detective."

"It's very hard for a beetle to understand," Sherlock said. "But you have to know how to make deductions. I'll try to explain how it works as we solve this crime. But, for my plan to work, we have to find out who went into the barn."

"That's easy," Bertha said. "Anyone who goes into the barn smells of oats. With one sniff I could tell if somebody went into that barn. Oat smell is very strong."

"Good," Sherlock said. "We'll find somebody who smells of oats, and we'll know who went into the barn."

- Listen: Sherlock thinks that he can figure out who stole the corn by finding someone who went into the barn.
- Anyone who goes into the barn will have a special smell. Everybody, what smell is that? (Signal.) *Oats.*
- Yes, there must be lots of oats in that barn, and anybody who goes in there smells of oats.

Just as they were approaching the barn, Sherlock spotted a red chicken. "Look over there," he said to Bertha. "Go over and take a sniff of that chicken. See if she's been in the barn."

So Bertha scurried over near the chicken and then scurried back.

Sherlock asked, "Well? Has she been in the barn?"

Bertha said, "Yep."

Sherlock said, "There, you see? We've solved the mystery already. That chicken took the corn."

"How do you know that?" Bertha said.

"Listen carefully to this deduction: Anybody who goes into the barn smells of oats. The red chicken went into the barn. So the red chicken smells of oats."

"I know that," Bertha said. "I didn't need a deduction to figure that out. I could smell her a mile away."

"Don't interrupt," Sherlock said, "because that's only the **first** deduction. Here's the **next** deduction: The corn thief went into the barn. The red chicken went into the barn. So the red chicken is the corn thief."

- I think there's something fishy about that deduction. Listen:

The corn thief went into the barn. The red chicken went into the barn. So the red chicken is the corn thief.

- That is not right. But let's see what happened.

Bertha didn't agree with that deduction. She couldn't shake her head the way you and I would do. So she rocked her little body from side to side as she said, "No, no, no. That still doesn't sound right to me."

- Here's what that beetle was trying to do with her head. (Shake your head no.) But the beetle couldn't do it that way. Show me how she did it. (Praise students who rock their body from side to side.)

Sherlock said, "You may not understand how I figured it out. But you can't question the deduction. I solved the crime, and now I'll be getting double corn. Good for me. I'm so smart."

The beetle looked at him and rocked her body from side to side again.

- What is she trying to say when she does that? (Signal.) *No, no, no.*

Sherlock said, "Let's go back and tell the others." And they went back to the pack.

Then Sherlock jumped up on an old oak stump and said, "I have an announcement to make. Everybody, listen." The other rats gathered around.

Sherlock stood up very tall and pushed out his little chest as far as it would go. Then, in a very important-sounding voice, he said, "I have solved the mystery. I know who has been taking corn from the barn."

"Who? Who? Who?" all the rats shouted.

"Calm down, please," Sherlock said. When all the rats were very, very quiet, he said, "The red chicken on Goober's farm is the one who took the corn."

"How do you know that?" the wise old rat said.

"Simple," Sherlock said. Then he repeated his deductions. First the one about anybody who goes into the barn smells of oats.

- Listen: I remember that deduction. See if you remember the last sentence: Anybody who goes into the barn smells of oats. The red chicken went into the barn. So . . .
  Your turn: (Signal.) *The red chicken smells of oats.*
- I remember the other deduction, too: The corn thief went into the barn. The red chicken went into the barn. So . . .
  Your turn: (Signal.) *The red chicken is the corn thief.*
- That's that fishy deduction.

When Sherlock finished, some of the rats scratched their head. Some of them nodded yes-yes. Some of them shook their head no-no. Bertha just rocked from side to side.

- What was she trying to say? (Signal.) *No, no, no.*

At last a brown rat said, "I don't know. I've never heard so much talk to figure something out. Maybe he's right." Bertha rocked back and forth faster and harder.

The wise old rat smiled and said to Bertha, "You don't agree with the gray rat's deductions. Tell me why you don't agree."

"Well," Bertha said slowly, "I don't know much about deductions, but . . . " She was getting embarrassed. She'd never talked before a large group of rats before.

"Go on," the wise old rat said.

She looked down and said, "Well, the gray rat—I mean Sherlock—said that the red chicken did it because she smelled of oats, which means she'd been in the barn. There's just one small problem."

"What's that? What's that?"

"Every single one of you rats smells of oats."

- Oh-oh. Why do they all smell of oats? (Call on a student. Idea: *Because they all went into the barn.*)
- Yes, they go into that barn every evening to get their dessert. If Sherlock's last deduction is right, every one of them could be the corn thief.
- Listen to that part again:

Bertha looked down and said, "Well, the gray rat—I mean Sherlock—said that the red chicken did it because she smelled of oats, which means she'd been in the barn. There's just one small problem."

"What's that? What's that?"

"Every single one of you rats smells of oats."

All the rats looked at each other. One of them said, "What does that mean? Does that mean we all stole the corn?"

Then the rats started pointing at each other and saying, "You're the one. You smell of oats. So you must have taken that corn."

"Not me. You smell of oats, too, you know. You're the one."

Fights started breaking out.

"Stop," the wise old rat said. He jumped up on the stump. "I don't know what's wrong with all of you. You must know that you've been in the barn. You've gone in there every evening after dinner. So of course you smell of oats."

"Yeah," one rat said. "We go in there every evening after dinner. Of course we smell of oats."

Then there was a long silence. At last the little black rat said, "If we all smell of oats and we've all been in the barn, how does that gray rat know that the red chicken is the one who took the corn? All he knows is that she went into the barn."

"Yeah, what does he know? All he does is talk a lot, come up with silly deductions and get all of us confused."

With that, nine or ten rats picked up the gray rat—I mean Sherlock—and tossed him into the pond again. By the time they reached the pond, the bloodbeetle was already home, and that's where she wanted to stay for a long time.

EXERCISE 5 Deductions

1. (Draw on the board:)

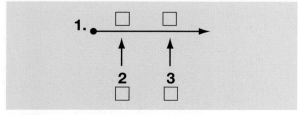

- I'll show you why Sherlock's deduction about who stole the corn doesn't work.

- For a good deduction, you do arrow 1, then arrow 2, then arrow 3. If you do the arrows in the wrong order, the deduction just doesn't work.
- Sherlock's deduction doesn't work because it does arrow 1, then arrow 3, then arrow 2.

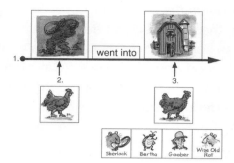

2. Everybody, find part D. ✔
   Touch arrow 1. ✔
   Here's the rule for that arrow: The corn thief went into the barn. Everybody, say that sentence. (Signal.) *The corn thief went into the barn.*
- Sherlock's first sentence says: The corn thief went into the barn. His next sentence should tell who the corn thief is. That's arrow 2. But he did arrow 3, not arrow 2. He told who went into the barn.
- Touch arrow 3. ✔
   Here's the statement for that arrow: The red chicken went into the barn.
- Touch arrow 2. ✔
   So the red chicken is the corn thief.
3. I'll say his whole deduction.
   Touch the arrows. ✔
- The corn thief went into the barn.
- The red chicken went into the barn.
- So the red chicken is the corn thief.
4. You say his whole deduction. I'll touch the arrows on the board.
- First sentence. (Touch arrow 1.) (Signal.) *The corn thief went into the barn.*
- Next sentence. (Touch arrow 3.) (Signal.) *The red chicken went into the barn.*
- Last sentence. (Touch arrow 2.) (Signal.) *So the red chicken is the corn thief.*
- That's wrong.

5. Below the arrows are some pictures of characters who went into the barn. Raise your hand if you can say the wrong deduction about Goober. (Call on a student. Touch arrows 1, 3, 2 on board as student says: *The corn thief went into the barn. Goober went into the barn. So Goober is the corn thief.*)
- Yes, that's not a good deduction.
- Raise your hand if you can say a wrong deduction about Sherlock. (Call on a student. Touch arrows on board as student says deduction.)
- Yes, that's a mixed-up deduction.

6. Sherlock's deduction is all mixed up. But listen to how silly it would sound if he put the sentences in the right order. I'll do arrows 1, 2 and 3 in the right order. Listen:
- (Touch arrow 1.) The corn thief went into the barn.
- (Touch arrow 2.) The red chicken is the corn thief.
- (Touch arrow 3.) So the red chicken went into the barn.
- No matter how you look at it, Sherlock is pretty mixed up.

Objectives

• Perform on master test of skills presented in lessons 31–39. (Exercise 1)
• Students vote on a story to be reread. (Exercise 2)
Exercises 3–5 provide instructions for marking the test and giving the students feedback.

WORKBOOK • LINED PAPER

EXERCISE 1 TEST
Writing Parallel Sentences

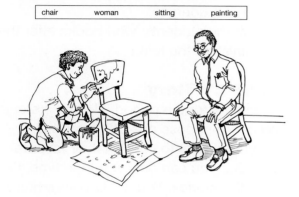

1. You're going to have a test to see how smart you are. You can't talk to anybody during the test or look at what anybody else does.
2. Open your workbook to lesson 40 and find part A. ✔
   You're going to write about this picture.
3. The picture shows what a woman and a man were doing.
   • What was the woman doing? (Call on a student. Idea: *Painting a chair.*)
   • What was the man doing? (Call on a student. Idea: *Sitting in a chair.*)
4. Listen: The woman was painting a chair. The man was sitting in a chair.
   • Everybody, say the whole sentence about the woman. (Signal.) *The woman was painting a chair.*
   • Say the whole sentence about the man. (Signal.) *The man was sitting in a chair.*
   • (Repeat sentences until firm.)
5. Look at the vocabulary box. These are some of the words you need: **chair . . . woman . . . sitting . . . painting.**
6. Say the sentence about the woman. (Signal.) *The woman was painting a chair.*
   • Say the sentence about the man. (Signal.) *The man was sitting in a chair.*

• Write both sentences.
   (Observe students and give feedback.)
7. **(Optional:)** Skip a line on your paper and write both sentences again.
   (Observe students and give feedback.)

Map—Movement To/From

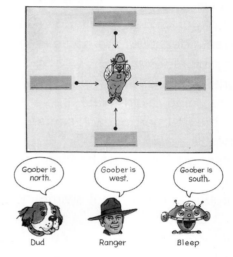

1. Everybody, find part B. ✔
2. You're going to write names on the map to show where different characters are standing.
   • Who is that in the middle of the map? (Signal.) *Goober.*
   • Touch Dud. ✔
     Dud is saying. "Goober is north."
   • Touch the ranger. ✔
     The ranger is saying, "Goober is west."
   • Touch Bleep. ✔
     Bleep is saying, "Goober is south."
3. Write the names on the map to show where they would have to be standing to make their statements about where Goober is. Raise your hand when you're finished.
   (Observe students but do not give feedback.)

Temporal Sequencing—After

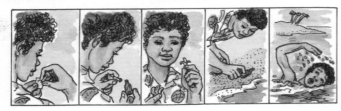

1. Find part C. ✔
   These pictures show what Owen did first, next, and next, and so forth.
   - Touch the first picture. ✔
     Everybody, what did Owen do in that picture? (Signal.) *Wrote a note.*
   - Next picture. What did he do there? (Signal.) *Put the note in a bottle.*
   - Next picture. What did he do? (Signal.) *Ate bananas.*
   - Next picture. What did he do? (Call on a student. Ideas: *Put the bottle in the water.*)
   - Last picture: Everybody, what did he do? (Signal.) *Went swimming.*
2. You're going to complete the sentences. I'll read the first part of each sentence. Follow along.
   - Sentence 1: Owen ate bananas after he . . . blank.
   - Sentence 2: Owen went swimming after he . . . blank.
   - Sentence 3: Owen put a note in the bottle after he . . . blank.
3. Write the words that go in the blank. If you're not sure about how to spell a word, do the best you can. Raise your hand when you're finished.
   (Observe students.)

Identifying the Larger Class

1. boys	children
2. animals	cows
3. fruit	apples

1. Find part D. ✔
   For each item, you'll circle the word for the bigger class. Remember, the bigger class has a larger number of things in it.
2. Touch item 1. ✔
   The classes are **boys** and **children.** Circle the name that tells about the larger class—boys or children. Raise your hand when you're finished.
   (Observe students.)
   - Touch item 2. ✔
     The classes are **animals** and **cows.** Circle the name that tells about the larger class—animals or cows. Raise your hand when you're finished.
     (Observe students.)
   - Touch item 3. ✔
     The classes are **fruit** and **apples.** Circle the name that tells about the larger class—**fruit** or **apples.** Raise your hand when you're finished.
     (Observe students.)
3. (Collect the student's workbooks after they have finished the test.)

EXERCISE 2 Story

1. For the rest of the period, I'll read a story. You get to choose one of the stories.
   - Everybody gets to vote on their favorite story. But you can only vote one time. I'll name the stories. You hold up your hand if you want that story. But remember, you can only hold up your hand one time.
   - Listen: Goober. Who wants to hear the story about Goober again?
     (Count the student's raised hands.)
   - Listen: Owen and the Little People. Who wants to hear the last part of that story again?
     (Count the student's raised hands.)
   - Listen: Dot and Dud. Who wants to hear the last part of that story again?
     (Count the student's raised hands.)
   - Listen: Zelda the Artist. Who wants to hear the last part of that story again?
     (Count the student's raised hands.)
2. (Read the chosen story. If time permits, read the story for the second choice.)

   Key: Lesson 15 for Goober;
   Lesson 23 for Owen (part 6);
   Lesson 37 for Dot and Dud (part 3);
   Lesson 36 for Zelda (part 3).

EXERCISE 3   Marking The Test

1. (Mark the test before the next scheduled language lesson. Use the *Language Arts Answer Key* to check the test.)
2. (Write the number of errors each student made in the test scorebox at the top of the test page.)
3. (Enter the number of errors each student made on the Summary for Test 4. A Reproducible Summary Sheet is at the back of the *Language Arts Teacher's Guide*.)

EXERCISE 4   Feedback On Test 4

1. (Return the students' workbooks after they are marked.)

- Everybody, open your workbook to lesson 40. Look at how I marked your test page.
- 2. I wrote a number at the top of your test. That number tells how many items you got wrong on the whole test.
- Raise your hand if I wrote **0** or **1** at the top of your test. **Those are super stars.**
- Raise your hand if I wrote **2** or **3**. Those are pretty good workers.
- If I wrote a number that's more than 3, you're going to have to work harder.

EXERCISE 5   Test Remedies

- (See the *Language Arts Teacher's Guide* for a general discussion of remedies.)

LESSON 41

Objectives

- Compose and write a parallel sentence pair based on a single picture. (Exercise 1)
- Identify where characters are on a map based on assertions about the direction of a common object. (Exercise 2)
- Edit ambiguous sentences to show how a character interpreted them. (Exercise 3)
- Listen to part 3 of a story and answer comprehension questions. (Exercise 4)
- Make a picture consistent with details of a story. (Exercise 5)

WORKBOOK • LINED PAPER

EXERCISE 1 Writing Parallel Sentences

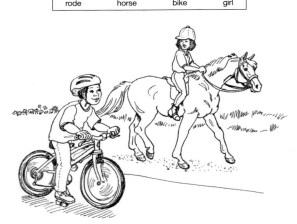

| rode | horse | bike | girl |

1. Open your workbook to lesson 41 and find part A. ✔
   You're going to write about this picture.
2. The picture shows what a boy and a girl did.
- What did the boy do? (Call on a student. Idea: *Rode a bike.*)
- What did the girl do? (Call on a student. Idea: *Rode a horse.*)
3. Listen: The boy rode a bike. The girl rode a horse.
- Say the whole sentence about the boy. (Signal.) *The boy rode a bike.*
- Say the whole sentence about the girl. (Signal.) *The girl rode a horse.*
- (Repeat sentences until firm.)
4. Look at the vocabulary box. These are some of the words you need: **rode . . . horse . . . bike . . . girl.**
5. Say the sentence about the boy. (Signal.) *The boy rode a bike.*
- Say the sentence about the girl. (Signal.) *The girl rode a horse.*

- Write both sentences.
  (Observe students and give feedback.)
6. **(Optional:)** Skip a line on your paper and write both sentences again.
   (Observe students and give feedback.)

EXERCISE 2 Map Directions

Relative Direction

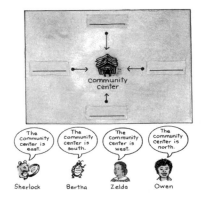

1. Find part B. ✔
   Here's a map, and below the map are characters from different stories. They are disagreeing about where the community center is.
- Touch Sherlock. ✔
  Sherlock is saying, "The community center is east."
- Touch Bertha. ✔
  Bertha is saying, "The community center is south."
- Touch Zelda. ✔
  What's Zelda saying? (Signal.) *The community center is west.*
- Touch Owen. ✔
  What's Owen saying? (Signal.) *The community center is north.*

2. The characters are saying different things, because they are all in different places. Sherlock is saying that the community center is east, because Sherlock would have to go east to get to the community center.

- Why is Bertha saying, "The community center is south"? (Call on a student. Idea: *Because Bertha would have to go south to get to the community center.*)

3. Listen: Write Sherlock's name to show where Sherlock must be. Raise your hand when you're finished.
   (Observe students and give feedback.)

- (Write on the board:)

Sherlock ⟶

- Here's the arrow you should have for Sherlock. That arrow has to point east. Raise your hand if you got it right.

4. Your turn: Write the names to show where Bertha, Zelda and Owen must be. Raise your hand when you're finished.
   (Observe students and give feedback.)

5. (Add to show:)

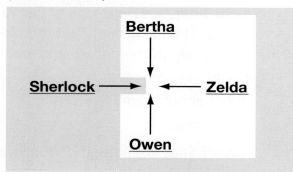

- Here's what you should have. Raise your hand if you got all the names in the right place.

EXERCISE 3 Interpreting Ambiguous Sentences

1. Aunt Mary put her pie near the stool and Wilber sat on it.

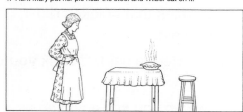

2. Uncle Henry talked to little Billy as he shaved.

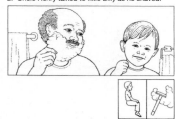

1. Everybody, find part C. ✔
   Remember that silly story about Zelda and Mrs. Hudson? Here are more things that Mrs. Hudson wrote.

- You're going to fix up the sentences to show what Zelda thought they meant. Then you're going to fix up the picture the way Zelda would do it.

- Remember, you need to find the word that confused Zelda.

- Touch number 1. ✔
  I'll read it twice. Raise your hand when you know the word that confused Zelda. Aunt Mary put her pie near the stool and Wilber sat on it.

- Listen again: Aunt Mary put her pie near the stool and Wilber sat on it.

- Raise your hand when you know what word would confuse Zelda. Everybody, what word? (Signal.) *It.*

- Mrs. Hudson wrote that Wilber sat on it. What did Wilber sit on? (Signal.) *The stool.*

- What would Zelda think Wilber sat on? (Signal.) *The pie.*

2. Cross out the word **it** and write the words that Zelda thought were correct. Raise your hand when you're finished. ✔

- You should have written these words above the word **it: the pie.** Raise your hand if you got it right.

3. Touch number 2. ✔

- I'll read it. Uncle Henry talked to little Billy as he shaved. Raise your hand when you know the word that confused Zelda.

- Listen again: Uncle Henry talked to little Billy as he shaved.

- Everybody, what word would confuse Zelda? (Call on a student.) *He.*

- Who did Mrs. Hudson mean when she wrote: As **he** shaved? (Signal.) *Uncle Henry.*

- Who did Zelda think shaved? (Signal.) *Little Billy.*

4. Cross out the word **he** and write the words that Zelda thought were correct. Raise your hand when you're finished. ✔

- You should have written these words above **he: little Billy.** Raise your hand if you got it right.

5. There's a box at the bottom of the page.

- Touch the first picture. ✔
  It shows Wilber sitting.

- Touch the next picture. ✔
  That's a razor.

6. Later, you can draw Wilber in picture 1 and fix up little Billy in picture 2 so he's holding a razor. You can also put soap on Billy's face.

EXERCISE 4 The Case of the Missing Corn *Part 3*

Storytelling

- I'm going to continue with Sherlock and the case of the missing corn, but first let's review what's happened.
- At the end of the last story, where was Sherlock? (Signal.) *In the pond.*
- Why did the rats throw him into the pond again? (Call on a student. Idea: *He didn't solve the crime; He came up with a silly deduction.*)
- Where was Sherlock's bloodbeetle? (Signal.) *At home.*
- Why was she at home? (Signal.) *She didn't want to get thrown into the pond.*
- How long did she plan to stay there? (Signal.) *A long time.*
- Listen:

The next day, the gray rat—I mean Sherlock—spent over half an hour bending over the entrance to Bertha's home, trying to talk her into coming out and working on the mystery again. He said, "We can't quit now. For some reason my deductions didn't work out the way they should have, but we can still solve this mystery if you'll come out and work with me."

"I don't think so," Bertha said. "Your deductions don't make a lot of sense to me."

"Of course they make sense. Just ask me where Benny the bluebird is right now, and I'll tell you the answer by using a deduction."

Bertha said, "I can tell you where he is right now without using a deduction."

"You can't either."

"I can too."

"Okay, let's see you do it."

Bertha peeked out of her hole and said, "He's in the berry bushes with the other bluebirds."

"Yeah, but how did you know that?" Sherlock asked.

"Well, that's simple: In the morning, all the bluebirds are in the berry bushes. Benny is a bluebird, so he's in the berry bushes."

"You used a **deduction,**" Sherlock shouted. He shouted so loudly that Bertha ducked back into her hole.

At last, she peeked out again and said, "I guess I did use a deduction, didn't I?"

"Of course you did. And that's all I was doing when I tried to solve the mystery of the missing corn. I just put a couple of deductions together."

Bertha crawled out of her hole and scratched her head with one of her very front legs. Then she said, "But there's something about the deductions you used that . . ."

"What about them?"

"They stink."

"Stink? They were great deductions."

"No," Bertha said. "They really stink."

"Why do you say a nasty thing like that?"

"Well, because you could use your deductions to show that everybody who went into the barn stole the corn."

"I still think that chicken did it," Sherlock said.

"Well," Bertha said. "I think **you** did it."

"How can you say anything as ridiculous as that?"

"I'll just say what **you** said." And Bertha did just that. First she said the deduction about the corn thief smelling of oats. Then she said, "The corn thief went into the barn. Sherlock went into the barn. So . . . "

- Everybody, what's the last sentence? (Signal.) *Sherlock is the corn thief.*

Bertha said, "So you must be the corn thief."

"No, no," Sherlock said. "I went into the barn, and I smell of oats, but I'm not the corn thief."

Bertha smiled and said, "That's why your deductions stink."

"You mean I spent all this time learning deductions and now I can't even use them?"

Bertha scratched her head again and then said, "I think I know the problem with your deductions. You want to figure out the **only** person who could have taken the corn. But **your** deductions tell you about a whole bunch of people."

"But how can I make a deduction that tells about the **only** person who could have taken the corn if I don't know who that person is?"

"Clues," Bertha said.

"What do you mean, clues?" Sherlock asked.

"I'm just a beetle," Bertha said. "But I think you need some clues that will tell about the **only** person who could have taken the corn."

"But I don't know how to make up good clues," Sherlock said. He was getting very nervous.

Bertha said, "Let me think about it. Come back in an hour. Maybe I'll have an idea by then."

So Sherlock went away and tried to think of a plan himself. But he didn't know much about how clues worked and how to get clues, so he didn't come up with any good plan.

An hour later, he went back to Bertha's place. She rushed up to him and said, "I've got it all worked out. Tonight the rats won't go to the barn to get their dessert."

"Oh, no," Sherlock said. "They'll get very upset if they don't get their dessert."

"Stop interrupting," Bertha said. "They'll get their dessert. But you'll bring it to them so they won't have to go to the barn. Then we'll fix up the rest of the corn in the barn so that anybody who goes into the barn will not only smell of oats; that person will also smell of pine needles."

Sherlock shook his head. "I don't know how we could do that. There aren't any pine needles near that barn. And I . . . "

"Stop interrupting," Bertha said. "If you turn around, you'll see a large tree behind you."

Sherlock turned around and looked at the tree. "So?" he said.

"So, what do you see growing all over that tree?"

"Pine needles," he said.

"And what do you see all over the ground under that tree?"

"More pine needles."

"Well, all we need to do is gather up a few bags of those pine needles and take them to the barn. Then we'll make a circle of pine needles all the way around the corn. Anybody who goes after that corn will have to go through the pine needles. So we'll just find the person who has a strong smell of oats **and** a strong smell of pine needles. That's the one who's been stealing the corn."

- Listen: Bertha's idea is to put a circle of something around the corn in the barn. What are they going to make that circle out of? (Signal.) *Pine needles.*
- Yes, pine needles, **and** the corn is inside the circle. So anybody who takes the corn will have to go through the pine needles. That person will have two smells.
- What are the two smells? (Signal.) *Oats and pine needles.*
- Does that sound like a pretty good plan? (Accept responses.)

> "But . . . " Sherlock said. "But . . . won't **we** smell of oats and pine needles when we're all done?"
>
> "Yes," said Bertha.
>
> "So how will we know that **we** didn't steal the corn?"
>
> Bertha looked at him and shook her little body from side to side. Then she said, "I'll watch you and you'll watch me. Then we'll know if we are guilty."
>
> "This is getting pretty hard to understand," Sherlock said. "I'm not sure . . . "
>
> "You don't have to be sure. I am. Let's get to work and solve this crime."
>
> So they did.

EXERCISE 5 Details

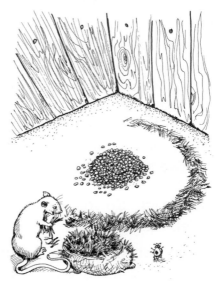

1. Find part D. ✔
   When the story ended, Sherlock and Bertha were going to gather up pine needles and take them to the barn.
- They were going to make a circle of needles around the corn.
2. In the picture, you can see the pile of corn.
- Touch that pile of corn. ✔
- Sherlock is making a circle of pine needles. You can see he has a whole big bag full of them.
- Touch that bag. ✔
- The pine needles look like little lines. Listen: Complete the circle of pine needles. Remember, you want a great wide circle of pine needles all the way around that corn, so anybody who goes to that corn has to go through the pine needles.
- Make little lines in a circle all the way around the corn. Use lots of pine needles and make sure that in your picture nobody would get to that corn without going through the pine needles. Raise your hand when you're finished.
   (Observe students and give feedback.)
3. Later you can color the picture.

Objectives

- Compose and write a parallel sentence pair based on a single picture. (Exercise 1)
- Edit an ambiguous sentence to show how a character interpreted it. (Exercise 2)
- Listen to the conclusion of a 4-part story and answer comprehension questions. (Exercise 3)
- Make a picture consistent with details of a story. (Exercise 4)

WORKBOOK • LINED PAPER

EXERCISE 1   Writing Parallel Sentences

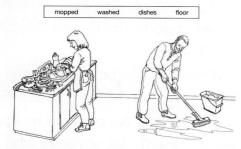

1. Open your workbook to lesson 42 and find part A. ✔
   You're going to write about this picture.
2. The picture shows what a woman and a man did.
- What did the woman do? (Call on a student. Idea: *Washed dishes.*)
- What did the man do? (Call on a student. Idea: *Mopped the floor.*)
3. Listen: The woman washed dishes. The man mopped the floor.
- Everybody, say the whole sentence about the woman. (Signal.) *The woman washed dishes.*
- Say the whole sentence about the man. (Signal.) *The man mopped the floor.*
- (Repeat sentences until firm.)
4. Look at the vocabulary box. These are some of the words you need: **mopped . . . washed . . . dishes . . . floor.**
5. Say the sentence about the woman. (Signal.) *The woman washed dishes.*
- Say the sentence about the man. (Signal.) *The man mopped the floor.*
- Write both sentences.
   (Observe students and give feedback.)
6. **(Optional:)** Skip a line on your paper and write both sentences again.
   (Observe students and give feedback.)

EXERCISE 2   Interpreting Ambiguous Sentences

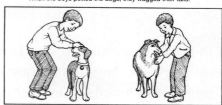

When the boys petted the dogs, they wagged their tails.

1. Everybody, find part B. ✔
   Here's another sentence that Mrs. Hudson wrote.
- You're going to fix up the sentence to show what Zelda thought it meant.
- Touch the sentence. ✔
   I'll read it twice. Raise your hand when you know the word that confused Zelda. When the boys petted the dogs, they wagged their tails.
- Listen again: When the boys petted the dogs, they wagged their tails.
- Listen: Draw a line under the word that confused Zelda. Raise your hand when you're finished. ✔
- Everybody, what word would confuse Zelda? (Signal.) *They.*
- Who did Mrs. Hudson mean when she wrote: **They** wagged their tails? (Signal.) *The dogs.*
- Who would Zelda think wagged their tails? (Signal.) *The boys.*
2. Cross out the word **they** and write the words that Zelda thought were correct above the word **they.** Raise your hand when you're finished. ✔
- You should have written these words above **they: the boys.** Raise your hand if you got it right. ✔
- That's what Zelda thought. Fix up your picture the way Zelda would have done it. Raise your hand when you're finished. ✔
- Later you can color the picture.

EXERCISE 3 The Case of the Missing Corn *Part 4*

Storytelling

- I'm going to finish the story: **The Case of the Missing Corn.** Let's review what has already happened.

> The little beetle had a plan for figuring out who took the corn from the barn. That plan involved pine needles.

- What were Sherlock and his bloodbeetle going to do with the pine needles? (Call on a student. Idea: *Put them around the corn.*)

> If the plan worked, somebody would have two smells. And any person who had both those smells must have gone into the barn **and** through the pine needles.

- What were those two smells? (Signal.) *Oats and pine needles.*
- Let's find out what happened.

> All afternoon, Sherlock and his bloodbeetle collected pine needles and carried them to the barn. Then they counted two kernels of corn for every rat in the pack. They put that corn outside the barn. Then they took the pine needles and made a great circle of pine needles around the pile of corn that was still in the barn.
>
> When they were done, Bertha said, "Now we'll go back and tell the rats about our plan. Then we'll wait until tomorrow and go hunting for the person who smells of pine needles **and** oats."
>
> They carried the corn that they had taken out of the barn back to the stump and called all the other rats. Sherlock stood on the stump.
>
> The rats looked at each other and asked, "What's all that corn doing out here?"

> "Quiet please," Sherlock said. "Everybody quiet."
>
> Sherlock cleared his throat—"ahem, ahem"—and stood up very straight. In his most important voice, he said, "I won't bother trying to tell you how we're going to find out who is stealing the corn, because it's very difficult to understand. But we've brought enough corn out here so every rat can have dessert tonight without going near the barn. We have very cleverly fixed the pile of corn that's still in the barn so that anybody who goes to the corn will give us a very good clue. But it's difficult to explain."
>
> "What kind of clue?" one of the rats asked.
>
> Bertha said, "We put pine needles all around the corn. So anybody who goes to the corn will smell of pine needles."
>
> "Now that makes sense," one of the rats said. Then other rats agreed and nodded their head up and down. "Yeah, if somebody smells of oats **and** pine needles, that's the guilty person."
>
> "Yeah, that's smart," the rats agreed.

- Did the rat pack have any trouble understanding the plan? (Signal.) *No.*

> So the rats had dinner and ate their dessert. Then they did what rats do in the evening—they went to sleep. Sherlock didn't sleep with the other rats. He had to sleep outside Bertha's place where she could keep an eye on him.

- Why would she have to keep an eye on him? (Call on a student. Idea: *To be sure he wasn't the one stealing the corn.*)

> The next morning, Bertha woke Sherlock up by tickling his nose with her little front legs. Then she said, "Let's go find the corn thief." And away they went.

They went all around, greeting every animal they saw and getting close enough for Bertha to get a good sniff.

- Remember, she had to sniff for two things. What were they? (Signal.) *Oats and pine needles.*

After they greeted Cora the crow, Bertha said, "She smells of pine needles."

"She did it," Sherlock said.

"No, she didn't do it," Bertha said. "She doesn't smell of oats."

"Oh," Sherlock said. He wasn't really too good at figuring things out.

After they greeted the red chicken, Bertha said, "She smells of oats."

"She did it," Sherlock said.

"No, she didn't do it," Bertha said. And then she explained why.

- Raise your hand if you know why Bertha knows the red chicken didn't do it. (Call on a student. Idea: *Because she didn't smell of pine needles.*)

At last they greeted Myron the mouse. Bertha took a good sniff. Then she walked away as Sherlock followed. Bertha stopped and whispered, "Myron smells of oats and he smells of pine needles."

Sherlock said, "Let's haul him back to the rat pack. He's the one who did it."

"I'm not really sure," Bertha said.

"Why not?" Sherlock asked.

"Something is missing," Bertha said. "Let's look around a little bit more."

- I wonder what could be missing. Myron smells of pine needles and smells of oats. I wonder why Bertha thinks something is missing. Maybe we'll find out.

So Sherlock and Bertha greeted frogs and toads and snakes and snails. They greeted chipmunks and skunks and sparrows and ducks. At last, they came to Cyrus the squirrel. He was leaning against a tree, yawning and stretching. After Sherlock and Bertha greeted him, they walked away. Then Bertha stopped and whispered, "Cyrus smells of oats and he smells of pine needles. He's the one who's been stealing the corn. Ask him."

- Wait a minute. Bertha is sure that Cyrus did it, but she wasn't sure that Myron did it. I wonder why.
- Listen to that part again:

Bertha whispered, "Cyrus smells of oats and he smells of pine needles. He's the one who's been stealing the corn. Ask him."

"Okay," Sherlock said. He walked over and said, "Been near the barn lately?"

"Not me," Cyrus said and yawned again.

"Been stealing any corn from that barn?"

"Who me?" Cyrus asked. "I know that corn is for the rat pack. I wouldn't take any of that corn."

"So you didn't steal the corn from the barn?"

"Absolutely not," he said and yawned again.

Sherlock shrugged and went back to Bertha. "He said he didn't do it."

Bertha got so angry that she started to quiver all over. She said, "We will see about that."

She charged over to Cyrus and said, "If you didn't go into the barn, why is it that you smell of fresh pine needles?"

"I'm a squirrel," he said. "I climb pine trees all the time."

"Okay, if you didn't go into the barn, why do you smell of oats?"

"There's an oat field on the other side of the pond. I was walking around there early this morning."

"Oh yeah?" Bertha said. "Well if you didn't go into the barn, why does your breath smell of corn?"

- That's it. Now I know what Bertha was doing. She was sniffing for **three** smells, not two smells. What were they? (Call on a student, Idea: *Oats, pine needles and corn.*)
- How did she know that Myron the mouse wasn't guilty? (Call on a student. Idea: *He had only two smells; there was no corn on his breath.*)
- Listen to that part again:

Bertha charged over to Cyrus and said, "If you didn't go into the barn, why is it that you smell of fresh pine needles?"

"I'm a squirrel," he said. "I climb pine trees all the time."

"Okay, if you didn't go into the barn, why do you smell of oats?"

"There's an oat field on the other side of the pond. I was walking around there early this morning."

"Oh yeah?" Bertha said. "Well if you didn't go into the barn, why does your breath smell of corn?"

"I, uh, I . . . well . . . "

Bertha said, "Your breath is so strong I could smell the corn every time you yawned. You're a liar and you stole the corn. Admit it."

"Well, I . . . uh . . . that is . . . I . . . "

"Stop trying to make excuses. You stole the corn. Admit it."

"Okay, okay. I admit it."

"Well, you'd better figure out some way of paying the pack back and you'd better think fast."

"I'm thinking. I'm thinking," Cyrus said.

Later that day, Cyrus, Sherlock and Bertha went to the stump. Cyrus was carrying a large sack filled with something that would interest all the rats. Sherlock called the other rats. "Attention, attention," he said. "I have an announcement to make." He was talking in his important voice. "We have found the guilty party. It was Cyrus the squirrel, and he admitted it."

"Let's throw him into the pond."

"No, no," Sherlock said. "Cyrus has promised to bring us a special dessert every night for the next two weeks—that dessert is your very favorite nut."

The rats all stared at Sherlock. Then one of them said, "You don't mean hazelnuts, do you?"

"Yes, hazelnuts," Sherlock said. "Everybody gets a big hazelnut every night for two weeks."

Great cheers went up from the rat pack. "What a deal," they shouted. "Corn is good, but hazelnuts are the best!"

The rats crowded around Sherlock and patted him on the back. One of them said, "Yeah, Cyrus can steal all the corn he wants as long as he pays us back with hazelnuts."

Other rats told Sherlock how smart he was. "You did a great job," they said. "We didn't think you knew what you were doing, but you really figured it out."

They shook his hand, patted him on the back and gave him great hugs. Some of the pretty little girl rats even gave him a kiss. One of them said,

> "You're so big and smart. And you solved this crime all by yourself."
>
> Sherlock said, "Oh, well, I had a little bit of help from Bertha."

- Everybody, did he get a little help or a lot of help from Bertha? (Signal.) *A lot.*

EXERCISE 4   Details

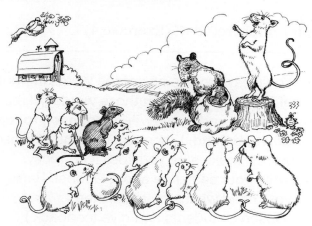

- Everybody, find part C. ✔
  This picture shows something that happened in the story.

- Sherlock is standing on that stump. Why is he standing up so straight and tall like that? (Call on a student. Idea: *He's talking in his important voice.*)
- Who is that character with the big sack? (Signal.) *Cyrus.*
- What's in that sack? (Signal.) *Hazelnuts.*
- What is Sherlock telling the rat pack? (Call on a student. Idea: *Who stole the corn.*)
- The way Sherlock tells the story it sounds as if one character figured everything out. Who is that character? (Signal.) *Sherlock.*
- But actually, another character did all the important figuring. Who was that? (Signal.) *Bertha.*
- Where is Bertha in the picture? (Call on a student. Idea: *Next to the stump.*)
- She's not in a very important place. Where do you think she should be? (Call on a student. Idea: *On the stump with Sherlock.*)
- Later you can color the picture.

Materials: Each student will need an orange crayon.

Objectives

- **Write a group of sentences that are thematically related.** (Exercise 1)
- Identify where characters are on a map based on assertions about the direction of a common object. (Exercise 2)
- Listen to part of a familiar story. (Exercise 3)
- Edit an ambiguous sentence to show how a character interpreted it. (Exercise 4)

WORKBOOK • LINED PAPER

EXERCISE 1 Sentence Writing

Note: For this activity students will need lined paper. Pass out paper. Direct students to write their name on the top line.

1. Find the page titled **Story words** at the front of your workbook. ✔
- Today you're going to write sentences that make up little stories. You're going to write your sentences on lined paper.
2. (Write on the board:)

> **Everybody hid.**

- This says: Everybody hid.
- Copy that sentence on the second line of your paper. Remember the capital and the period. Raise your hand when you've copied the sentence.
(Observe students and give feedback.)
3. (Write to show:)

> **Everybody hid.**
> **Goober hid _____.**

- Here's the first part of the sentence you'll write next. Goober hid blank. Complete the sentence for Goober. He hid in one of the places that you see in part B.

- You'll have to use one of the words in front of the pictures. Touch those words. I'll read them: **in, under, between, on, over, to, up, down, behind.** When you use one of those words, make sure you spell it correctly.
- Write your sentence about Goober. Raise your hand when you're finished.
(Observe students and give feedback.)
- (Call on individual students to read their sentence for Goober.)
4. (Write to show:)

> **Everybody hid.**
> **Goober hid _____.**
> **Bertha _____.**
> **I _____.**

- You're going to write more sentences. One will tell about Bertha and where she hid. The other will tell about you and where you hid.
- Your turn: Write both sentences. Remember the period at the end of each sentence. Raise your hand when you're finished.
(Observe students and give feedback.)
- (Call on individual students.) Read your sentence about Bertha. Read your sentence about where you hid.

EXERCISE 2   Map Directions

Relative Direction

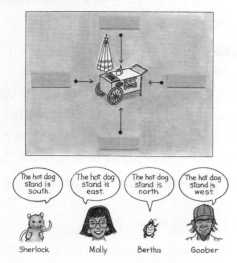

1. Open your workbook to lesson 43 and find part A. ✔
   Here's another map. Below the map are different people disagreeing about where the hot dog stand is.
   • Touch Sherlock. ✔
   Sherlock is saying, "The hot dog stand is south."
   • Touch Molly. ✔
   Molly is saying, "The hot dog stand is east."
   • Touch Bertha. ✔
   What's Bertha saying? (Signal.) *The hot dog stand is north.*
   • Touch Goober. ✔
   What's Goober saying? (Signal.) *The hot dog stand is west.*

2. They are saying different things because they are all in different places. Molly is saying that the hot dog stand is east because Molly would have to go east to get to the hot dog stand.
   • Why is Sherlock saying, "The hot dog stand is south"? (Call on a student. Idea: *Because Sherlock would have to go south to get to the hot dog stand.*)

3. Yes, Sherlock is saying, "The hot dog stand is south," because he would have to go south to get to the hot dog stand. Write **Sherlock** to show where Sherlock must be standing. Raise your hand when you're finished.

   • (Write on the board:)

   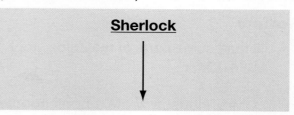

   • Here's the arrow you should have for Sherlock. That arrow has to point south. Raise your hand if you got it right.

4. Your turn: Touch Molly. ✔
   Molly is saying, "The hot dog stand is east."
   • Listen: Write **Molly** to show where Molly must be standing. Raise your hand when you're finished.
   • (Write on the board:)

Molly ⟶

   • Here's the arrow you should have for Molly. That arrow points east. Raise your hand if you got it right.

5. Touch Goober. ✔
   Goober is saying, "The hot dog stand is west."
   • Listen: Write **Goober** to show where Goober must be standing. Raise your hand when you're finished. ✔
   • (Write on the board:)

⟵ **Goober**

   • Here's the arrow you should have for Goober. That arrow points west. Raise your hand if you got it right.

6. Touch Bertha. ✔
   Bertha is saying, "The hot dog stand is north." Write **Bertha** to show where Bertha must be standing. Raise your hand when you're finished. ✔
   • (Write on the board:)

   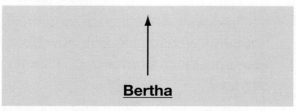

   • Here's the arrow you should have for Bertha. That arrow points north.

7. Raise your hand if you got all the arrows right.

EXERCISE 3   Zelda the Artist

Review

- I'll read some parts of the Zelda story again. Listen:

Mrs. Hudson wrote a book about some of the interesting things that happened to her. At least **she** thought they were interesting. Actually, they were very, very boring.

Mrs. Hudson had seen some of the fine work that Zelda had done, so she called Zelda on the phone and asked Zelda if she'd be interested in doing twenty illustrations for the book.

Zelda thought about it for a few moments. Then she said, "Yes, I'd like to do that."

Mrs. Hudson said, "Good. I'll bring over the book. I've marked parts of the book to let you know what you should illustrate."

Later that day, Mrs. Hudson drove over to Zelda's place and showed Zelda how she'd circled all the parts of the story that Zelda was to illustrate.

Mrs. Hudson turned to the second page of the book and said, "Listen to this part: **'That spring, the apple trees were covered with white flowers, and their branches were black.'**"

After Mrs. Hudson read that part, Zelda said, "That may be hard to illustrate."

"Why is that?"

"Well, it says that the trees were covered with white flowers and their branches were black. But, how do you draw black branches on little tiny flowers?"

Mrs. Hudson looked at Zelda for a long moment. Mrs. Hudson blinked two times. Then she broke into laughter. "Ho, ho," she laughed. "That's very funny.

I didn't catch the joke right away, but that's very funny—black branches on the flowers."

Mrs. Hudson turned to the next part of the book that was circled.

She said, "Listen to this part: **'When we were on the farm, my brother and my sister had pet pigs. They just loved to roll around in the mud.'**"

After Mrs. Hudson read, "They just loved to roll around in the mud," Zelda said, "They did?"

Mrs. Hudson said, "Oh, yes, they just loved it."

Zelda said, "Didn't they get their clothes all muddy?"

Mrs. Hudson looked at Zelda and blinked. Then she broke into laughter again: "Ho, ho, ho. My," she said, "you are very clever—'didn't they get their clothes all muddy?' Very funny."

Mrs. Hudson flipped to the next part that was circled. "Here's one of my favorite parts," she said. "Listen to this: **'Every day the children rode their horses through the valley. Their tails flew in the wind.'**"

After Mrs. Hudson read the part, "Their tails flew in the wind," Zelda shook her head and said, "They **all** had them?"

"Had what?"

"Tails."

"Well of course, long, flowing tails."

"Golly," Zelda said.

"The youngest one had the longest tail. He was gray and white."

Zelda said, "Really?"

"Yes," Mrs. Hudson said. "He was just **covered** with gray and white spots."

"Poor boy," Zelda said.

Mrs. Hudson flipped to one more place that was marked in the book. She said, "This is a little different. This was something inside the farm house. Listen: **'We always kept a glass on top of the refrigerator. We kept it full of water.'"**

Zelda said, "Didn't it spill out when you opened the door?"

Blink, blink—"Ho, ho, ho, ho. Oh, my dear, you have such a clever wit."

Mrs. Hudson patted Zelda on the knee and handed her the book. She said, "Well, I'll leave this with you, my dear. You can read through it and see what to show for the other parts I've marked. If you have any questions, you can give me a call."

Zelda said, "I have one big question."

"What's that my dear?"

"Is this book about very strange things?"

"Well," Mrs. Hudson said, "I suppose not many people have had the kinds of experiences I've had."

"You can say that again," Zelda said.

"All right," Mrs. Hudson said, "I suppose not many people have had the kinds of experiences I've had."

After Mrs. Hudson left, Zelda read through the book. Then she drew her first illustration. It was for the part that said, "When we were on the farm, my brother and my sister had pet pigs. They just loved to roll around in the mud."

Zelda made a beautiful picture of Mrs. Hudson's brother and sister rolling around in the mud next to the barn.

In the picture that Zelda drew, the pet pigs were standing there, looking at the students in the mud. When Zelda finished that picture, she said, "That woman must have a very strange family."

Then she did the next illustration. That one was for the part that said, "Every day the children rode their horses through the valley. Their tails flew in the wind."

Zelda didn't know how many children to draw or how long to make their "tails." But at last she decided to show three children riding horses. She gave each of the children a long tail. She gave the horses regular horse tails. After she finished the illustration, she said, "That woman knows some very strange people."

Then she went on to the next part. It said: "We always kept a glass on top of the refrigerator. We kept it full of water."

Zelda decided to show a picture of somebody opening the refrigerator and water pouring out. She said to herself, "I don't know any other way to show that it was full of water."

The part that was marked for the next illustration said this: "Our car stopped on top of the mountain. It was out of gas."

Zelda read that part again and again. At last she called Mrs. Hudson and asked her, "How am I going to show it was out of gas? I can't illustrate this picture."

"I see what you mean, my dear. Just looking at the picture, you wouldn't really know that it was out of gas, would you?"

"I sure wouldn't," Zelda said.

"Well, what if you sort of showed the inside of it, and we could see the gas gauge?"

"The gas gauge?"

"Yes, my dear. We could see that we were on top of the mountain. We could be looking inside the window and could see the gas gauge."

"Looking inside the window?"

"Of course."

"It has a window?"

"Well, certainly. It has windows all the way around."

"Wow," Zelda said. "I'll draw it, but I've never seen one with windows before."

"Well, the next time I go over to your place, I'll show you a picture of it."

Zelda said, "I'll take your word for it."

After Zelda hung up the phone, she did the illustration of a great mountain with a car parked on top. The mountain had windows all the way around, and inside the mountain was a great huge gas gauge.

Zelda looked at the picture and said, "That woman has sure been to some strange places."

The next part of the book that was marked said this: "Our car went down the dirt road, leaving a dust cloud behind. Soon, it floated away on the breeze."

Zelda read the part to herself two times. Then she shook her head and made the illustration. It showed a car floating through the air over a dirt road.

Zelda said to herself, "That woman sure has some strange vehicles, too."

- We'll finish the rest of the story next time.

EXERCISE 4 Interpreting Ambiguous Sentences

The children caught butterflies. They had orange wings.

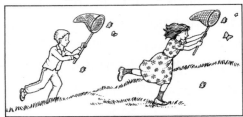

1. Everybody, find part B. ✔
   Here is something else that Mrs. Hudson wrote.
- You're going to fix up one of the sentences to show what Zelda thought **they** meant. Then you're going to fix up the picture the way Zelda would do it.
- Remember to find the word that confused Zelda.
- Touch the sentences.
  I'll read them twice. Raise your hand when you know the word that confused Zelda. The children caught butterflies. They had orange wings.
- Listen again: The children caught butterflies. They had orange wings.
- Everybody, what word would confuse Zelda? (Signal.) *They.*
- What did Mrs. Hudson mean when she wrote: **They** had orange wings? (Signal.) *The butterflies.*
- What would Zelda think had orange wings? (Signal.) *The children.*
2. Cross out the word **they** and write the words that Zelda thought were correct above the word **they.** Raise your hand when you're finished. ✔
- You should have written these words above **they: The children.** Raise your hand if you got it right.
- That's what Zelda thought. Use your orange crayon and fix up your picture the way Zelda would have done it. Raise your hand when you're finished.
  (Observe students and give feedback.)
- That's pretty silly. Later you can color the rest of the picture.

Objectives

- Construct sentences for different illustrations. (Exercise 1)
- Construct deductions to answer questions. (Exercise 2)
- Listen to the conclusion of a familiar story. (Exercise 3)
- Make a picture consistent with details of a story. (Exercise 4)

WORKBOOK

EXERCISE 1 Sentence Construction

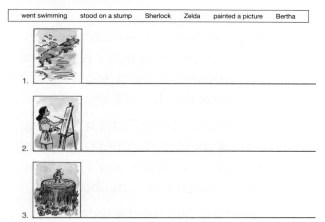

| went swimming | stood on a stump | Sherlock | Zelda | painted a picture | Bertha |

1.

2.

3.

1. Everybody, open your workbook to lesson 44 and find part A. ✔
   You're going to write sentences. You're going to use the words in the boxes to make up your sentences. I'll read the words that are in the boxes.
- Touch the first word box. ✔
  It says: went swimming.
- Next box: Sherlock.
- Next box: painted a picture.
- Next box: stood on a stump.
- Next box: Zelda.
- Last box: Bertha.
- Those are the words you'll use for your sentences.
2. Touch picture 1. ✔
   Your sentence for that picture will start out by naming the character in the picture. Who is in the picture? (Signal.) *Sherlock.*
- So your sentence will start with Sherlock.
- Touch picture 2. ✔
  Your sentence for that picture will start out by naming the character. Who is in the picture? (Signal.) *Zelda.*
- So your sentence will start with Zelda.

- Touch picture 3. ✔
  Who is in that picture? (Signal.) *Bertha.*
- So what will your sentence start with? (Signal.) *Bertha.*
3. Touch picture 1 again. ✔
   Who is in that picture? (Signal.) *Sherlock.*
- So what will your sentence start with? (Signal.) *Sherlock.*
- Then your sentence will tell what Sherlock did in that picture. What did he do? (Signal.) *Went swimming.*
- Touch the two boxes that have the words for that sentence.
- The words are: **Sherlock** and **went swimming.**
- I'll say the sentence. See if you're touching the right boxes. Sherlock. . .(pause). . .went swimming.
  (Observe students and give feedback.)
- Your turn: Write the sentence on the line for picture 1. Remember the capital and the period. Raise your hand when you're finished.
  (Observe students and give feedback.)
- (Write on the board:)

Sherlock went swimming.

- Here's what you should have for the first picture. Raise your hand if you got everything right.
4. Touch picture 2. ✔
   Who is in that picture? (Signal.) *Zelda.*
- So what will your sentence start with? (Signal.) *Zelda.*
- Then your sentence will tell what Zelda did in that picture. What did she do? (Signal.) *Painted a picture.*
- Touch the two boxes that have the words for that sentence.
  (Observe students and give feedback.)

- Your turn: Write the sentence that tells what Zelda did. Raise your hand when you're finished.
  (Observe students and give feedback.)
- (Write on the board:)

> **Zelda painted a picture.**

- Here's what you should have for picture 2. Raise your hand if you got everything right.
5. Touch picture 3. ✔
  Who is in that picture? (Signal.) *Bertha.*
- So what will your sentence start with? (Signal.) *Bertha.*
- Then your sentence will tell what Bertha did in that picture. What did she do? (Signal.) *Stood on a stump.*
- Listen: Touch the two boxes that have the words for that sentence.
  (Observe students and give feedback.)
- Your turn: Write the sentence for picture 3. Raise your hand when you're finished.
  (Observe students and give feedback.)
- (Write on the board:)

> **Bertha stood on a stump.**

- Here's what you should have. Raise your hand if you got everything right.

EXERCISE 2 Deduction Writing

Where is Fred the frog in the afternoon?

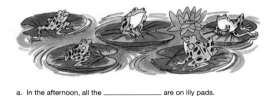

a. In the afternoon, all the _____ are on lily pads.

b. Fred is a _____ .

c. So in the afternoon, _____

1. Everybody, find part B. ✔
  This picture shows the pond in the afternoon.
- You can see the lily pads on the pond, and you can see the frogs on the lily pads.
2. Touch the question above the picture. ✔
  Follow along as I read it: Where is Fred the frog in the afternoon?
- What does that question say? (Signal.) *Where is Fred the frog in the afternoon?*
3. Listen big: Here's the rule. In the afternoon, all the frogs are on lily pads.
- Listen again: In the afternoon, all the frogs are on lily pads.

4. Your turn: Answer the question by completing the deduction below the picture. Raise your hand when you're finished.
  (Observe students and give feedback.)
5. Here's what you should have: In the afternoon, all the frogs are on lily pads. Fred is a frog. So, in the afternoon, Fred is on a lily pad. Raise your hand if you got it right. ✔

EXERCISE 3 Zelda the Artist
Review

- Today we'll finish the rest of the Zelda story.

Zelda worked on the illustrations week after week. And every week Mrs. Hudson would call Zelda and remind her that the book had to be finished soon.

"Remember, Zelda," she would say, "This book must go to the publisher by March. I certainly hope you'll be done with all the illustrations by then."

Every time Mrs. Hudson called to remind Zelda about getting the book ready for the publisher, Zelda would say, "I'm working as fast as I can, but some of these illustrations are not very easy."

Then, in the middle of February, Mrs. Hudson called and started to say, "Remember, Zelda, this book must go to the publisher before. . ."

"I'm done with the illustrations," Zelda said.

"How perfectly wonderful!" Mrs. Hudson said. "How marvelous! Isn't this just grand?"

She told Zelda that she would be right over and she was. She was still talking about how wonderful everything was. "This is just perfect," she said. "I can hardly wait to see your illustrations, my dear."

Then Mrs. Hudson saw Zelda's illustrations. She looked at the first one, and her eyes got wide, and her face became very serious and stiff. Her face stayed that way as she looked at the next illustration, and the next illustration and the next illustration. She wasn't saying anything like, "How wonderful this is." She wasn't saying **anything.** She was just staring at those illustrations with wide eyes and a very stiff face.

At last, she dropped the illustrations on the floor and said to Zelda, "What have you done to my wonderful book? These illustrations are awful. They are terrible. They are unbelievable. They are . . ." (She had run out of bad words.)

Zelda said, "Well, I did the best I could. I had never seen any of the things your book told about. Like the picture of the children with their tails flying in the wind. I didn't know if they should have monkey tails, lion tails or short little bunny tails."

"Stop it," Mrs. Hudson said. "I do not find your wit one bit funny. And I find your illustrations terrible, awful, unbelievable and simply. . ." (She'd run out of bad words again.)

"Well," Zelda said, "I'm sorry. I don't have time to redo them now, but I could . . ."

"No," Mrs. Hudson said, "this book must be at the publisher by March. If it's not at the publisher by March, it doesn't get published."

So Mrs. Hudson picked up the illustrations, picked up her book and marched out of Zelda's place.

Nobody was very happy.

Mrs. Hudson sent her book and Zelda's illustrations to the publisher. She wrote a note. It said:

Dear Publisher,

I am not completely pleased with the illustrations for this book, and I apologize for them. But I'm sure you'll find the writing very interesting. The book tells about one enjoyable experience after another.

She signed the note: Sincerely, Mrs. R. R. Hudson.

In the meantime, Zelda was trying to forget about that book. She was working on illustrations for an animal book. She tried to keep her mind on the animals she was drawing, but she couldn't help thinking about Mrs. Hudson's book. "I worked a long time on that book," she told herself, "and I did the best job I could. I can't help it if I drew the wrong kind of windows on that mountain. And how do I know what kind of gas gauges mountains have? That Mrs. Hudson shouldn't have been so mean to me."

Weeks went by. Zelda heard nothing from Mrs. Hudson. Mrs. Hudson heard nothing from the publisher.

But things were very busy at the publisher. The publisher read the book and laughed so hard that her ribs hurt for three days. She read about each of Mrs. Hudson's boring experiences. Then she would look at the picture and almost die from laughter.

She called in other people who worked at the publishing company to read the book and they all had the same reaction. They all ended up with sore ribs for three days.

One of the persons who read the book made a suggestion to the publisher. She said, "What you should do is make each of these illustrations two full pages big. Then underneath you could have the sentences from the book that tell about the illustration."

And that's just what the publisher did. When the publishing company was finished with the book and it was ready to be printed, the picture of the children riding their horses was two full pages. Below the picture, it said: "Every day, the children rode their horses through the valley. Their tails flew in the wind."

The picture of the car on the mountain was two full pages. Below the picture it said: "Our car stopped on top of the mountain. It was out of gas."

And all the other pictures were also two pages, with Mrs. Hudson's sentences written below each picture.

Mrs. Hudson didn't really like the book as much as she thought she would. She thought that the pictures were far, far too large. She said to herself, "Huh, they made the pictures more important than my wonderful experiences."

Zelda was very happy. She was even happier when she read the note the publisher sent to her. The note said:

Dear Zelda,

I find your pictures superb. You have taken a very boring book and made it exciting and wonderfully funny. Thank you so much.

And, when the bookstores got their copies of Mrs. Hudson's book, they didn't keep them very long. Within a few weeks, thousands of copies of the book were sold. Within three months, that book was the fastest selling best-seller book in the world. Newspaper articles raved about the book. One report said this:

R. R. Hudson may be the greatest wit of the century. When you first read the book, you get the idea that she doesn't know how to write clearly. She makes up sentences that could have more than

one meaning. And as you read about her boring experiences, you begin to wonder: Does this woman have anything to say? But then, you'll come across an illustration that makes everything clear. The only way to describe the illustrations is to get the book. And that's just what **a lot** of people are doing.

After the book became so popular, Mrs. Hudson sort of pretended that she had planned it that way. She told reporters, "Yes, my good friend Zelda and I planned it that way. I selected the parts of the book she was to illustrate, and I might add that I selected them very carefully. Then Zelda did those quaint illustrations."

So Mrs. Hudson became very famous. And very rich.

And the book also made another person very rich and very popular. That person was Zelda. But Zelda never really understood why people found the book so funny.

She told reporters, "I just did the best I could with the sentences Mrs. Hudson gave me."

And the reporters would laugh so hard that their ribs hurt for three days.

EXERCISE 4   Details

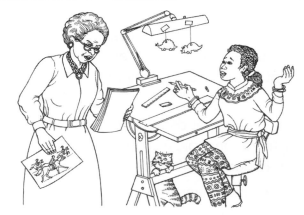

- Find part C in your workbook. ✔
  There's Mrs. Hudson looking upset over the illustrations.
- Everybody, is this picture before or after Zelda got a nice letter from the publisher? (Signal.) *Before.*
- Right. You may color your picture now.

Objectives

- Compose and write a parallel sentence pair based on a single picture. (Exercise 1)
- Construct sentences for different illustrations. (Exercise 2)
- Edit an ambiguous sentence to show how a character interpreted it. (Exercise 3)
- Construct deductions to answer questions. (Exercise 4)
- Listen to part of a familiar story. (Exercise 5)

WORKBOOK • LINED PAPER

EXERCISE 1   Writing Parallel Sentences

| its | gray | scratched | chased | rabbit | ear |

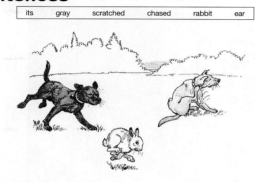

1. Open your workbook to lesson 45 and find part A. ✔
   You're going to write about this picture.
2. The picture shows what a black dog and a gray dog did.
- What did the black dog do? (Call on a student. Idea: *Chased the rabbit.*)
- What did the gray dog do? (Call on a student. Idea: *Scratched its ear.*)
3. Listen: The black dog chased a rabbit. The gray dog scratched its ear.
- Everybody, say the whole sentence about the black dog. (Signal.) *The black dog chased a rabbit.*
- Say the whole sentence about the gray dog. (Signal.) *The gray dog scratched its ear.*
- (Repeat sentences until firm.)
4. Look at the vocabulary box. These are some of the words you need: **its . . . gray . . . scratched . . . chased . . . rabbit . . . ear.**
5. Say the sentence about the black dog. (Signal.) *The black dog chased a rabbit.*
- Say the sentence about the gray dog. (Signal.) *The gray dog scratched its ear.*

- Write both sentences.
  (Observe students and give feedback.)
6. **(Optional:)** Skip a line on your paper and write both sentences again.
   (Observe students and give feedback.)

EXERCISE 2   Sentence Construction

| Goober | Paul | painted a pot | fed the pigs | sat on an apple | Fizz and Liz |

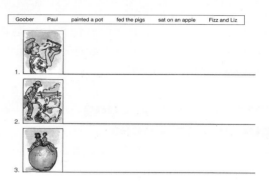

1. Find part B. ✔
   You're going to write sentences for the pictures. The words you'll use are in the boxes. I'll read those words.
- Touch the first word box. ✔
  It says: Goober.
- Next box: painted a pot.
- Next box: sat on an apple.
- Next box: Paul.
- Next box: fed the pigs.
- Last box: Fizz and Liz.
- Those are the words you have to use for your sentences.
2. Touch picture 1. ✔
   Who is in that picture? (Signal.) *Paul.*
- So what will your sentence start with? (Signal.) *Paul.*
- Then your sentence will tell what Paul did in that picture.
3. Touch the two boxes that have the words for that sentence.
   (Observe students and give feedback.)

- I'll say the sentence.
  Paul . . . (pause) . . . painted a pot.
- Your turn: Write the sentence on the line for picture 1. Remember the capital and the period. Raise your hand when you're finished.
  (Observe students and give feedback.)
- (Write on the board:)

> **Paul painted a pot.**

- Here's what you should have. Raise your hand if you got it right.
4. Your turn: Write the sentence for picture 2. Then write the sentence for picture 3. Use the words in the boxes. Raise your hand when you're finished.
   (Observe students and give feedback.)
5. (Write on the board:)

> **2. Goober fed the pigs.**
> **3. Fizz and Liz sat on an apple.**

- Here's what you should have for picture 2 and picture 3. Raise your hand if you got them right. That's great.

EXERCISE 3   Interpreting Ambiguous Sentences

The girls had pet goats. One of them had very long horns.

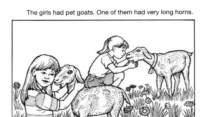

1. Everybody, find part C. ✔
   These are things that Mrs. Hudson wrote.
- You're going to fix up the sentence to show what Zelda thought they meant. Then you're going to fix up the picture the way Zelda would do it.
- Touch the sentences: I'll read them twice. Raise your hand when you know the word that confused Zelda. The girls had pet goats. One of them had very long horns.
- Listen again: The girls had pet goats. One of them had very long horns.
- Everybody, what word would confuse Zelda? (Signal.) *Them.*
- Who was Mrs. Hudson referring to when she wrote: One of **them** had very long horns? (Signal.) *A goat.*

- Who would Zelda **think** had very long horns? (Call on a student. Idea: *One of the girls.*)
2. Cross out the word **them** and write the words that Zelda thought were correct above the word **them.** Raise your hand when you're finished. ✔
- You should have written these words above the word **them: the girls.** Raise your hand if you got it right. ✔
- That's what Zelda thought. Later you can fix up the picture the way Zelda would have done it.

EXERCISE 4   Deduction Writing

Where is Sherlock after dinner?

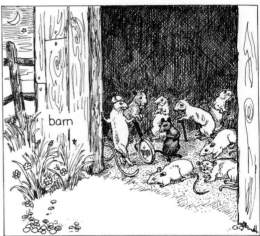

1. After dinner, all the rats are _____
2. Sherlock _____
3. So after dinner, _____

1. Find part D. ✔
   This picture shows something that happens after dinner.
2. Here's the rule: After dinner, all the rats are in the barn. Listen again: After dinner, all the rats are in the barn.
3. There's a question above the picture.
- Touch it. ✔
   I'll read it: Where is Sherlock after dinner?
- Everybody, what does that question say? (Signal.) *Where is Sherlock after dinner?*
- You're going to tell about Sherlock by completing the deduction below the picture. Raise your hand when you're finished. ✔
4. Let's check your work. Here's what you should have: After dinner, all the rats are in the barn. Sherlock is a rat. So after dinner, Sherlock is in the barn.
5. Later you can color this picture.

EXERCISE 5 The Case of the Missing Corn

Review

• I'm going to re-read some parts of **The Case of the Missing Corn.**

At first Sherlock wasn't very good at deductions, but he worked hard until he could figure out the answer faster than any rat in the pack. If somebody said, "Where's Martha the moth?" he'd say, "In the afternoon, all the moths are sleeping in the shed. Martha is a moth. So Martha is sleeping in the shed."

The gray rat was so good at deductions that he said, "Now I'm ready to be a detective. And I'll solve crimes."

He looked through some books to learn more about detectives. He learned that some of them have hound dogs called bloodhounds that can follow the scent of people.

It didn't make much sense for a rat to have a great big bloodhound on a leash, but the gray rat knew a shy little beetle with a very good nose. Her name was Bertha. He went to Bertha and talked her into being his bloodbeetle.

Then he got a large magnifying glass. All the detectives in the books had large magnifying glasses, so the rat got one, too. The magnifying glass was so large that the rat could hardly lift it.

Now the only thing the rat needed to become a complete detective was a name. He thought and thought, and at last he decided to name himself Sherlock.

Just about the time that he was ready to start being a detective, a great problem came up in the rat pack. There was a very special pile of corn in the corner of Goober's barn. This corn was in a place where none of the horses or cows could get it.

Every day after dinner, the rats would go to the barn, and each rat would have two kernels of corn—only two.

But lots of corn was missing from the pile, and the rats were getting mad at each other. Some of the rats even said that the wise old rat was eating it.

This was the greatest argument that had ever taken place in the rat pack. Everybody was angry because, when that pile of corn was gone, nobody would have any dessert until next year.

"Well," Sherlock said to himself, "this is a perfect spot for a detective." He put his bloodbeetle on her leash, stood up very straight and walked out to where the other rats were arguing.

"Calm down," he said loudly. "Listen to me. I have an announcement to make."

Before Sherlock could continue, five rats pointed to him and said, "You stole that corn."

"No, no, I didn't steal any . . . "

Poor Sherlock wasn't able to finish what he was trying to say. "You're the corn stealer," the rats shouted. Nine or ten rats picked him up, carried him to the pond and threw him in. Splash. Bertha saw what happened to Sherlock and ran home the fast way.

As Sherlock waded out of the pond, he said, "I can use my skill at making deductions, and I can track anybody with my bloodbeetle."

The wise old rat said, "Listen to what he has to say. Maybe he can solve this mystery."

The rats argued for a while, and then they told Sherlock that, if he solved the mystery, he could get two times as much dessert as anybody else. And one rat said, "But, if you don't solve this mystery pretty quick, nobody's going to have **any** dessert. That corn is disappearing fast."

Sherlock had to talk his bloodbeetle into working for him again.

He went to Bertha's home—which was a big hole in the ground. He called to her, but she didn't want to come out. She kept saying, "I don't like this job. I saw what they did to you." She was talking about the other rats throwing Sherlock into the pond.

"That was a mistake," Sherlock said. "Everything is straightened out now. All the rats agreed to let me solve the mystery."

Sherlock talked and talked. At last he agreed to give Bertha part of all the extra corn he'd get if he solved the mystery.

Now Sherlock and Bertha were ready to go to work. They went to Goober's barn. On the way, Sherlock explained the plan. "I have everything figured out," he said. "The corn thief went into the barn. So all we have to do is to find somebody who goes into the barn and we'll know who the corn thief is."

Bertha gave Sherlock a funny look. She said, "That doesn't sound right to me, but you're the detective."

"It's very hard for a beetle to understand," Sherlock said. "But, for my plan to work, we have to find who went into the barn."

"That's easy," Bertha said. "Anyone who goes into the barn smells of oats. With one sniff I could tell if somebody went into that barn. Oat smell is very strong."

"Good," Sherlock said. "We'll find somebody who smells of oats, and we'll know who went into the barn."

Just as they were approaching the barn, Sherlock spotted a red chicken. "Look over there," he said to Bertha. "Go over and take a sniff of that chicken. See if she's been in the barn."

So Bertha scurried over near the chicken and then scurried back.

Sherlock asked, "Well? Has she been in the barn?"

The beetle said, "Yep."

Sherlock said, "There, you see? We've solved the mystery already. That chicken took the corn."

"How do you know that?" Bertha asked.

"Listen carefully to this deduction: Anybody who goes into the barn smells of oats. The red chicken went into the barn. So the red chicken smells of oats."

"I know that," Bertha said. "I didn't need a deduction to figure that out. I could smell her a mile away."

"Don't interrupt," Sherlock said, "because that's only the **first** deduction. Here's the **next** deduction: The corn thief went into the barn. The red chicken went into the barn. So the red chicken is the corn thief."

Bertha didn't agree with that deduction. She moved her body from side to side as she said, "No, that still doesn't sound right to me."

Sherlock said, "You can't question the deduction. I solved the crime, and now I'll be getting double corn. Good for me. I'm so smart."

Bertha looked at him and rocked her body from side to side again.

Sherlock said, "Let's go back and tell the others." And they did.

Sherlock jumped up on an old oak stump. He stood up very tall and pushed out his little chest as far as it would go. Then in a very important-sounding voice, he said, "I have solved the mystery. I know who has been taking corn from the barn."

"Who? Who? Who?" all the rats shouted.

"Calm down, please," Sherlock said. When all the rats were very, very quiet, he said, "The red chicken on Goober's farm is the one who took the corn."

"How do you know that?" the wise old rat said.

"Simple," Sherlock said. Then he repeated his deductions. First the one about anybody who goes into the barn smells of oats.

When Sherlock finished, some of the rats scratched their head. Some of them nodded yes-yes. Some of them shook their head no-no. Bertha just rocked from side to side.

At last a brown rat said, "I don't know. I've never heard so much talk to figure something out. Maybe he's right." Bertha rocked back and forth faster and harder.

The wise old rat smiled and said to Bertha, "You don't agree with the gray rat's deductions. Tell me why you don't agree."

"Well," Bertha said slowly, "I don't know much about deductions, but . . . " She was getting embarrassed. She'd never talked before a large group of rats before. She looked down and said, "Well, the gray rat—I mean Sherlock— said that the red chicken did it because she smelled of oats, which means she'd been in the barn. There's just one small problem."

"What's that? What's that?"

"Every single one of you rats smells of oats."

All the rats looked at each other. One of them said, "What does that mean? Does that mean we all stole the corn?"

Then the rats started pointing at each other and saying, "You're the one. You smell of oats. So you must have taken that corn."

"Not me. You smell of oats, too, you know. You're the one."

Fights started breaking out. "Stop," the wise old rat said.

He jumped up on the stump. "I don't know what's wrong with all of you. You must know that you've been in the barn. You've gone in there every evening after dinner. So of course you smell of oats."

"Yeah," one rat said. "We go in there every evening after dinner. Of course we smell of oats."

Then there was a long silence. At last the black rat said, "If we all smell of oats and we've all been in the barn, how does that gray rat know that the red chicken is the one who took the corn? All he knows is that she went into the barn."

"Yeah, what does he know? All he does is talk a lot, come up with silly deductions and get all of us confused."

With that, nine or ten rats picked up the gray rat—I mean Sherlock—and tossed him into the pond again. By the time they reached the pond, Bertha was already home, and that's where she wanted to stay for a long time.

- We'll continue the rest of the story next time.

Objectives

- Write a group of sentences that are thematically related. (Exercise 1)
- Identify the characters on a map by their assertions about relative direction. (Exercise 2)
- Construct sentences for different illustrations. (Exercise 3)
- Listen to part of a familiar story. (Exercise 4)
- **Indicate the order of story events shown in 3 pictures. (Exercise 5)**

WORKBOOK • LINED PAPER

EXERCISE 1 Sentence Writing

> **Note:** For this activity students will need lined paper. Pass out paper. Direct students to write their name on the top line.

1. Find the page titled **Story words** at the front of your workbook.
- (Write on the board:)

> **Everybody bought something.**

- This says: Everybody bought something.
- Copy that sentence on the second line of your paper. Remember the capital and the period. Raise your hand when you've copied the sentence.
(Observe students and give feedback.)
2. (Write to show:)

> **Everybody bought something.**
> **Owen** _____.

- Here's the first part of the sentence you'll write next. Owen blank. Complete the sentence for Owen. He bought one of the things shown on the page with **Story words.**
- Write your sentence about Owen. Raise your hand when you're finished.
(Observe students and give feedback.)
- (Call on individual students to read their sentence about Owen.)
3. (Write to show:)

> **Everybody bought something.**
> **Owen** _____.
> **Mrs. Hudson** _____.
> **I** _____.

- You're going to write more sentences. One will tell about Mrs. Hudson and what she bought. The other will tell about you and what you bought.
- Your turn: Write both sentences. Remember the period at the end of each sentence. Raise your hand when you're finished.
(Observe students and give feedback.)
- (Call on individual students to read their sentence about Mrs. Hudson. Then call on individual students to read their sentence about themselves.)

EXERCISE 2 Map Directions

Relative Direction

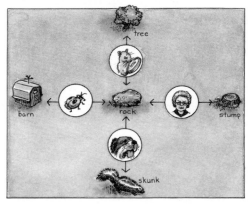

1. Bertha said, "The rock is _____ of me and the
   _____ is _____ of me."

2. Mrs. Hudson said, "The rock is _____ of me and the
   _____ is _____ of me."

3. Sherlock said, "The rock is _____ of me and the
   _____ is _____ of me."

1. Open your workbook to lesson 46 and find part A. ✔
   I'll tell you what different characters said. You're going to be a detective and figure out who could have said that.
- Here's what one character said: "The rock is west of me and the stump is east of me."

- Listen again: "The rock is west of me and the stump is east of me." Raise your hand when you know who said that.
- Everybody, who said, "The rock is west of me and the stump is east of me"? (Signal.) *Mrs. Hudson.*
- Yes, Mrs. Hudson.
- Here's what another character said: "The rock is north of me and the skunk is south of me."
- Listen again: "The rock is north of me and the skunk is south of me." Raise your hand when you know who said that.
- Everybody, who said, "The rock is north of me and the skunk is south of me"? (Signal.) *Dud.*
- Yes, Dud.
- Here's what the last character said: "The rock is east of me and the barn is west of me."
- Listen again: "The rock is east of me and the barn is west of me." Raise your hand when you know who said that.
- Everybody, who said, "The rock is east of me and the barn is west of me"? (Signal.) *Bertha.*

2. You're going to complete the items. They are tough. They all start by telling about the rock. But they have a lot of blanks.
- Touch item 1. ✔
  I'll read: Bertha said, "The rock is blank of me and the blank is blank of me."
- The first part of the sentence is: The rock is blank of me. Write the word for the direction. Raise your hand when you're finished. ✔
- The first part should say: Bertha said, "The rock is **east** of me."
- Then she says that something is in another direction. Name the object that is in the other direction and write the direction. Raise your hand when you're finished. ✔
- Here's what item 1 should say: Bertha said, "The rock is east of me and the **barn** is **west** of me." Raise your hand if you got it right.

3. Touch item 2. ✔
  I'll read: Mrs. Hudson said, "The rock is blank of me and the something else is blank of me."

- Complete the statement. Raise your hand when you're finished. ✔
- Here's what Mrs. Hudson said: "The rock is **west** of me and the **stump** is **east** of me." Raise your hand if you got it right.

4. Touch item 3. ✔
  Sherlock said, "The rock is blank of me and the something else is blank of me." Complete the statement. Raise your hand when you're finished. ✔
- Here's what Sherlock said: "The rock is **south** of me and the **tree** is **north** of me." Raise your hand if you got it right.
- Raise both hands if you got all those items right. I guess some of you are ready to be detectives.

EXERCISE 3 Sentence Construction

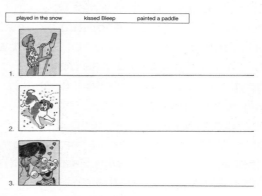

| played in the snow | kissed Bleep | painted a paddle |

1.

2.

3.

1. Find part B. ✔
  The pictures show the sentences you'll write. The words in the boxes tell about the last part of each sentence. You'll have to figure out the first part of each sentence. Remember, that's the name of the character in the picture.

2. Touch picture 1. ✔
  Who is in that picture? (Signal.) *Paul.*
- So how will your sentence start out? (Signal.) *Paul . . .*
- (Write on the board:)

Paul

3. Touch picture 2. ✔
  Who is in that picture? (Signal.) *Dud.*
- So how will your sentence start out? (Signal.) *Dud . . .*
- (Write on the board:)

Dud

4. Touch picture 3. ✔
   Your sentence for that picture will start with Molly.
- (Write on the board:)

> **Molly**

5. I'll read the words that are in the boxes.
- Touch the top word box. ✔
  It says: Played in the snow.
- Next box: Kissed Bleep.
- Last box: Painted a paddle.
6. Listen: Raise your hand when you can say the whole sentence for picture 1. Remember, your sentence has to start with the name of the character and then tell what the character did.
- Everybody, say the sentence for picture 1. (Signal.) *Paul painted a paddle.*
7. Touch picture 3. ✔
   Listen: Raise your hand when you can say the whole sentence for that picture. Remember, your sentence has to start with Molly and then tell what she did.
- Everybody, say the sentence. (Signal.) *Molly kissed Bleep.*
8. Your turn to write the sentences.
   Listen: Write your sentence for picture 1, just picture 1. Start with **Paul.** Use the words in the boxes for the rest of your sentence. Remember the period at the end of the sentence. Raise your hand when you're finished.
   (Observe students and give feedback.)
- (Write to show:)

> **Paul** painted a paddle.

- Here's what you should have for picture 1. Raise your hand if you got it right.
9. Your turn: Write your sentence for picture 2. Remember to use the words in the boxes for part of that sentence. Raise your hand when you're finished.
   (Observe students and give feedback.)
- (Write to show:)

> **Dud** played in the snow.

- Here's what you should have for picture 2. Raise your hand if you got everything right.
10. Write your sentence for picture 3. Remember, start out with the name of the character. Then tell what the character did. Raise your hand when you're finished.

(Observe students and give feedback.)
- (Write to show:)

> **Molly** kissed Bleep.

- Here's what you should have for picture 3.
11. Raise your hand if you got everything right.
- You're writing some pretty tough sentences.

EXERCISE 4   The Case of the Missing Corn

Review

- I'm going to read some more of the Sherlock story.
- Listen: At the end of the last part, Sherlock was in the pond and Bertha was at home. She planned to stay there for a long time.

The next day, Sherlock spent over half an hour bending over the entrance to Bertha's home, trying to talk her into coming out and working on the mystery again. He said, "We can still solve this mystery if you'll come out and work with me."

"I don't think so," Bertha said. "Your deductions don't make a lot of sense to me."

"Of course they make sense."

Bertha said, "But there's something about the deductions you used that . . . "

"What about them?"

"They really stink."

"Why do you say a nasty thing like that?"

"Well, because you could use your deductions to show that **everybody** who went into the barn stole the corn—even you."

"No, no," Sherlock said. "I went into the barn, and I smell of oats, but I'm not the corn thief."

Bertha smiled and said, "That's why your deductions stink. You want to figure out the **only** one who could have taken the corn. But your deductions tell you about a whole bunch of people."

"But how can I make a deduction that tells about the **only** one who could have taken the corn if I don't know who it is?"

"Clues," Bertha said.

Then Bertha said, "Let me think about it. Come back in an hour. Maybe I'll have an idea by then."

An hour later, Sherlock went back to Bertha's place. She rushed up to him and said, "Tonight the rats won't go to the barn to get their dessert."

"Oh, no," Sherlock said. "They'll get very upset if they don't get their dessert."

"Stop interrupting," Bertha said. "They'll get their dessert. But you'll bring it to them so they won't have to go to the barn. Then we'll fix up the rest of the corn in the barn so that anybody who goes into the barn will not only smell of oats; that person will also smell of pine needles."

Sherlock shook his head. "There aren't any pine needles near that barn. And I . . . "

"Stop interrupting," Bertha said. "If you turn around, you'll see a large tree behind you. And what do you see all over the ground under that tree?"

"Pine needles."

"Well, all we need to do is gather up a few bags of those pine needles and take them to the barn."

All afternoon, Sherlock and Bertha collected pine needles and carried them to the barn. Then they counted two kernels of corn for every rat in the pack. They put that corn outside the barn. Then they took the pine needles and made a great circle of pine needles

around the pile of corn that was still in the barn.

When they were done, they carried the corn back to the stump and called all the other rats.

Sherlock stood on the stump. "Quiet please," he said. "Everybody quiet."

The rats looked at each other and asked, "What's all that corn doing out here?"

Sherlock cleared his throat—"ahem, ahem"—and stood up very straight.

In his most important voice, he said, "I won't bother trying to tell you how we're going to find out who is stealing the corn because it's very difficult to understand. But we've brought enough corn out here so every rat can have dessert tonight without going near the barn. We have very cleverly fixed the pile of corn that's still in the barn so that anybody who goes to the corn will give us a very good clue. But it's difficult to explain."

"What kind of clue?" one of the rats asked.

Bertha said, "We put pine needles all around the corn. So anybody who goes to the corn will smell of pine needles."

"Now that makes sense," one of the rats said. Then other rats agreed and nodded their heads up and down. "Yeah, if somebody smells of oats and pine needles, that's the guilty person."

"Yeah, that's smart," the rats agreed.

So the rats had dinner and ate their dessert. Then they did what rats do in the evening—went to sleep.

Sherlock didn't sleep with the other rats. He had to sleep outside Bertha's place where she could keep an eye on him.

The next morning, Bertha woke him up by tickling his nose with her little front legs. Then she said, "Let's go find the corn thief." And away they went.

- We'll finish the story next time.

EXERCISE 5 Temporal Sequencing

Story Events

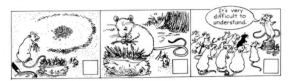

1. Find part C. ✔
   These pictures show three things that happened in the story, but the things are not in the right order.
2. Touch the picture of Sherlock and Bertha spreading pine needles. That's one of the things that happened.
   - Touch the picture of Sherlock and Bertha gathering pine needles. That's another thing that happened.
   - Touch the picture of Sherlock making a speech. He is saying, "It's very difficult to understand." The rats are looking at him with unhappy expressions.

3. Listen: Think of the story. Put number 1 in the picture that happened first. Put number 2 in the picture that happened next. Put number 3 in the picture that happened last.
   - Everybody, write 1 in the picture of the first thing, 2 in the picture of the next thing and 3 in the picture of the last thing. Raise your hand when you're finished.
   (Observe students and give feedback.)
4. What is happening in the picture for number 1? (Call on a student. Idea: *Sherlock and Bertha are gathering pine needles.*)
   - What is happening in the picture for number 2? (Call on a student. Idea: *Sherlock and Bertha are spreading pine needles.*)
   - What is happening in the picture for number 3? (Call on a student. Idea: *Sherlock is telling the rats, "It's very difficult to understand."*)
5. Later you can color the pictures.

Objectives

- Identify the characters on a map by their assertions about relative direction. (Exercise 1)
- Construct sentences for different illustrations. (Exercise 2)
- **Rewrite unambiguous sentence pairs so the second sentence is ambiguous.** (Exercise 3)
- Listen to part of a familiar story. (Exercise 4)
- **Put on a play to show part of a familiar story.** (Exercise 5)

WORKBOOK

EXERCISE 1   Map Directions

Relative Direction

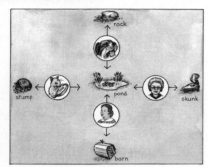

1. Zelda said, "The pond is _____ of me and the

   _____ is _____ of me."

2. Sherlock said, "The pond is _____ of me and the

   _____ is _____of me."

3. Mrs. Hudson said, "The pond is _____ of me and the

   _____ is _____ of me."

1. Open your workbook to lesson 47 and find part A. ✔

    I'll tell you what different characters said. You're going to play detectives again and figure out who could have said that.

- Here's what one character said: "The pond is east of me and the stump is west of me." Raise your hand when you know who said that.
- Everybody, who said that? (Signal.) *Sherlock.*
- Yes, Sherlock.

2. Here's what another character said: "The pond is north of me and the barn is south of me." Raise your hand when you know who said that.

- Everybody, who said that? (Signal.) *Zelda.*
- Yes, Zelda.

3. Here's what the third character said: "The pond is west of me and the skunk is east of me." Raise your hand when you know who said that.

- Everybody, who said that? (Signal.) *Mrs. Hudson.*

4. You're going to complete the items. They are tough. They all start by telling about the pond. But they have a lot of blanks.

- Touch item 1. ✔
  I'll read: Zelda said, "The pond is blank of me and the blank is blank of me."
- The first part of the sentence is: The pond is blank of me. Write the word for the direction. Raise your hand when you're finished. ✔
- The first part should say: Zelda said, "The pond is **north** of me."
- Then she said that something else is in another direction. Name the object that is in the other direction and write the direction. Raise your hand when you're finished. ✔
- Here's what item 1 should say: Zelda said, "The pond is north of me and the **barn** is **south** of me." Raise your hand if you got it right.

5. Touch item 2. I'll read: Sherlock said, "The pond is blank of me and the something else is blank of me."

- Complete the statement. Raise your hand when you're finished. ✔
- Here's what Sherlock said: "The pond is **east** of me and the **stump** is **west** of me." Raise your hand if you got it right.

6. Touch item 3. ✔
   Mrs. Hudson said, "The pond is blank of me and the something else is blank of me."
   - Complete the statement. Raise your hand when you're finished. ✔
   - Here's what Mrs. Hudson said: "The pond is **west** of me and the **skunk** is **east** of me." Raise your hand if you got it right.
7. Raise your hand if you got all those items right.

EXERCISE 2 Sentence Construction

1. Find part B. ✔
   The pictures show the sentences you'll write. The words in the boxes tell about the last part of each sentence. You'll have to figure out the first part of each sentence. Remember, that's the name of the character in the picture.
2. Touch picture 1. ✔
   Who is in that picture? (Signal.) *Goober.*
   - (Write on the board:)

   Goober

   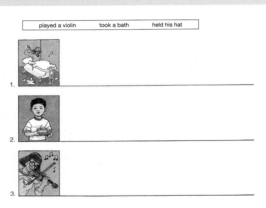

   - So how will your sentence start out? (Signal.) *Goober.*
3. Touch picture 2. ✔
   Who is in that picture? (Signal.) *Roger.*
   - (Write on the board:)

   Roger

   - So how will your sentence start out? (Signal.) *Roger.*
4. Touch picture 3. ✔
   Who is in that picture? (Signal.) *Molly.*
   - (Write on the board:)

   Molly

   - So how will your sentence start out? (Signal.) *Molly.*

5. I'll read the words that are in the boxes.
   - Touch the top box. ✔
   It says: played a violin.
   - Next box: took a bath.
   - Last box: held his hat.
6. Listen: Raise your hand when you can say the whole sentence for the top picture. Remember, your sentence has to start with the name of the character and then tell what the character did.
   - Everybody, say the sentence for the top picture. (Signal.) *Goober took a bath.*
7. Touch picture 2. ✔
   Listen: Raise your hand when you can say the whole sentence for that picture. Remember, your sentence has to start with the name of the character and then tell what the character did.
   - Everybody, say the sentence. (Signal.) *Roger held his hat.*
8. Your turn to write the sentences.
   Listen: Write your sentence for picture 1. Remember the period at the end of the sentence. Raise your hand when you're finished.
   (Observe students and give feedback.)
   - (Write on the board:)

   Goober took a bath.

   - Here's what you should have for picture 1. Raise your hand if you got everything right.
9. Your turn: Write your sentence for picture 2. Raise your hand when you're finished.
   (Observe students and give feedback.)
   - (Write on the board:)

   Roger held his hat.

   - Here's what you should have for picture 2. Raise your hand if you got everything right.
10. Listen: Write your sentence for picture 3. Remember, start out with the name of the character. Then tell what the character did. Raise your hand when you're finished.
    (Observe students and give feedback.)
    - (Write on the board:)

    Molly played a violin.

    - Here's what you should have. Molly played a violin. Raise your hand if you got everything right.

11. Raise both hands if you got all the sentences right. You're writing some pretty tough sentences.

EXERCISE 3　Creating Ambiguous Sentences

1. The boys played with dogs. The dogs had short tails.
2. The girls went in boats. The boats were made of wood.
3. The truck went up a hill. The truck had a flat tire.

1. Everybody, find part C. ✔
   Each item has two sentences. The sentences are **not** confusing. You're going to fix them up so they **are** confusing. You're going to pretend that you're Mrs. Hudson.
2. Touch the sentences for item 1. ✔
   I'll read: The boys played with dogs. The dogs had short tails.
- Those sentences are not confusing. Here's what you'll do to make them confusing. You'll change the way the second sentence starts out.
- Touch the second sentence in item 1. ✔
  That sentence starts out by naming something. Raise your hand when you know what it names.
- Everybody, what does the second sentence name? (Signal.) *The dogs.*
- Listen: Cross out the words **the dogs** in the second sentence.
  (Observe students and give feedback.)
3. Touch the sentences for item 2. ✔
   I'll read: The girls went in boats. The boats were made of wood.
- Those sentences are not confusing. To make them confusing, you'll change the way the second sentence starts out.
- Touch the second sentence in item 2. That sentence starts out by naming something. Raise your hand when you know what it names.
- Everybody, what does the second sentence name? (Signal.) *The boats.*

- Listen: Cross out the words **the boats** in the second sentence.
  (Observe students and give feedback.)
4. Touch the sentences for item 3. I'll read: The truck went up a hill. The truck had a flat tire.
- Those sentences are not confusing. To make them confusing, you'll change the way the second sentence starts out. That sentence starts out by naming something. Raise your hand when you know what it names.
- Everybody, what does the second sentence name? (Signal.) *The truck.*
- Listen: Cross out the words **the truck** in the second sentence.
  (Observe students and give feedback.)
5. (Write on the board:)

He　She　It　They

- To make the sentences confusing, you use one of these words. The words are **he, she, it, they.**
- You have to pick the right word to start the second sentence in each item.
- Touch item 1. ✔
  Everybody, what did you cross out in the second sentence? (Signal.) *The dogs.*
- You can use one of the words on the board to tell about the boys or the dogs. Raise your hand when you know which word that is.
- Everybody, which word? (Signal.) *They.*
- Yes, **they.** Write the word **they** above the crossed-out words.
  (Observe students and give feedback.)
- I'll read what item 1 should say now: The boys played with dogs. **They** had short tails.
- Now we don't know who had short tails. Maybe it was the dogs. Maybe it was . . . (pause) . . . **the boys.**
6. Item 2: The girls went in boats. The boats were made of wood.
- What did you cross out in the second sentence? (Signal.) *The boats.*
- You can use one of the words on the board to tell about the girls or the boats. Raise your hand when you know which word that is.

- Everybody, which word? (Signal.) *They.*
- Yes, **they.** Write the word **they** above the crossed-out words. Raise your hand when you're finished.
- I'll read what item 2 should say now: The girls went in boats. **They** were made of wood.
- Now we don't know what was made of wood. Maybe it was the boats. Maybe it was . . . (pause) . . . **the girls.**

7. Item 3: The truck went up a hill. The truck had a flat tire.
- What did you cross out in the second sentence? (Signal.) *The truck.*
- You can use one of the words on the board to tell about the truck or the hill. Raise your hand when you know which word that is.
- Everybody, which word? (Signal.) *It.*
- Yes, **it.** Write the word **it** above the crossed-out words. Raise your hand when you're finished.
- I'll read what item 3 should say now: The truck went up a hill. **It** had a flat tire.
- Now we don't know what had a flat tire. Maybe it was the truck. Maybe it was . . . (pause) . . . **the hill.**

8. There is a big box at the bottom of the page.
- Later you can draw a picture in that box to show how Zelda might illustrate one of those items.

EXERCISE 4   The Case of the Missing Corn

Review

- I'm going to read the last part of the story about Sherlock and **The Case of the Missing Corn.** That's the part where Bertha and Sherlock meet Cyrus the squirrel.
- Listen very carefully because we're going to act out this part. We'll have a play.
- Somebody will play Bertha. That person will have to remember the three questions.
- Another person will play Cyrus. That person will have to remember all of Cyrus's excuses about why he smells of pine needles and why he smells of oats.
- A third person will have to play the part of Sherlock. Sherlock is going to ask Cyrus

questions before Bertha launches into Cyrus. The person who plays Sherlock will have to remember all of Sherlock's questions.
- Remember what happened. Bertha and Sherlock have been greeting different animals so that Bertha can get close enough to sniff them. She's really trying to find out if they have three smells.
- What are they? (Call on a student. Idea: *Pine needles, oats and corn.*)
- Listen to the story:

At last they greeted Myron the mouse. Bertha took a good sniff. Then she walked away as Sherlock followed.

Bertha stopped and whispered, "Myron smells of oats and he smells of pine needles."

Sherlock said, "Let's haul him back to the rat pack. He's the one who did it."

"I'm not really sure," Bertha said.

"Why not?" Sherlock asked.

"Something is missing," Bertha said. "Let's look around a little bit more."

So they greeted more frogs and toads and snakes and snails. They greeted more chipmunks and skunks and sparrows and ducks. At last, they came to Cyrus the squirrel. He was leaning against a tree, yawning and stretching. After Sherlock and Bertha greeted him, they walked away. Then Bertha stopped and whispered, "He smells of oats and he smells of pine needles. He's the one who's been stealing the corn. Ask him."

"Okay," Sherlock said. He walked over and said, "Been near the barn lately?"

"Not me," Cyrus said and yawned again.

"Been stealing any corn from that barn?"

"Who me?" Cyrus asked. "I know that corn is for the rat pack. I wouldn't take any of that corn."

"So you didn't steal the corn from the barn?"

"Absolutely not," he said and yawned again.

Sherlock shrugged and went back to Bertha. "He said he didn't do it."

Bertha got so angry that she started to quiver all over. She said, "We will see about that."

She charged over to Cyrus and said, "If you didn't go to the barn, why is it that you smell of fresh pine needles?"

"I'm a squirrel," he said. "I climb pine trees all the time."

"Okay, if you didn't go into the barn, why do you smell of oats?"

"There's an oat field on the other side of the pond. I was walking around there early this morning."

"Oh yeah?" Bertha said. "Well if you didn't go into the barn, why does your breath smell of corn?"

"I . . . uh . . . I . . . "

Bertha said, "Your breath is so strong, I could smell the corn every time you yawned. You're a liar and you stole the corn. Admit it."

"Well, I . . . uh . . . that is . . . I . . . "

"Stop trying to make excuses. You stole the corn. Admit it."

"Okay, okay. I admit it."

"Well, you'd better figure out some way of paying the pack back and you'd better think fast."

"I'm thinking. I'm thinking," Cyrus said.

Later that day, Cyrus, Sherlock and Bertha went to the stump. Sherlock called the other rats. "Attention, attention," he said. "I have an announcement to make." He was talking in his important voice. "We have found the guilty party. It was Cyrus the squirrel, and he admitted it."

"Let's throw him into the pond."

"No, no," Sherlock said. "Cyrus has promised to bring us a special dessert every night for the next two weeks. That dessert is your very favorite nut."

The rats all stared at Sherlock. Then one of them said, "You don't mean hazelnuts, do you?"

"Yes, hazelnuts," Sherlock said. "Everybody gets a big hazelnut every night for two weeks."

Great cheers went up from the rat pack. "What a deal," they shouted. "Corn is good, but hazelnuts are the best!"

The rats crowded around Sherlock and patted him on the back.

One of them said, "Yeah, Cyrus can steal all the corn he wants as long he pays us back with hazelnuts." Other rats told Sherlock how smart he was. "You did a great job," they said. "We didn't think you knew what you were doing, but you really figured it out."

They shook his hand, patted him on the back and gave him great hugs. Some of the pretty little girl rats even gave him a kiss. One of them said, "You're so big and smart. And you solved this crime all by yourself."

Sherlock said, "Oh well, I had a little bit of help from Bertha."

EXERCISE 5　Play

The Case of the Missing Corn

1. (Write on the board:)

Sherlock

- For the first part of our play, Sherlock asks questions. Who remembers the first question he asks Cyrus? (Call on a student. Idea: *Been near the barn lately?*)
- And what does Cyrus say? (Signal.) *Not me.*
- Then what does Sherlock ask? (Call on a student. Idea: *Been stealing any corn from the barn?*)
- And what does Cyrus say? (Signal.) *Absolutely not.*
- Then Sherlock goes back to Bertha and says, "He said he didn't do it."

2. (Write on the board:)

Bertha

- Then Bertha gets very angry. She charges over to Cyrus and asks him a whole bunch of questions. All of them start the same way, "If you didn't go into the barn . . ."
- Who remembers what she asks first? (Call on a student. Idea: *If you didn't go into the barn, why do you smell of pine needles?*)
- Her next question is, "If you didn't go into the barn, why do you smell of oats?"
- Her last question is, "Well, if you didn't go into the barn, why does your breath smell of corn?"
- Who can ask all three of those questions? (Call on a student. Praise appropriate questions.)

3. (Write on the board:)

Cyrus

- Cyrus gives an excuse for the first question. What does he say to explain why he smells of pine needles? (Call on a student. Idea: *I'm a squirrel. I climb pine trees all the time.*)
- Then Bertha says, "If you didn't go into the barn, why do you smell of oats?"
- And Cyrus gives another excuse. What does he say? (Call on a student. Idea: *There's an oat field on the other side of the pond. I was walking around there early this morning.*)

- Then Bertha says, "Oh yeah, well, if you didn't go into the barn, why does your **breath** smell of corn?"
- And Cyrus doesn't have an excuse. He just tries to make up something, and all he says is "I . . . uh . . . well . . ."
- Then Bertha keeps questioning and telling him to admit it. Finally he admits it, and Bertha says, "Well, you'd better figure out some way of paying the pack back, and you'd better think fast."
- Then Cyrus tells how he'll pay the pack back. How will he do that? (Call on a student. Idea: *Give them hazelnuts.*)
- Yes, he'll give the pack enough hazelnuts so that every member of the pack will have a hazelnut every night for two weeks.

4. When we put on this play, the person who has to remember the most things to say is Bertha. That will be a tough part. Who thinks they can play Bertha and remember to do all the things Bertha did? (Assign Bertha.)

5. The person who plays Cyrus will have to remember a lot of excuses and also remember what he'll do to pay the pack back. Who thinks they can play Cyrus? (Assign Cyrus.)

6. And who wants to play Sherlock? (Assign Sherlock.)

7. (Arrange students so that Cyrus is about 10 feet from Sherlock and Bertha.)

- Bertha and Sherlock are going to greet Cyrus. Then Bertha is going to get close enough to get a good sniff. Then she'll go over and tell Sherlock he did it.
- Let's do that part. Remember, Cyrus is yawning a lot. Cyrus: start yawning. Sherlock and Bertha: start greeting. (Students act out parts.)

8. (After students greet and walk away, say:) Now the next part is Sherlock's turn. Bertha is going to tell him to ask Cyrus if he stole the corn. Then Sherlock will ask his questions.

- Go Sherlock. (Students act out parts.)

9. (After Sherlock's questions, say:) Now it's Bertha's turn to ask Cyrus her questions.

- Go Bertha. (Students act out parts.)

10. (After Bertha's questions, say:) We did a pretty good job. Maybe we can do it again later with different people playing Bertha, Sherlock and Cyrus.

Objectives

- Compose and write a parallel sentence pair based on a single picture. (Exercise 1)
- **Combine subjects and predicates to construct sentences about familiar characters.** (Exercise 2)
- Listen to part 1 of a story and answer comprehension questions. (Exercise 3)
- Edit words to correct dialect. (Exercise 4)

WORKBOOK • LINED PAPER

EXERCISE 1 Writing Parallel Sentences

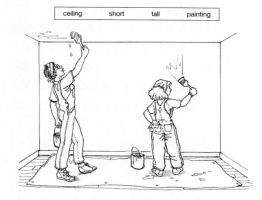

| ceiling | short | tall | painting |

1. Open your workbook to lesson 48 and find part A. ✔
   You're going to write about this picture.
2. The picture shows what a tall woman and a short woman were doing.
- What was the tall woman doing? (Call on a student. Idea: *Painting the ceiling.*)
- What was the short woman doing? (Call on a student. Idea: *Painting the wall.*)
3. Listen: The tall woman was painting the ceiling. The short woman was painting the wall.
- Say the whole sentence about the tall woman. (Signal.) *The tall woman was painting the ceiling.*
- Say the whole sentence about the short woman. (Signal.) *The short woman was painting the wall.*
- (Repeat sentences until firm.)
4. Look at the vocabulary box. These are some of the words you need: **ceiling . . . short . . . tall . . . painting.**
5. Say the sentence about the tall woman. (Signal.) *The tall woman was painting the ceiling.*

- Say the sentence about the short woman. (Signal.) *The short woman was painting the wall.*
- Write both sentences. (Observe students and give feedback.)
6. Skip a line on your paper and write both sentences again. (Observe students and give feedback.)

EXERCISE 2 Sentence Construction

Bleep	rolled in the mud
Dud	sat on Roger
Zelda	played in the snow
Mrs. Hudson	chased a skunk
	said silly things

1. _____
2. _____
3. _____

1. Find part B. ✔
   There are two big boxes with words in them.
- Touch the first box. ✔
   Those are the names you'll start your sentences with. I'll read the names.
- Touch the top name. ✔
   It says: Bleep.
- Next name: Dud.
- Next name: Zelda.
- Last name: Mrs. Hudson.
- Remember those are the names you'll start your sentences with. The other box tells what the characters did.
- Touch the top words. ✔
   They say: rolled in the mud.
- Next words: sat on Roger.
- Next words: played in the snow.
- Next words: chased a skunk.
- Last words: said silly things.

2. Listen: Your first sentence will tell about the first character.

- Touch the name of the first character. ✔ Everybody, what name are you touching? (Signal.) *Bleep.*
- Your first sentence will start with **Bleep,** and it will tell something that Bleep did in a story. Raise your hand when you've found one of the parts that tell something that Bleep did in a story.
- Everybody, what did Bleep do in a story? (Signal.) *Said silly things.*
- Write your sentence about what Bleep did on line 1. Remember to start with a capital and end with a period. Raise your hand when you're finished.
  (Observe students and give feedback.)
- (Write on the board:)

Bleep said silly things.

- Here's what you should have. Raise your hand if you got everything right.
3. Your next sentence will tell about the next character.
- Touch the name of the next character. ✔ Everybody, what name are you touching? (Signal.) *Dud.*
- Your sentence will start with **Dud,** and it will tell something that Dud did in a story. Raise your hand when you've found one of the parts that tells something that Dud did in a story.
- Everybody, what did Dud do in a story? (Signal.) *Played in the snow.*
- Write your sentence about what Dud did on line 2. Raise your hand when you're finished.
  (Observe students and give feedback.)
- (Write on the board:)

Dud played in the snow.

- Here's what you should have. Raise your hand if you got everything right.
4. Your next sentence will start with one of the names you haven't used. It can start with Zelda or Mrs. Hudson. And that sentence **won't** tell what happened in a story you've heard. That sentence will tell something you would like to happen in a story. I think we're going to have some pretty silly sentences.

- Your turn: Start with **Zelda** or **Mrs. Hudson.** Complete the sentence with any part you want. Raise your hand when you're finished.
  (Observe students and give feedback.)
- I'll call on three individual students to read their sentence 3. I'll write those sentences on the board.
  (Call on 3 students:) Read your sentence. (Write sentences on board.)
5. There's a big box at the bottom of the page. Later, you can draw a picture of your sentence 3 in that box.

EXERCISE 3   Bleep Visits West Town *Part 1*

- This is a story that took place before the little girl from West Town started bringing Goober pig soap and clean clothes.
- When this story took place, the smell from Goober's farm was going to West Town because a steady wind was blowing from the east to the west. That wind blew through Goober's farm and carried the smells of his pigs. Phew.

It was the middle of summer, so the people in West Town had their doors and windows open. Usually a summer wind carries smells of freshly mowed lawns and summer flowers and barbecues. The wind that blew into West Town that summer carried those smells, but the people couldn't really smell them because there was a smell that just overpowered all the others.

- What smell was that? (Call on a student. Idea: *Goober's farm; Goober's pigs.*)

Well, just after the wind started blowing from the east, all the people in West Town who lived within a mile of Goober's farm put a clothespin on their nose, and they talked as if they had a very bad cold. They couldn't say two sounds.

- What sounds are those? (Call on a student. Idea: *N and M sounds.*)

Instead of saying, "Let's buy some ham," they said, "Let's buy sub hab."

Instead of saying, "The sun is shining," they said, "The sud is shydig."

Well, you'll never guess who came to visit somebody in West Town just after everybody put their clothespin on. It was Bleep.

Molly had to go to California. She didn't want to leave Bleep at her house, so she asked her sister Holly if she needed some help around her house.

Molly told Holly that Bleep could be a very big help. Holly needed some yard work done and the fence painted, so she liked the idea of Bleep staying at her place for a couple of weeks.

A few days later, a truck delivered a great wooden box to Holly's place. When Holly opened it, Bleep rolled out, looked at Holly and said, "My name is Bleep."

Holly was wearing a clothespin on her nose. So she said, "By dabe is Holly."

Bleep looked at her and said, "Blurp?" He didn't understand what she was trying to say.

Holly said, "I dote dough what blurp beads."

- What was she trying to say? (Call on a student. Idea: *I don't know what blurp means.*)
- Listen to that part again:

Holly said, "I dote dough what blurp beads."

Bleep looked at her and said, "Blurp, blurp."

Holly scratched her head. She didn't know why Bleep was saying "blurp."

Bleep scratched his head. He didn't know what Holly was trying to say.

Later that day, Bleep was working away at painting the fence. Holly, of course, had had some trouble trying to explain to Bleep what she wanted him to do.

He didn't understand her when she said, "Paidt the fedts."

He just looked at her and said that word again.

- What word is that? (Signal.) *Blurp.*

She finally showed him what she wanted him to do, and he started at one end of the fence and began painting. When he was about half way finished with the fence, a couple of little children came by, a boy and a girl. Of course, they both had a clothespin on their nose.

The girl said, "Hello. Who are you?"

Bleep said, "Bleep."

The girl pointed to herself and said, "I'b Berry."

Bleep said, "Hello, I'b Berry."

"Dough," she said. "Dot I'b Berry. Just Berry."

Bleep said, "Hello, just Berry."

"Dough, dough," she said, and the two children started to laugh.

- She said, "I'b Berry." Berry is not a very common girl's name. What do you think she was trying to say when she said, "I'b Berry"? (Call on a student. Idea: *I'm Mary.*)

Then the little boy pointed to himself and said, "I'b Dick."

Bleep said, "Hello, I'b Dick."

"Dough, dough," he said. "Dick."

Bleep said, "Hello, Dick."

"Dot Dick," the boy said, "**Dick.**"

Bleep said, "Blurp."

- The boy didn't like when Bleep called him Dick. Maybe his name wasn't really Dick. What do you think it was? (Call on a student. Idea: *Nick.*)

The children laughed again. They left giggling and snickering.

Pretty soon, the mailman came by. "Hello," he said. "You bust be dew aroud here."

Bleep didn't say anything. He just kept on painting, but he was doing a lot of thinking.

The mailman asked Bleep, "Is it all right for be to give you the bail?"

Bleep said, "Blurp."

- Listen to what the mailman said: "Is it all right for be to give you the bail?"
- What was he trying to say? (Call on a student. Idea: *Is it all right for me to give you the mail?*)

The mailman handed Bleep a bunch of letters and said, "Bake sure that Holly gets these letters."

Bleep was beginning to think that everybody in this town was crazy. Why did they all have sticks on their faces? And why did they talk so funny?

The smell of Goober didn't bother Bleep because he couldn't smell, so he didn't really understand why people had sticks on their faces.

- Everybody, what were those sticks? (Signal.) *Clothespins.*

Bleep wondered whether people thought the sticks made them look better.

The next day, Bleep figured out what people were trying to say. By then he had heard lots of people talk.

He heard the neighbors talking to each other. He heard Holly. He heard children. He even heard the garbage collector. Of course, all these people wore a clothespin, including the garbage collector.

And, after hearing enough people talk, Bleep figured out some things. The first thing was that people couldn't say the sound for M or the sound for N.

Bleep also figured out what they said instead of M and what they said instead of N.

- What did they say instead of the sound for M? (Signal.) *B.*
- What did they say instead of the sound for N? (Signal.) *D.*

Another thing that Bleep figured out was that he didn't look like everyone else. He figured that it would be easy enough to fix himself up so he looked like the other people. He'd just get one of those sticks and put it on his face. He didn't really have a nose, but he figured that he could put the stick somewhere in the middle of his face.

Fixing the way he talked was a bigger problem. He thought about that for a long time. Here's the way he reasoned: The people around here must know how to speak correctly. I do not speak the way they do. So I don't speak correctly.

That evening, Bleep decided that he had to fix himself up. So he took off the top of his head and started adjusting screws. At last he found the right screws for the M sound and the N sound, and he adjusted those screws so he was saying something else for M and something else for N.

When he was done, he went into the living room, where Holly was reading a book.

Bleep said, "I fixed byself so I say thigs the right way."

Holly laughed. Then she said, "I thik it's fuddy. But I dote thik Bolly will fide it very fuddy."

- We'll find out next time.

EXERCISE 4 Correcting Non-nasal Speech

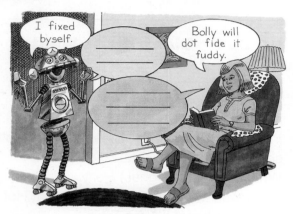

1. Find part C. ✔
   This is a picture of Bleep talking to Holly.
- Touch the words that Bleep is saying. ✔
   He's saying "I fixed byself."
- Everybody, what is he trying to say? (Signal.) *I fixed myself.*
- Touch the words that Holly is saying. ✔
   She is saying, "Bolly will dot fide it fuddy."
- Everybody, what is she trying to say? (Signal.) *Molly will not find it funny.*

2. See if you can write the words so they show what the characters are **trying** to say. Write the words Bleep is trying to say in the empty balloon for Bleep. Write the words Holly is trying to say in the empty balloon for Holly. Remember the periods. Raise your hand when you're finished. (Observe students and give feedback.)
- (Write on the board:)

> **I fixed myself.**
> **Molly will not find it funny.**

- Here's what you should have for Bleep and for Holly. Bleep is trying to say: I fixed myself. Holly is trying to say: Molly will not find it funny. Raise your hand if you wrote both sentences correctly.

3. Later you can fix up that picture. Neither character is wearing a clothespin. That's wrong. Holly should have one and Bleep should have some kind of stick in the middle of his face. See what you can do for him.

Objectives

- Compose and write a parallel sentence pair based on a single picture. (Exercise 1)
- Listen to the conclusion of a 2-part story and answer comprehension questions. (Exercise 2)
- Edit words to show dialect. (Exercise 3)
- Write a group of sentences that are thematically related. (Exercise 4)

WORKBOOK • LINED PAPER

EXERCISE 1 Writing Parallel Sentences

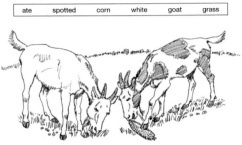

| ate | spotted | corn | white | goat | grass |

1. Open your workbook to lesson 49 and find part A. ✔
   You're going to write about this picture.
2. The picture shows what a white goat and a spotted goat ate.
- What did the white goat eat? (Signal.) *Grass.*
- What did the spotted goat eat? (Call on a student. *Idea: Corn.*)
3. Listen: A white goat ate grass.
- Everybody, say the whole sentence about a white goat. (Signal.) *A white goat ate grass.*
- (Repeat the sentence until firm.)
4. Look at the vocabulary box. These are some of the words you need: **ate . . . spotted . . . corn . . . white . . . goat . . . grass.**
5. Write both sentences.
   (Observe students and give feedback.)
6. Check your sentences. (Call on several students to read both sentences. Idea: *A white goat ate grass. A spotted goat ate corn.*)
- Raise your hand if you got both of them right. ✔
7. **(Optional:)** Skip a line on your paper and write both sentences again.
   (Observe students and give feedback.)
8. (Collect and correct papers.)

EXERCISE 2 Bleep Visits West Town *Part 2*

Storytelling

- It's story time.
  In the last Bleep story, Bleep went to visit somebody.
- Who was that? (Signal.) *Holly.*
- What was the name of the town that Holly lived in? (Signal.) *West Town.*
- Things were not very good in West Town when Bleep got there. What was the problem? (Call on a student. Idea: *A big wind was blowing from the east; the smell from Goober's farm was bad.*)
- The people in West Town were wearing things that puzzled Bleep. What were they wearing? (Signal.) *Clothespins.*
- And the people were talking very strangely. What sounds couldn't they say? (Call on a student. Idea: *N and M sounds.*)
- Why did Bleep think that he was not speaking properly? (Call on a student. Idea: *Nobody else talked the way he did.*)
- What did he do about it? (Call on a student. Idea: *Adjusted his screws.*)

Bleep stayed with Holly for two weeks. During that time, he mowed the lawn, planted the garden, cleaned out the garage and, of course, painted the fence.

During those two weeks something else happened. That great wind that had been blowing from east to west died down. The air was still, with no wind at all, not even a small breeze.

When the air was still, the smell from Goober's farm didn't blow this way or that way, it just kept hanging like a great cloud over his farm.

All the animals on the farm were very upset because they hated that smell. But the people in West Town were very happy because they could take their clothespins off and talk normally.

Well, almost all of them could talk normally.

Bleep was mowing the lawn for the second time when the wind stopped. He was wearing a clothespin on his face. He felt silly wearing it, but he thought that he was doing the right thing.

Shortly after the wind died, Holly came out of the house. She was not wearing her clothespin. She spread her arms out to the side and said, "What a wonderful, wonderful day."

Bleep looked up from the lawn mowing and said, "Yes, it's a dice day."

Holly said, "It's not just nice. It's wonderful. Ah, smell that fine air."

Bleep said, "I cad dot sbell."

- What's he trying to say? (Signal.) *I cannot smell.*

Holly said, "How nice it is to get that clothespin off my nose."

Bleep looked up and saw that Holly wasn't wearing her clothespin. He said, "Should I take bide off, too?"

"Sure," she said. "Take it off. The air is now as sweet as honey."

Bleep noticed that Holly was talking differently, and he really didn't know why. And he didn't know that everybody else was talking normally again. But he found out.

The two children came by.

Bleep said, "Hello, Berry. Hello, Dick."

Mary said, "Hi, Bleep. Isn't it a wonderful day?"

"Yes," Bleep said. "It's a good day to bow the lawd."

Nick said, "You talk silly. But we can talk normally again. What a wonderful day."

Bleep said to himself, "These people are strage. First they talk wud way; thed they talk adother way. I wish they would bake up their bide."

Just then a car pulled up. It was Molly's car. She got out, greeted Holly with a great big hug and asked Holly, "Has Bleep been behaving himself?"

"Yes and no," Holly said.

Molly put her hands on her hips and said, "What's Bleep been up to now?"

Holly chuckled and said, "Why don't you ask him yourself?"

So Molly walked over to Bleep and said, "It's good to see you Bleep. Have you been behaving yourself?"

He said, "Yes, I have."

Molly asked, "Bleep, could you get my suitcase from the car and take it inside?"

"Okay, baby."

- Everybody, has Bleep talked funny to Molly yet? (Signal.) *No.*
- So does Molly know what the problem is? (Signal.) *No.*

Bleep went over to the car and took the suitcase inside. While he was doing that, Molly walked over to Holly and said, "He told me that he's been behaving himself. What's the problem?"

"Why don't you talk to him some more? Maybe you'll find out."

Molly shook her head. "What should I talk to him about?"

Holly said, "Anything. Just talk to him for a while."

Molly said, "Okay, baby."

She went inside and said, "Bleep, come here. I want to talk to you. Have you been doing everything that Holly tells you to do?"

"Yes, I have."

"Have you been telling the truth?"

"Yes, I have."

"Did you plant that pretty garden out there?"

"Yes, I did."

"What did you plant in that garden?"

"Peas, celery, lettuce, squash and radishes."

- That Bleep **still** hasn't said any words that have **M** or **N.** Molly must be very puzzled about what his problem could be.

Molly shook her head. She couldn't find any problem with Bleep.

She said, "Are those the only things you planted in the garden?"

Bleep looked at her and then said in a big voice, "Yes, Holly wadded to pladt beads but there was dough roob for theb."

"What?" Molly said. "What did you say?"

"I said, Holly wadded to pladt beads but there was dough roob for theb."

- I guess Molly found out what the problem was. Listen to that part again:

She said, "Are those the only things you planted in the garden?"

Bleep looked at her and then said in a big voice, "Yes, Holly wadded to pladt beads but there was dough roob for theb."

- What was Bleep trying to say? (Call on a student. Idea: *Holly wanted to plant beans but there was no room for them.*)

Molly said, "Bleep, have you been messing with your screws again?"

Bleep said, "Dot all of theb."

"I'll bet you adjusted the pink one and the green one, didn't you?"

Bleep said, "Yes, pick and greed."

"Well, I'm just going to have to adjust them back the way they were."

And she did just that.

The next day, Molly and Holly went shopping, and Bleep started straightening out all the boxes that were in Holly's basement.

Suddenly the great wind started to blow from the east again. The great cloud of smell that had been over Goober's farm moved to the west. People who lived in West Town ran for their clothespins. Bleep didn't know about the wind or about the clothespins because he was working in the basement.

He got his first clue that something had changed when Holly and Molly came back from shopping. Molly opened the door to the basement. Bleep could not see her, and she could not see him.

So she called down, "Bleep, are you albost fidished?"

Bleep shook his head and said, "Blurp."

- That's the end of the story.

EXERCISE 3 Writing Non-nasal Speech

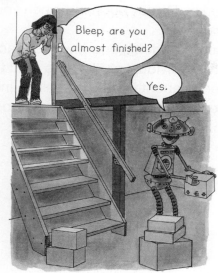

Bleep, are you almost finished?

Yes.

1. Find part B. ✔
   This picture shows what would have happened if the big wind hadn't started blowing from the east at the end of the story.
   • Molly is at the top of the basement stairs. See if you can read what she's saying.
   • What is Molly saying? (Call on a student.) *Bleep, are you almost finished?*
   • And Bleep is answering. Everybody, what is Bleep saying? (Signal.) *Yes.*
   • That's what would have happened if the great wind hadn't started blowing.
   • But when the wind started blowing, Molly had to wear something to protect her from the smell. What's that? (Signal.) *A clothespin.*
   • And when she wore the clothespin, she couldn't say some of the words the right way. Raise your hand when you know which words she couldn't say.
   • What's the first word she couldn't say? (Signal.) *Almost.*
   • What's the next word she couldn't say? (Signal.) *Finished.*
2. Underline the word **almost** and the word **finished.** Then fix up those words so they say what Molly actually said with the clothespin on her nose. Cross out the letters she can't say. Write the letter she said above it.

• (Write on the board:)

> b   d
> al~~m~~ost fi~~n~~ished

• Here's what you should have.
3. Raise your hand if you remember what Bleep always said when he heard people talking in that strange way. Everybody, what did he say? (Signal.) *Blurp.*
4. Fix up Bleep so he says **blurp.**
   • Cross out the word **yes** and write **blurp.** Raise your hand when you're finished.
   • (Write on the board:)

> **Blurp**

• Here's what you should have.
• Later you can fix up that picture so it shows a clothespin on Molly's nose.

LINED PAPER

EXERCISE 4 Sentence Writing

1. Find the page titled **Story words** at the front of your workbook.
   • (Write on the board:)

> **Everybody hugged.**

• This says: Everybody hugged.
• Copy that sentence on the second line of your paper. Remember the capital and the period. Raise your hand when you've copied the sentence.
  (Observe students and give feedback.)
2. (Write to show:)

> **Everybody hugged.**
> **Roger** _____.

• Here's the first part of the sentence you'll write next. Roger blank. Complete the sentence for Roger. He hugged one of the characters shown on the page with **Story words.**
• Write your sentence about Roger. Raise your hand when you're finished.
  (Observe students and give feedback.)
• (Call on individual students to read their sentence about Roger.)

3. (Write to show:)

> **Everybody hugged.**
> **Roger** _____ .
> **Fizz** _____ .
> **I** _____ .

- You're going to write more sentences. One will tell about Fizz and who he hugged. The other will tell about you and who you hugged.

- Your turn: Write both sentences. Remember the period at the end of each sentence. Raise your hand when you're finished.
  (Observe students and give feedback.)

- (Call on individual students to read their sentence about Fizz. Then call on individual students to read their sentence about themselves.)

Objectives

- Perform on mastery test of skills presented in lessons 41–49. (Exercise 1 and 2)
- Students vote on a story to be reread. (Exercise 3)
  Exercises 4–6 provide instructions for marking the test and giving the students feedback.

WORKBOOK

EXERCISE 1   Test
Sentence Construction

Molly	ran home
Bertha	sat on a cake
Owen	kissed Goober
Mrs. Hudson	fixed Bleep
	fed the pigs
	picked up Owen

1. _____
2. _____
3. _____

1. Everybody, open your workbook to lesson 50 and find part A. ✔
   There are two big boxes with words in them.
- Touch the first box. ✔
  Those are the names you'll start your sentences with. I'll read the names.
- Touch the top name. ✔
  It says: Molly.
- Next name: Bertha.
- Next name: Owen.
- Last name: Mrs. Hudson.
- Remember, those are the names you'll start your sentences with. The other box tells what the characters did.
2. Touch the top words of the second box. ✔
   They say: ran home.
- Next words: sat on a cake.
- Next words: kissed Goober.
- Next words: fixed Bleep.
- Next words: fed the pigs.
- Last words: picked up Owen.
3. Listen: Your first sentence will tell about the first character.
- Touch the name of the first character. ✔
  Everybody, what name are you touching? (Signal.) *Molly.*

- Your first sentence will start with Molly, and it will tell something that Molly did in a story. Write your first sentence. Remember to start with a capital and end with a period. Raise your hand when you're finished.
  (Observe students and give feedback.)
- (Write on the board:)

> **Molly fixed Bleep.**

- Here's what you should have. Raise your hand if you got everything right.
4. Your next sentence will tell about the next character.
- Touch the name of the next character. ✔ Everybody, what name are you touching? (Signal.) *Bertha.*
- That sentence will start with Bertha, and it will tell something that Bertha did in a story. Write your sentence about Bertha. Raise your hand when you're finished.
  (Observe students and give feedback.)
- (Write on the board:)

> **Bertha ran home.**

- Here's what you should have. Raise your hand if you got everything right.
5. Your next sentence will start with one of the names you haven't used. It can start with Owen or Mrs. Hudson. And that sentence **won't** tell what happened in a story you've heard. That sentence will tell something you would like to happen in a story.
- Your turn: Start with **Owen** or **Mrs. Hudson.** Complete your sentence with any of the parts you want. Raise your hand when you're finished.
  (Observe students and give feedback.)
- I'll call on 3 individual students to read their sentence 3. I'll write the sentences on the board.

(Call on 3 students:) Read your sentence. (Write sentences on board.)

6. There's a big box at the bottom of the page. Later, you can draw a picture of sentence 3 in that box.

EXERCISE 2 Test

Map—Relative Direction

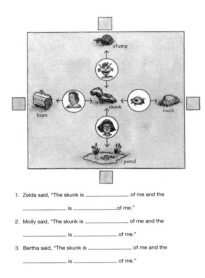

1. Zelda said, "The skunk is _____ of me and the _____ is _____ of me."
2. Molly said, "The skunk is _____ of me and the _____ is _____ of me."
3. Bertha said, "The skunk is _____ of me and the _____ is _____ of me."

1. You're going to have a test to see how smart you are. You can't talk to anybody during the test or look at what anybody else does.
- Find part B. ✔
2. Put the letters for north, south, east and west in the boxes around this map. Raise your hand when you're finished. ✔
- Different people are telling where they are. Everybody starts out by telling about the skunk.
3. Touch item 1. ✔
Follow along: Zelda said, "The skunk is blank of me and the something else is blank of me."
- Complete item 1. Raise your hand when you're finished.
(Observe students but do not give feedback.)
4. Touch item 2. ✔
Molly said, "The skunk is blank of me and the something else is blank of me."
- Complete item 2. Raise your hand when you're finished.
(Observe students.)

5. Touch item 3. ✔
Bertha said, "The skunk is blank of me and the something else is blank of me."
- Fill in the blanks. Raise your hand when you're finished.
(Observe students.)

EXERCISE 3 Story

1. For the rest of the period, I'll read a story. You get to choose one of the stories.
- Everybody gets to vote on their favorite story. But you can only vote one time. I'll name the stories. You hold up your hand if you want that story. But remember, you can only hold up your hand one time.
- Listen: Dot and Dud. Who wants to hear the last part of that story again?
(Count the students' raised hands.)
- Listen: Zelda the Artist. Who wants to hear the last part of that story again?
(Count the students' raised hands.)
- Listen: The Case of the Missing Corn. Who wants to hear the last part of that story again?
(Count the students' raised hands.)
- Listen: Bleep Visits West Town. Who wants to hear the last part of that story again?
(Count the students' raised hands.)
2. (Read the chosen story. If time permits, read the story for the second choice.)

Key: Lesson 37 for Dot and Dud (part 3);

Lesson 42 for The Case of the Missing Corn (part 4);

Lesson 44 for Zelda the Artist (part 2);

Lesson 49 for Bleep Visits West Town (part 2).

EXERCISE 4   Marking the Test

1. (Mark the test before the next scheduled language lesson. Use the *Language Arts Workbook Answer Key* to check the test.)
2. (Write the number of errors each student made in the test scorebox at the beginning of the test.)
3. (Enter the number of errors each student made on the Summary for Test 5. A Reproducible Summary Sheet is at the back of the *Language Arts Teacher's Guide*.)

EXERCISE 5   Feedback on Test 5

1. (Return the students' workbooks after they are marked.)

- Everybody, open your workbook to lesson 50. Look at how I marked your test page.
2. I wrote a number at the top of your test. That number tells how many items you got wrong on the whole test.
- Raise your hand if I wrote **0** or **1** at the top of your test.
  Those are super stars.
- Raise your hand if I wrote **2** or **3**. Those are pretty good workers.
- If I wrote a number that's more than 3, you're going to have to work harder.

EXERCISE 6   Test Remedies

- (See the *Language Arts Teacher's Guide* for a general discussion of remedies.)

Objectives

- Compose and write a parallel sentence pair based on a single picture. (Exercise 1)
- **Write sentences that use the word after and tell what an illustrated character did.** (Exercise 2)
- Rewrite unambiguous sentence pairs so the second sentence is ambiguous. (Exercise 3)
- Listen to part 1 of a story and answer comprehension questions. (Exercise 4)
- **Complete a deduction used in the story.** (Exercise 5)

WORKBOOK • LINED PAPER

EXERCISE 1 Writing Parallel Sentences

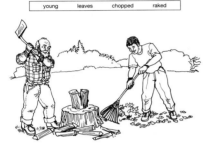

| young | leaves | chopped | raked |

1. Open your workbook to lesson 51 and find part A. ✔
   You're going to write about this picture.
2. The picture shows what an old man and a young man did.
- What did the old man do? (Call on a student. Idea: *Chopped wood.*)
- What did the young man do? (Call on a student. Idea: *Raked leaves.*)
3. Listen: An old man chopped wood.
- Everybody, say the whole sentence about an old man. (Signal.) *An old man chopped wood.*
- (Repeat the sentence until firm.)
4. Look at the vocabulary box. These are some of the words you need: **young . . . leaves . . . chopped . . . raked.**
5. Write both sentences.
   (Observe students and give feedback.)
6. Check your sentences. (Call on several students to read both sentences. Idea: *An old man chopped wood. A young man raked leaves.*)
- Raise your hand if you got both of them right. ✔
7. **(Optional:)** Skip a line on your paper and write both sentences again.
   (Observe students and give feedback.)

EXERCISE 2 Sentence Writing

Temporal Sequencing

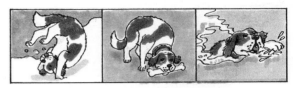

1. _____

   after he played in the snow.
2. Dud _____

   _____.

1. (Write on the board:)

> **Dud he after snow the ate went in ham bone played swimming**

- Find part B. ✔
  The pictures show Dud doing three things.
- Touch the first thing Dud did. ✔
  What did Dud do first? (Signal.) *Played in the snow.*
- Touch the next thing Dud did.
  What did Dud do after he played in the snow? (Signal.) *Ate a ham bone.*
- Touch the last thing Dud did.
  What did Dud do after he ate a ham bone? (Signal.) *Went swimming.*
2. You're going to complete sentences that tell what Dud did after he played in the snow and what he did after he ate a ham bone.
- (Point to the words on the board.) Here are some words you may use.
  (Touch each word as you say:) **Dud, he, after, snow, the, ate, went, in, ham bone, played, swimming.** If you use any of those words, make sure you spell them correctly.

3. Touch number 1. ✔
- On that line, you'll write what Dud did after he played in the snow.
- Touch the picture that shows what Dud did after he played in the snow. ✔
- Start your sentence with **Dud** and tell what he did after he played in the snow. Raise your hand when you're finished.
  (Observe students and give feedback.)
4. (Write on the board:)

> **Dud ate a ham bone after he played in the snow.**

- Here's what you should have for your first sentence: Dud ate a ham bone after he played in the snow. Raise your hand if you wrote everything correctly.
5. Touch number 2. ✔
- You'll write the whole sentence that tells what Dud did after he ate a ham bone.
- Touch the picture that shows what Dud did after he ate a ham bone. ✔
- The word **Dud** is already written. Tell what Dud did in the last picture. Then tell when he did it. Remember, Dud went swimming **after** he ate a ham bone. Raise your hand when you're finished.
  (Observe students and give feedback.)
6. (Write on the board:)

> **Dud went swimming after he ate a ham bone.**

- Here's what you should have for your second sentence.
- Raise your hand if you wrote everything correctly and if you put a period at the end of the sentence.

EXERCISE 3 Creating Ambiguous Sentences

1. Aunt Martha pulled a turnip out of the dirt.

   The turnip tasted good.

2. The ranger led the dogs toward the mountains.

   The mountains were covered with snow.

1. Everybody, find part C. ✔
   (Write on the board:)

> **He   She   It   They**

- The sentences in each item are not confusing. You're going to make them confusing. This could be funny. I'll read each item.
- Item 1: Aunt Martha pulled a turnip out of the dirt. The turnip tasted good.
- Item 2: The ranger led the dogs toward the mountains. The mountains were covered with snow.
2. Touch item 1. ✔
   You're going to change the second sentence in item 1. The second sentence starts out by naming something. Raise your hand when you know what it names.
- Everybody, what does the second sentence name? (Signal.) *The turnip.*
- Listen: Cross out the words **the turnip.**
- Use one of the words on the board to tell about the turnip or the dirt. Find that word and write it above the crossed-out words. Raise your hand when you're finished.
  (Observe students and give feedback.)
- (Touch the word **It** on the board.)
  Here's the word you should have written: **It.**
- I'll read what your item 1 should say now: Aunt Martha pulled a turnip out of the dirt. **It** tasted good.
- Now we don't know what tasted good. Maybe it was the turnip. Maybe it was . . . (Signal.) *The dirt.*
3. Item 2: The ranger led the dogs toward the mountains. The mountains were covered with snow.
- You're going to change the second sentence in item 2. The second sentence starts out by naming something. Raise your hand when you know what it names.
- Everybody, what does the second sentence name? (Signal.) *The mountains.*
- Listen: Cross out the words **the mountains.**
- Use one of the words on the board to tell about the mountains or the dogs. Find that word and write it above the crossed-out words. Raise your hand when you're finished.
  (Observe students and give feedback.)
- (Touch the word **They.**)
  Here's the word you should have written: **They.**

- I'll read what your item 2 should say now: The ranger led the dogs toward the mountains. **They** were covered with snow.
- Now we don't know what was covered with snow. Maybe it was the mountains. Maybe it was . . . (Signal.) *The dogs.*

4. Later you can draw a picture for item 1 or 2 the way Zelda might do it. Some of those pictures will probably be very silly.

EXERCISE 4 The Case Of The Squashed Squash *Part 1*

Storytelling

- The title of this story is **The Case of the Squashed Squash.**

One day in late autumn, when the leaves were red and the weather was getting cooler, the rat pack was getting ready for their great squash feast. Every year, the rats would find the biggest and the yellowest and the best squash on Goober's farm. They would roll that big yellow squash to a hiding place in the berry bushes, where it would be safe.

There were lots of bluebirds in the berry bushes, and they loved squash, but they couldn't eat squash unless it was squashed. Then they could get to the inside and eat away.

But the squash was safe in the berry bushes because the squash was not squashed.

Finally it was the day before the great feast. Everything was almost ready. The rats had gathered apples and corn and walnuts and seeds of all kinds.

The wise old rat sent four young rats to go to the berry bushes and roll the great big squash back to the meeting grounds, where the feast would be held.

So four young rats dashed off to the berry bushes, but soon they came running back.

"The squash is gone," they said. "We looked all over for it, and we can't find it."

The rats became very excited. They rushed to the berry bushes and looked here and there, but they didn't find even a scrap of squash.

"Somebody took that squash," one of the rats said.

Sherlock said, "Or maybe somebody ate it."

The rats started to argue. Some of them were saying, "Somebody **took** that squash."

Others were saying, "No, somebody **ate** it."

The argument went on for a while. Then Sherlock put his little chest out as far as it would go, stood up very straight and said, "I know a way to find out whether somebody took that squash or somebody ate it."

"How can you find out?" all the rats asked.

So Sherlock told them.

- Raise your hand if you know how Sherlock could find out if somebody ate the squash.
- (Call on a student. Idea: *Have Bertha sniff to see if anybody has squash breath.*)

Sherlock went to Bertha's place and told her that he had an important detective job. She told him that she was tired of doing detective work, but finally he talked her into working with him.

Before Bertha agreed, she made Sherlock promise her that she could be an honorary rat and could join in all the feasts and dinners the rats had.

Sherlock agreed.

So Bertha went with Sherlock back to the berry bushes and started sniffing animals. After a lot of sniffing, she said, "None of the rats ate that squash."

After a lot more sniffing, she said, "None of the rabbits or squirrels or gophers ate that squash."

> After even more sniffing, she said, "All the bluebirds have squash on their breath."
>
> Sherlock said, "Anybody who has squash on their breath ate squash. The bluebirds have squash on their breath. So . . . "

- What's the last part of the deduction? (Signal.) *So the bluebirds ate squash.*

> Sherlock said, "Those bluebirds. I never did trust them. Imagine, they ate the squash that we were saving for our great fall feast."

- We'll read more of the story next time.

EXERCISE 5   Deduction Writing

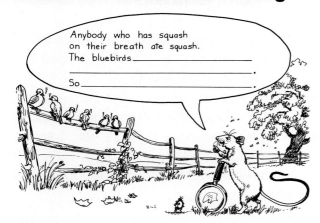

1. Find part D. ✔
   The picture shows Sherlock, Bertha, and a bunch of bluebirds. Those marks coming from the bluebirds' beaks show a smell. Everybody, what smell is coming from their beaks? (Signal.) *Squash.*
- Yes, they all have squash on their breath.
- And Sherlock is saying the deduction about the bluebirds. But only the first sentence of the deduction is complete.

2. Touch the words as I read them: **Anybody . . . who . . . has . . . squash . . . on . . . their . . . breath . . . ate . . . squash.**
- The first part of the next sentence is written: The bluebirds . . . That sentence is not complete.
- Listen to what is written again: Anybody who has squash on their breath ate squash. The bluebirds . . .

3. Tell the fact that you know about the bluebirds. Complete the second sentence. Raise your hand when you're finished. (Observe students and give feedback.)
- Here's what your second sentence should say: The bluebirds **have squash on their breath.** Raise your hand if you got it right.

4. Now your deduction says: Anybody who has squash on their breath ate squash. The bluebirds have squash on their breath. So . . .
- Complete the deduction. Raise your hand when you're finished.
   (Observe students and give feedback.)
- Here's what your last sentence should say: So **the bluebirds ate squash.** Raise your hand if you got it right.

5. Who can start with "Anybody who has squash on their breath ate squash," and say the whole deduction? (Call on a student. Praise complete deduction.)
- It's tough.

6. Later you can color that picture.

LESSON 52

WORKBOOK

EXERCISE 1 Sentence Construction

Temporal Sequencing

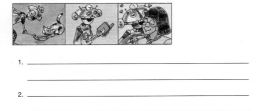

1. _____
   _____
2. _____
   _____

1. (Write on the board:)

> after Molly Bleep sat kissed read
> fed book cat he

- Open your workbook to lesson 52 and find part A. ✔
  The pictures show Bleep doing three things.
- Touch the first thing Bleep did. ✔
  What did Bleep do first? (Signal.) *Fed a cat.*
- Touch the next thing Bleep did. ✔
  What did Bleep do after he fed a cat?
  (Signal.) *Read a book.*
- Touch the last thing Bleep did. ✔
  What did Bleep do after he read a book?
  (Signal.) *Kissed Molly.*
- (Point to the words on the board:) Here are some words you may use.
  (Touch each word as you say:)
  after . . . Molly . . . Bleep . . . sat . . . kissed . . . read . . . fed . . . book . . . cat . . . he.
- If you use any of these words, make sure you spell them correctly.
2. Touch number 1. ✔
  On that line you'll write what Bleep did after he fed a cat.
- Touch the picture that shows what Bleep did after he fed a cat. ✔
- The second picture shows what Bleep did after he fed a cat.

- Listen: Start your sentence with **Bleep** and tell what he did in the second picture. Don't write the whole sentence. Just tell **what** Bleep did in the second picture. Raise your hand when you've written that much.
  (Observe students and give feedback.)
- (Write on the board:)

> **Bleep read a book**

- Here's what you should have so far: Bleep read a book.
- Now you'll complete your sentence by telling **when** he read a book. He read a book **after** he fed a cat.
- So you'll complete your first sentence by writing these words: after he fed a cat.
- Complete sentence 1. Raise your hand when you're finished.
  (Observe students and give feedback.)
- (Write to show:)

> **Bleep read a book** after he fed the cat.

- Here's what sentence 1 should say: Bleep read a book after he fed a cat.
- Raise your hand if you wrote everything correctly and remembered the period.
3. Touch number 2. ✔
  On that line you'll write what Bleep did **after** he read a book.
- Touch the picture that shows what Bleep did after he read a book. ✔
- Start your sentence with **Bleep** and tell what he did in the last picture. Don't write the whole sentence. Just tell **what** Bleep did in the last picture. Raise your hand when you've written that much.
  (Observe students and give feedback.)
- (Write on the board:)

> **Bleep kissed Molly**

- Here's what you should have so far: Bleep kissed Molly.
- Now you'll complete your sentence by telling **when** he kissed Molly. When did he do that? (Signal.) *After he read a book.*
- Yes, he kissed Molly after he read a book.
- Complete your sentence. Raise your hand when you're finished.
  (Observe students and give feedback.)
- (Write to show:)

Bleep kissed Molly after he read a book.

- Here's what sentence 2 should say: Bleep kissed Molly after he read a book.
4. Raise your hand if you wrote everything correctly.

EXERCISE 2   The Case Of The Squashed Squash *Part 2*

Storytelling

- I'll read the next part of the story: **The Case of the Squashed Squash.**
  In the part I read last time, the squash was missing from the berry bushes. That squash was important. Why? (Call on a student. Idea: *It was needed for the feast.*)
- When Sherlock and Bertha went to the berry bushes, Sherlock figured out that somebody ate squash. Who ate squash? (Signal.) *The bluebirds.*
- How did Sherlock know that the bluebirds ate squash? (Call on a student. Idea: *They had squash on their breath.*)
- Sherlock made the deduction: Anybody who has squash on their breath ate squash. The bluebirds have squash on their breath. So . . . (Signal.) *The bluebirds ate squash.*

Sherlock said, "Those bluebirds. I never did trust them. Imagine, they ate the squash that we were saving for our great fall feast."

"But . . . " Bertha said.

Sherlock interrupted. "I'd better make an announcement about who ate that squash. I don't know what the rats will do to get even with those thieving bluebirds."

"But . . . " Bertha said.

"There are no buts about it," Sherlock said. "We found out who is guilty."

"Wrong," Bertha said. "You found out who ate squash, but you have one problem."

"What's that?"

"Well," Bertha said, "Bluebirds can't eat squash that is not squashed. If the bluebirds ate your squash, what do you know about your squash?"

Sherlock said, "Our squash must have been squashed when the bluebirds ate it."

"Right," Bertha said.

Bonnie the bluebird had been listening to Sherlock and Bertha discuss the squash.

She said, "It was squashed, all right. We didn't know it was your squash. We just saw that squashed squash under the berry bushes, and we ate it up. It was good, too."

Bertha started pacing around very fast. She said, "We might be able to figure out who squashed the squash if we knew **how** the squash got squashed."

Sherlock said, "What?"

"Never mind," Bertha said. Then she asked Bonnie, "What did the squashed squash look like? Did it have a great big bear footprint in the middle of it?"

"No."

"Did it have a deer footprint in it?"

"No."

"Did it have a big human footprint in the middle of it?"

"No, but . . ."

"Yes, yes?"

Bonnie said, "It looked like it had a human seat print in the middle of it."

"What's a seat print?" Sherlock asked.

Bonnie said, "Well, you know the kind of marks that humans leave when they sit on something soft."

"Yes."

"Well, I'm not sure, but that's the kind of print that was in the middle of the squash."

Then Bonnie added, "And if you look over there, near the berry bushes, you can see some great big human footprints."

- Listen: You're going to figure out what Bertha and Sherlock did next. Figure out what you could find out from the footprints. And figure out what kind of clue you'd look for to find whether somebody sat on that squash.
- If you sat on the squash, you might have something on the seat of your pants.
- Your turn: Figure out what Sherlock and Bertha will do with the footprints and what they'll do to check out humans to see whether they squashed the squash. Raise your hand when you can tell what they'll do about the footprints and the seat print.
- (Call on individual students. Praise ideas: *Follow footprints; Match shoes with footprints; Look for somebody with squash on the seat of the pants*.)
- Next time we'll see what Sherlock and Bertha did.

EXERCISE 3   Deduction Writing

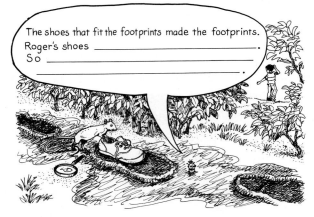

> The shoes that fit the footprints made the footprints.
> Roger's shoes _____.
> So _____
> _____.

1. Everybody, find part B. ✔
   Touch Sherlock.
   He's got one of Roger's shoes in a footprint by the berry bushes.
- Does that shoe fit the footprint? (Signal.) *No.*
- That shoe is way too small to make those footprints.
- Bertha is saying the deduction, but parts are missing. I'll read what she says. Follow along: The shoes that fit the footprints made the footprints. Roger's shoes . . .
- Listen: What do you know about Roger's shoes and the footprints? (Call on a student. Idea: *Roger's shoes do not fit the footprints*.)
- So here are the first two sentences of the deduction. The shoes that fit the footprints made the footprints. Roger's shoes do not fit the footprints. So . . .
2. Your turn: Complete the deduction. Raise your hand when you're finished.
   (Observe students and give feedback.)
- I'll read the whole deduction: The shoes that fit the footprints made the footprints. Roger's shoes do not fit the footprints. So Roger's shoes did not make the footprints.
- Raise your hand if you got everything right.
3. You can color the picture later. If you look very closely at the picture, you may be able to find Roger. I think he's looking for one of his shoes. Poor Roger.

Objectives

- Complete a letter. (Exercise 1)
- Write sentences that use the word **after** and tell what an illustrated character did. (Exercise 2)
- Complete a deduction used in the story. (Exercise 3)
- Listen to the conclusion of a 3-part story and answer comprehension questions. (Exercise 4)
- Make a picture consistent with the details of a story. (Exercise 5)

WORKBOOK

EXERCISE 1 Letter Writing

1. Open your workbook to lesson 53 and find part A. ✔
   You're going to complete a letter. It is a make-believe letter that tells about what you saw when you went to a zoo. If you've never been to a zoo, you can imagine what a trip to the zoo might be like.

- At the top of the page is a box. There are some words in the box that you may want to use when you write your letter. Touch the first part of the box. ✔
- Follow along while I read the words. **Zoo . . . friends . . . class . . . family.**
- Touch the second part of the box. ✔
- You may want to use the names of these animals when you write your letter. Follow along while I read the names of the animals. **Elephants . . . lions . . . tigers . . . bears . . . monkeys . . . giraffes . . . parrots.**
- If you use any of these words when you write your letter, be sure to spell them correctly.

2. Touch the word **Dear.** ✔

- In the space after the word, **Dear,** you'll write the name of the person whom you're writing to. If you're writing a letter to your mom, you'll write **Mom.** If you're writing a letter to a friend named Ted, you'll write, **Ted.** What would you write if your letter was going to a man named Mr. Wilson? (Signal.) *Mr. Wilson.*
- Pick somebody whom you want to write to and write the name in the space after the word **Dear.** Raise your hand when you've filled in the first space of the letter. (Observe students and give feedback.)
- (Call on several students to read their greeting.)

3. I'll read the next part of the letter and you'll follow along. **Yesterday, I went to the blank.** Everybody, what word goes in the blank? (Signal.) *Zoo.*
   Yes, zoo. Write the word, **zoo,** in the blank space. ✔

- There's more to that sentence. Listen: **Yesterday, I went to the zoo with my blank.** The missing word could be friends, class, or family. You could even put another name in the blank if you wish. Write whom you went with in the blank space. ✔

4. The next sentence says, **We saw blank, blank, and blank.** You have three spaces to write the names of three kinds of animals. Write the names of three kinds of animals in the blank spaces. Remember to look at the words in the picture box so that you can spell the names correctly. ✔

5. The next sentence says, **My favorite animals were the blanks.** Fill in the blank and then stop. ✔

6. (Call on several students to read the part of their letter as it is completed thus far. Praise letters that have appropriate names and words in the blanks.)

7. The last sentence of the letter says, **I hope that I can go back to the blank soon.** The very end of the letter says **From, blank.** You are the one the letter is from. So you write your name in the last blank. Complete your letter by filling in the last two blank spaces.
   (Observe students and give feedback. Students who are finished early may wish to draw a picture to go with their letter.)

8. (Call on several students to read their complete letter. Praise letters that have appropriate names and words in the blanks.)

EXERCISE 2 Sentence Construction

Temporal Sequencing

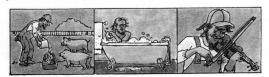

1. (Write on the board:)

   > after   a violin   pigs   took
   > played   bath   fed

- Find part B. ✔
  These pictures show Goober doing three things.
- Touch the first thing Goober did. ✔
  What did Goober do first? (Signal.) *Fed the pigs.*
- Touch the next thing Goober did. ✔
  What did Goober do after he fed the pigs? (Signal.) *Took a bath.*
- Touch the last thing Goober did. ✔
  What did Goober do after he took a bath? (Signal.) *Played a violin.*
- (Point to words on the board:)
  Here are some words you may use.
  (Touch each word as you say:)
  after . . . a violin . . . pigs . . . took . . . played . . . bath . . . fed.

2. You're going to write two sentences. The first sentence will tell what Goober did after he fed the pigs. Touch the picture that shows what he did after he fed the pigs. ✔
- How will your sentence start out? (Signal.) *Goober.*
- Start sentence 1 with **Goober** and tell what he did after he fed the pigs. Raise your hand when you've written that much.
  (Observe students and give feedback.)
- (Write on the board:)

  > **Goober took a bath.**

- Here's what you should have so far for sentence 1: Goober took a bath.
- Now complete that sentence by telling when he did that. He did that just after he did something else.
- (Write to show:)

  > **Goober took a bath after**

- Write the word **after** and then tell when Goober took a bath. Raise your hand when you're finished.
  (Observe students and give feedback.)
- (Write to show:)

  > **Goober took a bath after he fed the pigs.**

- Here's the whole first sentence: Goober took a bath after he fed the pigs. Raise your hand if you got everything right.

3. Now you'll write a sentence that tells what Goober did after he took a bath.
- Touch the picture that shows what he did after he took a bath. ✔
- Start your sentence with **Goober.** Tell what he did after he took a bath. Then tell when he did that. Raise your hand when you're finished.
  (Observe students and give feedback.)
- (Write on the board:)

  > **Goober played a violin after he took a bath.**

- Here's what you should have for your second sentence: Goober played a violin after he took a bath. Raise your hand if you got everything right.

EXERCISE 3 Deduction Writing

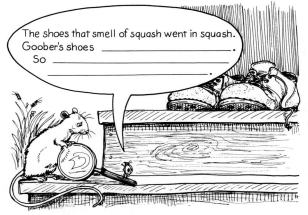

1. Everybody, find part C. ✔
   The picture shows Sherlock and Bertha at Goober's farm. They're looking at Goober's shoes. Bertha is saying the right deduction about the shoes. The first part is already written. Touch the words as I read them: The shoes that smell of squash went in squash.
- The first part of the next sentence is written: Goober's shoes . . .

2. Tell the fact about the shoes and the smell. Complete the second sentence. Raise your hand when you're finished.
(Observe students and give feedback.)
- Here's what your second sentence should say: Goober's shoes smell of squash. Raise your hand if you got it right.
- Now your deduction says: The shoes that smell of squash went in squash. Goober's shoes smell of squash. So . . .
- Complete the deduction. Raise your hand when you're finished.
(Observe students and give feedback.)
- Here's what your last sentence should say: So Goober's shoes went in squash. Raise your hand if you got it right.
3. Listen: Start with this statement: The shoes that smell of squash went in squash. Then say the rest of the deduction. (Call on a student. Praise complete deductions.)
- It's tough.
4. Later you can color that picture.

EXERCISE 4 The Case Of The Squashed Squash *Part 3*

Storytelling

- We're going to continue with **The Case of the Squashed Squash.**
- Sherlock knew that the squash had been squashed. He knew what kind of print was in the squash when it was squashed.
- Everybody, what kind of print? (Signal.) *A seat print.*
- He also knew that there were other prints around the berry bushes.
- Everybody, what kind of prints? (Signal.) *Footprints.*
- Let's find out what happened.

So Sherlock had some good ideas about how to find out who squashed the squash. He told Bertha, "The shoes that fit those footprints made those footprints. So, if we find the shoes that fit those footprints, we'll know who made the footprints."

Bertha rocked her little body from side to side. Then she said, "That's not completely true. If you find the shoes that fit the footprint, you won't

know **who** made the footprints. You'll just know which **shoes** made those footprints."

"Well," Sherlock said. "I think you're being too fussy. If we find the shoes, we'll know **who** made the footprints."

Bertha didn't say anything, but she rocked her little body again.

- Bertha doesn't believe that if you find the shoes that made the footprints you'll know who made the footprints. I'm not sure I understand the problem she sees. How would it be possible that somebody's shoes made the footprints but that the person who owns those shoes didn't make the footprints?
(Call on a student. Idea: *Somebody else was wearing the shoes.*)

Sherlock said, "And, once we find the person who made the footprints, we can check that person's pants. We know that pants with squash on them sat on the squash. So, if we find pants with squash on them, we'll know who sat in the squash."

"No, no," Bertha said. She was rocking from side to side like crazy. "If you find the pants with squash on them, you won't know **who** sat in the squash. You'll know which **pants** sat in the squash."

"Oh, stop that fussy talk," Sherlock said. "If we find the shoes and the pants, we'll know who did it. Trust me."

Bertha's little body was still rocking from side to side.

- Everybody, show me how Bertha rocked. (Praise good rockers.)
- Bertha has that same problem again. She doesn't believe that the squash on the pants lets you know **who** sat on the squash. But how would it be possible for somebody's pants to have squash on the seat when the person who owns those pants didn't sit on the squash?
(Call on a student. Idea: *Somebody else was wearing the pants.*)

Then Bertha said, "Those footprints tell you something about the person who made them."

"What's that?" Sherlock said.

"Well," Bertha said, "footprints go where the person goes."

"So what?"

"So, if we follow the footprints, we'll find out where the person who made them went."

Sherlock scratched his head. Then he said, "Yes, I guess that's right. The footprints would have to go where the person went. So let's just follow those footprints and find out where they go."

"That's easy," Bertha said. "I'll just sniff those footprints and pick up the trail."

And she did just that. She sniffed around and then she took off, running just as fast as her little legs would take her. Sherlock followed.

Bertha went through the berry bushes, across two fields, under three fences and, at last, she came to Goober's barn.

"The footprints go into that barn," she said.

Sherlock snuck around and peeked into the barn. Then he snuck around to the back of the barn where there was a clothesline. On that clothesline were some clean clothes. One of the things on the line was a large pair of overalls. They were still wet.

Sherlock whispered to Bertha, "I'll bet those are the pants that sat in the squash, but I can't prove it. They've already been washed."

"I can prove it," Bertha said. "Help me up. I'll crawl up and sniff the seat. If that seat had squash on it, I'll still be able to smell it."

"Okay," Sherlock said. He crouched down. Bertha crawled up his back. Then she could reach the bottom of one of the pants legs. She crawled up the leg, sniffed the seat and said, "Yep. These overalls had squash on the seat."

"I knew it," Sherlock said. "Those are Goober's overalls. So he sat in our squash."

"You don't know that," Bertha said as she climbed down the pants leg. "All you know is that these are the pants that sat in the squash."

"Oh, stop that fussy talk." Then Sherlock said, "Now let's see if we can find a shoe that matches the footprints near the berry bushes."

Sherlock and Bertha snuck around to the back door of Goober's house. There was a pair of big shoes on the porch.

Sherlock said, "I think those are the shoes that made the prints. But we'll have to take one of those back to the berry bushes and see if it matches the footprints."

"Wrong," Bertha said. "There's a much faster way."

"What's that?" Sherlock asked.

So Bertha told him.

- What do you think her fast plan was for finding out if the shoes had been in the berry bushes? (Call on a student. Idea: *Sniff*.)

Then she climbed up to the porch, sniffed the shoes a couple of times and said, "Yep, these shoes made the footprints. These shoes have been in the berry bushes, all right. They smell of squashed berries **and** of squashed squash."

"Those are Goober's shoes," Sherlock said. "So we know who did it. It was Goober."

"No, no," Bertha said. "You only know that Goober's shoes made those footprints."

"Stop that fussy talk."

Just then, the door to the house opened and Goober stepped out. By the time he stepped out onto the porch, Bertha and Sherlock were hiding under the porch.

Goober was talking to somebody. He was saying, "Well, let's hope you don't fall down again today."

"Yeah," the other man said. "That was pretty bad. I got your new overalls all messed up with squash. When that rabbit jumped out in front of me, I jumped, and the next thing I knew I was on the seat of my pants—I mean, I was on the seat of **your** pants, right on that squash."

- Now we know how the squash got squashed and who squashed it.
- Listen to that part again:

The other man said, "That was pretty bad. I got your new overalls all messed up with squash. When that rabbit jumped out in front of me, I jumped, and the next thing I knew I was on the seat of my pants—I mean, I was on the seat of **your** pants, right on that squash."

- Who sat on the squash? (Call on a student. Idea: *The other man*.)
- Why did that man sit on the squash? (Call on a student. Idea: *A rabbit scared him and he fell on the squash*.)
- Everybody, whose overalls was that man wearing? (Signal.) *Goober's.*

The two men walked down the stairs, toward the barn. Bertha whispered, "I recognize that man who's with Goober. That's Goober's brother."

Goober said, "Well, the next time you come and visit me, you'll have to bring your own overalls and work shoes, so you can mess up your own clothes."

The men laughed. Then they went inside the barn.

Bertha said, "See? I told you. I wasn't just being fussy. Goober wasn't wearing those shoes and those overalls. And I knew that all along."

"How did you know that?"

So Bertha told him. She explained that the overalls and the shoes smelled of a person that was **not** Goober.

Just then, the men came out of the barn. Each of them was carrying a great big, yellow squash.

Goober was saying, "We'd better put these squashes back in the berry bushes. You know, every year those silly rats take one of the squashes for their fall feast. They'd be pretty upset if they found out that their squash got squashed." Goober laughed.

Then he continued, "I'll bet those rats will be very puzzled trying to figure out how two squashes got in the berry bushes."

"Yeah," his brother said, "very puzzled."

So Goober and his brother took the two sqashes and put them in the berry bushes. And, on the next day, the rats had their fall feast with the best-tasting yellow squash they ever had.

Bertha was an honorary member of the rat pack. So she sat with the wise old rat and Sherlock at the head table.

After the feast was over and everybody was so full of squash and walnuts and apples and berries and seeds and corn that they couldn't eat any more, the wise old rat stood up and said, "We can thank the gray rat—I mean Sherlock—for this fine feast. He figured out how the squash got squashed, and somehow he fixed things up so that there were two great squashes in our berry patch—not just one."

Sherlock stood up as straight as he could. He cleared his throat and said, "Well, this was a very difficult job. A detective without my skill would have been confused. That person would have used the wrong deductions. That detective would have figured out that Goober did it. After all, Goober's shoes made the footprints in the berry bushes, and Goober's overalls sat in the squash. Because I'm so good at deductions, I knew how to do them the right way. I knew that, if Goober's **shoes** made the footprints, you couldn't say that **Goober** made the footprints. All you could say is that Goober's **shoes** made the footprints. I also knew that, if Goober's overalls sat on the squash, you couldn't say that Goober sat in the squash. All you could . . ."

"Enough talking," the wise old rat said. He was looking at Bertha. Her little body was rocking very fast, and it was easy to see that she was very, very unhappy.

- Why was she unhappy? (Call on a student. Idea: *Sherlock was lying.*)

The wise old rat said to her, "I can see that you don't agree with everything that Sherlock is saying."

She said, "Well . . ."

"Tell it the way it was," the wise old rat said.

"Yeah," the other rats shouted. "Tell it the way it was."

So she did just that. She told what had really happened.

- Oh, my. Everybody, did her story sound very much like Sherlock's? (Signal.) *No.*
- I'll bet Sherlock felt pretty embarrassed. Let's see.

As she talked, the other rats started staring at Sherlock with very unfriendly expressions. And Sherlock started to slouch. At first he slouched just a little bit. Then a little bit more. And finally he slouched right down into his chair.

When Bertha was finished, one of the rats said, "That Sherlock is a dirty liar."

"Yeah," another rat said. "A dirty liar. Let's clean him up."

So they rushed to Sherlock, picked him up, carried him to the pond and splash.

And, while they were cleaning up Sherlock, the bluebirds moved into the feast area.

They said, "Wow, there are all kinds of squash and other good things to eat here."

And there was. There were lots of things that bluebirds love. So the bluebirds ate and ate. They ate walnuts and berries and corn and seeds and lots of yellow squash. Those bluebirds had their first annual fall feast.

Bertha said, "This is a fall feast for everybody." And she was almost right. But there was one person who wasn't very happy with the feast.

- Who wasn't very happy? (Signal.) *Sherlock.*
- Why not? (Call on a student. Idea: *He wasn't very popular.*)

EXERCISE 5   Details

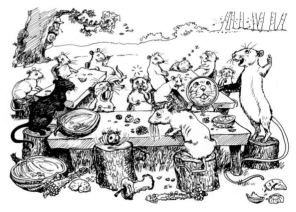

1. Everybody, find part D. ✔
   This picture shows the rat pack and their annual fall feast.
- Sherlock is making a speech. Look closely for Bertha. What is Bertha doing? (Signal.) *Rocking.*
- Yes, she's very, very unhappy.
2. If you look carefully at that picture, you may be able to find Goober and his brother. And there are bluebirds in the tree.
- What's going to happen right after this picture? (Call on a student. Idea: *Bertha tells her story; the rats take Sherlock to the pond; and the bluebirds have a feast.*)
- I think you'll have a lot of fun coloring this picture.

Objectives

- Complete a letter. (Exercise 1)
- **Complete directions for going to different locations on a map.** (Exercise 2)
- Rewrite unambiguous sentence pairs so the second sentence is ambiguous. (Exercise 3)
- Listen to part of a familiar story. (Exercise 4)
- Put on a play to show part of a familiar story. (Exercise 5)

WORKBOOK

EXERCISE 1 Letter Writing

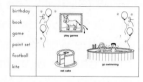

1. Open your workbook to lesson 54 and find part A. ✔
   You're going to complete another letter. It is a make-believe letter that tells about what you are going to do on your birthday.
   - At the top of the page is a box. There are some words in the box that you may want to use when you write your letter. Touch the first part of the box. ✔
   - Follow along while I read the words. **Birthday . . . book . . . game . . . paint set . . . football . . . kite.**
   - Touch the second part of the box. ✔
   - These pictures show some things you may want to do on your birthday. Follow along while I read the words. **Play games . . . go swimming . . . eat treats.**
   - If you use any of these words when you write your letter, be sure to spell them correctly.
2. Touch the word **Dear.** ✔
   - In the space after the word **Dear,** you'll write the name of the person whom you're writing to. Raise your hand when you've filled in the first space of the letter. (Observe students and give feedback.)
   - (Call on several students to read their greeting.)
3. I'll read the next part of the letter and you'll follow along. **Next week I will be blank years old.** How many years old are you going to be on your next birthday? (Call on several students.) Fill in the blank. ✔

4. The next sentence says, **I am going to have a blank party.** Fill in the missing word. Remember to look at the words in the picture box so that you can spell your words correctly.
   (Observe students and give feedback.)
5. The next sentence says, **My friends and I will blank and blank.** Write two things you would like to do at your party—play games, go swimming, or eat treats.
   (Observe students and give feedback.)
6. The rest of the letter says, **The birthday present I want the most is a blank. I hope I get it.** Finish your letter and sign your name. (Observe students and give feedback. Students who are finished early may wish to draw a picture to go with their letter.)
7. (Call on several students to read their complete letter. Praise letters that have appropriate names and words in the blanks.)

EXERCISE 2 Map Directions

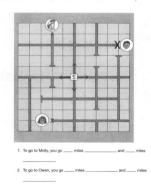

1. To go to Molly, you go ____ miles _____ and ____ miles

2. To go to Owen, you go ____ miles _____ and ____ miles
_____

1. Find part B. ✔
   This is a map. Each square is one mile. That's a long distance.
   - You're going to complete the directions for going to different places. For each set of directions you'll start at the start box. That's the box with the **S** in it.

- You can see different things on the map.
- Touch the little **X** that marks where Molly is. ✔
- Touch the big **X** that marks where Owen is. ✔

2. Touch description 1. ✔
   It says: To go to Molly, you go blank miles blank and blank miles blank.
   - Start at the start box and figure out the route for going to Molly. Then complete the description. Remember, tell the number of miles and the direction for each part of the description. Raise your hand when you're finished.
   (Observe students and give feedback.)
   - Here's what your description should say: To go to Molly, you go **four** miles **south** and **two** miles **west.** Four miles south and two miles west. Raise your hand if you got it right.

3. Touch description 2. ✔
   It says: To go to Owen, you go blank miles blank and blank miles blank.
   - Start at the start box and figure out the route for going to Owen. Then complete the description. Tell the number of miles and the direction for each part of the description. Raise your hand when you're finished.
   (Observe students and give feedback.)
   - Here's what your description should say: To go to Owen, you go **three** miles **north** and **four** miles **east.** Three miles north and four miles east. Raise your hand if you got it right.

4. Later on, you may want to write the description about how to get to Dud. That looks pretty hard.

EXERCISE 3 Creating Ambiguous Sentences

1. Three ladies picked berries.

   The berries were blue.

2. Our chicken laid an egg.

   The egg was no bigger than a stone.

3. We used a shovel to plant the flower.

   The flower grew all summer long.

1. Everybody, find part C. ✔
   (Write on the board:)

   He   She   It   They

- The sentences in each item are not confusing. You're going to make them confusing. I'll read each item.
- Item 1: Three ladies picked berries. The berries were blue.
- Item 2: Our chicken laid an egg. The egg was no bigger than a stone.
- Item 3: We used a shovel to plant the flower. The flower grew all summer long.

2. Touch item 1. ✔
   You're going to change the second sentence in item 1. That sentence starts out by naming something. Raise your hand when you know what it names.
   - Everybody, what does the second sentence name? (Signal.) *The berries.*
   - Listen: Cross out the words **the berries.** Then use one of the words on the board to tell about the berries or ladies. Find that word and write it above the crossed-out words. Raise your hand when you're finished. ✔
   - (Touch the word **They.**)
   Here's the word you should have written: **They.**
   - I'll read what your item 1 should say now: Three ladies picked berries. **They** were blue.
   - Now we don't know what was blue. Maybe it was the berries. Maybe it was . . . (Signal.) *The ladies.*

3. Item 2: Our chicken laid an egg. The egg was no bigger than a stone.
   - You're going to change the second sentence in that item. That sentence starts out by naming something. Raise your hand when you know what it names. ✔
   - Everybody, what does the second sentence name? (Signal.) *The egg.*
   - Listen: Cross out the words **the egg.** Then use one of the words on the board to tell about the egg or the chicken. Find that word and write it above the crossed-out words. Raise your hand when you're finished. ✔
   - (Touch the word **It.**)
   Here's the word you should have written: **It.**
   - I'll read what your item 2 should say now. Our chicken laid an egg. **It** was no bigger than a stone. Now we don't know what was no bigger than a stone. Maybe it was the egg. Maybe it was . . . (Signal.) *The chicken.*

4. Item 3: We used a shovel to plant the flower. The flower grew all summer long.

- You're going to change the second sentence. That sentence starts out by naming something. Raise your hand when you know what it names.
- Everybody, what does the second sentence name? (Signal.) *The flower.*
- Listen: Cross out the words **the flower.** Then find the word that could tell about the flower or the shovel and write that word above the crossed-out words. Raise your hand when you're finished. ✔
- (Touch the word **It**.) Here's the word you should have written: **It.**
- I'll read what your item 3 should say now: We used a shovel to plant the flower. **It** grew all summer long.
- Now we don't know what grew all summer. Maybe it was the flower. Maybe it was . . . (Signal.) *The shovel.*

5. Later you can draw a picture for item 3 the way Zelda might do it. You can show a shovel growing very large.

EXERCISE 4   The Case Of The Squashed Squash

Review

- I'm going to re-read the last part of **The Case of the Squashed Squash.** Listen very carefully to the things that happen because we're going to put on a play.

After the feast was over and everybody was so full of squash and walnuts and apples and berries and seeds and corn that they couldn't eat any more, the wise old rat stood up and said, "We can thank the gray rat—I mean Sherlock—for this fine feast. He figured out how the squash got squashed, and somehow he fixed things up so that there were two great squashes in our berry patch—not just one."

Sherlock stood up as straight as he could. He cleared his throat and said, "Well, this was a very difficult job. A detective without my skill would have been confused. That person would

have used the wrong deductions. That detective would have figured out that Goober did it. After all, Goober's shoes made the footprints in the berry bushes, and Goober's overalls sat in the squash. Because I'm so good at deductions, I knew how to do them the right way. I knew that, if Goober's **shoes** made the footprints, you couldn't say that **Goober** made the footprints. All you could say is that Goober's **shoes** made the footprints. I also knew that, if Goober's overalls sat on the squash, you couldn't say that Goober sat in the squash. All you could . . ."

"Enough talking," the wise old rat said. He was looking at Bertha. Her little body was rocking very fast, and it was easy to see that she was very, very unhappy.

The wise old rat said to her, "I can see that you don't agree with everything that Sherlock is saying."

She said, "Well . . ."

"Tell it the way it was," the wise old rat said.

"Yeah," the other rats shouted. "Tell it the way it was."

So she did just that. She told what had really happened.

As she talked, the other rats started staring at Sherlock with very unfriendly expressions. And Sherlock started to slouch. At first he slouched just a little bit. Then a little bit more. And finally he slouched right down into his chair.

When Bertha was finished, one of the rats said, "That Sherlock is a dirty liar."

"Yeah," another rat said. "A dirty liar. Let's clean him up."

So they rushed to Sherlock, picked him up, carried him to the pond and splash.

And, while they were cleaning up Sherlock, the bluebirds moved into the feast area.

They said, "Wow, there are all kinds of squash and other good things to eat here."

And there was. There were lots of things that bluebirds love. So the bluebirds ate and ate. They ate walnuts and berries and corn and seeds and lots of yellow squash. Those bluebirds had their first annual fall feast.

Bertha said "This is a fall feast for everybody." And she was almost right. But there was one person who wasn't very happy with the feast.

EXERCISE 5   Play

The Case of the Squashed Squash

1. Now we're going to put on a play. This play will take place during the fall feast. Sherlock will tell his version of what happened. Then Bertha will tell what really happened. Then the rats will carry Sherlock off to clean him up.
   - We need somebody to play the wise old rat. (Identify the student.)
   - We need somebody to play the part of Sherlock. This is a big part because Sherlock has to brag on and on about how he solved The Case of the Squashed Squash. (Identify the student.)
   - We need somebody to play the part of Bertha. This is a very tough part because the story doesn't tell what Bertha said to the rat pack. (Identify the student.)
   - The rest of us will play the part of the rat pack. At the end, some of us are going to rush over to Sherlock and take him away. We won't really pick Sherlock up. (Identify 4 or 5 students to take Sherlock away.)
2. (Arrange Sherlock, Bertha and the wise old rat at the "head table.")
   - The wise old rat starts out by saying that we can thank Sherlock for this fine feast.
   - Then Sherlock stands up very straight and tells how **he** wasn't fooled and how **he** made all the right deductions. While he's talking, Bertha gets madder and madder.
   - Then the wise old rat interrupts Sherlock and asks Bertha why she doesn't agree with Sherlock.
   - She tells what really happened. Then the rats call Sherlock a dirty liar and say that he should be cleaned up.
   - Remember, the feast is over and everybody is full of squash.
3. Is everybody ready?
   - Wise old rat, start. (Prompt students if necessary.)
     (Cue: Sherlock to brag.)
     (Cue: Wise old rat to interrupt.)
     (Cue: Bertha to tell what happened.)
     (Cue: Rats to call Sherlock a dirty liar.)
4. That was pretty good. Maybe we can do that part again some time with different actors.

Note: Data are collected in exercise 5. These data will be referred to in lesson 56.

Objectives

- Complete a letter. (Exercise 1)
- Complete directions for going to different locations on a map. (Exercise 2)
- **Construct deductions that are formally incorrect.** (Exercise 3)
- Listen to part 1 of a story and predict the outcome. (Exercise 4)
- **Identify the illustrator of ambiguous sentences.** (Exercise 5)

WORKBOOK

EXERCISE 1 Letter Writing

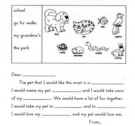

1. Open your workbook to lesson 55 and find part A. ✔
   You're going to complete another letter. It is a make-believe letter that tells about the pet you would like to have the most. If you already have a pet, you may want to write about that pet.
   - At the top of the page is a box. There are some words in the box that you may want to use when you write your letter. Touch the first part of the box. ✔
   - Follow along while I read the words. **School . . . go for walks . . . my grandma's . . . the park.**
   - Touch the second part of the box. ✔
   - These pictures show some animals you may want for a pet. Follow along while I read the words. **Dog . . . cat . . . fish . . . parrot . . . turtle . . . hamster . . . snake . . . bunny.**
   - Remember to spell any of these words correctly.
2. Touch the word **Dear.** ✔
   - In the space after the word, **Dear,** you'll write the name of the person whom you're writing to. Raise your hand when you've filled in the first space of the letter.
   - (Call on several students to read their greeting.)
3. I'll read the next part of the letter and you'll follow along. **The pet that I would like the most is a blank.** Write what kind of pet you would like the most. ✔

4. The next sentence says, **I would name my pet blank and I would take care of my blank.** Fill in the missing words. (Observe students and give feedback.)
5. The rest of the letter says, **We would have a lot of fun together. I would take my pet to blank and to blank. I would love my blank and my pet would love me.** Write the name of 2 places you would take your pet. Write what kind of pet you would love. Then remember to write your name at the end of the letter. (Observe students and give feedback. Students who are finished early may wish to draw a picture to go with their letter.)
6. (Call on several students to read their complete letter. Praise letters that have appropriate names and words in the blanks.)

EXERCISE 2 Map Directions

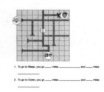

1. Find part B. ✔
   This is a map. Each square is one mile.
   - You're going to complete the directions for going to different places. For each set of directions you'll start at the start box.
   - Touch the start box. ✔
   - You can see different things on the map.
   - Touch the little **X** that marks where Bleep is. ✔
   - Touch the big **X** that marks where Owen is. ✔
2. Touch description 1. ✔
   It says: To go to Bleep, you go blank miles blank and blank miles blank.

- Start at the start box and figure out the route for going to Bleep. Then complete the description. Remember, tell the number of miles and the direction for each part of the description. Raise your hand when you're finished.
  (Observe students and give feedback.)
- Here's what your description should say: To go to Bleep, you go **two** miles **north** and **four** miles **west.** Two miles north and four miles west. Raise your hand if you got it right.
3. Touch description 2. ✔
  It says: To go to Owen, you go blank miles blank and blank miles blank.
- Start at the start box and figure out the route for going to Owen. Then complete the description. Tell the number of miles and the direction for each part of the description. Raise your hand when you're finished.
  (Observe students and give feedback.)
- Here's what your description should say. To go to Owen, you go **three** miles **north** and **three** miles **east.** Three miles north and three miles east. Raise your hand if you got it right.
4. Later on, you may want to write the description about how to get to Fizz and Liz. That looks pretty hard.

EXERCISE 3 Deductions

Good/Bad

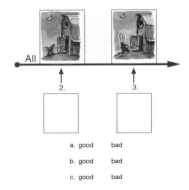

1. Everybody, find part C. ✔
  Sherlock made some pretty bad deductions. Remember, if the deduction isn't about arrow 1, arrow 2 and arrow 3, the deduction is bad. Some of Sherlock's deductions told about arrow 1, then arrow 3, then arrow 2. Boo.
- (Write on the board:)

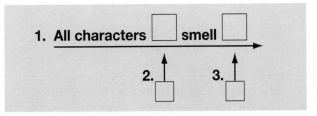

- I'll say the rule for arrow 1: All characters who go into the barn smell of oats.
2. Everybody, say the rule for arrow 1. (Signal.) *All characters who go into the barn smell of oats.*
- (Repeat step 2 until firm.)
3. So the next part of the deduction should tell who **went into the barn,** not who **smells of oats.**
- I'll say a deduction. You tell me if it's a good deduction or a bad deduction. Listen: All characters who go into the barn smell of oats. The red hen smells of oats. So the red hen went into the barn. Is that a good deduction or a bad one? (Signal.) *Bad.*
- It's bad because it goes from arrow 1 to arrow 3.
- I'll touch the arrows. Watch.
- (Touch arrow 1.)
  All characters who go into the barn smell of oats.
- (Touch arrow 3.)
  The red hen smells of oats.
- (Touch arrow 2.)
  So the red hen went into the barn.
4. I'll say some deductions. You'll circle **good** or **bad.**
- Here's deduction A. Listen: All characters who go into the barn smell of oats. Sherlock went into the barn. So Sherlock smells of oats. Circle **good** or **bad** for deduction A. Raise your hand when you're finished. ✔
- Everybody, what did you circle for deduction A? (Signal.) *Good.*
5. Here's deduction B: All characters who go into the barn smell of oats. Bertha smells of oats. So Bertha went into the barn. Circle **good** or **bad** for deduction B. Raise your hand when you're finished. ✔
- Everybody, what did you circle for deduction B? (Signal.) *Bad.*
6. Here's deduction C: All characters who go into the barn smell of oats. Bertha went into the barn. So Bertha smells of oats. Circle **good** or **bad** for deduction C. Raise your hand when you're finished. ✔

- Everybody, what did you circle for deduction C? (Signal.) *Good.*
- Raise your hand if you completed that deduction. Just remember, that's a silly deduction.

EXERCISE 4   Mrs Hudson Writes Another Book *Part 1*

Storytelling

1. I'm going to read a story about Mrs. Hudson. The title of this story is **Mrs. Hudson Writes Another Book.**

- Listen:

Mrs. Hudson decided to write another book. This book was about gardening. Mrs. Hudson loved to grow things in her garden, and she had lots of experiences to tell about. Of course, they were as boring as the experiences she told about in her first book.

But, as Mrs. Hudson wrote her new book, she kept thinking about her first book and about Zelda.

Mrs. Hudson knew that her first book was very popular and that people really liked it, but she was still a little upset because they thought the book was funny.

She hadn't meant to write a funny book, but Zelda's illustrations made it funny.

As Mrs. Hudson thought about that book, she decided that she didn't want Zelda to illustrate her new book.

She said to herself, "I don't want people who read this book to see silly pictures and think the book is funny. I want them to enjoy my wonderful experiences and look at pictures that show those experiences."

So, when Mrs. Hudson finished her book, she didn't take it to Zelda to be illustrated. She found another illustrator. His name was Henry.

Henry was a good illustrator, not as good as Zelda, but good. And Henry didn't misunderstand the parts of the stories that Mrs. Hudson marked for her illustrations.

One place that was marked for an illustration said this: "My two sisters pulled out the morning glories. They were climbing all over the fence."

- Listen again to what Mrs. Hudson wrote:

"My two sisters pulled out the morning glories. They were climbing all over the fence."

If Zelda made an illustration for that part, she would get things mixed up. She would show something climbing all over the fence, but it wouldn't be morning glories.

Henry didn't have that problem. He knew that the morning glories were climbing all over the fence, and that's what his illustration showed.

It showed two sweet little girls pulling out morning glories. They were smiling.

- Get a picture of that illustration. Two sweet little girls pulling out morning glories. They were smiling.
- Who was smiling? (Call on a student. Idea: *The little girls.*)
- If Zelda illustrated that sentence, who would be smiling? (Call on a student. Idea: *The morning glories.*)

Naturally, Mrs. Hudson went over every illustration with Henry before he drew anything. She wanted to make very sure that he understood what he would show in each picture.

Mrs. Hudson would turn to each part that was marked for an illustration. Then she'd read something like this: "Uncle George picked berries with my sisters. He liked them because they were so big and blue."

- Listen to what Mrs. Hudson wrote:

> "Uncle George picked berries with my sisters. He liked them because they were so big and blue."
>
> Mrs. Hudson would ask questions because she didn't want the kind of picture that Zelda might make. We know what would be big and blue in Zelda's picture, and it wouldn't be the berries.

- What would it be? (Signal.) *The sisters.*

> Henry would answer Mrs. Hudson's questions, and he'd explain how he planned to illustrate each part.
>
> He'd say things like this: "Well, I thought I would show these wonderfully plump blue berries. The girls would be very close to them, smiling. Perhaps, one of the girls would have a slight blue line on her lower lip to show that she'd been eating berries as she picked them. Uncle George would be standing in the background, smiling at the girls and at the berries."
>
> That's how every illustration went. Henry would always end up making a happy picture, with everybody smiling and everything just wonderful.
>
> And that made Mrs. Hudson feel just wonderfully marvelous. She thought that Henry's illustrations were just what she needed to give her exciting stories even more excitement.
>
> Henry worked on the illustrations for three months. At last, he was finished.
>
> The next day, Mrs. Hudson called the publisher and said, "I'm sending you my latest book. I think it's wonderful. It's delightful. It's deliciously entertaining, and it's wonderfully educational. It's just superbly . . ." She had run out of **good** words this time.
>
> The publisher said, "Well, I'll be looking forward to reading it. If it's half as good

as your last book, you'll have another best seller."

> "Oh," Mrs. Hudson said. "I'm sure you'll find this book perfectly delightful and absolutely marvelous and completely . . ." She'd run out of good words again.
>
> She sent the book and the illustrations to the publisher and she waited for a phone call. She expected the publisher to call her and tell her how perfectly excited she was, how totally thrilled, how absolutely . . . But the call didn't come. Three weeks later, Mrs. Hudson received a large package from the publisher.

2. That's the end of this part. Next time, we'll find out what happens. But first, we'll see who is good at figuring out what will happen.
- (Draw on the board:)

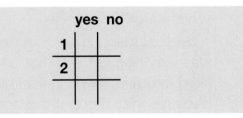

- I'll ask questions. Then I'll count the number of hands raised. You're going to have to close your eyes for this part so you can't see what other students are doing.
3. Everybody gets to vote for each question. But don't say anything or do anything until I tell you to.
- Here's question 1: Do you think the publisher will like the new book with Henry's illustrations?
- Listen again: Do you think the publisher will like the new book with Henry's illustrations?
- Everybody, close your eyes and keep them closed. Raise your hand if you think the publisher will like the new book with Henry's illustrations. (Count raised hands and write the number under **yes** for **1.**)
- Hands down.

- Raise your hand if you think the publisher won't like the new book with Henry's illustrations. **(Count raised hands and write the number under no for 1.)**
- Open your eyes. Here's the vote for whether the publisher will like the new book. ___ students think the publisher will like the new book. ___ students think the publisher won't like the new book.
4. Here's question 2: Do you think Zelda will end up illustrating this new book before it's published?
- Everybody, close your eyes and keep them closed. Raise your hand if you think that Zelda will end up illustrating this new book before it's published. **(Count raised hands and write the number under yes for 2.)**
- Hands down.
- Raise your hand if you think that Zelda won't end up illustrating this new book before it's published. **(Count raised hands and write the number under no for 2.)**
- Open your eyes. Here's the vote for whether Zelda will illustrate the new book. ___ students think she will. ___ students think she won't.
5. Next time, we'll see who's right.

> *Note:* Save data for lesson 56.

EXERCISE 5 Character

Extrapolation

1. Three little boys picked strawberries. They were as big as apples.

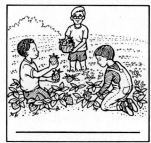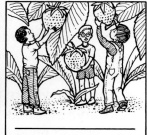

2. Before the children pulled up the tulips, my sister watered them with the hose.

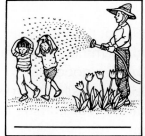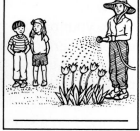

1. Find part D. ✔
   The sentences show parts from Mrs. Hudson's second book. Below each part are two pictures. One was done by Henry, and one was done by Zelda. You have to write the name of the illustrator on the blank line in each picture.
2. Touch number 1. ✔
   I'll read that part: Three little boys picked strawberries. They were as big as apples.
- One of the pictures below that part was drawn by Zelda. One was drawn by Henry.
- (Write on the board:)

Zelda	Henry

- Write the correct names in the top two pictures. Raise your hand when you're finished.
   (Observe students and give feedback.)
- Touch the first picture for part 1. ✔
   Some things are as big as apples in that picture. What are as big as apples? (Signal.) *Strawberries.*
- Who made that illustration? (Signal.) *Henry.*
- Raise your hand if you wrote **Henry** in the blank for the first picture.
- Touch the other picture for part 1. ✔
   What are as big as apples in that picture? (Signal.) *Little boys.*
- Who made that illustration? (Signal.) *Zelda.*
3. Touch number 2. ✔
   I'll read what it says: Before the children pulled up the tulips, my sister watered them with a hose.
- Write the correct names in the bottom two pictures. Raise your hand when you're finished.
   (Observe students and give feedback.)
- Touch the first picture for part 2. ✔
   What's getting watered in the picture? (Signal.) *The children.*
- Who made that illustration? (Signal.) *Zelda.*
- Touch the other picture for part 2. What's getting watered in that picture? (Signal.) *The tulips.*
- Who made that illustration? (Signal.) *Henry.*
4. Later, you can color the pictures.

Objectives

- **Write 2 good clues for a mystery sequence.** (Exercise 1)
- **Indicate whether statements about a picture report** or **do not report.** (Exercise 2)
  Note: Statements do not report if they do not tell about details that can be touched in the picture.
- **Listen to the conclusion of a 2-part story and answer comprehension questions.** (Exercise 3)
- **Make a picture consistent with the details of a story.** (Exercise 4)

WORKBOOK

EXERCISE 1 Mystery Arrow

Generating Clues

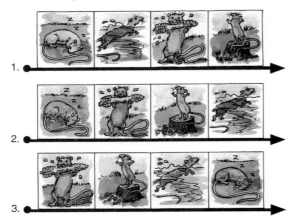

1. Open your workbook to lesson 56 and find part A. You're going to make up clues that tell about the mystery arrow.
- (Write on the board:)

> **Sherlock**
> **went to sleep**
> **went swimming**
> **ate corn**
> **stood on a stump**

- Here are words that you'll use to write your clues.
2. Touch arrow 3.
   That's the mystery arrow.
- Touch the first picture on that arrow. What did Sherlock do first?
  (Signal.) *Ate corn.*
- What did he do after he ate corn? (Signal.) *Stood on a stump.*
- What did he do after he stood on a stump? (Signal.) *Went swimming.*
- What did he do after he went swimming? (Signal.) *Went to sleep.*

3. Look at the first two pictures on arrow 3. They show Sherlock standing on the stump after he ate corn.
- Look at all the arrows.
  Circle the pictures on any arrow that show Sherlock standing on the stump just after he ate corn. Raise your hand when you're finished.
  (Observe students and give feedback.)
4. Did you circle pictures on arrow 1?
   (Signal.) *Yes.*
- Did you circle pictures on arrow 2?
  (Signal.) *Yes.*
- Did you circle pictures on arrow 3?
  (Signal.) *Yes.*
- All the arrows show Sherlock standing on the stump just after he ate corn. So a clue about Sherlock standing on the stump is not a good clue because it tells about all the arrows.
5. Look at arrow 3 again.
   What did Sherlock do after he stood on the stump? (Signal.) *Went swimming.*
- Look at all the arrows. Draw a circle around any picture that shows Sherlock swimming just after he stood on a stump. Raise your hand when you're finished.
  (Observe students and give feedback.)
6. You should have circled pictures on arrows 2 and 3.
- You should not have circled any picture on arrow 1.
- Raise your hand if you got it right.
7. Listen: Sherlock went swimming after he stood on a stump. That's a good clue because it doesn't tell about all the arrows.
- Listen again: Sherlock went swimming after he stood on a stump.

8. Everybody, say that. (Signal.) *Sherlock went swimming after he stood on a stump.*
   • (Repeat step 8 until firm.)
9. Your turn: Write that clue on line 1. Raise your hand when you're finished.
   (Observe students and give feedback.)
10. (Write on the board:)

> **Sherlock went swimming after he stood on a stump.**

   • Here's what you should have for clue 1: Sherlock went swimming after he stood on a stump.
   • If you told somebody that clue, they'd be able to cross out one of the arrows. Raise your hand when you know which arrow they would cross out.
   • Which arrow could be crossed out? (Signal.) *Arrow 1.*
   • Cross out arrow 1. That arrow could not be the mystery arrow.
11. Look at arrow 3 again.
    What did Sherlock do just after he went swimming? (Signal.) *Went to sleep.*
   • Look at the arrows that are not crossed out. Draw a circle around any picture that shows Sherlock sleeping just after he went swimming. Raise your hand when you're finished.
    (Observe students and give feedback.)
12. You should have circled the picture on arrow 3. That's the only arrow left that shows that Sherlock went to sleep after he went swimming. So the clue about when Sherlock went to sleep is a good clue.
   • Listen: Sherlock went to sleep after he went swimming.
13. Write that clue on line 2. Raise your hand when you're finished.
    (Observe students and give feedback.)
14. (Write on the board:)

> **Sherlock went to sleep after he went swimming.**

   • Here's what you should have for clue 2: Sherlock went to sleep after he went swimming. Raise your hand if you got it right.
15. If you gave somebody both your clues, they'd be able to find the mystery arrow.

   • Here's clue 1: Sherlock went swimming after he stood on a stump.
   • That clue would let you know that one of the arrows could not be the mystery arrow. Which arrow is that? (Signal.) *Arrow 1.*
   • Here's clue 2: Sherlock went to sleep after he went swimming. That clue would let you know that another arrow could not be the mystery arrow. Which arrow is that? (Signal.) *Arrow 2.*
   • The only arrow left is arrow 3. That's the mystery arrow.

EXERCISE 2   Reporting

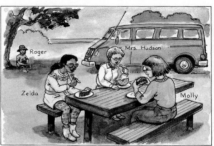

1. Zelda drove a van to the picnic.	reports	does not report
2. Three people sat at a picnic table.	reports	does not report
3. Everybody was going to swim later that day.	reports	does not report
4. Roger wore a hat.	reports	does not report
5. Zelda ate more than anybody else.	reports	does not report
6. A van was close to the picnic tables.	reports	does not report
7. Zelda sat next to Mrs. Hudson.	reports	does not report

1. Find part B in your workbook. ✔
   Look at the picture in part B.
   You're going to learn about sentences that report on the picture.
   • Listen: If a sentence tells about something that you can touch in the picture, the sentence **reports** on the picture. If the sentence does not tell about something you can touch, the sentence **does not report.**
   • Remember: If the sentence tells you something you can touch in the picture, the sentence **reports.**
2. Listen: Roger was sitting under a tree. That sentence reports.
   • Touch the part of the picture that shows Roger sitting under a tree. ✔
3. Listen: Zelda was wearing a swimsuit. Everybody, does that sentence report? (Signal.) *No.*
   • Right, the picture does not show Zelda wearing a swimsuit.
4. This is tricky. Listen: Mrs. Hudson loved watermelon. Everybody, does that sentence report? (Signal.) *No.*

- Right, the sentence doesn't report because the picture doesn't show whether Mrs. Hudson loved watermelon. The picture shows that she was eating watermelon, but maybe she doesn't like it very much.

5. Listen: Molly ate a hamburger. Everybody, does that sentence report? (Signal.) *Yes.*
- Touch the part of the picture that shows Molly eating a hamburger. ✔

6. Listen: Zelda wore sunglasses. Everybody, does that sentence report?(Signal.) *Yes.*

7. Listen: Roger was not hungry. Everybody, does that sentence report? (Signal.) *No.*
- Right, the sentence doesn't report because we don't know whether Roger was hungry. Maybe he was very hungry. All the picture shows is that he wasn't eating.
- Under the picture are sentences. After each sentence are the words **reports** and **does not report.**

8. Everybody, touch sentence 1. Sentence 1. ✔
- I'll read sentence 1: Zelda drove a van to the picnic. Everybody, does that sentence report? (Signal.) *No.*
- The sentence does not report, so circle the words **does not report.** Find the words **does not report** on the same line as sentence 1. Then make a circle around those words. ✔

9. Everybody, touch sentence 2. I'll read sentence 2: Three people sat at a picnic table. Everybody, does that sentence report? (Signal.) *Yes.*
- The sentence reports, so circle the word **reports** on the same line as sentence 2. Find the word **reports** and circle it. ✔

10. Touch sentence 3. I'll read sentence 3: Everybody was going to swim later that day. Everybody, does that sentence report? (Signal.) *No.*
- That sentence does not report. So what words are you going to circle for sentence 3? (Signal.) *Does not report.*
- Do it. Circle **does not report.**

11. I'll read the rest of the sentences. Touch each sentence as I read it. Don't circle anything. Just touch the sentences.

- Sentence 4: Roger wore a hat.
- Sentence 5: Zelda ate more than anybody else.
- Sentence 6: A van was close to the picnic table.
- Sentence 7: Zelda sat next to Mrs. Hudson.

12. Your turn: Circle the right words for the sentences. Read each sentence to yourself. If the sentence reports, circle **reports.** If the sentence does not report, circle **does not report.** Raise your hand when you're finished.
(Observe students and give feedback.)

13. Let's check your work. Make an **X** next to any item you missed. I'll read each sentence. You tell me whether you circled **reports** or **does not report.**
- Sentence 4: Roger wore a hat. What did you circle? (Signal.) *Reports.*
- Sentence 5: Zelda ate more than anybody else. What did you circle? (Signal.) *Does not report.*
- Sentence 6: A van was close to the picnic table. What did you circle? (Signal.) *Reports.*
- Sentence 7: Zelda sat next to Mrs. Hudson. What did you circle? (Signal.) *Reports.*

14. Raise your hand if you got no items wrong. Great job.
- Raise your hand if you got only 1 item wrong. Good work.
- Listen: Fix up any mistakes you made in part B. Do it now. Circle the right words for any items you missed.
(Observe students and give feedback.)

EXERCISE 3   Mrs. Hudson Writes Another Book *Part 2*

Storytelling

- Last time, you voted on how you thought the story about Mrs. Hudson would end. I'll read the ending. We'll see who was right.
- Listen:

Last time, Mrs. Hudson sent her boring book to the publisher with Henry's illustrations. All of them were hap, hap, happy pictures showing nice things. They were as boring as the book.

Mrs. Hudson waited for a phone call from the publisher. But the call didn't come. Three weeks later, she received a large package from the publisher.

It was her book and the illustrations. There was also a note from the publisher. It said:

Dear Mrs. Hudson,

Thank you for sending us your latest book. Unfortunately, our company will not be able to publish it. We read it and we all agree that it doesn't have the same kind of spark and humor that your first book had. Frankly, Mrs. Hudson, this book is a little boring. And the illustrations are, frankly, a little boring too.

At the bottom of the letter was a note that said this: "Maybe the book would be more lively if Zelda did the illustrations."

Mrs. Hudson was crushed. She was completely saddened. She was so thoroughly disappointed that she cried.

She stopped crying by the next day. She had decided to take the publisher's advice. So she took the book to Zelda and said, "I've marked the places where you can make illustrations. Just do the pictures the way you think they should be."

Zelda read the book. After she read this part: "Uncle Rover's rosebush grew next to the garage. It was made of red brick," she said to herself, "That man sure has strange plants in his garden."

A few months later, Zelda finished the illustrations, and Mrs. Hudson sent them with her book to the publisher. This time, she didn't have to wait weeks to receive a letter from the publisher.

The publisher called two days later. She said, "It's great. It's just great. It's so funny and so humorous and so delightful and just so . . ." **She** had run out of good words.

And, of course, she was right. And Mrs. Hudson had a best-selling book again. But, when she looked through it, she still had trouble appreciating Zelda's illustrations.

Under each picture was the part of the story that was illustrated. Mrs. Hudson would read those parts and then shake her head sadly when she looked at the illustration that Zelda had drawn.

Here is what it said under one of the illustrations: "Donna and her mother watched the tiny spiders. They were upside down in their web."

Mrs. Hudson did not like Zelda's picture at all.

- Listen to what Mrs. Hudson wrote:

Donna and her mother watched the tiny spiders. They were upside down in their web.

- What do you think Zelda's illustration showed? (Call on a student. Idea: *Donna and her mother upside down in a spider web*.)
- That's not what Mrs. Hudson meant, was it? (Signal.) *No.*

Another picture made Mrs. Hudson particularly unhappy. That was the picture for this part: "Uncle George and Billy raked the leaves. The wind kept blowing them into the garage."

"No, no, no, no," Mrs. Hudson would say to herself every time she looked at that picture.

- Listen to the words again:

Uncle George and Billy raked the leaves. The wind kept blowing them into the garage.

- What do you think Zelda's illustration showed blowing into the garage? (Call on a student. Idea: *Uncle George and Billy*.)

- That's not what Mrs. Hudson meant, was it? (Signal.) *No.*

> But the picture that made Mrs. Hudson most unhappy was the picture for this part of the story: "The birds watched my sisters plant the new garden. They wore red sweaters and perky little caps."
>
> "No, no, no, no," Mrs. Hudson would say to herself.

- Listen to the words:

> The birds watched my sisters plant the new garden. They wore red sweaters and perky little caps.

- Who do you think Zelda's illustration showed wearing red sweaters and perky little caps? (Call on a student. Idea: *The birds.*)
- That's not what Mrs. Hudson meant, was it? (Signal.) *No.*

> But the book sold a lot of copies and made lots of money. It also made Mrs. Hudson even more famous than her first book did.
>
> And everybody thought that she was the funniest writer in the whole world.

EXERCISE 4 Ambiguous Sentences

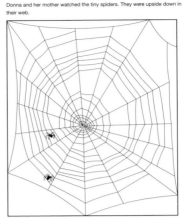

Donna and her mother watched the tiny spiders. They were upside down in their web.

- Find part C. ✔
  I'll read what it says. You follow along: Donna and her mother watched the tiny spiders. They were upside down in their web.
- Part of the picture is already drawn. There's a great web, and I can see a couple of tiny spiders in that web. But, I don't see Donna and her mother.
- You're going to fix up this picture the way Zelda would do it. In her illustration, where would Donna and her mother be? (Signal.) *In the spider web.*
- And would they be right-side up or upside down? (Signal.) *Upside down.*
- Yes, Donna and her mother would be upside down in the spider web. Fix up the picture to show that.

Note: For exercise 5, students will work in 3 teams.

Materials: Each student will need a piece of lined paper.

Objectives

- Indicate whether statements about a picture **report** or **do not report.** (Exercise 1)
- **Write sentences that report on what pictures show.** (Exercise 2)
- Listen to part 1 of a new story and answer comprehension questions. (Exercise 3)
- Edit words to show a character's dialect. (Exercise 4 and 5)
- **Work cooperatively to write 2 clues for a mystery sequence.** (Exercise 5)

WORKBOOK

EXERCISE 1 Reporting

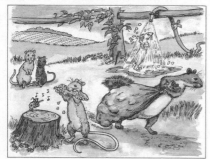

1. Sherlock ate too much corn.	reports	does not report
2. Bertha was mad at Sherlock.	reports	does not report
3. Cyrus pulled a large sack.	reports	does not report
4. Bertha played a violin.	reports	does not report
5. The wise old rat was dirty.	reports	does not report
6. The sack was full of hazelnuts.	reports	does not report
7. The wise old rat was wet.	reports	does not report

1. Open your workbook to lesson 57 and find part A. ✔

   Look at the picture in part A. Remember, if a sentence tells about something that you can touch in the picture, the sentence **reports** on the picture. If the sentence does not tell about something you can touch, the sentence **does not report.**

2. Listen: Bertha played a violin.
   That sentence reports. Touch the part of the picture that shows: Bertha played a violin. ✔

- Listen: Cyrus was mad at Sherlock. Everybody, does that sentence report? (Signal.) *No.*

- Right, nothing in the picture shows: Cyrus was mad at Sherlock.

3. Listen: The sack that Cyrus was pulling belonged to Sherlock. Everybody, does that sentence report? (Signal.) *No.*

- The picture doesn't show who the sack belongs to.

- Listen: Two rats were sitting. Everybody, does that sentence report? (Signal.) *Yes.*

- Touch the part of the picture that shows: Two rats were sitting. ✔

- Listen: The wise old rat was taking a shower. Everybody, does that sentence report? (Signal.) *Yes.*

- Listen: Bertha was playing a pretty tune. Everybody, does that sentence report? (Signal.) *No.*

- It doesn't report because the picture doesn't show the music is a pretty tune. Maybe she's just making squeaking sounds.

4. Everybody, touch sentence 1 below the picture. Sentence 1.
   I'll read sentence 1: Sherlock ate too much corn. Everybody, does that sentence report? (Signal.) *No.*

- The sentence does not report, so circle the words **does not report.** Find the words **does not report** on the same line as sentence 1 and circle them. ✔

5. Everybody, touch sentence 2.
   I'll read sentence 2: Bertha was mad at Sherlock. Everybody, does that sentence report? (Signal.) *No.*

- The sentence does not report, so circle the words **does not report** on the same line as sentence 2.

6. I'll read the rest of the sentences. Touch each sentence as I read it. Don't circle anything. Just touch the sentences.

- Sentence 3: Cyrus pulled a large sack.

- Sentence 4: Bertha played a violin.
- Sentence 5: The wise old rat was dirty.
- Sentence 6: The sack was full of hazelnuts.
- Sentence 7: The wise old rat was wet.

7. Your turn: Circle the right words for the sentences. Read each sentence to yourself. If the sentence reports, circle **reports.** If the sentence does not report, circle **does not report.** Raise your hand when you're finished.
   (Observe students and give feedback.)

8. Let's check your work. Look at the picture. Make an **X** next to any item you missed. I'll read each sentence. You tell me whether you circled **reports** or **does not report.**
   - Sentence 3: Cyrus pulled a large sack. What did you circle? (Signal.) *Reports.*
   - Sentence 4: Bertha played a violin. What did you circle? (Signal.) *Reports.*
   - Sentence 5: The wise old rat was dirty. What did you circle? (Signal.) *Does not report.*
   - Sentence 6: The sack was full of hazelnuts. What did you circle?
     (Signal.) *Does not report.*
   - Sentence 7: The wise old rat was wet. What did you circle? (Signal.) *Reports.*

9. Raise your hand if you got no items wrong. Great job.
   - Raise your hand if you got only 1 item wrong.
     Good work.
   - Listen: Fix up any mistakes you made in part A. Do it now. Circle the right words for any items you missed.
     (Observe students and give feedback.)

LINED PAPER

EXERCISE 2   Sentence Writing

Reporting-Main Idea

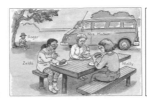

1. Find part B. ✔
   (Pass out lined paper to students.)

- Everybody, you're going to write sentences on lined paper. Your sentences will report on the main thing that people in the pictures did. The vocabulary box has words you may use.
- Touch the words on the top line. What do they say? (Signal.) *Ate a burger.*
- Next line. (Signal.) *Sat under a tree.*
- Next line. (Signal.) *Drove a van.*
- Next line. (Signal.) *Went fishing.*
- Next line. (Signal.) *Ate watermelon.*
- Next line. (Signal.) *Sat on a table.*
- Next line. (Signal.) *Ate pie.*

2. (Write on the board:)

   > **Molly** _____.

- Your turn: Write a sentence that reports on the main thing Molly did in the picture. Start your sentence with Molly. Remember to end the sentence with a period. Raise your hand when you're finished.
  (Observe students and give feedback.)

3. I'll call on individual students to read their sentence about Molly. (Call on individual students to complete the sentence on the board. Praise sentences such as: *Molly ate a burger.*)

4. (Write on the board:)

   > **Roger** _____.

- Now write a sentence about Roger. Tell the main thing he did in the picture. Raise your hand when you're finished.
  (Observe students and give feedback.)

5. I'll call on individual students to read their sentence about Roger. (Call on individual students to complete the sentence on the board. Praise sentences such as: *Roger sat under a tree.*)

6. (Write on the board:)

   > **Zelda** _____.
   >
   > **Mrs. Hudson** _____.

- For your last sentence, you can report on the main thing Zelda did or the main thing Mrs. Hudson did. Start your sentence with the name you want and report on the main thing that person did. Raise your hand when you're finished.
  (Observe students and give feedback.)

7. I'll call on individual students to complete their sentence about Zelda or Mrs. Hudson. (Call on students. Praise sentences such as: *Zelda ate pie; Mrs. Hudson ate watermelon*.)

EXERCISE 3 More Silly Bleep-Talk
Part 1

Storytelling

* I'm going to read the first part of a story. It's another story about Bleep.
* Here's the first part.

Molly had to fix up Bleep so he would talk correctly. After she fixed him up, she told him, "Don't ever take the top of your head off again and mess around with those screws."

And Bleep was good—for a while. But then one day he bonked his head while cleaning up the basement. It happened when he was piling some boxes. One box was under the stairs. He bent over and went under the stairs, but then he didn't stay bent over. He stood up. Bonk. He hit his head on the stairs.

Bleep went over to a mirror and looked at himself. He had a dent right on the top of his head.

"That doesn't look good," he said to himself. So he took off the top of his head, took a hammer and pounded out the dent.

He was ready to put the top of his head on when he looked in the mirror again and said to himself, "I wonder what all those screws do."

In the back of his mind, he could hear Molly saying, "Don't ever mess around with those screws." But those screws looked very interesting—all those different colors. So, before he really knew what he was doing, he touched the yellow screw, then the black screw, then the pink screw. And, before he knew what he was doing, he turned the pink screw—not very much, but just enough to change the way he said the sound the letter **a** makes in words like **as** or **hat** or **sand.**

He could say all the other sounds. He could say the sound the letter **a** makes in words like **take** and **ate** and **cake.** But he couldn't say that other sound. Instead of saying **"at,"** he would say "ut." Instead of saying **"Sam,"** he would say "Sum." Instead of saying **"ran,"** he would say "run."

Well, Bleep put the top of his head back on and finished piling the boxes. Just as he was piling the last box, Molly came downstairs.

"Hi, Bleep," she said.

"Hi, Molly," Bleep said.

"You're really working hard, aren't you?"

* And that's where the story stops, right in the middle.

EXERCISE 4 Correcting Bleep-Talk
1. In the next lesson, you're going to make up an ending to the story. Your ending will tell some of the funny things that Bleep says. Then Molly will fix Bleep up.
* Before you work on your ending, you'll fix up some sentences to show what Bleep would say.
2. (Write on the board:)

1. and	2. bad	3. cat

* Here are some words that Bleep cannot say.
* Word 1 is **and.** What would Bleep say instead of **and**? (Signal.) *Und.*
* (Write to show:)

1. a̶nd (u)	2. bad	3. cat

* Word 2 is **bad.** What would Bleep say instead of **bad**? (Signal.) *Bud.*
* (Write to show:)

1. a̶nd (u)	2. ba̶d (u)	3. cat

* Word 3 is **cat.** What would Bleep say instead of **cat?** (Signal.) *Cut.*

- (Write to show:)

u	u	u
1. ~~a~~nd	2. b~~a~~d	3. c~~a~~t

EXERCISE 5 Writing Bleep-Talk

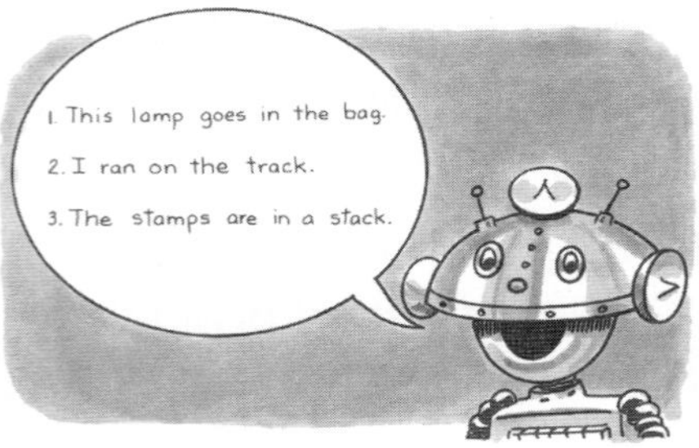

1. Find part C in your workbook. ✔
   These sentences have words that Bleep cannot say. You're going to fix up the sentences to show how Bleep would say them.
2. Sentence 1. He's supposed to say "This lamp goes in the bag." Two words have sounds that Bleep cannot say. Cross out the letters he cannot say. Write the letters he says above them. Then read the sentence to yourself and figure out what Bleep says instead of "This lamp goes in the bag." Raise your hand when you've fixed up sentence 1.
   (Observe students and give feedback.)
3. Sentence 2. Here's what Bleep is trying to say, "I ran on the track." Two words have sounds that Bleep cannot say. Cross out the letters he cannot say. Write the letters he says above them. Then read the sentence to yourself and figure out what Bleep says instead of "I ran on the track." Raise your hand when you're finished.
   (Observe students and give feedback.)
4. Sentence 3. Here's what Bleep is trying to say, "The stamps are in a stack." Fix up the sentence. Raise your hand when you're finished.
   (Observe students and give feedback.)
5. Let's see some of the funny things Bleep says.
   - Sentence 1. He's trying to say "This lamp goes in the bag." What does he say instead of that? (Signal.) *This lump goes in the bug.*
   - Sentence 2. Bleep is trying to say "I ran on the track." What does he say instead of that? (Signal.) *I run on the truck.*
   - Sentence 3. Bleep is trying to say "The stamps are in a stack." What does he say instead of that? (Signal.) *The stumps are in a stuck.*
6. Remember, next time you're going to make up an ending to this story. So think of some other silly things that Bleep might say because you'll use them in your ending.
7. Later you can color Bleep.

EXERCISE 6 Mystery Arrow

Generating Clues

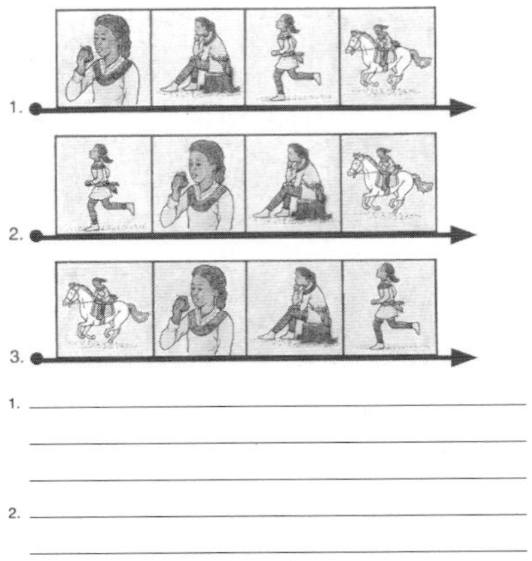

> ***Note:*** Form three teams of students—A, B and C. Team members sit together, apart from the other teams. All members of a team will write the same set of clues.

1. Find part D. ✔
   You're going to work in teams to figure out the mystery arrow. Each team will have a different mystery arrow. The members of each team are going to write two clues that tell about their mystery arrow. Then they'll give clues to everybody else. We'll see if we can find their arrow.
2. (Secretly circle the arrow number to show each team which arrow they are to write about.)
   Key for Team A: Arrow 1.
   Key for Team B: Arrow 2.
   Key for Team C: Arrow 3.
   - (Whisper to each group:) Remember, that's **your** mystery arrow.
   - (Write on the board:)

Zelda
went jogging
ate an apple
rode a horse
sat on a stump

- Here are words that you'll use to write your two clues.
- Listen: Both your clues have to tell about two pictures that are together on your arrow. The first clue must tell about the first two pictures that are not together on **all** the arrows. So you start at the beginning of your arrow and look at the first two pictures. If they are together on all the arrows, you go to the next two pictures. If they are not together on all the arrows, circle them. That's your first clue.
- Find the first two pictures on **your arrow** that are together and are not on all three arrows. You can whisper to your teammates, but do not talk so other teams can hear you. When you find the first two pictures on your arrow that are not together on all three arrows, circle the pictures. Raise your hand when you've circled the pictures for your first clue.
  (Observe students and give feedback.)
3. (For acceptable clues, direct all members of the team to write clue 1:) The clue tells about the circled pictures. It tells what Zelda did after she did something else.
   Key A: Zelda went jogging after she sat on a stump. (Arrow 1.)
   Key B: Zelda ate an apple after she went jogging. (Arrow 2.)
   Key C: Zelda ate an apple after she rode a horse. (Arrow 3.)
4. Now figure out your clue 2. Find the next two pictures on your arrow that are not shown together on all three arrows. Remember, you can talk to your teammates, but not too loudly. Raise your hand when everybody in your team has circled the picture for clue 2.
   (Observe students and give feedback.)
5. (For acceptable clues, direct all members of the team to write clue 2:) The clue tells about the circled pictures. It tells what Zelda did after she did something else.
   Key A: Zelda rode a horse after she went jogging.
   Key B: Zelda rode a horse after she sat on a stump.
   Key C: Zelda went jogging after she sat on a stump.

6. Everybody, read both clues to yourself and make sure your clues tell about your arrow and no other arrow.
   (Observe students and give feedback.)
7. Now we'll have somebody from each team tell the clues for their mystery arrow. The other teams will see if they can find the right arrow.
   - (Call on a member from team A:) Tell your first clue. *Zelda went jogging after she sat on a stump.*
   - Tell your second clue. (Signal.) *Zelda rode a horse after she went jogging.*
   - Everybody on the other teams, which arrow is the mystery arrow for that team? (Signal.) *Arrow 1.*
8. (Call on a member from team B:) Tell your first clue. *Zelda ate an apple after she went jogging.*
   - Tell your second clue. (Signal.) *Zelda rode a horse after she sat on a stump.*
   - Everybody in the other teams, which arrow is the mystery arrow for that team? (Signal.) *Arrow 2.*
9. (Call on a member from team C:) Tell your first clue. *Zelda ate an apple after she rode a horse.*
   - Tell your next clue. (Signal.) *Zelda went jogging after she sat on a stump.*
   - Everybody in the other teams, which arrow is the mystery arrow for that team? (Signal.) *Arrow 3.*
10. You're getting good at giving clues.

Materials: Each student will need a piece of lined paper.

Objectives

- Write sentences that report on what pictures show. (Exercise 1)
- Cooperatively compose an episode (ending) involving familiar story grammar. (Exercises 2 and 3)

Note: This lesson may take more than the allotted time. Permit students to complete the discussions and planning called for in exercise 3 before presenting lesson 59. For exercise 3, students will work in 3 groups.

WORKBOOK • LINED PAPER

EXERCISE 1 **Sentence Writing**

Reporting—Main Idea

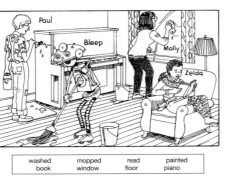

| washed | mopped | read | painted |
| book | window | floor | piano |

1. Open your workbook to lesson 58 and find part A. ✔
   (Pass out lined paper.)
- You're going to write sentences that report on the main thing that each character did in this picture. Each sentence you'll write will name the character and then tell what the character did.
2. Touch Bleep. ✔
- Raise your hand when you know the main thing Bleep did.
- Everybody, what did Bleep do? (Signal.) *Mopped the floor.*
- Here's the whole sentence for Bleep: Bleep mopped the floor. Everybody, say that sentence. (Signal.) *Bleep mopped the floor.*
3. Touch Molly. ✔
- Raise your hand when you can say the whole sentence that tells what Molly did. Remember, start with Molly and tell what she **did.**

- (Call on a student.) Say the sentence for Molly. (Idea: *Molly washed the window.*)
- Here's the sentence for Molly: Molly washed the window. Everybody, say that sentence. (Signal.) *Molly washed the window.*
4. Touch Paul. ✔
- Raise your hand when you can say the whole sentence that tells what Paul did.
- (Call on a student.) Say the sentence for Paul. (Idea: *Paul painted a piano.*)
- Here's the sentence for Paul: Paul painted a piano. Everybody, say that sentence. (Signal.) *Paul painted a piano.*
5. Touch Zelda. ✔
- Raise your hand when you can say the whole sentence that tells what Zelda did.
- (Call on a student.) Say the sentence for Zelda. (Idea: *Zelda read a book.*)
- I wonder if she's reading Mrs. Hudson's book.
- Here's the sentence for Zelda: Zelda read a book. Everybody, say that sentence. (Signal.) *Zelda read a book.*
6. Touch the vocabulary box.
   That's the box with the words in it. These are words that you will use when you write your sentences. I'll read the words: **washed . . . mopped . . . read (red) . . . painted . . . book . . . window . . . floor . . . piano.**
7. Your turn: Write your sentence for Bleep. Start your sentence with Bleep. Tell what he did. Remember to spell the words correctly and end your sentence with a period. Raise your hand when you're finished.
   (Observe students and give feedback.)

- (Write on the board:)

  Bleep mopped the floor.

- Here's what you should have for your sentence that reports on Bleep.
8. Your next sentence will report on the main thing Molly did. Remember, start with Molly. Tell the main thing she did. Raise your hand when you're finished.
   (Observe students and give feedback.)
- (Write on the board:)

  Molly washed the window.

- Here's what you should have for Molly.
9. Your next sentence will report on the main thing Paul did. Start with Paul and tell the main thing he did. Raise your hand when you're finished.
   (Observe students and give feedback.)
- (Write on the board:)

  Paul painted a piano.

- Here's what you should have for Paul.
10. Your next sentence will report on the main thing Zelda did. Start with Zelda and tell the main thing she did. Raise your hand when you're finished.
    (Observe students and give feedback.)
- (Write on the board:)

  Zelda read a book.

- Here's what you should have for Zelda.
11. Raise your hand if you got all the sentences right. Good for you.
- Later you can color the picture. I wonder what color Paul painted the piano.

EXERCISE 2 More Silly Bleep-Talk

Storytelling

> *Note:* Form three groups of students.

1. We're going to work in groups to figure out a good ending to the story about Bleep. I'll read the first part again. Then we'll go over some of the questions you should answer when your group makes up the ending to the story.
- Here's the Bleep story again.

After Molly fixed up Bleep, she told him, "Don't ever take the top of your head off again and mess around with those screws."

And Bleep was good—for a while. But then one day he bonked his head while cleaning up the basement. It happened when he was piling some boxes. One box was under the stairs. He bent over and went under the stairs, but then he didn't stay bent over. He stood up. Bonk. He hit his head on the stairs.

Bleep went over to a mirror and looked at himself. He had a dent right on the top of his head.

"That doesn't look good," he said to himself. So he took off the top of his head, took a hammer and pounded out the dent.

He was ready to put the top of his head on when he looked in the mirror again and said to himself, "I wonder what all those screws do."

In the back of his mind, he could hear Molly saying, "Don't ever mess around with those screws." But those screws looked very interesting—all those different colors. So, before he really knew what he was doing, he touched the yellow screw, then the black screw, then the pink screw. And, before he knew what he was doing, he turned the pink screw— not very much, but just enough to change the way he said the sound the letter **a** makes in words like **as** or **hat** or **sand**.

He could say all the other sounds. He could say the sound the letter **a** makes in words like **take** and **ate** and **cake**. But he couldn't say that other sound. Instead of saying **"at,"** he would say "ut." Instead of saying **"Sam,"** he would say "Sum." Instead of saying **"ran,"** he would say "run."

Well, Bleep put the top of his head back on and finished piling the boxes.

Just as he was piling the last box, Molly came downstairs.

"Hi, Bleep," she said.

"Hi, Molly," Bleep said.

"You're really working hard, aren't you?"

- And that's where the story stops, right in the middle.

EXERCISE 3 Team Story Construction

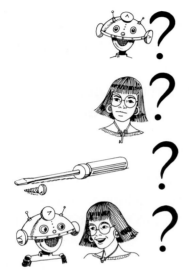

1. Find part B. ✔
   These pictures and question marks show the things you'll have to tell about when you make up your ending to the story.
2. The first picture shows Bleep talking. The question mark shows that you'll have to tell some of the things that Bleep said. That's where Bleep could say some funny things.
3. The question mark by Molly shows that you'll have to tell some of the things she said.
- I wonder what Molly said when she found out that Bleep had messed with some screws. I'll bet she asked why Bleep did it.
4. Touch the screwdriver and the screw. The question mark shows that you'll tell what Molly did.
- Did she fix Bleep up?
- Did she know which screw to turn?

5. The last picture shows Bleep and Molly looking very happy. But there's a question mark. Did Molly fix Bleep up? Were they really happy at the end of the story? Or was Molly mad at Bleep for messing with the screws?
6. Get together with your group. Discuss each question and how your story ending is going to answer the question.
- Start with the question about what Bleep says. Remember, he's got to say some things that let Molly know there's a problem. Figure out what you want Bleep to say. Maybe you'll want to write down some of the things Bleep will say so that you'll remember them. You can write them on this page. Raise your hand when your group has figured out how you're going to answer the first question.
   (Observe groups. When groups raise their hands, direct them to whisper some of the things they plan to have Bleep say. Praise good sentences.)
7. Now figure out the answer to the next question. That's the question about what Molly said when she found out that Bleep had troubles. She'll probably ask Bleep a lot of questions about how he could have done such a silly thing. You can also figure out how Bleep will answer these questions. Raise your hand when your group has figured out what Molly is going to say to Bleep.
   (Observe groups. When groups raise their hands, direct them to whisper to you some of the things they plan to have Molly say. Praise good sentences.)
8. Figure out answers to the rest of the questions. Figure out what Molly did with that screwdriver. You can color the screw the right color for your answer. Then tell how your story will end. Raise your hand when you've got your whole story worked out.
   (Observe groups.)
9. Next time, you'll figure out how your group will tell the ending to the story. Maybe your group will decide to act out the ending.
10. Later you can color the pictures.

Materials: Each student will need a piece of lined paper.

Objectives

- Write sentences that report on what pictures show. (Exercise 1)
- Present a cooperatively developed episode based on familiar story grammar. (Exercise 2)
- Make a picture consistent with details of a story by writing sentences that show dialect. (Exercise 3)

WORKBOOK • LINED PAPER

EXERCISE 1 Sentence Writing

Reporting—Main Idea

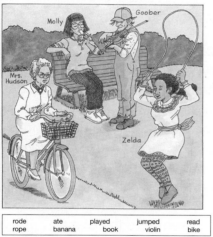

rode	ate	played	jumped	read
rope	banana	book	violin	bike

1. Open your workbook to lesson 59 and find part A. ✔
(Pass out lined paper to students.)
You're going to write sentences that report on the main thing that characters did in this picture. Each sentence you'll write will name the character and then tell what the character did.
2. Touch Mrs. Hudson. ✔
- Raise your hand when you know the main thing Mrs. Hudson did.
- Everybody, what did Mrs. Hudson do? (Signal.) *Rode a bike.*
- Here's the whole sentence for Mrs. Hudson: Mrs. Hudson rode a bike. Everybody, say that sentence. (Signal.) *Mrs. Hudson rode a bike.*
3. Touch Zelda. ✔
- Raise your hand when you can say the whole sentence that tells what Zelda did.

Remember, start with Zelda and tell what she **did.**
- (Call on a student.) Say the sentence for Zelda.
(Idea: *Zelda jumped rope.*)
- Here's the sentence for Zelda: Zelda jumped rope. Everybody, say that sentence. (Signal.) *Zelda jumped rope.*
4. Touch Molly. ✔
- Raise your hand when you can say the sentence that tells what Molly did.
- (Call on a student.) Say the sentence for Molly.
(Idea: *Molly ate a banana.*)
- Here's the sentence for Molly: Molly ate a banana. Everybody, say that sentence. (Signal.) *Molly ate a banana.*
5. Touch Goober. ✔
- Raise your hand when you can say the sentence that tells what Goober did.
- (Call on a student.) Say the sentence for Goober.
(Idea: *Goober played the violin.*)
- Here's the sentence for Goober: Goober played the violin. Everybody, say that sentence. (Signal.) *Goober played the violin.*
6. Touch the vocabulary box.
That's the box with the words in it.
These are the words that you will use when you write your sentences. I'll read the words:
rode . . . ate . . . played . . . jumped . . . read (red) . . . rope . . . banana . . . book . . . violin . . . bike.

7. Your turn: Write your sentence for Mrs. Hudson. Start your sentence with **Mrs. Hudson.** Tell what she did. Remember to spell the words correctly and end your sentence with a period. Raise your hand when you're finished.
(Observe students and give feedback.)

• (Write on the board:)

> **Mrs. Hudson rode a bike.**

• Here's what you should have for your sentence that reports on Mrs. Hudson.

8. Your next sentence will report on the main thing Zelda did. Remember, start with **Zelda.** Tell the main thing she did. Raise your hand when you're finished.
(Observe students and give feedback.)

• (Write on the board:)

> **Zelda jumped rope.**

• Here's what you should have for Zelda.

9. Your next sentence will report on the main thing Molly did. Start with **Molly** and tell the main thing she did. Raise your hand when you're finished.
(Observe students and give feedback.)

• (Write on the board:)

> **Molly ate a banana.**

• Here's what you should have for Molly.

10. Your next sentence will report on the main thing Goober did. Start with Goober and tell the main thing he did. Raise your hand when you're finished.
(Observe students and give feedback.)

• (Write on the board:)

> **Goober played the violin.**

• Here's what you should have for Goober.

11. Raise your hand if you got all the sentences right.
Good for you.

EXERCISE 2 Story Construction
More Silly Bleep-Talk—Group Read

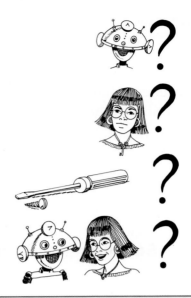

> **Note:** Divide the class into its three story-construction groups.

1. Everybody, turn to part B in lesson 58. ✔ Remember, these pictures ask questions about important parts of your story.

• Today, we're going to hear stories about Bleep and Molly from the different groups. Before we do that, the groups have to figure out how they'll tell their story.

2. Practice your story in your group before you present it to the class.

• If individual students are telling different parts, they should each practice telling their part. The other members of the group should listen carefully and make sure that each storyteller is telling it the right way.

• You may want to put on a play that shows your ending. If you do that, make sure that your play answers all the questions.

• Talk quietly so that the other groups can't hear your story. Raise your hand when your group is ready.
(Observe groups and give feedback. Praise groups who practice and comment on the storyteller's rendition.)

• I'll read the first part of the story; then we'll have the groups tell their endings or put on a play to show their ending.

• Here's the Bleep story again.

After Molly fixed up Bleep, she told him, "Don't ever take the top of your head off again and mess around with those screws."

And Bleep was good—for a while. But then one day he bonked his head while cleaning up the basement. It happened when he was piling some boxes. One box was under the stairs. He bent over and went under the stairs, but then he didn't stay bent over. He stood up. Bonk. He hit his head on the stairs.

Bleep went over to a mirror and looked at himself. He had a dent right on the top of his head.

"That doesn't look good," he said to himself. So he took off the top of his head, took a hammer and pounded out the dent.

He was ready to put the top of his head on when he looked in the mirror again and said to himself, "I wonder what all those screws do."

In the back of his mind, he could hear Molly saying, "Don't ever mess around with those screws." But those screws looked very interesting—all those different colors. So, before he really knew what he was doing, he touched the yellow screw, then the black screw, then the pink screw. And, before he knew what he was doing, he turned the pink screw—not very much, but just enough to change the way he said the sound the letter **a** makes in words like **as** or **hat** or **sand.**

He could say all the other sounds. He could say the sound the letter **a** makes in words like **take** and **ate** and **cake.** But he couldn't say that other sound. Instead of saying **"at,"** he would say "ut." Instead of saying **"Sam,"** he would say "Sum." Instead of saying **"ran,"** he would say "run."

Well, Bleep put the top of his head back on and finished piling the boxes.

Just as he was piling the last box, Molly came downstairs.

"Hi, Bleep," she said.

"Hi, Molly," Bleep said.

"You're really working hard, aren't you?"

- And that's where the story stops, right in the middle.
3. (Call on a group. Say:) Group ___, is your ending a story or a play?
- Everybody, listen to the ending from group ___.

    (Praise stories or plays that tell about all details suggested by the pictures.)
    (Repeat step 3 with each group.)

> **Note:** If not all the groups are able to present, tell the class that the storytelling will be continued to the next lesson.

EXERCISE 3   Writing Bleep-Talk

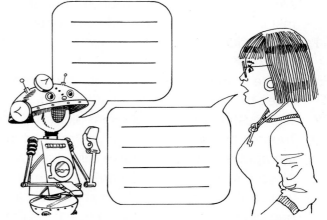

1. Everybody, turn to lesson 59, part B. ✔ This picture shows part of your story about Bleep. Bleep is saying something that really shocks Molly. Then Molly is saying something back to Bleep.
- I'll bet Bleep is saying some of those silly words that let Molly know there's a problem.
2. Write the best thing you can think of for Bleep to say, and write what Molly is saying back. Later you can color the picture, and we'll put up some of the better pictures.

LESSON **60**—Test **6**

Materials: Each student will need a piece of lined paper.

Objectives

- Perform on mastery test of skills presented in lessons 51–59. (Exercise 1)
- Present a cooperatively developed episode based on familiar story grammar. (Exercise 2)
  Exercises 3–5 provide instructions for marking the test and giving the students feedback.

WORKBOOK • LINED PAPER

EXERCISE 1 Test—Writing Sentences

Generating Clues

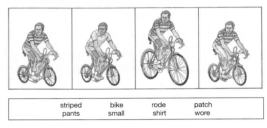

striped pants	bike small	rode shirt	patch wore

- This lesson is a test to see how smart you are. You can't talk to anybody during the test or look at what anybody else does.
1. Open your workbook to lesson 60 and find part A. ✔
   You're going to use lined paper and write clues that tell about the mystery man.
2. The mystery man is in the first picture.
- Touch that man. Make sure you're touching the right man or you'll make silly clues.
- All your clues should tell something that you can't say about all the men. Here's a bad clue: The man rode a bike. Why is that a bad clue? (Call on a student. Idea: *All the men rode a bike.*)
- Here's a good clue: The man had a patch on his pants. Why is that a good clue? (Call on a student. Idea: *Not all the men had a patch on their pants.*)
- Who can say another good clue? (Call on a student. Accept clues such as: *The man rode a small bike; The man wore a striped shirt.*)

3. (Write on the board:)

   The man _____.

- You're going to write three clues. Somebody who reads all three clues would know exactly which man was the mystery man.
- Each clue will start with the words **the man.** Each clue will tell what the man wore or did.
- Touch the vocabulary box below the picture. I'll read the words: **striped . . . bike . . . rode . . . patch . . . pants . . . small . . . shirt . . . wore.**
- If you use any of those words, spell them correctly. Write your three clues. Remember the capital at the beginning and the period at the end of each sentence. Raise your hand when you're finished. (Observe students and give feedback.)
4. (Call on several students to read their set of clues. For each student, say:)
- Read your first clue. (Student reads.)
- Read your next clue. (Student reads.)
- Read your last clue. (Student reads.)
- (For each student, ask:)
  Everybody, do those three clues let you know which man is the mystery man? (Students respond.)
- (Praise good sets of clues.)
  Key: Good sets contain these 3 ideas in any order.
  The man rode a small bike.
  The man wore a striped shirt.
  The man had a patch on his pants.

Writing Bleep-Talk

can	cake	corn	rat	tack	bend

1. Everybody, find part B. ✔
   These are words. Bleep could not say some of them after he adjusted the pink screw.
   - Touch the words as I read them: **can . . . cake . . . corn . . . rat . . . tack . . . bend.**
2. Fix up the words Bleep could not say. Cross out the letter he couldn't say. Write the letter for the sound he did say. Raise your hand when you're finished.
   (Observe students but do not give feedback.)

Reporting

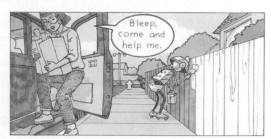

1. Bleep was holding a can of paint.	reports	does not report
2. Only part of the fence was painted.	reports	does not report
3. Bleep did not hear Molly.	reports	does not report
4. Molly is getting irritated with Bleep.	reports	does not report
5. Molly's car door was open.	reports	does not report
6. Molly called for Bleep's help.	reports	does not report

1. Find part C. ✔
   You're going to circle the words **report** or **does not report** for each item.
   - Look at the picture. You can see that Bleep was painting the fence. Molly was getting out of her car, carrying groceries. She was calling to Bleep, "Bleep, come and help me."
2. Item 1: Bleep was holding a can of paint. Circle **reports** or **does not report.** ✔
   - Item 2: Only part of the fence was painted. Circle **reports** or **does not report.** ✔
   - Item 3: Bleep did not hear Molly. Circle **reports** or **does not report.** ✔
   - Item 4: Molly was getting irritated with Bleep. Circle **reports** or **does not report.** ✔
   - Item 5: Molly's car door was open. Circle **reports** or **does not report.** ✔
   - Item 6: Molly called for Bleep's help. Circle **reports** or **does not report.** ✔

EXERCISE 2   Story Construction

More Silly Bleep-Talk—Group Read

- (If time permits, listen to plays or stories involving Bleep-talk.)

EXERCISE 3   Marking The Test

1. (Mark the test before the next scheduled language lesson. Use the *Language Arts Answer Key* to check the test.)
2. (Write the number of errors each student made in the test scorebox at the beginning of the test.)
3. (Enter the number of errors each student made on the Summary for Test 6. A Reproducible Summary Sheet is at the back of the *Language Arts Teacher's Guide.*)

EXERCISE 4   Feedback On Test 6

1. (Return the students' workbooks after they are marked.)
   - Everybody, open your workbook to lesson 60. Look at how I marked your test page.
2. I wrote a number at the top of your test. That number tells how many items you got wrong on the whole test.
   - Raise your hand if I wrote **0** or **1** at the top of your test.
     Those are super stars.
   - Raise your hand if I wrote **2** or **3.** Those are pretty good workers.
   - If I wrote a number that's more than 3, you're going to have to work harder.

EXERCISE 5   Test Remedies

- (See the *Language Arts Teacher's Guide* for a general discussion of remedies.)

Materials: Each student will need a piece of lined paper.

Objectives

- Complete statements of relative direction based on a map. (Exercise 1)
- Write 3 sentences to identify the mystery character. (Exercise 2)
- Listen to part 1 of a story and answer comprehension questions. (Exercise 3)
- Rewrite a passage so that it unambiguously reports on what a picture sequence shows. (Exercise 4)

WORKBOOK

EXERCISE 1 Map Directions

Relative Direction

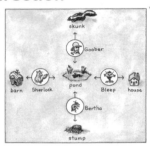

_____ said, "The pond is _____ of me and the
_____ is _____ of me."

_____ said, "The pond is _____ of me and the
_____ is _____ of me."

_____ said, "The pond is _____ of me and the
_____ is _____ of me."

_____ said, "The pond is _____ of me and the
_____ is _____ of me."

1. Open your workbook to lesson 61 and find part A. ✔
   This is a map. Below it are statements that different characters are saying. But the names of the characters are blank. You're going to fill in the blanks.
   - Touch item 1. ✔
     Somebody said, "The pond is blank of me, and the something else is blank of me."
   - Look at item 2.
     It says the same thing: Somebody said, "The pond is blank of me, and the something else is blank of me."
   - And that's what item 3 says, too.
2. Your turn: Pick three of the characters and complete the items. Put in the name of your character at the beginning of the sentence. Remember to start your sentence with a capital. Then fill in the other blanks. Raise your hand when you've written about all three characters. ✔

3. Who wrote an item about Sherlock?
   Everybody who wrote about Sherlock should have this: Sherlock said, "The pond is east of me, and barn is west of me."
   - Who wrote about Goober?
     Everybody who wrote about Goober should have this: Goober said, "The pond is south of me, and the skunk is north of me."
   - Who wrote about Bertha?
     Everybody who wrote about Bertha should have this: Bertha said, "The pond is north of me, and the stump is south of me."
   - Who wrote about Bleep?
     Everybody who wrote about Bleep should have this: Bleep said, "The pond is west of me, and the house is east of me."
4. Raise your hand if you got your three sentences right.

LINED PAPER

EXERCISE 2 Writing Sentences

Generating Clues

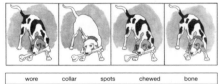

| wore | collar | spots | chewed | bone |

1. Find part B. ✔
   You're going to use lined paper and write clues that tell about the mystery dog. The mystery dog is in the first picture.
   - Touch that dog. ✔
     Each clue should say something you can't say about **all** the dogs.
2. Here's a bad clue: The mystery dog chewed a bone. Why is that a bad clue?
   (Call on a student. Idea: _All the dogs chewed a bone._)

- Here's a good clue: The mystery dog chewed a big bone. That's a good clue because it doesn't tell about **all** the dogs.
3. (Write on the board:)

   The dog

- You're going to write three clues. Somebody who reads all three clues should know exactly which dog is the mystery dog. Each clue will start with the words **the dog.**
- Touch the vocabulary box below the picture. I'll read the words: **wore . . . collar . . . spots . . . chewed . . . bone.**
- If you use any of those words, make sure you spell them correctly.
4. Write your three clues. Remember the capital at the beginning of each sentence and the period at the end. Raise your hand when you're finished.
   (Observe students and give feedback.)
5. (Call on several students to read their clues. For each student say:)
- Read your first clue. (Student reads.)
- Read your next clue. (Student reads.)
- Read your last clue. (Student reads.)
- Those clues should tell about only one dog. Everybody, do those three clues let you know which dog is the mystery dog? (Students respond.)
6. (Praise good sets of clues.)
   Key: Good sets contain these 3 ideas in any order.
   The dog wore a collar.
   The dog had spots.
   The dog chewed a big bone.

EXERCISE 3   Zena and Zola *Part 1*

Storytelling

- I'm going to tell a story about Zena and Zola. Listen:

Zelda the artist had two sisters—Zena and Zola. They didn't draw or paint or make statues. They were reporters. They worked for a newspaper and reported on news stories. And they always worked together. The reason they

worked together was that they had a problem similar to Zelda's problem.

Neither Zena nor Zola could write things clearly. If Zena wrote something by herself, she'd do a good job of telling what somebody or something did, but she'd forget to name the person or thing. She'd write something like this: "He robbed the convenience store on the corner of Elm and Oak Streets." Zena wouldn't tell who did it.

Zola always told who did something, but she wouldn't tell what the person did. She'd write something like this: "A short, masked bandit carrying a large bag did **it**." But she wouldn't tell what that person did.

- Remember, one sister doesn't clearly name the person or thing. Who is that? (Signal.) *Zena.*
- One sister doesn't tell clearly what the person **did.** Which sister is that? (Signal.) *Zola.*

When Zena and Zola worked together, they would write wonderful reports. Zola would tell who was doing the action and Zena would tell what the person did. Here's the kind of sentence they'd write together: "A short, masked bandit carrying a large bag robbed the convenience store on the corner of Elm and Oak Streets."

Things went fine for years. When important news stories would break, the chief at the newspaper would send Zena and Zola out to cover the story. They'd work together and write a very complete report. Everybody was happy.

That is, they were happy until Zena and Zola had a terrible argument and decided that they would not work with each other any more.

Zena said, "I don't need to work with you. I can write great reports without all those needless words you write."

"Oh, yeah," Zola said. "You're the one who writes the words that are not necessary."

So one day, Zena and Zola went to the chief at the newspaper and told him that they didn't want to work on the same reporting assignments any more. Zena said, "Don't send me out to work with her any more."

"That goes double for me," Zola said. "If I work alone, I'll write reports that don't have a lot of unnecessary words."

The chief said, "Two big stories just broke. So I can send Zola to cover one and Zena to cover the other."

And that's just what the chief did. He sent Zola out to write about the Queen of Garbo. She was arriving at the airport, and it was the first time a queen from Garbo had visited North America.

The other story was about an inventor who had just invented a bicycle that folded up to the size of a book. Zena went out to cover that story.

Later that day, both women returned to the newspaper with their reports. The chief started to read Zena's report about the folding bicycle.

The chief read the first part. Here's the title:

"It Folds Up."

Here's the report:

It was regular sized with two full-sized wheels. Then it folded up to the size of a book.

She said, "I got the idea when I talked to him. I decided, if it can get small and get big, why can't **it** get small and get big?"

So she invented a model . . .

The chief shook his head and said, "I don't know what Zena's writing about. She doesn't name what it is or who is talking."

- Listen to Zena's report again. See if you could tell what she's writing about.

It Folds Up

It was regular sized with two full-sized wheels. Then it folded up to the size of a book.

She said, "I got the idea when I talked to him. I decided, if it can get small and get big, why can't **it** get small and get big?"

So she invented a model . . .

- Would you know what that report is telling about? (Signal.) *No.*

Next the chief read the report that Zola wrote about the Queen of Garbo.

Here's the title:

"The Stylish Queen of Garbo Visits It."

Here's the report:

A delightful queen, who had refreshing new ideas on many topics, arrived at it. The queen, who is officially named Dessera the Fourth, stepped off it and talked to them. Her four greyhounds, each wearing a diamond collar, were also . . .

The chief scratched his head. "I don't understand this at all," he said. "Zola's sentences start out very good. They really name the person or thing. But the rest of her sentences are bad. They don't clearly tell what each person or thing did."

The chief called Zola and Zena in. Then he said, "Listen. These are the two worst reports I've ever read in my whole life." Then he said, "If you want to continue to work for this newspaper, you'll have to work together. If you can't do that, you're both **fired.**"

Zena looked at Zola, and Zola looked at Zena. "Fired?" they both said.

Then Zena said, "Well, actually, working with Zola is not all that bad. She puts in a lot of words, but maybe some of them help make the report better."

Zola said, "I agree with Zena. Some of the words she puts in the report may make the story easier to understand."

The sisters gave each other a little smile. They knew that their reports were not very good.

The chief said, "Well, you'd better get moving if you expect to write stories about the Queen of Garbo and about that new folding bicycle."

The sisters dashed out of the chief's office, wrote their reports and had them on the chief's desk two hours later.

The chief read them and said, "Now that's what I call a couple of very good reports."

Everybody was happy again.

EXERCISE 4 Rewriting Ambiguous Passage

It Folds Up

It was regular-sized with two full-sized wheels.

Then it folded up to the size of a book.

She said "I got the idea when I talked to him."

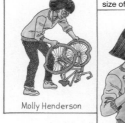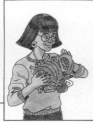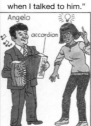

1. Find part C. ✔
   The pictures show some of the things that Zena reported on.
   - Who is in the first picture? (Signal.) *Molly.*
   - She's the person who invented that folding bike. In the first picture, she's folding it up.
   - Look at the next picture. You can see the bike is now the size of a book.
   - Touch the last picture. ✔
   The person in that picture is Angelo, the accordion player. He's playing away, and Molly is getting an idea. That lightbulb over her head shows her idea.

2. Above the pictures is the first part of the report Zena wrote. It tells what happened, but it doesn't do a good job of naming anybody or anything.
   - You're going to fix up the report so it names the right people or things.
   - The title says: It Folds Up. You have to tell what **it** is. What folds up? (Signal.) *A bike.*
   - So a good title would be: **A Bike** Folds Up.

3. The first-sentence of the story says: It was regular-sized with two full-sized wheels. What was regular-sized with two full-sized wheels? (Signal.) *The bike.*
   - Yes, the bike. That sentence should say: **The bike** was regular-sized with two full-sized wheels.

4. Next sentence: Then it folded up to the size of a book. What folded up to the size of a book? (Signal.) *The bike.*
   - So that sentence should say: Then **the bike** folded up to the size of a book.

5. Listen to the next sentence: She said, "I got the idea when I talked to him."
   - Who is she? (Signal.) *Molly Henderson.*
   - Molly Henderson is the inventor of this bike. The sentence should begin: **Molly Henderson** said.
   - She got the idea for the folding bike by talking to the person in the picture. Who is that person? (Signal.) *Angelo.*
   - What is that thing he's playing? (Signal.) *An accordion.*
   - So the whole sentence should say this: Molly Henderson said, "I got the idea when I talked to Angelo, the accordion player."

6. Your turn: Use lined paper. Write the first part of the report the way it would be written after both Zena and Zola worked on it.

Materials: Each student will need a piece of lined paper.

Objectives

- Write 3 sentences to identify the mystery character. (Exercise 1)
- Complete statements of relative direction based on a map. (Exercise 2)
- **Apply a rule about moving south and north to a map of North America.** (Exercise 3)
- Listen to the conclusion of a 2-part story. (Exercise 4)
- **Edit ambiguous sentences in a passage.** (Exercise 5)

WORKBOOK • LINED PAPER

EXERCISE 1　Sentences

Generating Clues

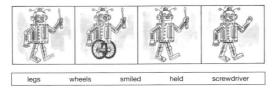

| legs | wheels | smiled | held | screwdriver |

1. Everybody, open your workbook to lesson 62 and find part A. ✔
   You're going to use lined paper and write clues that tell about the mystery robot. The mystery robot is in the first picture.
   - Touch that robot. ✔
     Each clue should say something that you can't say about **all** the robots.
2. (Write on the board:)

   > **The robot**

   - You're going to write three clues. Somebody who reads all three clues should know exactly which robot is the mystery robot.
   - Each clue will start with the words, **The robot.**
3. Touch the vocabulary box below the picture. I'll read the words: **legs . . . wheels . . . smiled . . . held . . . screwdriver.**
   - If you use any of those words, make sure you spell them correctly.
4. Write your three clues. Remember the capital at the beginning of each sentence and the period at the end. Raise your hand when you're finished.
   (Observe students and give feedback.)

5. (Call on several students to read their set of clues. For each student, say:)
   - Read your first clue. (Student reads.)
     Read your next clue. (Student reads.)
     Read your last clue. (Student reads.)
   - Those clues should tell about only one robot. Everybody, do those clues tell about more than one robot or only one robot? (Students respond.)
   - (Praise good sets of clues.)
     Key: Good sets contain these 3 ideas in any order.
     The robot smiled.
     The robot held a screwdriver.
     The robot had legs.

EXERCISE 2　Map Directions

Relative Direction

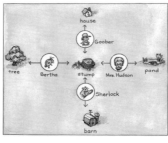

_____ said, "The stump is _____ of me and the
_____ is _____ of me."

_____ said, "The stump is _____ of me and the
_____ is _____ of me."

_____ said, "The stump is _____ of me and the
_____ is _____ of me."

_____ said, "The stump is _____ of me and the
_____ is _____ of me."

1. Everybody, find part B. ✔
   The names of the characters are missing in the items. You're going to write what three of the characters on the map said.
   - Touch item 1. ✔
     Somebody said, "The stump is blank of me, and the something else is blank of me."

- Look at item 2.
  It says the same thing: Somebody said, "The stump is blank of me, and the something else is blank of me."
- And that's what item 3 says, too.

2. Your turn: Pick three of the characters and complete the items. Remember, put in the name of your character at the beginning of the sentence. Then fill in the other blanks. Raise your hand when you've finished all three sentences.
   (Observe students and give feedback.)

3. Who wrote an item about Sherlock? Everybody who wrote about Sherlock should have this: Sherlock said, "The stump is north of me, and the barn is south of me."

- Who wrote about Goober?
  Everybody who wrote about Goober should have this: Goober said, "The stump is south of me, and the house is north of me."
- Who wrote about Bertha?
  Everybody who wrote about Bertha should have this: Bertha said, "The stump is east of me, and the tree is west of me."
- Who wrote about Mrs. Hudson?
  Everybody who wrote about Mrs. Hudson should have this: Mrs. Hudson said, "The stump is west of me, and the pond is east of me."

4. Raise your hand if you got your three sentences right.

EXERCISE 3   Map

North America

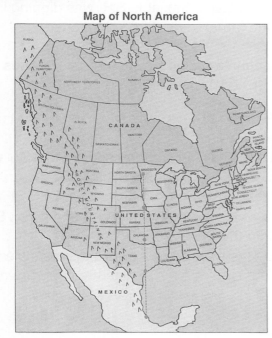

Map of North America

1. Find part C. ✔
   That's a map of North America.
2. (Write the name of your state or province on the board.)
- This is the name of our state (province).
- (Hold up a workbook and show the students where your state or province is on the map.)
- Here's ___ on the map.
3. In the next lesson, you're going to learn about the migration of ducks.
- (Write on the board:)

Minnesota

- This says Minnesota. It's a state at the north part of the United States.
- (Hold up a workbook and show the students where Minnesota is.)
- Everybody, touch Minnesota. ✔
  That's where some ducks go for the summer. Other ducks spend the summer farther north in Canada.
4. Remember, in the summer, the ducks are in the north. The ducks go south for the winter.
- (Hold up a workbook and trace the route shown on the map.)
- Some ducks go down into Mexico.
- Your turn: Touch where the ducks go for the winter. ✔
5. I'll name a season. You touch where the ducks would be.
- Listen: Summer. Touch where the ducks would be. ✔
  You should be touching Minnesota or Canada.
- Winter. Touch where the ducks would be. ✔
  You should be touching Mexico.
6. Listen: When the spring comes and the ducks are in Mexico, which direction do they fly for the summer? (Signal.) *North.*
- When the ducks are in Minnesota and the winter comes, which direction do they fly for the winter? (Signal.) *South.*
- (Repeat step 6 until firm.)
7. Remember those facts.

EXERCISE 4   Zena and Zola Part 2

Storytelling

- Last time, you listened to a story about Zelda's sisters. One of them did a good job of naming. The other sister did a good job of telling what somebody did.
- Listen: Who did the good job of naming? (Signal.) *Zola.*
- Who did the good job of telling what somebody did? (Signal.) *Zena.*
- Last time, the sisters went out and fixed up their report about **It Folds Up.** You worked with that report last time. The sisters also rewrote their report about **The Queen of Garbo.**
  Here's what happened:

Zena could not understand Zola's report about the Queen of Garbo. So the sisters decided that both of them should talk to the queen. The queen had left the airport and was at her hotel with her four greyhounds.

Zena and Zola had to argue with guards and police officers before they would allow the sisters to visit with the queen. Finally, the guards took the sisters into the queen's room. The sisters asked the queen questions and wrote down the answers. Then they compiled the report.

Zola's first report had the title: "The Stylish Queen of Garbo Visits It." The new title said: "The Stylish Queen of Garbo Visits North America."

Zola's first report said this: "A delightful queen, who had refreshing new ideas on many topics, arrived at it." The new sentence said: "A delightful queen, who had many refreshing new ideas on many topics, arrived at National Airport."

The first report said: "The queen, who is officially named Dessera the Fourth, stepped off it and talked to them." The new report said: "The queen, who is officially named Dessera the Fourth, stepped off the plane and talked to a large crowd of people."

Then the new report told about the queen's plans. Here's what the report said:

Four greyhounds, each wearing a diamond collar, were also with the queen. According to the queen, they are the fastest and most talented dogs in the world.

The queen planned to visit different parts of the United States and Canada. She planned to take her four greyhounds with her. The queen was particularly interested in visiting the Rocky Mountains. She said, "In our country, we have no snow and no large mountains. I'm looking forward to skiing and mountain climbing in the Rockies."

When the chief read the report, he was very pleased. He told the sisters, "We'll have to do another story on that Queen of Garbo. A lot of people are interested in her."

- That's the end of the story, but we may be hearing some more about the Queen of Garbo.

EXERCISE 5   Editing Ambiguous Passage

Linda Carry was at it. She was digging in it. She found them. She sold them.

**beach   rooster   gold   coins   bushes
trees   ten   sand   turkeys   money**

1. Everybody, turn back to lesson 62 and find part C. ✔
   This is part of a different report that Zola did all by herself.
- I'll read the report: "Linda Carry was at it. She was digging in it. She found them. She sold them."
- Each sentence has a word that is unclear. You're going to underline the unclear words.

2. First sentence: Linda Carry was at it. Underline the unclear word. Raise your hand when you're finished. ✔
- Everybody, Linda Carry was at it. Which word is unclear? (Signal.) *It.*
- Yes, we don't know where Linda was.
- Next sentence: She was digging in it.
- Listen again: She was digging in it.
- The word **she** is not unclear because we know she is Linda. But there is an unclear word in that sentence. Underline the unclear word. Raise your hand when you're finished. ✔
- Everybody, which word is unclear? (Signal.) *It.*
- Next sentence: She found them. Underline the unclear word. Raise your hand when you're finished. ✔
- Everybody, which word is unclear? (Signal.) *Them.*
- **Them** is unclear because we don't know what she found.
- Last sentence: She sold them. Underline the unclear word. Raise your hand when you're finished. ✔
- Everybody, which word is unclear in the last sentence? (Signal.) *Them.*
3. The story doesn't tell what she found or where she was digging when she found them. If the underlined words were clear words, we'd know where she was and what she found.
- What do you think she found when she was digging? (Call on individual students. Accept reasonable ideas.)
4. Everybody, turn to page 195 in your workbook and find the picture for lesson 62.

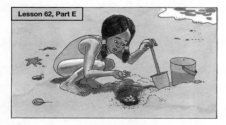

- There's a picture that shows where Linda was digging and what she found. I think those are gold coins. And I count ten of them.
- I'll say the first sentence the way Zola wrote it. Then we'll see who can say a clear sentence.

- First sentence: Linda Carry was at it. Who can say a sentence that's clear? (Call on a student. Idea: *Linda Carry was at the beach.*)
- Next sentence: She was digging in it. Who can say a sentence that's clear? (Call on a student. Idea: *She was digging in the sand.*)
- Next sentence: She found them. Who can say a clear sentence that tells what she found and how many there were? (Call on a student. Idea: *She found ten gold coins.*)
- Last sentence: She sold them. Who can say a sentence that's clear? (Call on a student. Idea: *She sold the coins.*)
5. Everybody, turn back to lesson 62 and find part D.
- I'll read the words in the vocabulary box: **beach . . . rooster . . . gold coins . . . bushes . . . trees . . . ten . . . sand . . . turkeys . . . money.**
- You can use some of those words when you fix up the sentences.
6. Listen: Cross out every underlined word in part C and write any words you need to make the sentences clear. Raise your hand when you're finished. (Observe students and give feedback.)
7. I'll read a very clear report. Follow along: Linda Carry was at the beach. She was digging in the sand. She found ten gold coins. She sold the coins.

Materials: Each student will need a piece of lined paper and a red, a blue and a yellow crayon.

Objectives

- Complete sentences of the form: Blank happened **after** blank. (Exercise 1)
- Write 3 sentences to identify the mystery character. (Exercise 2)
- Listen to part 1 of a story. Relate the details to a map. (Exercise 3)
- **Use rules about relative direction to indicate why specific places on a map are not the correct places.** (Exercise 4)

WORKBOOK

EXERCISE 1   Temporal Sequencing

After

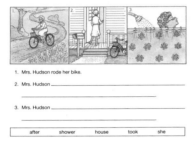

1. Mrs. Hudson rode her bike.

2. Mrs. Hudson _____

3. Mrs. Hudson _____

| after | shower | house | took | she |

1. Open your workbook to lesson 63 and find part A. ✔
    These pictures show three things that Mrs. Hudson did.

- Touch the first picture. ✔
  What did she do first? (Call on a student. Idea: *Rode a bike.*)

- Yes, Mrs. Hudson rode a bike.

- Touch picture 2.
  That picture shows what she did after she rode a bike. What did she do? (Call on a student. Idea: *She went into her house.*)

- Touch picture 3.
  That picture shows what she did after she went into her house. What did she do? (Call on a student. Idea: *Took a shower.*)

2. The sentence for picture 1 is already written. It says: Mrs. Hudson rode her bike.

- The first part of sentence 2 is written. It says: Mrs. Hudson. Finish the sentence so it tells what she did in picture 2 and tells when she did it. She did it after she rode her bike.

- Write sentence 2. Be sure to tell what Mrs. Hudson did and when she did it. You might find some of the words you need in the vocabulary box. Raise your hand when

you've completed the whole sentence for picture 2.
(Observe students and give feedback.)

- Check your sentence for picture 2. You could have written a sentence like this: Mrs. Hudson went into her house after she rode her bike. (Call on several students to read the sentence they wrote. Praise acceptable sentences.)

3. The first part of sentence 3 is written. It says: Mrs. Hudson. Finish the sentence so it tells what she did in picture 3 and tells when she did it. She did it after she went into her house. Raise your hand when you've completed the whole sentence for picture 3.
(Observe students and give feedback.)

- Check your sentence for picture 3. You could have written a sentence like this: Mrs. Hudson took a shower after she went into her house. (Call on several students to read the sentence they wrote. Praise acceptable sentences.)

LINED PAPER

EXERCISE 2   Writing Sentences

Generating Clues

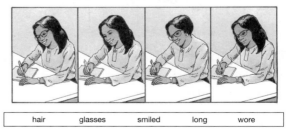

| hair | glasses | smiled | long | wore |

1. Everybody, find part B. ✔
    You're going to use lined paper and write clues that tell about the mystery woman. The mystery woman is in the first picture.

- Touch that woman. ✔
  Each clue should say something that you can't say about **all** the women.
2. (Write on the board:)

> **The woman**

- You're going to write three clues. Somebody who reads all three clues should know exactly which woman is the mystery woman.
- Each clue will start with the words: **The woman.**
3. Touch the vocabulary box below the picture. I'll read the words: **hair . . . glasses . . . smiled . . . long . . . wore.**
- If you use any of those words, make sure you spell them correctly.
4. Write your three clues. Remember the capital at the beginning of each sentence and the period at the end. Raise your hand when you're finished.
  (Observe students and give feedback.)
5. (Call on several students to read their set of clues. For each student say:)
- Read your first clue. (Student reads.)
- Read your next clue. (Student reads.)
- Read your last clue. (Student reads.)
- Those clues should tell about only one woman. Everybody, do those clues tell about more than one woman or only one woman?
  (Students respond.)
- (Praise good sets of clues.)
  Key: Good sets contain these 3 ideas in any order.
  The woman wore glasses.
  The woman had long hair.
  The woman smiled.

EXERCISE 3 Dooly The Duck *Part 1*
Storytelling

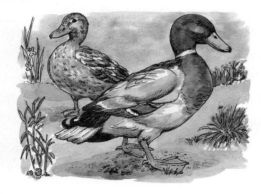

- Everybody, find part C. ✔
  We're going to start a new story today. It's about a mallard duck. The picture shows a male mallard and a female mallard. The male mallard is the one with the green head and the bright colored feathers. As you'll learn from the story, the male mallard duck loses those feathers during the summertime and cannot fly. Losing the feathers is called **molting.**
- Here's the story:

> Dooly was a duck. He wasn't a wood duck or a pintail duck. He wasn't a black duck or a red-headed duck. He was a mallard duck, and like other mallard ducks he went south for the winter and north for the summer. He spent his summers sunning and swimming in some wonderful lakes in Minnesota. Then, when fall approached, he'd fly south with the other ducks, down through the states of Nebraska, Oklahoma and Texas, and down into Mexico, where he'd spend the winter swimming and sunning in some wonderful lakes near the ocean.

- (Write on the board:)

> **Nebraska**
> **Oklahoma**
> **Texas**
> **Mexico**

- These names are: **Nebraska, Oklahoma, Texas and Mexico.** Nebraska, Oklahoma and Texas are states. **Mexico** is a country south of the United States.
- Turn to the map of North America on page 184 of your workbook. ✔
- I'll read that part of the story again. See if you can follow the route south from Minnesota.
- Touch Minnesota. ✔
- Listen:

> When fall approached, Dooly would fly south with the other ducks, down through the states of Nebraska, Oklahoma and Texas, and down into Mexico.

- Follow the flight path from Minnesota to Nebraska. Raise your hand when you've found Nebraska on the flight path.
(Observe students and give feedback.)
- Now go to Oklahoma. Raise your hand when you've found it.
(Observe students and give feedback.)
- Now go to Texas. Raise your hand when you've found it.
(Observe students and give feedback.)
- Now go to the south end of the flight path in Mexico. Raise your hand when you've found it.
(Observe students and give feedback.)
- Listen to that part again. See if you can start with Minnesota and touch the places that are named in the story.

Dooly spent his summers sunning and swimming in some wonderful lakes in Minnesota. Then, when fall approached, he'd fly south with the other ducks, down through the states of **Nebraska, Oklahoma** and **Texas,** and down into **Mexico,** where he'd spend the winter swimming and sunning in some wonderful lakes near the ocean.

This year was different. Dooly had a molting problem. It was very embarrassing. Male mallard ducks molt during the summer. When they molt, they lose a lot of feathers. They not only look kind of silly, they **are** silly because they can't fly. Imagine a duck that can't fly and has to waddle around until his feathers grow in. Usually, the male mallards will have all their lovely new winter feathers in time for their migration to the south. When the weather turns cold and the days start to get short, they will be ready to fly south with the rest of the ducks. That's usually what happens. But sometimes, for some unknown reason, a few male mallards will molt late.

If you're a male mallard and that happened to you, it would be very embarrassing. All the other ducks would look at you. Little ducks would point and ask their mother questions like, "Is that a baby duck, or is he just bald all over?"

"Hush," the mother duck would say. "And don't point."

Sometimes, you'd be waddling around and would meet a duck you hadn't seen for a while, and the duck would walk right past you before recognizing who you were. "Oh, golly," the duck would say. "I didn't even recognize you without your feathers. You're sure molting late this year, aren't you?"

Of course, lots of the ducks, particularly old grandmother ducks, would have ideas about why a duck might be molting late. They would say things like, "I told you not to eat those green berries, but you wouldn't listen. Now you're molting late."

Well, Dooly molted late during his third summer—very late. When the other male ducks lost their feathers, Dooly still had all of his feathers. When the other ducks were growing new feathers, Dooly was just starting to molt. And when the days were growing cold and the ducks were talking about their trip to the south, Dooly was getting concerned because his fall feathers were just starting to grow. When nobody was watching him, he tried to fly, but, no matter how hard he flapped his skinny little wings, with those tiny feathers, he couldn't fly—not even an inch.

The rest of the flock would sometimes discuss their flight plans in front of Dooly. Then they'd remember that he couldn't go with them. "Whoops," they would say, "We forgot that you'll be staying here for a while."

Some of the little ducks would ask their mother, "But Mom, why can't that funny looking bald duck go with us?"

"Hush. That's not a polite question."

The question might not have been polite, but it was one that concerned Dooly. "Yeah," he said to himself. "When am I going to fly south? When am I going to have enough feathers to fly? What did I do to deserve this punishment in the first place? I've always been a pretty good duck. Why do I have to molt late?"

Nobody seemed to know the answer to those questions. But the leader of the flock had a lot to say to Dooly. The leader's name was Horace, and he was a gruff old mallard. On the morning that the rest of the flock was to take off, he took Dooly aside and told him where to land on the way south.

"Listen carefully," he said. "There are some safe landing places along the flyway. There are other places that are not safe. The first safe place is in Nebraska. You fly to the lake that is the shape of a walnut. Just north of that lake is a hill. The safe place is south of the hill and north of the lake. Remember, south of the hill and north of the lake. Will you remember that?"

Dooly said, "Yes, south of the hill and north of the lake."

"Well," Horace said, "when your feathers grow in, take off and keep flying until you get to that place. Then you can land and spend the night there. There will be an old crow around by the name of Caw-Caw. She'll tell you about the next safe place along the flyway. Will you remember all that?"

"Yes," Dooly said. "Walnut-shaped lake. Land just south of the hill and north of the lake. Talk to Caw-Caw about the next safe landing place."

"That's it, then," Horace said. "If your feathers grow out before the great freeze comes and you don't freeze to death, we'll see you down in Mexico."

And with that, Horace waddled away, leaving poor Dooly all alone. A few moments later, the entire flock of ducks took off—young mallards, old ones, males, females, everybody except Dooly. This wasn't just embarrassing. This was getting scary.

For the next two weeks, the mornings got colder and colder. On one morning, the edge of the lake had a paper-thin sheet of ice on it. Brrr.

Every morning when Dooly woke up, he tried out his wings. Flap, flap, flap. But he couldn't take off. He looked at his little feathers and noticed that they were a teeny weeny bit bigger than they were the day before, but still not big enough or strong enough.

And every day, Dooly made sure he remembered the directions Horace had given him about the safe landing place.

- Let's see if you can remember all those details about the safe landing place.
- The safe landing place is in a state. Which state? (Signal.) *Nebraska.*
- The safe landing place is by a lake that is shaped like something else. What's the lake shaped like? (Signal.) *A walnut.*
- There's a hill north of the lake. The safe landing place is which direction from the hill? (Signal.) *South.*
- Which direction from the lake? (Signal.) *North.*
- Yes, south of the hill and north of the lake. (Repeat this series of questions if students have difficulty.)

Then fifteen days after the other ducks had left, Dooly woke up, flapped his wings, and **he took off.** It wasn't a great flight. He had to flap those wings awfully hard to stay up in the air, but he could do it. He practiced all that day. By the end of the day, he could actually fly pretty well. He told himself, "I'll get a good night's sleep tonight, and, in the morning, this duck is on his way to Nebraska and then on to Mexico."

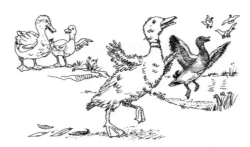

1. Turn to lesson 63 and find part D. ✔
   This picture shows Dooly while he was still molting. You can see him flapping his skinny little wings. In the background, you can see other mallards taking off. I also see a mother mallard and a young mallard. I think that young mallard is pointing at Dooly and asking his mother some questions about Dooly.
2. Later you can color the rest of the picture.

EXERCISE 4   Maps

Relative Direction

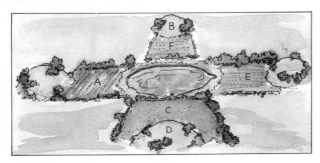

B is not the safe landing place because B is not

_____

C is not the safe landing place because C is not

_____

1. Find part E. ✔
   Here's a map that shows the walnut-shaped lake in Nebraska. There are some hills around the lake. The letters show different landing places. Not all of these places are safe.
   • You're going to circle the letter of the safe landing place. When you circle that letter, you'll show Dooly where to land. If you circle the wrong letter, you'll have him land in a place that is not safe.

2. Find the hill that's north of the lake. The safe landing place is south of that hill and north of the lake.
   • Once more: Find the hill that's north of the lake. The safe landing place is south of that hill and north of the lake. Circle the letter of the safe landing place. Raise your hand when you're finished.
   • Everybody, which letter did you circle? (Signal.) *F.*
   • If you circled any letter but F, you had poor Dooly land in a place that is not safe.
3. You're going to complete the statements below the map.
   • Touch statement 1. ✔
   It says: B is not the safe landing place because B is not blank. Look at B on the map and ask yourself: Is B south of the hill **and** north of the lake? Write which part of the directions is not true for B. Raise your hand when you're finished.
   (Observe students and give feedback.)
   • Everybody, tell me the answer. B is not the safe landing place because B is not . . . (Signal.) *South of the hill.*
4. Touch statement 2. ✔
   It says: C is not the safe landing place because C is not blank. Look at C on the map and ask yourself: Is C south of the hill **and** north of the lake? Write which part of the directions is not true for C. Raise your hand when you're finished.
   (Observe students and give feedback.)
   • Everybody, tell me the answer: C is not the safe landing place because C is not . . . (Signal.) *North of the lake.*
5. Raise your hand if you got everything right. You're pretty good navigators.

Materials: Each student will need a piece of lined paper.

Objectives

- **Write 4 sentences to identify the mystery character.** (Exercise 1)
- Listen to part 2 of a story and answer comprehension questions. (Exercise 2)
- **Connect specific story events to a map.** (Exercise 3)
- Complete a letter. (Exercise 4)

WORKBOOK • LINED PAPER

EXERCISE 1 Writing Sentences

Main Idea and Clues

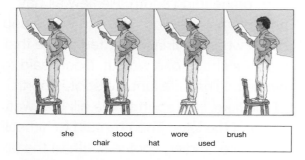

she   stood   wore   brush
chair   hat   used

1. Everybody, open your workbook to lesson 64 and find part A. ✔
   This is a new kind of clue game.

- You're going to write sentences that tell about the woman in the first picture, but you'll start with a sentence that tells the **main thing** that all the women did. Raise your hand when you can tell the main thing the women did. Don't tell what they are doing now. Tell what they did.

- What's the main thing all the women did? (Call on a student. Idea: *Painted a wall.*)

2. I'll say some sentences. You'll say whether each sentence tells about all the women, some of the women or none of the women.

- Listen: The woman stood on a chair. Does that tell about all the women, some of the women or none of the women? (Signal.) *Some of the women.*

- Listen: The woman sat on a chair. Does that tell about all the women, some of the women or none of the women? (Signal.) *None of the women.*

- Listen: The woman painted the wall. Does that tell about all the women, some of the women, or none of the women? (Signal.) *All the women.*

- (Write on the board:)

> **The woman painted a wall.**

- That's the first sentence you'll write. Then you'll write three more sentences that tell about the woman in the first picture. When you're all done, your report should give a clear picture of the woman in the first picture. Anybody who reads the report should know that the report tells about the woman in the first picture and no other woman.

3. I'll read the words in the vocabulary box. Follow along: **she . . . stood . . . wore . . . brush . . . chair . . . hat . . . used.**

4. (Write to show:)

> **The woman painted a wall.**
>
> **She**

- Listen: Your first sentence will say, the woman painted a wall. All your other sentences will start with the word **she.** Copy the first sentence on your lined paper. Then write three more sentences about the woman in the first picture. Raise your hand when you're finished.
   (Observe students and give feedback.)

5. (Call on several students to read their descriptions. For each student, say:)

- Read your whole description about the woman in the first picture.
   (Student reads.)

- (After each description, ask the students:) Everybody, does that description tell about the woman in the first picture or could it tell about somebody else, too?
   (Students respond.)

- (Praise descriptions that include all these sentences:)

  Key: The woman painted a wall.
  She stood on a chair.
  She wore a hat.
  She used a (paint) brush.

EXERCISE 2   Dooly The Duck *Part 2*

Storytelling

1. When we left Dooly, all the other ducks had gone to Mexico. His feathers had grown back, and he was going to take off the next morning. He was going to have a long day of flying.
- Turn to the map of North America on page 184 of your workbook. ✔
- Everybody, touch the state Dooly was leaving from.
  (Observe students and give feedback.)
- Everybody, what's the name of the state Dooly was leaving from? (Signal.) *Minnesota.*
- He was going to fly until he got to another state. Everybody, what state is that? (Signal.) *Nebraska.*
- Follow the flight path from Minnesota to Nebraska. That's a long, long distance for one day of flying.
- Then he was going to find a lake that was shaped like something. What was that lake shaped like? (Signal.) *A walnut.*
- There was a hill north of that lake. And there was a safe landing spot. Who remembers where the safe landing spot was? (Call on a student. Idea: *North of the lake and south of the hill.*)
- There are two ways to tell about the landing place. Here's one way: North of the lake and south of the hill.
- Here's another way of saying those directions: South of the hill and north of the lake.
2. Everybody, say it that way. (Signal.) *South of the hill and north of the lake.*
- (Repeat step 2 until firm.)
3. Here's the next part of the story:

> Dooly woke up early. There was a paper-thin sheet of ice near the edge of the lake. Dooly could see his breath when he breathed out. Brrr.

He tested his wings. They worked even better than the day before.

"I'm on my way to Nebraska," Dooly said, and he took off. He circled the lake and made sure his wings were working well. He tested his tail feathers, too, by doing some fancy turns. Then he turned south, stretched his neck straight ahead and flapped his wings at a good steady pace.

He flew, and he flew, and he flew. He passed over a lot of places that looked like good landing spots, but he remembered what Horace had told him, and he flew over those spots and just kept on heading south. He flew all day and into the evening. The sun was going down when he finally spotted a lake that was the shape of a walnut. Dooly said to himself, "The safe landing spot is north of the lake." He spotted the hill that was north of the lake. Then he said to himself, "The safe landing spot is south of the hill. I'll go to the hill and go south."

That's just what he did. He flew over the hill, and then he headed south. He kept saying, "South of the hill," and he flew south right over the lake.

His problem was that he didn't understand directions very well. After all, he'd never had to do this kind of thing before. On his earlier flights, he just did what the other ducks did. So he didn't know how to think about two directions at the same time. He could think about going south of the hill. But, when he did that, he couldn't think about going north of the lake. He flew south until he was way, way past the lake. Then he knew that something was wrong. So he went back and tried it again. But the same thing happened. So, he tried it two more times. But each time, the same thing happened. He'd get right over the hill, and then he'd say, "South of the hill." He'd fly south of the hill. But he wouldn't remember "north of the lake." So he'd just keep going right past that lake, again, and again, and again, until he was all pooped out. His little wings were so tired that he could hardly flap them.

- Everybody, turn to part B in lesson 64 and find the map. ✔

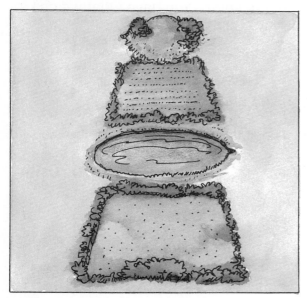

- Put your finger on that hill and pretend your finger is Dooly. He'd get right over the hill, and he'd fly south. Do it. Fly south from that hill. Fly right over the lake and then stop.
- Dooly would know something was wrong when he'd get over the lake, but he wouldn't know what to do about it. So he'd go back over the hill and do it again.
- Listen:

On his last trip south, he went all the way past the lake. He was south of the hill and south of the lake. Dooly knew that something was wrong, but he had to land. So he did. He landed in a field.

He sat there. Everything was quiet. The sun was setting in the west. The air was cool. Everything seemed safe. Then, suddenly, a large flock of very angry Canada geese came running toward Dooly. These geese were shouting and honking at Dooly, and it was easy to see they planned to bite him.

"Honk, honk. Get out of here, you lousy duck. Honk. Can't you see this is a field for Canada geese? Honk."

Although Dooly was tired, he found enough strength to take off, very fast. He flew above the lake and said to himself, "I don't know where that safe field is. It's somewhere north of this lake. So I'll just go north of the lake and land. I don't have enough strength to go any farther.

And that's just what he did. He went just north of the lake and landed. Well, the field he landed in was just south of the hill.

- Everybody, touch where Dooly landed. It's the place just north of the lake and south of the hill. ✔

Dooly didn't know he was in the field Horace had told him about, but he was. Dooly sat there and waited and watched. He didn't know whether some more Canada geese would attack him. He didn't know what would happen.

Nothing happened, except the sun went down and the sky turned a brilliant red in the west.

Then, suddenly, Dooly heard something in the tall grass of the field. Something was moving toward him. Dooly got ready to take off again if he had to. The movement in the grass came closer and closer. Then a big black crow hopped into view. "Howdy, howdy," the crow said. "I'm Caw-Caw. They told me to expect you, but they didn't tell me that you'd fly over this place a dozen times before you'd land."

"I got confused," Dooly said.

"That happens a lot with you late-molting ducks. You folks don't seem to know much about following directions or navigating."

Dooly was too tired to feel bad. He just looked at Caw-Caw and blinked.

Then Caw-Caw said, "Don't worry. I'll get you fixed up. If you look around this field, you'll find some good grain and berries. Eat up. Get a good night's sleep. Then see me in the morning. We'll get your directions straightened out."

So Dooly ate grain and berries. Then he snuggled up with his head tucked inside his warm feathers and had a good night's sleep.

In the morning, Caw-Caw woke him up with a poke of her beak. "Hey, Duck," she said. "I told you to get a good night's sleep. I didn't say to sleep all day. Wake up, and let's get to work."

The crow said, "Let's go make some maps in the sand."

"Maps?" Dooly said. "Sand?"

"Yeah, you know. Maps in the sand."

Dooly did not know maps or how they worked, but he soon found out. Caw-Caw went over to the edge of the walnut-shaped lake where the bank was sandy. Then she picked up a stick with her beak and scratched a map in the sand. On the map was a walnut-shaped lake. Then Caw-Caw picked up a little leaf with her beak and put the leaf on the map just north of the lake. "Okay," she said. "You see a leaf and a walnut-shaped lake, right?"

"Right."

"You do know north and south, right?"

"Right."

"Take your wing and show me which direction is north."

Dooly pointed north.

"Now show me south."

Dooly pointed south.

"Now take a stick and mark the place that is north of the lake and south of the leaf."

Dooly picked up a stick and said to himself, "North of the lake and south of the leaf." He moved the stick over the lake, and then he kept moving it north. But he moved it right past the leaf.

"There's your problem," Caw-Caw said. "You're going north, but you're not going south. You have what we call a one-track mind."

Dooly was embarrassed.

"Hey, don't worry, Duck. I'll get you fixed up."

• That's the end of this part of the story.

EXERCISE 3 Connecting Details

Story Events and Map

1. Find part B. ✔
   There are two pictures of things that happened in the story, and there's a map. Who remembers where the safe landing spot was? (Call on a student. Idea: *North of the lake and south of the hill.*)
   You're going to draw a line from each picture to the spot on the map where the picture took place.

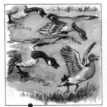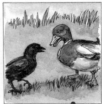

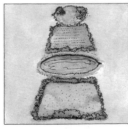

2. The first picture shows Dooly being chased by those Canada geese. Remember where he was when that happened. He flew south of the hill and south of the lake. When he got just south of the lake he landed. Draw a line from the picture to show where he was when the Canada geese chased him. Raise your hand when you're finished. (Observe students and give feedback.)

- You should have drawn a line from the picture to the field just south of the lake. Raise your hand if you got it right.

3. The other picture shows Caw-Caw and Dooly. Remember where that place was? That's the safe landing place. Draw a line from the picture to the safe landing place. Raise your hand when you're finished. **(Observe students and give feedback.)**

- You should have drawn a line from the picture to the field just north of the lake. Raise your hand if you got it right.

EXERCISE 4   Letter Writing

Dear _____,

    Here are a few of my favorite things. My favorite things to eat are _____ and _____. My favorite things to do are _____ and _____. My favorite people are _____ and _____.

                          From,

                           _____

1. Everybody, find part C. ✔
   You're going to complete another letter. It is a make-believe letter that tells about some of your favorite things.

- At the top of the page is a box. There are some words in the box that you may want to use when you write your letter. Touch the first part of the box. ✔

- These pictures show some things to eat that you might like. Follow along while I read the words. **Apples . . . pizza . . . burgers . . . ice cream . . . corn on the cob . . . macaroni and cheese.**

- Touch the second part of the box. ✔

- These pictures show some things you might enjoy doing. Follow along while I read the words. **Read a book . . . play in the park . . . draw.**

- Remember to spell any of these words correctly.

2. Touch the line at the top of the letter. ✔

- This is a line for the date. You'll write today's date in that space. (Ask the students to tell you the date. Write it on the board.)

- Write the date and write the name of the person to whom you're writing. Raise your hand when you're finished. **(Observe students and give feedback.)**

3. I'll read the next part of the letter and you'll follow along. "Here are some of my favorite things. My favorite things to eat are blank and blank." Write two of your favorite foods. **(Observe students and give feedback.)**

4. The next sentence says, "My favorite things to do are blank and blank." Write two things you like to do. **(Observe students and give feedback.)**

5. The rest of the letter says, "My favorite people are blank and blank. Write the names of two of your favorite people. Then sign your name to the letter. **(Observe students and give feedback. Students who are finished early may wish to draw a picture to go with their letter.)**

6. (Call on several students to read their complete letter. Praise letters that have appropriate names and words in the blanks.)

Materials: Each student will need a piece of lined paper.

Objectives

- Write 4 sentences to identify the mystery character. (Exercise 1)
- Listen to the conclusion of a 3-part story and answer comprehension questions. (Exercise 2)
- Make a picture consistent with details of the story. (Exercise 3)
- Complete a letter. (Exercise 4)

LINED PAPER

EXERCISE 1 Writing Sentences

Main Idea and Clues

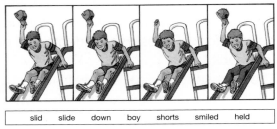

| slid | slide | down | boy | shorts | smiled | held |

1. Everybody, find part A. ✔
   You're going to use lined paper and write a description of the boy in the first picture. You'll start with a sentence that tells the main thing all the boys did.
2. I'll read the words in the vocabulary box. You follow along: **slid . . . slide . . . down . . . boy . . . shorts . . . smiled . . . held.**
3. Your turn to write the first sentence.
- (Write on the board:)

> **The boy**

- Start with **the boy** and tell the main thing the boy did. That's the same thing all the other boys did. Raise your hand when you've written your first sentence. Tell the main thing the boy did.
  (Observe students and give feedback.)
- (Write to show:)

> **The boy** slid down the slide.

- Here's the main thing the boy did. You could have told about the same thing with different words. You could have written: The boy went down the slide.
- (Call on individual students:) Read the sentence you wrote.

- (Direct students with inappropriate sentences [present tense verb or unacceptable expressions] to fix up their sentence.)
4. You've got a sentence that tells the main thing the boy in the first picture did. Now you'll write three more sentences that tell about the boy in the first picture. Remember, when you're done, your report should give a clear picture of the boy in the first picture. Anybody who reads the report should know who the report tells about.
- (Write to show:)

> **The boy slid down the slide.**
> **He**

- All the other sentences you'll write will begin with the word **he.** Write three sentences that tell about the boy in the first picture. Raise your hand when you're finished.
  (Observe students and give feedback.)
5. Check your work. (Call on several students to read their descriptions. For each student, say:)
- Read your whole description about the boy in the first picture. (Student reads.)
- (After each description, ask the students:) Does that description tell only about the boy in the first picture or could it tell about somebody else too? (Students respond.)
- (Praise good descriptions that include all these sentences:)
  Key: The boy slid down a slide.
  He smiled.
  He held a hat.
  He wore shorts.

EXERCISE 2 Dooly The Duck *Part 3*

Storytelling

- When we left Dooly, he was with Caw-Caw in the safe landing place.
- Here's the last part of the Dooly story. Listen:

Dooly knew that he had a problem understanding flight directions. Caw-Caw told Dooly, "You're going north, but you're not going south. You have what we call a one-track mind." Then Caw-Caw said, "I'll show you a whole bunch of different ways to get your mind working on two tracks at the same time. Here's a good way."

Caw-Caw hopped over to the map she'd scratched in the sand. The leaf was to her left and the lake was to her right.

- Get a picture of Caw-Caw in your mind. She was standing next to that map so that the leaf was to her left and the lake was to her right.
- Pretend you're Caw-Caw. Point to where the leaf would be from you. (Students point left with left hand.)
- Point to where the lake would be from you. (Students point right with right hand.)
- Listen to that part again:

Caw-Caw hopped over to the map she'd scratched in the sand. The leaf was to her left and the lake was to her right.

She said, "This is so easy I'll do it with my eyes closed." Then she closed her eyes and said, "You want to see how to find the place that's north of the lake and south of the leaf. Watch my wings."

Caw-Caw started to move her wings together. When the wings came together, she said, "There you have it. My wings are over a place that's north of the lake and south of the hill. Pretty difficult, huh?"

"No, that looks pretty easy. Let me try it." Dooly hopped over to the map, held his left wing over the leaf and his right wing over the lake. Then he moved his wings together. They met right in front of him. "Let's see what you do when I make it a little harder," Caw-Caw said. She dropped a stick on the map. The stick was north of the leaf.

Caw-Caw said, "Let's see you find the place that's north of the leaf and south of the stick."

"North of the leaf," Dooly said, "and south of the stick."

He put his left wing over the leaf and his right wing over the stick and moved his wings together. "There," he said. "My wings are right over a place that's north of the leaf and south of the stick."

"You're a pretty fast learner for a duck," Caw-Caw said.

Then Caw-Caw made another map. This map had an X and a stick on it. The X was east of the stick. Caw-Caw said, "Here's another way of thinking about flight directions. If I tell you that something is east of the stick and west of the X, it must be between the stick and the X. You know **between,** don't you?"

"Sure," Dooly said.

"Well, then these directions should be as easy as duck soup for you."

"We don't talk that way," Dooly said.

"Oh, I forgot," Caw-Caw said. "You ducks are sensitive about that expression."

- Why would Dooly be sensitive about the expression, "It's as easy as duck soup?" (Call on a student. Idea: *To make duck soup, somebody had to cook a duck.*)

"Caw-Caw made different maps for Dooly. Then she'd tell about places on the map and remind Dooly, "That description tells you that you're looking for something that's between two places on this map."

After a while, Dooly got pretty good at listening to those directions and going between the two places.

So Dooly and Caw-Caw practiced a while longer. It was still pretty early in the morning. Then Caw-Caw said, "Well, I don't know about you, but I'm getting tired of doing this."

"Me, too," Dooly said.

"Well then, I'll tell you about the next safe place to land. Here's what you do. You keep heading south and go right into Oklahoma. You'll follow a river until it runs into a lake that's shaped like a slug. To the east of the lake is a green barn. The safe landing place is east of the lake and west of the barn."

"I've got it," Dooly said. "Go to the lake that's shaped like a slug. There's a green barn to the east. The safe spot is east of the lake and west of the barn. So it's between the barn and the lake."

Caw-Caw said, "For a duck that molts late, you're really pretty smart. Good luck to you."

"Thank you," Dooly said, and he took off. With great confidence he flew south. He flew all day and into the late, late evening before he finally spotted the lake that was shaped like a slug. He flew over the lake and said to himself, "The safe place is east of the lake, but west of that barn over there." So he flew until he was between the barn and the lake. Then he swooped down and landed in the field. Within a few seconds, a crow hopped out of the weeds.

"Howdy," the crow said. "I'm Caw. I'm a second cousin of Caw-Caw."

The birds shook wings.

Then Caw said, "It's always a pleasure to watch a duck that knows something about navigation, and you obviously know a lot about navigation."

"Oh, it's nothing," Dooly said modestly.

But he did know a lot about navigation.

He spent the night in Oklahoma. In the morning, Caw told him directions for the next safe spot, and Dooly followed them. Dooly landed next in Texas. Caw's uncle, Caw-O-Caw, met Dooly and gave him directions for the last landing spot, which was in Mexico. The next morning, Dooly took off and flew, and flew, and flew over the ocean.

At last, he reached the great lake near the ocean where he would spend his winter with the rest of the ducks from his flock and with thousands and thousands of other ducks from other flocks. Dooly swooped down and showed off a little bit. Then he came in for a landing. One of the younger ducks asked her mother, "Who is that strong, handsome mallard that just landed?"

"I'm not sure," the mother duck said. "He looks something like Dooly, but he's far too handsome."

When they found out that it was Dooly, they were amazed. "What a flier," they said. "What a navigator." News of Dooly's amazing flight in record time spread through the duck community, and everybody wanted to shake his wing. Dooly was a hero, and a lot of very attractive female ducks were very interested in him.

The next spring, when it was time to fly back up to Minnesota, Horace assembled the flock and said, "Here's an announcement: All of you are going back, but I'm staying here."

"What?"

"That's right," Horace said. "This old bird is retiring."

"Then who will lead us back up the flyway?"

Horace shook his head. "Is that a dumb question, or what?" he said. "You want an experienced navigator and somebody who is smart. Am I right?" Everybody nodded.

"Well, there's only one duck for the job, and that's Dooly."

The ducks cheered, and Dooly was embarrassed. But he proved to be a very good choice. For the next four years, he led the flock up and down the flyway without losing one single duck.

Map Directions

1. Find the map of North America on page 184 of your workbook. ✔
   Let's go over the whole flight route.
   - (Write on the board:)

Oklahoma **Texas**

2. Everybody, start in Minnesota. ✔
   - Everybody, take off and fly to the first safe spot. Raise your hand when you've found it. ✔
   - Everybody, what state are you in? (Signal.) *Nebraska.*
   - Take off and go south to Oklahoma and land somewhere in that state along the flight path. Raise your hand when you're finished. ✔
   - Now Caw meets you and tells you the next landing place. Does anybody remember where that landing place is? (Call on a student. Idea: *Texas.*)
   - Fly and go south and go as far south as you can in Texas. Raise your hand when you're finished. ✔
   - Now you're going to have one long flight to get down to where the ducks are in Mexico. Get your wings ready and go. Raise your hand when you land near the ocean in Mexico. ✔
   - That's a long flight.

EXERCISE 3   Details

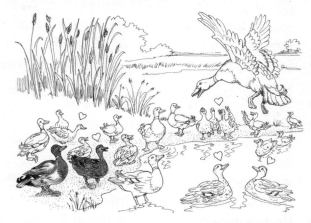

1. Turn back to lesson 65 and find part B. ✔
   That's a picture of Dooly in Mexico. Look at all those ducks.
   - Some of those female mallards have heart symbols above them. What do those heart symbols mean? (Call on a student. Idea: *They like Dooly.*)
   - Yes, they really like Dooly.
2. Later you can color the picture. Two of the ducks are already colored. Remember, those female mallards are brown and black. Male mallards have pretty green heads.

EXERCISE 4   Letter Writing

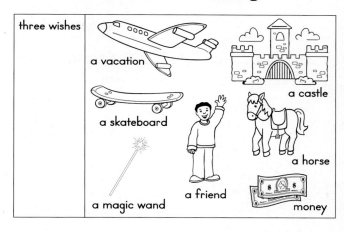

_____

Dear _____,

   This is what I would wish for if I had _____. First, I would

wish for _____. Next, I would wish for _____.

Last, I would wish for _____.

          From,

1. Everybody, find part C. ✔
   You're going to complete another letter. It is a make-believe letter that tells what you would wish for if you had three wishes.

- At the top of the page is a box. There are some words in the box that you may want to use when you write your letter. Touch the first part of the box. ✔
- Follow along while I read the words. **Three wishes.**
- Touch the second part of the box. ✔
- These pictures show some things you might wish for. Follow along while I read the words. **A vacation . . . a castle . . . a skateboard . . . a horse . . . a magic wand . . . money . . . a friend.**
- Remember to spell any of these words correctly.

2. Touch the line at the top of the letter. ✔
- This is a line for the date. You'll write today's date in that space. (**Ask the students to tell you the date. Write it on the board.**)
- Write the date and write the name of the person whom you're writing to. Raise your hand when you're finished. (**Observe students and give feedback.**)

3. I'll read the first part of the letter and you'll follow along. **This is what I would wish for if I had blank.** Write the words, **three wishes** in the blank.
   (**Observe students and give feedback.**)

4. The next sentence says, **First I would wish for blank.** Write one thing you would wish for. Maybe it's a skateboard, maybe it's a vacation somewhere, maybe it's something that you can't buy with money.
   (**Observe students and give feedback.**)

5. Read the sentence that tells the first thing you would wish for. (**Call on several students.**)

6. Complete the other sentences. They tell what you would wish for next and what you would wish for last. Remember to sign your name to the letter. Raise your hand when you're finished. (**Observe students and give feedback. Students who are finished early may wish to draw a picture to go with their letter.**)

7. (**Call on several students to read their complete letter. Praise letters that have appropriate names and words in the blanks.**)

Grade 2 Language Arts Curriculum Map

	Phonics/ Vocabulary	Comprehension	Grammar/ Usage/ Mechanics	Writing/ Composition/ Speaking	Study Skills
Lesson 1	Left, right: 2	Classification: 3, 4 Sequence: 5 Listening comprehension: 7 Recalling details: 8		Sentences: 6	
Lesson 2	Left, right: 2	True, false: 3, 7 Sequence: 4 Classification: 5 Listening comprehension: 6 Recalling details: 8		Sentences: 1	
Lesson 3	Left, right: 1	True, false: 2 Classification: 3 Listening comprehension: 5 Recalling details: 6		Sentences: 4	
Lesson 4		True, false: 2 Classification: 3 Listening comprehension: 4 Recalling details: 5		Sentences: 1	
Lesson 5	Left, right: 5	True, false: 3 Classification: 4 Listening comprehension: 6 Recalling details: 7		Sentences: 1	Cardinal directions: 2
Lesson 6		Classification: 3 Listening comprehension: 4	Correcting word usage errors: 5, 6	Sentences: 2	Cardinal directions: 1
Lesson 7		Classification: 2 Listening comprehension: 4	Correcting word usage errors: 5	Sentences: 3	Cardinal directions: 1
Lesson 8		If-then reasoning: 3 Deduction: 5 Listening comprehension: 6 Recalling details: 7	Correcting word usage errors: 4	Sentences: 2	Cardinal directions: 1
Lesson 9	Left, right: 4	If-then reasoning: 3 Deduction: 5 Listening comprehension: 6 Recalling details: 7		Sentences: 2	Cardinal directions: 1
Lesson 10	Left, right: 2	Listening comprehension: 3		Sentences: 1	
Lesson 11	Seasons: 4	Deduction: 2 Listening comprehension: 5 Recalling details: 6		Sentences: 3	Cardinal directions: 1
Lesson 12	Seasons: 1	Deduction: 3 Listening comprehension: 5	Correcting word usage errors: 6	Sentences: 4	Maps: 2
Lesson 13	Seasons: 1	Deduction: 3 Listening comprehension: 5	Correcting word usage errors: 6	Sentences: 4	Maps: 2
Lesson 14		Deduction: 4 Listening comprehension: 5 Recalling details: 6		Sentences: 1	Cardinal directions: 2 Maps: 3
Lesson 15	Initial letter substitution: 5	Deduction: 2 Listening comprehension: 4		Sentences: 3	Maps: 1

	Vocabulary	Comprehension	Grammar	Composition	Study Skills
Lesson 16		Listening comprehension: 4 True, false: 5		Sentences: 1	Cardinal directions: 2 Maps: 3
Lesson 17		Deduction: 2 Listening comprehension: 3 Comparisons: 4		Sentences: 1	
Lesson 18		Listening comprehension: 3 Comparisons: 4		Sentences: 1	Mazes directions: 2
Lesson 19		Listening comprehension: 3 Comparisons: 4		Sentences: 1	Maze directions: 2
Lesson 20		Listening directions: 3		Sentences: 1	Maps: 2
Lesson 21				Story sentences: 1	
Lesson 22	To, from: 2	Classification: 3 Deduction: 4 Listening comprehension: 5		Sentences: 1	
Lesson 23	To, from: 1	Classification: 3 Listening comprehension: 4		Sentences: 5	Maps: 2
Lesson 24		Classification, subclass: 2 Listening comprehension: 3	Correcting word usage errors: 4	Sentences: 1	
Lesson 25	To, from: 1	Listening comprehension: 2 Deduction: 3			Maps: 1
Lesson 26				Story sentences: 1	
Lesson 27	To, from: 1	Sequencing: 2 Classification, subclass: 3 Listening comprehension: 4		Fictional story: 5	Maps: 1
Lesson 28		Sequencing: 1 Deduction: 2		Fictional story: 3 Story presentation: 3	
Lesson 29		Deduction: 1 Listening comprehension: 3		Writing deductions: 1	Maps: 2, 4
Lesson 30	To, from: 2	Deduction: 2 Listening comprehension: 3		Sentences: 1	Maps: 2
Lesson 31				Story sentences: 1	
Lesson 32		Classification: 3 Listening comprehension: 4			Alphabetical order: 1 Maps: 2, 5
Lesson 33		Classification: 3 Listening comprehension: 4			Alphabetical order: 1 Maps: 2
Lesson 34		Classification: 1 Sequencing: 3 Listening comprehension: 4	Pronoun referents: 5	Sentences: 6	Maps: 2
Lesson 35		Classification: 3 Listening comprehension: 4	Pronoun referents: 5		Alphabetical order: 1 Maps: 2
Lesson 36		Following written directions: 3 Listening comprehension: 4	Pronoun referents: 5		Alphabetical order: 1 Maps: 2, 3
Lesson 37		Following written directions: 2 Deduction: 3 Listening comprehension: 5	Pronoun referents: 4	Story sentences: 1	

	Vocabulary	Comprehension	Grammar	Composition	Study Skills
Lesson 38		Listening comprehension: 4 Deduction: 5	Pronoun referents: 3		Alphabetical order: 1 Maps: 2
Lesson 39		Deduction: 2, 5 Listening comprehension: 4	Pronoun referents: 3		Alphabetical order: 1
Lesson 40		Sequencing: 2 Classification: 2 Listening comprehension: 3		Sentences: 1	Maps: 2
Lesson 41		Listening comprehension: 4 Recalling details: 5	Pronoun referents: 3	Sentences: 1	Maps: 2
Lesson 42		Listening comprehension: 3 Recalling details: 4	Pronoun referents: 2	Sentences: 1	
Lesson 43		Listening comprehension: 3	Pronoun referents: 4	Story sentences: 1	Maps: 2
Lesson 44		Deduction: 2 Listening comprehension: 3 Recalling Details: 4		Sentences: 1	
Lesson 45		Deduction: 4 Listening comprehension: 5	Pronoun referents: 3	Sentences: 1, 2	
Lesson 46		Listening comprehension: 4 Sequencing: 5		Story sentences: 1, 3	Maps: 2
Lesson 47		Listening comprehension: 4	Pronoun referents: 3	Sentences: 2 Dramatic activity: 5	Maps: 1
Lesson 48		Listening comprehension: 3	Correcting word usage errors: 4	Sentences: 1, 2	
Lesson 49		Listening comprehension: 2	Correcting word usage errors: 3	Sentences: 1 Story sentences: 4	
Lesson 50		Listening comprehension: 3		Sentences: 1	Maps: 2
Lesson 51		Sequencing: 2 Listening comprehension: 4 Deduction: 5	Pronoun referents: 3	Sentences: 1, 2 Deductive sentences: 5	
Lesson 52		Sequencing: 1 Listening comprehension: 2 Deduction: 3		Sentences: 1 Deductive sentences: 3	
Lesson 53		Sequencing: 2 Deduction: 3 Listening comprehension: 4 Recalling details: 5		Letter writing: 1 Sentences: 2 Deductive writing: 3	
Lesson 54		Listening comprehension: 4	Pronoun referents: 3	Letter writing: 1 Dramatic activity: 5	Maps: 2
Lesson 55		Deduction: 3 Listening comprehension: 4 Character extrapolation: 5		Letter writing: 1	Maps: 2
Lesson 56		Deduction: 1 Main idea: 2 Listening comprehension: 3	Pronoun referents: 4		
Lesson 57		Main idea: 1, 2 Listening comprehension: 3 Deduction: 5		Sentences: 2 Write an ending to a story: 4	
Lesson 58		Main idea: 1		Sentences: 1 Write an ending to a story: 2	

	Vocabulary	Comprehension	Grammar	Composition	Study Skills
Lesson 59		Main idea: 1 Listening comprehension: 2		Sentences: 1 Write an ending to a story: 2	
Lesson 60		Main idea: 1 Deduction: 2	Correcting word usage errors: 2	Sentences: 1 Write an ending to a story: 3	
Lesson 61		Listening comprehension: 3	Pronoun referents: 4	Sentences: 2	Maps: 1
Lesson 62		Listening comprehension: 4	Pronoun referents: 5	Sentences: 1	Maps: 2, 3
Lesson 63	After: 1	Sequencing: 1 Listening comprehension: 3		Sentences: 2	Maps: 4
Lesson 64		Main idea: 1 Listening comprehension: 2 Recalling details: 3		Sentences: 1 Letter writing: 4	Maps: 3
Lesson 65		Main idea: 1 Listening comprehension: 2 Recalling details: 3		Sentences: 1 Letter writing: 4	
Lesson 66		Main idea: 1 Deductions: 5 Listening Comprehension: 6	Subject of sentence: 2, 4 Capitalization: 3 Sentence punctuation: 3		
Lesson 67		Deduction: 6 Listening Comprehension: 7	Subject of sentence: 2, 3, 5		
Lesson 68		Deduction: 4 Main idea: 6 Listening Comprehension: 7	Subject of sentence: 2, 3, 5 Capitalization: 4		
Lesson 69	Suffix –ed: 2	Deduction: 3 Main idea: 5 Listening Comprehension: 7	Subject of sentence: 4, 6 Punctuation: 5		
Lesson 70	Suffix-ed: 2	Deduction: 4 Listening Comprehension: 7	Predicate of sentence: 5 Subject of sentence: 6 Irregular Verbs: 3		
Lesson 71		Deduction: 5 Main idea: 6, 7 Listening Comprehension: 8	Irregular verbs: 2 Verb tense: 3 Subject/predicate: 4	Editing: 3	
Lesson 72		Main idea: 5, 6 Listening Comprehension: 7	Subject/predicate: 2 Verb tense: 3 Pronouns: 4	Editing: 3	
Lesson 73		Deduction: 5 Main idea: 7 Listening Comprehension: 8	Subject/predicate: 2 Pronouns: 3 Verb tense: 4 Irregular verb: 6	Editing: 4	
Lesson 74		Main idea: 5 Listening Comprehension: 6	Pronouns: 2 Verb tense: 3 Subject/predicate: 4	Editing: 3	
Lesson 75		Main idea: 2 Listening Comprehension: 3	Irregular verbs: 4 Subject/predicate: 4 Verb tense: 4	Editing: 4	
Lesson 76		Main idea: 6, 7 Listening Comprehension: 8	Irregular verbs: 2 Subject/predicate: 3 Pronouns: 4 Verb tense: 5	Editing: 5	
Lesson 77		Deduction: 5 Main idea: 6, 7 Listening Comprehension: 8	Subject/predicate: 2 Irregular verbs: 3 Pronouns: 4		

	Vocabulary	Comprehension	Grammar	Composition	Study Skills
Lesson 78		Main idea: 6, 7 Listening Comprehension: 8	Verb tense: 2 Subject/predicate: 3 Pronouns: 4 Irregular verbs: 5	Editing: 2	
Lesson 79		Main idea: 6, 7 Listening Comprehension: 8	Pronouns: 2 Subject/predicate: 3 Verb tense: 4 Irregular verbs: 5	Editing: 4	
Lesson 80		Classification: 5 Main idea: 6 Listening Comprehension: 8	Pronouns: 2 Verb tense: 3 Subject/predicate: 4	Editing: 3 Paragraph copying: 7	
Lesson 81		Classification: 6 Main idea: 7 Listening Comprehension: 8	Verb tense: 2 Subject/predicate: 3 Pronouns: 4 Capitalization: 5 Punctuation: 5	Editing: 2 Paragraph copying: 5	
Lesson 82		Classification: 4 Main Idea: 6, 7 Listening Comprehension: 8	Pronouns: 2 Subject/Predicate: 3 Capitalization: 3, 5 Punctuation: 3, 5	Editing: 3 Paragraph copying: 5	
Lesson 83		Classification: 4 Main idea: 4, 6	Subject/Predicate: 2 Capitalization: 2 Punctuation: 2 Verb tense: 3	Editing: 2, 3 Paragraph copying: 5	
Lesson 84		Main idea: 5 Classification: 5 Listening Comprehension: 7	Subject/predicate: 2 Capitalization: 3, 6 Punctuation: 3, 6 Verb tense: 4	Editing: 3, 4 Paragraph writing: 6	
Lesson 85		Main idea: 3 Listening Comprehension: 3	Capitalization: 2, 3 Punctuation: 2, 3 Pronouns: 3 Past Time: 3 Clarity: 3	Paragraph writing: 2 Editing: 3	
Lesson 86		Main idea: 5	Capitalization: 2, 6 Punctuation: 2, 6 Subject/predicate: 3 Verb tense: 4 Irregular verbs: 4	Editing: 2 Paragraph writing: 6	
Lesson 87		Main idea: 6	Capitalization: 2, 7 Punctuation: 2, 7 Subject/Predicate: 3 Verb tense: 4 Irregular verbs: 5	Editing: 2, 4 Paragraph writing: 7	
Lesson 88		Main idea: 5, 7	Subject/Predicate: 2 Capitalization: 3, 6 Punctuation: 3, 6 Irregular verbs: 4 Verb tense: 4	Editing: 3 Paragraph writing: 6	
Lesson 89		Main idea: 5, 7	Capitalization: 2, 6 Punctuation: 2, 6 Subject/predicate: 3 Pronouns: 4	Editing: 2 Paragraph writing: 6	
Lesson 90		Main idea: 7	Capitalization: 2, 6 Punctuation: 2, 6 Pronouns: 3 Verb tense: 4 Irregular verbs: 4 Subject/predicate: 5	Editing: 2 Paragraph writing: 6	
Lesson 91			Capitalization: 2 Punctuation: 2 Verb tense: 3 Irregular verbs: 3 Pronouns: 4 Subject/predicate: 6	Editing: 2 Paragraph writing: 5 Sentences: 7	
Lesson 92		Main idea: 6	Subject/predicate: 2 Verb tense: 3 Irregular verbs: 3 Pronouns: 4	Sentences: 5 Paragraph writing: 7	

	Vocabulary	Comprehension	Grammar	Composition	Study Skills
Lesson 93		Main idea: 6	Capitalization: 2, 7 Punctuation: 2, 7 Subject/predicate: 3 Pronouns: 4 Verb tense: 5 Irregular verbs: 5	Editing: 2 Paragraph writing: 7	
Lesson 94		Main idea: 5	Capitalization: 2, 4, 7 Punctuation: 2, 6 Pronouns: 3 Verb tense: 6 Irregular verbs: 6	Editing: 2 Paragraph writing: 7	
Lesson 95	Prepositions: 2	Main idea: 2, 4	Verb tense: 3 Irregular verbs: 3 Subject/predicate: 4 Capitalization: 4 Punctuation: 4 Pronouns: 4	Editing: 4	
Lesson 96	Prepositions: 4	Main idea: 4	Capitalization: 1, 2 Punctuation: 2 Run-on sentences: 2 Verb tense: 3 Irregular verbs: 3 Subject/predicate: 5	Editing: 2 Paragraph writing: 6	
Lesson 97		Main idea: 5	Capitalization: 2, 4 Pronouns: 3 Punctuation: 4 Run-on sentences: 4 Subject/predicate: 6	Editing: 4, 5 Paragraph writing: 5	
Lesson 98			Capitalization: 2, 4 Pronouns: 3 Punctuation: 4 Subject/predicate: 5 Verb tense: 6 Irregular verbs: 6	Editing: 4 Revising for clarity: 7	
Lesson 99			Subject/predicate: 2 Capitalization: 3, 5 Punctuation: 3 Pronouns: 4	Editing: 3 Revising for clarity: 6, 7 Sentences: 8	
Lesson 100			Capitalization: 2 Pronouns: 3 Verb tense: 4 Irregular verbs: 4 Subject/predicate: 6	Editing: 3 Revising for clarity: 6, 7 Sentences: 8	
Lesson 101			Capitalization: 2, 5 Verb tense: 3 Irregular verbs: 3 Pronouns: 4 Punctuation: 5	Editing: 2 Revising for clarity: 4 Paragraph writing: 6	
Lesson 102			Capitalization: 2 Pronouns: 4 Verb tense: 5 Irregular verbs: 5	Editing: 2, 3 Revising for clarity: 4 Sentences: 6 Paragraph writing: 7	
Lesson 103		Supporting facts: 5	Subject/predicate: 2 Capitalization: 3 Verb tense: 4 Irregular verbs: 4	Editing: 3 Paragraph writing: 6	
Lesson 104		Main idea: 5	Capitalization: 2 Punctuation: 2 Run-on sentences: 3 Pronouns: 4	Editing: 2, 3 Revising for clarity: 4 Sentences: 6 Paragraph writing: 7	
Lesson 105			Run-on sentence: 2 Verbs: 3 Predicates: 3 Capitalization: 4 Pronouns: 4 Subject/predicate: 4	Editing: 2	
Lesson 106			Pronouns: 1 Run-on sentences: 2 Verbs: 3, 4 Subject/Predicate: 4 Capitalization: 5	Editing: 2, 5 Paragraph writing: 6	

	Vocabulary	Comprehension	Grammar	Composition	Study Skills
Lesson 107			Subject/predicate: 2 Run-on sentences: 3 Verb tense: 4 Irregular verbs: 4 Pronouns: 5	Editing: 3 Paragraph writing: 6	
Lesson 108		Main ideas: 5	Subject/predicate: 2 Run-on sentence: 3 Pronouns: 4, 5	Editing: 3 Paragraph writing: 6	
Lesson 109		Main ideas: 5	Run-on sentences: 2 Verbs: 3 Possessives: 4	Sentences: 5 Paragraph writing: 6	
Lesson 110		Main ideas: 5	Run-on sentences: 2 Verbs: 3 Possessives: 4 Compound predicate: 6	Sentences: 5 Paragraph writing: 7	